Clinical Disorders of Balance, Posture and Gait

Clinical Disorders of Balance, Posture and Gait

Second edition

Edited by

Adolfo M. Bronstein MD PhD FRCP
Professor of Neuro-Otology and
Honorary Consultant Neurologist
Imperial College of Science and Technology,
Charing Cross Hospital, London, UK

Thomas Brandt MD FRCP
Professor, Department of Neurology
Ludwig-Maximilians University, Munich, Germany

Marjorie H. Woollacott PhD
Professor, Department of Exercise and Movement Science
Institute of Neuroscience, University of Oregon, Eugene,
Oregon, USA

and

John G. Nutt MD
Professor, Departments of Neurology and
Physiology & Pharmacology
Oregon Health Sciences University, Portland, Oregon, USA

A member of the Hodder Headline Group
LONDON

First published in Great Britain in 1996 by Arnold
Reprinted in 1998
This second edition published in 2004 by
Arnold, a member of the Hodder Headline Group,
338 Euston Road, London NW1 3BH

http://www.arnoldpublishers.com
Distributed in the United States of America by
Oxford University Press Inc.,
198 Madison Avenue, New York, NY10016
Oxford is a registered trademark of Oxford University Press

Whilst the advice and information in this book are believed to be true and
accurate at the date of going to press, neither the authors nor the publisher
can accept any legal responsibility or liability for any errors or omissions
that may be made. In particular (but without limiting the generality of the
preceding disclaimer) every effort has been made to check drug dosages;
however, it is still possible that errors have been missed. Furthermore,
dosage schedules are constantly being revised and new side-effects
recognized. For these reasons the reader is strongly urged to consult the
drug companies' printed instructions before administering any of the drugs
recommended in this book.

British Library Cataloguing in Publication Data
A catalogue record for this book is available from the British Library

Library of Congress Cataloging-in-Publication Data
A catalog record for this book is available from the Library of Congress

ISBN   0 340 80657 5

1 2 3 4 5 6 7 8 9 10

Commissioning Editor: Joanna Koster
Development Editor: Sarah Burrows
Project Editor: Wendy Rooke
Production Controller: Deborah Smith
Cover Design: Lee-May Lim

Typeset in 10/12 pt Minion by Phoenix Photosetting, Chatham, Kent
Printed and bound in the UK by Butler & Tanner Ltd, Frome, Somerset

What do you think about this book? Or any other Arnold title?
Please send your comments to feedback.arnold@hodder.co.uk

Contents

Contributors

Bernard Amblard
Institute of Physiological and Cognitive Neurosciences (INPC),
National Center of Scientific Research (CNRS), Marseille, France

Lynne Armstrong
Consultant in Elderly Care, Craigavon Area Hospital, Craigavon,
Northern Ireland, UK

Christine Assaiante
Institute of Physiological and Cognitive Neurosciences (INPC),
National Center of Scientific Research (CNRS), Marseille, France

Kailash Bhatia MD FRCP
University Department of Clinical Neurology, Institute of
Neurology and National Hospital for Neurology, London, UK

Bastiaan R. Bloem MD PhD
Assistant Professor of Neurology, Department of Neurology,
University Medical Centre St Radboud, Nijmegen, The
Netherlands

Thomas Brandt MD FRCP
Professor, Department of Neurology, Ludwig-Maximilians-
Universität München, Klinikum Grosshadern, Munich, Germany

Adolfo M. Bronstein MD PhD FRCP
Academic Department of Neuro-Otology, Division of
Neuroscience & Psychological Medicine, Imperial College of
Science, Technology and Medicine, Faculty of Medicine,
Charing Cross Hospital, London, UK

Marianne Dieterich MD
Professor of Neurology, Department of Neurology,
Johannes-Gutenberg University, Mainz, Germany

V. Dietz MD FRCP
Paraplegic Centre, University Hospital Balgrist, Zurich,
Switzerland

J. Gert van Dijk MD PhD
Department of Neurology and Clinical Neurophysiology, Leiden
University Medical Centre, Leiden, The Netherlands

Joseph M. Furman MD PhD
Departments of Otolaryngology, Neurology, Bioengineering, and
Physical Therapy, University of Pittsburgh School of Medicine,
Pittsburgh, PA, USA

Michael A. Gresty
MRC Spatial Disorientation Group, Academic Department of
Neuro-otology, Division of Neurosciences and Psychological
Medicine, Imperial College of Science and Medicine, Medical
School at Charing Cross Hospital, London, UK

Richard S. Hallam MSc PhD
Reader in Psychology, University of East London,
London, UK

Stefan Hesse MD
Klinik Berlin, Department of Neurological Rehabilitation, Free
University Berlin, Berlin, Germany

Fay B. Horak PhD
Neurological Sciences Institute and Department of Neurology
and Physiology & Pharmacology, Oregon Health & Science
University, Portland, Oregon, USA

Rolf G. Jacob MD
Departments of Psychiatry and Otolaryngology, University of
Pittsburgh School of Medicine, Pittsburgh, PA, USA

Marjan Jahanshahi MPhil (Clin Psychol) PhD
Honorary Reader in Cognitive Neuroscience, Institute of
Neurology, University College London, London, UK

Kenton R. Kaufman PhD PE
Associate Professor of Bioengineering, Director, Biomechanics
Laboratory, Consultant, Department of Orthopedic Surgery,
Mayo Clinic/Mayo Foundation, Rochester, MN, USA

Rose Anne Kenny MD FRCP FRCPI
Professor and Consultant in Cardiovascular Research, Royal
Victoria Infirmary, Newcastle-upon-Tyne, UK

José C. Masdeu MD PhD
Professor and Chairman, Department of the Neurological
Sciences, University of Navarre Medical School, CUN,
Pamplona, Spain

Jean Massion
Institute of Physiological and Cognitive Neurosciences (INPC),
National Center of Scientific Research (CNRS), Marseille, France

Karl-Heinz Mauritz MD
Professor and Chairman, Klinik Berlin, Department of Neurological
Rehabilitation, Free University Berlin, Berlin, Germany

Louw van Niekerk MBChB(Pret), FRCS(Ed) FRCS (Orth)
Consultant Orthopaedic Sports Surgeon, Friarage Duchess of
Kent Military Hospital, Northallerton, North Yorkshire, UK

John G. Nutt MD
Department of Neurology and Physiology & Pharmacology,
Oregon Health & Sciences University, Portland, OR, USA

Sebastiaan Overeem PhD
Department of Neurology and Clinical Neurophysiology, Leiden
University Medical Centre, Leiden, The Netherlands

Peter Overstall MB FRCP
Consultant in Geriatric Medicine, County Hospital,
Hereford, UK

Aftab Patla
Gait and Posture Laboratory, Department of Kinesiology,
University of Waterloo, Ontario, Canada

John H. Patrick MB FRCS
Orthotic Res & Locomotor Assessment Unit, Robert Jones &
Agnes Hunt Hospital, Oswestry, Shropshire, UK

Marousa Pavlou BA PT
Lecturer, Department of Physiotherapy, King's College London,
London, UK

Peter Rudge
Institute of Neurology, National Hospital for Neurology &
`Neurosurgery, London, UK

Anne Shumway-Cook
Northwest Physical Therapy Services, Seattle, WA, USA

Lewis Sudarsky MD
Department of Neurology, Brigham and Women's Hospital,
Harvard Medical School, Boston, MA, USA

Pei-Fang Tang PhD, PT
Assistant Professor, School and Graduate Institute of Physical
Therapy, College of Medicine, National Taiwan University,
Taipei, Taiwan

Philip D. Thompson MB PhD FRACP
University Department of Medicine, University of Adelaide, and
Department of Neurology, Royal Adelaide Hospital, South
Australia

Cordula Werner
Junior Researcher, Klinik Berlin, Department of Neurological
Rehabilitation, Free University Berlin, Berlin, Germany

Marjorie H. Woollacott PhD
Professor, Department of Exercise and Movement Science,
University of Oregon, Eugene, Oregon, USA

Lucy Yardley MSc PhD
Reader in Health Psychology, Department of Psychology,
University of Southampton, Southampton, UK

Preface to the second edition

The reasons for writing a second edition of this book are rooted in the first one. First, disorders of balance and gait are on the increase, as might be expected with our longer lifespan. Second, the first edition was so well received by colleagues and reviewers that we felt it our duty to keep this multidisciplinary effort alive. Problems with balance, gait and posture are produced by such a diversity of disorders, in so many disparate systems, that a book attempting to bring various disciplines together is a rewarding and necessary task.

The seven-year gap between the first and second editions means that the book has been almost completely rewritten. John Nutt, who has specific expertise in movement disorders and related problems of gait, has joined the editorial team. New chapters dealing with critical issues such as classification of balance and gait disorders, objective assessment of posture and gait, cerebrovascular disease and hydrocephalus have been incorporated. The important topic of syncope related falls is now covered in two chapters, including one specifically devoted to this

problem in the elderly. Fifteen new authors have brought new expertise and complementary view points to the different chapters. Examples are the chapters on psychiatric aspects of imbalance, where neurologists and psychiatrists present complementary views, and the chapter on drop attacks, syncope-related falls and their mimics, where neurologists and autonomic nervous system specialists address these problems together.

As before, we did not intend to produce a mammoth book exhausting the field (and the reader). Our intention was to bring together basic scientists and various clinical specialists in order to present the range of problems and to help busy clinicians to manage their patients. We hope we have succeeded.

Adolfo M. Bronstein
Thomas Brandt
Marjorie H. Woollacott
John G. Nutt

Preface to the first edition

A crucial issue facing clinicians is the management of the patient who has critically impaired walking abilities. Patients face the reality of being unable to look after themselves and the resultant pressure is transmitted to relatives and social services. The magnitude of this problem has already begun to increase as the mean age of the population in industrialized societies has risen. Unfortunately, the mechanisms underlying the production of human locomotion are complex and the nature of the disorders affecting locomotion are varied. Thus a simple solution to the problem of managing gait disorders is not available to us.

The diagnosis and management of the patient with abnormal balance, posture and gait presents the clinician with a formidable challenge. In no other set of disorders is it more genuine to think that what is wrong with the patient can be due to impairments ranging from the top of the head to the tip of the toes! For example, disorders may include various components of the motor system, the vestibular system, and the musculoskeletal apparatus, giving rise to gait disorders or a sensation of unsteadiness. In addition, psychological dysfunction can result from, or present to the clinician, as a balance and gait problem. In older adults the involvement of multiple systems in balance and gait disorders is most typical.

This book has been conceived with this multidisciplinary concept in mind. Although biased towards a clinical audience, we have attempted to provide a strong physiological basis for a better understanding of mechanisms underlying balance and gait disorders. We have divided the text into four sections dealing with normal and developmental aspects, assessment, disorders and rehabilitation of balance and gait plus a separate section devoted to the problems of the elderly. The contributors comprise neurologists, orthopedic surgeons, neuro-otologists, geriatricians, psychologists, physiotherapists and physiologists who have been encouraged to tread across frontiers as is appropriate for such an interdisciplinary task. It is therefore unavoidable that some overlap may occur, but we believe that the reader will be enriched by witnessing the way similar topics are dealt with from a variety of viewpoints.

The aim of this book is not to exhaust any specific disease resulting in impairment of gait, balance or posture. Such diseases will remain in the domain of the appropriate specialist but general guidelines and references are provided for those interested. It is not our intention to create a new balance and gait specialist. Rather, we hope to emphasize that whoever is dealing with patients with balance and gait disorders can benefit from broadening the horizon of his or her own speciality.

Adolfo M. Bronstein
Thomas Brandt
Marjorie H. Woollacott
1996

1

Posture and equilibrium

JEAN MASSION AND MARJORIE H. WOOLLACOTT

INTRODUCTION

There are two different types of motor ability critical for motor coordination: the first involves voluntary motor control and includes activities such as eye–hand coordination function, and the second involves postural or equilibrium control. The latter is really the foundation for all voluntary motor skills, with almost every movement that an individual makes being made up of both (1) postural components, which stabilize the body, and (2) the prime mover components which relate to a particular movement goal.

Although clinicians understand the importance of postural control for activities such as standing, walking and manipulation skills, there is no universal definition of postural control, or a clear consensus on the mechanisms that underlie postural and balance functions. In this chapter we will first offer a broad definition of postural control and then discuss research on the contributions of different body systems to the control of balance or posture.

In order to understand postural control as a behavior, we first need to understand its task. Initially, this involves the maintenance of the alignment of body posture and the adoption of an appropriate vertical relationship between body segments to counteract the forces of gravity and thus allow the maintenance of upright stance. Postural muscle tone is a primary contributor to the maintenance of vertical stance.

Once this alignment is achieved, the position of the body's center of mass must be maintained within specific boundaries in space, or stability limits, related to the individual's base of support. Thus, a second part of the task of postural control is the maintenance of equilibrium.

Posture is also a key component of all perception–action systems and serves to maintain bodily orientation to the environment. For example, an individual's posture can be considered a primary support for the exploration of the surrounding space in terms of perceptual analysis and motor action. For this exploration, the nervous system must have an accurate picture of the position of the body segments with respect to each other and with respect to space. The internal postural image or postural body schema provides this information and it is monitored by multisensory inputs. On the basis of this representation and according to the perception–action task, the orientation of one or several body segments (head, trunk, arm, etc.) will be selected as a reference frame for the organization of the corresponding action.

Finally, posture also serves as a mechanical support for action. It organizes the coupling between the different segments as a function of the task and adjusts the joint stiffness dynamically during the movement.

We begin this chapter with a discussion of postural control in relation to body alignment and the maintenance of bodily orientation to the environment. We will then discuss the control of stability or balance control. Finally, we will consider posture as a mechanical support for action.

POSTURAL CONTROL DURING QUIET STANCE

Erect posture in humans is achieved by the superposition of body segments (head, trunk and legs) along the longitudinal axis. This superposition is such that it should fulfil the two functions of posture. The first is the *antigravity function*. The superposition of segments is performed against the force of gravity and the associated ground reaction forces. The postural tone, which is predominantly distributed among the extensor muscles, plays an important role in this antigravity function.

There is an additional constraint, which is equilibrium maintenance. This means that the positioning of body segments (which is only restricted by the mechanical limits of joint movement) should be such that the projection of the center of gravity (CG) remains inside the support base under static conditions.

A second function of posture is to serve as an interface with the external world for perception and action. It means that the orientation with respect to space of given body segments such as the head, the trunk or the arm are used as a reference frame. The reference frame may be used either to perceive the position of the body's movement with respect to the external world or to organize movements toward a target in external space.

Taking into account the functions of posture according to the context and the task, two modes of postural organization have been proposed.

First, a global organization of posture is mainly related to equilibrium control. It is represented by the inverted pendulum model described by Nashner and McCollum.[1] The reference value to be regulated for equilibrium control is still a matter of discussion. Balance, *stricto sensu*, is preserved when the center of pressure (CP) remains inside the support base (i.e. the surface under the feet). Under static conditions this corresponds to the projection of the CG.

However, under dynamic conditions, as, for example, initiation of gait, the CG is accelerated by a torque at the level of the ankle joint created by activating muscles controlling that joint; this causes a shift of the CP, which moves away from the CG projection. Thus, both CP position and CG projection onto the support base should be taken into account for equilibrium control in dynamic conditions. According to the modeling of Païand Patton,[2] the border of the stability limits can be predicted in dynamic conditions by a combination of three parameters: the CP position, the CG horizontal position and the CG velocity.

In order to regulate the CG position, which is located at the level of the pelvis, the whole body can be moved as an inverted pendulum around the ankle joint. However, as will be commented on later, these oscillations are very slow (frequency around 0.2 Hz) because of the high inertia of the body. In case of fast perturbations, fast corrections are required. Other body segments with lower inertia (trunk around the hip, thigh around the knee) are then moved for fast corrections.[3]

Interestingly, the constraints related to body inertia are not only important for equilibrium control. They are also a key characteristic for the organization of movements. For example, it is possible to couple a set of joints by increasing the corresponding joint stiffness. This results in creating a new ensemble with an increased inertia corresponding to that of the whole set of segments coupled together. Droulez and Berthoz[4] introduced the concept of topological organization of posture in order to describe this reorganization of body inertia. They provided two examples. When reading a paper

while walking, stiffness of the arm, trunk and head is increased in order to create a new high inertial ensemble that will reduce the movements of the arms with respect to the head. Conversely, unlocking the arm from the trunk occurs in tasks where the stability of the hand position in space should be preserved independently from the trunk oscillations, as when the subject is walking holding a full glass in the hand.

A second mode of organization is modular organization, which is used for orienting segments such as the head and trunk (which serve as a reference frame for perception and action) with respect to space. The various segments of the kinematic chain from the feet to the head are not controlled as a single functional unit, but as a superposition of individual 'modules'. Each module is tied to the next one by a set of muscles which has its own central and peripheral control, aimed at maintaining the reference position of the module. Martin[5] has reported that postencephalitic patients that had lost the ability to maintain the head axis vertical during normal life held the head permanently inclined on the trunk. When asked to raise the head by a voluntary movement, they were able to do so for some time. There was thus dissociation between an automatic regulation of the head position, which was lost, and its voluntary control, which was preserved.

The head is the site of different categories of sensors, such as the retina, the labyrinthine afferents and the neck muscle proprioceptors. Each category of receptors has been shown to be able to stabilize the head. The head can be stabilized with respect to gaze,[6] verticality[7] and to the trunk.[8] Orientation and stabilization of the trunk axis, which is the largest axis of any body segment, is critical.[9] Stabilization of the trunk has also been observed with respect to vertical in the frontal plane during leg movement[10] and during locomotion[11] or during oscillatory movements of the supporting platform.[12] Interestingly, maintaining equilibrium through the global organization of posture and preserving the orientation of body segments with respect to space may be conflicting in given motor acts through the modular control of posture. For example, there will be a conflict between equilibrium maintenance and holding a full glass of wine by the hand (local posture) when a postural disturbance occurs that endangers balance. In this case, the subject will lose balance, take a support with the other hand and keep the glass full. The modular organization of posture can serve to regulate posture itself. The stabilization of the head in space during locomotion is used as a navigational inertial platform for the evaluation of the visual or labyrinthine inputs. These inputs signal changes of body position with respect to the external world.[13]

Another important role of this modular organization of posture is to serve as an egocentric reference frame for the organization of movement. For example, during a reaching task, head and trunk axes are reference values for the calculation of the target position with respect to the body (as shown by neck vibration experiments)[14] and for the calculation of the hand trajectory.[15] Also, during manipulation of heavy objects, the forearm position is stabilized and serves as a reference frame for this task.[9]

How the various modes of postural organization are centrally controlled has been a matter of discussions and two main models have been proposed, the 'genetic model' and the 'hierarchical model.'

GENETIC MODEL OF POSTURE CONTROL

In a classical view of postural control, based on the work of Magnus[16] and Rademaker,[17] each animal species is considered to have a reference posture or stance, which is genetically determined. According to this view, postural control and its adaptation to the environment is based on background postural tone and on the postural reflexes or reactions. These reactions are considered to originate from inputs from the visual and vestibular systems (localized at the level of the head) and from the somatosensory system, with inputs at the level of the different body segments.

According to this classical view, the main constraint for building up the reference posture, which is stance, is considered to be the effect of gravity on the body segments. The gravity vector is considered to serve as a reference frame, the so-called geocentric reference frame,[18] for the positioning of the different body segments with respect to each other and to the external world.

Three main functions are identified in the genetic model of posture: (1) an antigravity function; (2) body segment orientation with respect to gravity; (3) the adaptation of posture to the body orientation in space.

Antigravity function

The antigravity function provides a support for the body segments against the contact forces exerted by the ground due to gravity and contributes to equilibrium maintenance.

Postural tone is the main tool for building the antigravity posture. It is predominantly observed at the level of the limbs, back and neck extensor muscles and the masseter muscle of the jaw. The main force vector of these muscles counteracts the effect of gravity when the subject is standing on a support surface. Decerebrate rigidity, which is observed after midcollicular decerebration in animals, is a caricature of this background postural tone.[19]

Interestingly, postural tone depends on the integrity of the myotatic reflex loop and is suppressed by section of the dorsal roots. Therefore, decerebrate rigidity has been called 'gamma' rigidity, in contrast to the 'alpha' rigidity observed in the quadruped after cerebellar anterior lobe lesions, which is preserved after dorsal root section. Since postural tone is under the control of the myotatic reflex loop, one possible mechanism for controlling erect posture is the stretch reflex, which would be able to oppose any deviation from the initial posture, as pointed out by Lloyd.[20] However, recent research indicates that normal young adults typically do not show monosynaptic stretch reflex responses when responding to threats to balance during quiet stance[21–23] and that higher levels of control are involved.

A series of postural reflexes contribute to the antigravity function: they adapt muscle force to body weight. Examples include the myotatic reflexes and the positive supporting reactions which adjust the leg and trunk muscle tone to the body weight.

The postural reactions are aimed at restoring balance in face of an internal disturbance. According to Forssberg,[24] they are based on a set of inborn reactions that are selected and shaped during ontogenesis.

Orientation of the body segments with respect to the gravity vector

The gravity sensors of the lateral line organ, together with light-sensitive afferents, serve to orient the longitudinal body axis of fish with respect to gravity. In mammals, where the body is segmented into head, trunk and legs, the otoliths and vision serve for orienting the head with respect to the gravity axis. The orientation is horizontal in the cat and vertical in humans; the orientation of the other segments is a function of that of the head. The righting reflexes described by Rademaker[17] are an illustration of this concept. As first shown by Etienne-Jules Marey, when a cat falls from an inverted position, the head is first reoriented along the horizontal plane, then the trunk orientation with respect to the head is restored and finally the leg axis becomes vertical. The head orientation in space is stabilized by the vestibulocollic reflexes, which play an important role during locomotion.

Other reflexes serve to orient the foot with respect to the support. These include the placing reactions. There are three placing reactions: the tactile placing reaction, which causes flexion followed by extension of the leg in response to cutaneous stimulation; and the visual and labyrinthine placing reactions, both eliciting extension of the forelimbs when the animal is dropped toward the ground. Other reflexes such as the hopping reaction, are aimed at reorienting the leg with respect to the gravity axis.[25]

Adaptation of the antigravity posture to the body segment posture or movement

A third function of the genetic organization is to adjust antigravity posture to ongoing activity. Examples of this are the labyrinthine reflexes, which adjust the postural tone as a function of the head position in the frontal or sagittal plane. For example, when the whole body is inclined toward one side, the otolith inputs from that side induce an increased postural tone on the same side. The neck and labyrinthine reflexes illustrate another example of adaptation of posture to ongoing activity. They orient the leg and trunk posture as a function either of the neck orientation in space or of the pelvis orientation in space. For example, turning the head toward the right induces an extension of the fore and hind limbs toward the same side and a flexion of the limbs of the opposite side. In contrast, turning the trunk toward the same side provokes a flexion of the ipsilateral forelimb and an extension of the ipsilateral hindlimb (Fig. 1.1).[26]

Tonic neck reflex

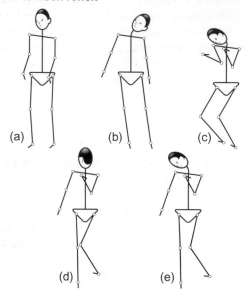

Tonic lumbar reflex

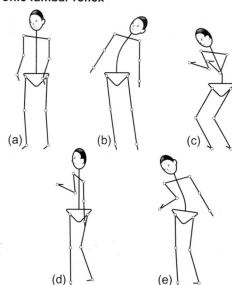

(a) Stance
(b) Dorsiflexion
(c) Ventroflexion
(d) Rotation right
(e) Deviation right

Figure 1.1 *Comparison between neck and lumbar reflexes. Reproduced from Tokizane T, Murao M, Ogata T, Kondo T. Electromyographic studies on tonic neck, lumbar and labyrinthine reflexes in normal persons. Jpn J Physiol 1951;2:130–46, with permission from the Center for Academic Publications, Japan.*

Summary

To conclude, the three main functions of the genetic organization of erect posture (i.e. the support of the body against gravity, the orientation of the body with respect to the gravity vector and the adaptation of the body posture to the ongoing head and trunk movement) are critical for adapting erect posture to the environment and to ongoing activity. These functions are controlled by spinal cord (propriospinal circuits) and brainstem pathways. Some reflexes, such as the tactile placing reaction include motor cortex pathways.

HIERARCHICAL MODEL OF POSTURAL ORGANIZATION

The genetic model of posture has been challenged for several reasons. First, the postural reactions to stance disturbance have been shown to be flexible.[1,27] For example, when a balance disturbance occurs while standing, the main muscles involved in the correction are the leg muscles. If the subject holds on to an additional support with the hands, the postural reactions will involve mainly the arm muscles. These, and other observations are not compatible with a reflex organization and suggest a spatio-temporal flexibility of the response according to task constraints.

Second, postural control has been analysed in a behavioral context during the performance of voluntary movements. Anticipatory postural adjustments have been described during the performance of goal-directed movements. They are aimed at both preserving balance and the orientation of body segments during the performance of the movement and at assisting the movement in terms of force and velocity.[28] Interestingly, anticipation means prediction of the postural disturbance because of the movement. This prediction would depend on internal models built by the brain, which would map the surrounding space, the body characteristics and their interaction. This idea was proposed by Bernstein[29] on the basis of his observations on motor learning and were extended to posture by Gurfinkel and co-workers.[30–32]

The hierarchical model of posture proposes that two levels of control exist. The first is a level of representation or postural body schema; the second is a level of implementation for postural control.

The concept of body schema was first proposed by Head.[33] In its adaptation to posture, the internal representation of body posture, or body schema has been hypothesized to be partly genetically determined and partly acquired by learning. It includes three main aspects: (1) a representation of the body geometry, (2) a representation of body kinetics, mainly related to the conditions of support, and (3) a representation of the body orientation with respect to gravity (vertical).

Geometric representation of the body

Research suggests that the individual's geometric representation of the body depends mainly on the information provided by the proprioceptive Ia afferent inputs. Studies using minivibrators to excite eye, neck and ankle muscles afferents[34,35] have explored the contributions of proprioceptive inputs from these muscles both to perception of body sway and to actual posture control during quiet stance. It was found that vibration to the eye muscles, the neck muscles or the ankle muscles of a standing subject with eyes closed produced body sway, with the sway direction depending on the muscle vibrated. When these muscles were vibrated simultaneously, the effects were additive, with no clear domination of one proprioceptive influence over another. When the body was prevented from moving during the tendon vibration, it created an illusion of movement.

This suggests that proprioception from all parts of the body plays an important role in the maintenance of quiet stance body posture. The experiments also suggest that, when an individual is standing, there is a kinematic chain formed by the Ia inputs from muscles around each joint, informing the nervous system about the position of each joint with respect to the remaining parts of the body. It is interesting that vibration of the ocular muscles also induced postural reactions. This indicates that they monitor the position of the eyes with respect to the head and thus are able to estimate the position of a visual target in terms of head coordinates.

The output of the spindle primary afferent inputs is interpreted differently by the central nervous system depending on such factors as the selected reference frame of the subject (for example, is the body the reference frame, or are three-dimensional environmental coordinates the reference frame) and the presence of gravity. As mentioned above, when an individual is standing and when body weight is exerted on a supporting surface, the proprioceptive Ia afferent inputs monitor both body displacement and velocity of displacement. The effect of Achilles tendon vibration when the eyes are closed is to cause postural sway in response to the erroneous Ia input that mimics the displacement of the limb. However, under microgravity conditions[36] or when an individual is sitting, tendon vibration produces no postural reactions. This means that the monitoring of body posture by proprioceptive inputs depends a great deal on graviceptors.

It is also interesting that the postural response induced by galvanic stimulation of vestibular receptors depends on the body geometry and the postural body schema.[32,37] For example, it has been demonstrated that when a subject is standing normally, cathodic stimulation of one labyrinth elicits a shift of the center of gravity in the frontal plane toward the same side. However, when the head is turned to the right, the same stimulation elicits a displacement of the center of gravity backwards. The result shows that the postural response depends on the head position with respect to the trunk. The same change in the direction of the postural response is observed when head and trunk together are rotated to the right.

How is the head and trunk position monitored with respect to the legs? Vibration of the right gluteus maximus with the trunk fixed induces an illusory rotation of the head–trunk segment to the right. When galvanic vestibular stimulation is performed during right gluteus maximus vibration, it provokes a backward sway as if the head (and trunk) was actually rotated to the right. This observation elucidates the role of the Ia proprioceptive inputs stimulated by vibration in reorienting the postural reaction and thus monitoring the head–trunk position with respect to the legs (Fig. 1.2).

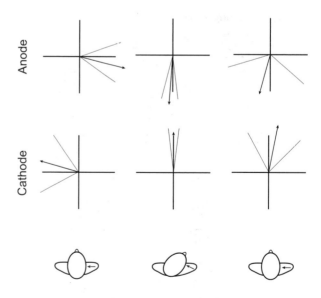

Figure 1.2 *Galvanic stimulation of the right labyrinth. The arrow indicates the stimulated side. Center of pressure recorded from a force platform (according to ref. 32). When the head is straight, the postural reaction to anodic stimulation is oriented to the right. When the head (or head and trunk) is turned to the right, the postural reaction to the same stimulus is oriented backward. The same backward-oriented postural reaction is obtained by galvanic stimulation during a vibration of the gluteus maximus, which provokes an illusion of head–trunk rotation to the right.*

Representation of body kinetics

Two issues concerning body kinetics should be mentioned: (1) the nervous system's evaluation of the support conditions (this concerns the orientation of body segments with respect to the gravity axis; see next section), and (2) the calculation under dynamic conditions of the inertia of different body segments, providing an accurate estimation of the center of gravity position.

During stance, reaction forces are exerted by the supporting platform on the body. They are the main basis for the maintenance of the erect posture. It is generally concluded that stance results from a 'bottom up' (that is, support surface oriented) maintenance of balance, on the basis of these reaction forces. Whether these reaction forces are perceived and how they might be perceived is still partly unanswered. The foot sole receptors together with proprioceptive inputs monitoring the ankle joint angle play an important role in this respect.[38]

Several studies have shown that the organization of postural reactions depends on the conditions of support. For example, when the standing subject is holding a lever with the hands, the postural reactions previously seen in the leg muscles now move to the arm extensors.[39] Thus, when part of the body support is taken by the hand, the postural reactions to a stance disturbance involve mainly the arm extensor muscles in place of the leg muscles. When the body weight is absent, as under water, the postural reactions tend to disappear.[40] There is thus an internal representation of the support conditions, which selects the appropriate actuators for optimizing the equilibrium maintenance.

A second aspect of body kinetics involves the inertial properties of the segments. These properties are automatically taken into account for the regulation of balance. For example, after adding a 10 kg load on the shoulder, the regulation of the center of gravity during an upper-trunk bending is just as efficient as without a load.[41] There is also evidence indicating that perception of body inertia does exist.[42] This would explain why a regulation of the body center of mass still exists in microgravity during multisegmental movements such as trunk bending.[43]

Orientation with respect to vertical

The orientation of the body with respect to vertical in the frontal plane and in the sagittal plane is a primary constraint for erect posture in a world in which the effects of gravity must be taken into account. Which sensors indicate that the body posture is appropriately oriented with respect to vertical and which ones are used for stabilizing the selected orientation? There are no static sensors that directly monitor the center of gravity projection to the ground. The body orientation with respect to vertical in the frontal and sagittal plane is reg-

ulated by sensors located in the head and in other body segments.

As mentioned earlier, body posture results from the superposition of multiple segments from the feet to the head. How is the orientation of the segments with respect to the vertical calculated and how is the orientation of the individual segments controlled in order to maintain equilibrium? In this respect, according to Mergner and Rosemeier,[44] there are two main modes of representation of the body segments with respect to the external world, depending on the reference value selected for this calculation.

In a top-down mode, the labyrinthine information from the otoliths is used as a reference value for calculating the head orientation with respect to the vertical. The calculation of the position of the trunk, pelvis, leg and feet segments in space is performed with respect to the head position in space. This mode is the first to emerge during ontogenesis, with the early stabilization of the head in space.[24] A second mode, a bottom-up mode, uses the support surface (under the feet) as a reference value for the calculation of the pelvic position in space. This mode is mainly related to equilibrium control. It emerges later during ontogenesis, with stance and locomotion.

Four sources of information regarding orientation with respect to verticality are the labyrinthine and visual sensors located in the head, the haptic sensors and the body graviceptors.

LABYRINTHINE SENSORS

Information about the gravity vector is provided by the otoliths. The vertical orientation of the head in the dark is generally attributed to their activity.[16,17] The distribution of the otoliths in the vertical and horizontal plane provides information on the inclination of the head with respect to vertical both in the sagittal and in the frontal plane. Since the otolith receptors also monitor the linear acceleration along the horizontal and the vertical axes, the information about the gravity vector is biased when the subject (or the head) is moving. It is still unclear to what extent these sensors contribute to the determination of vertical.

The labyrinthine receptors also play an important role in stabilizing the head and in body orientation. Linear acceleration is monitored by the otoliths and angular acceleration (pitch, roll and yaw) by the three pairs of semicircular canals.

VISUAL SENSORS

Visual static input, involving the vertical or horizontal structure of the visual frame (the objects within the visual field), is used for orienting the body axis.[45] Research has shown that providing a biased visual frame modifies both the perception of vertical and postural orientation.

The stabilization of orientation on the basis of visual input depends mainly on visual inputs detecting movement. Through this information the visual system monitors head and body displacement with respect to the external world. This type of information is called vection. The linear displacement of the visual frame within the peripheral visual field provokes body sway in the direction of the displacement of the visual frame, with the intensity of the sway depending on the velocity and on the spatial frequency of the visual frame.[46]

Sinusoidal displacements of the visual frame are associated with sinusoidal postural sway, with no phase shift between the two, indicating a coupling between both oscillations.[47] Circular vection in the frontal plane causes body inclination toward the direction of the vection.[48,49] The direction of postural reactions can be interpreted in the following ways. The displacement of the visual scene backwards when the subject is standing mimics the situation of the body falling forward, in a direction opposite to the moving scene. The backward postural sway in the direction of the moving scene thus mimics the normal compensatory reactions that would occur when the subject was actually falling forward.

The visual and labyrinthine inputs are located in the head and they help to orient the head position. However, as the position of the head with respect to the trunk is not fixed, their influence on body posture and, more specifically, on balance control depends on the evaluation of head position with respect to the trunk. As mentioned earlier, this evaluation is made by the neck muscle proprioceptors.

HAPTIC SENSORS

A simple contact of the hand or of the fingers with an external surface can be used as a reference frame for calculating the body oscillations with respect to that surface and to correct the oscillations with a latency of around 50 ms. Haptic cues are very efficient in stabilizing posture, especially by handicapped patients when using a cane. Interestingly, when the support on which the hand is in contact is rhythmically moving, some subjects show body sway at the same frequency without phase shift, indicating a feed-forward control.[50]

BODY GRAVICEPTORS

A fourth category of sensors that serve for the orientation with respect to verticality is represented by the 'so-called' body graviceptors. The existence of body graviceptors was first proposed by Gurfinkel et al.[12] in order to explain the ability of subjects to stabilize the trunk when the support surface was moving sinusoidally and by Mittelstaedt[51] who provides evidence for graviceptors in the area around the kidney. Riccio et al.,[52] using a specific set-up to dissociate the axis for balance control from the vertical axis, indicated that the perceived orientation of the body depends both on the gravity vector and on the orientation of the ground reaction force exerted by the subject to control balance.

Indirect evidence concerning the role of body graviceptors on body orientation was provided by experiments on the postural orientation of divers when under water. It was shown that, when under water, the body orientation was always tilted forward with respect to vertical, suggesting incorrect information from body graviceptors contributing to the body's orientation under this abnormal weight condition.[53]

Experiments by Dietz and colleagues[54,55] have also provided evidence in favor of body graviceptors. When a subject standing on a platform under water in a pool is given support surface perturbations to balance, postural reactions are absent. Since the water pressure cancels normal body weight, the researchers compensated for the lack of body weight in the subjects by adding loads at the level of the different joints. Under these conditions, the postural corrective reactions in response to a disturbance of the support platform returned as a function of the weight added at each joint.

Further experiments were performed in which horizontal loads were placed on subjects lying supine, thus creating forces on joints equivalent to standing vertically. Under these conditions, the subjects showed postural reactions similar to those observed during quiet standing, when the support surface to which the feet were attached was disturbed. Dietz et al.[55] suggested that graviceptors were monitoring the force exerted by the subject to oppose the external forces. In normal stance, these graviceptors would monitor the force vector exerted at each joint to oppose gravity and this information would contribute to an internal representation of the vertical axis. A putative candidate for the monitoring of this sensory information is the Golgi tendon organ, which measures the number of active motor units at a given time in each muscle used in postural control.[56]

In addition to specific graviceptors, the stabilization of balance by body sensors depends mainly on cutaneous foot sole sensors which monitor the amplitude and the direction of the contact forces exerted by the body onto the ground. Experiments that support these conclusions have shown that replacing a firm support surface by a foam surface or cooling the foot sole results in postural instability,[45,57,58] whereas vibration of the foot sole restricted to front or back parts induces postural sway[38] in a direction that would oppose the swaying of the person toward the front or the back part of the feet.

MULTISENSORY CONVERGENCE AND BALANCE CONTROL

The use of sensory information from multiple sources, including the visual, vestibular and somatosensory systems, is a key feature of the neural control of both body orientation with respect to vertical and stabilization against external disturbances.

There are two opposite interpretations concerning the role of the multisensory afferents. According to one view, the multiple sensory afferents are used to build up the vertical reference value on which the body will be aligned. This hypothesis has been put forward by Hlavacka et al.[59] to explain the postural reorientation that is observed after combined proprioceptive and vestibular stimulation. The misperception of the body midline when unilateral neck muscles are vibrated or when unilateral vestibular galvanic stimulation is performed supports this interpretation.[60]

Another interpretation is that the multiple sensory inputs serve for monitoring the error of the actual posture with respect to a reference value defined by other sensors. The forward sway of the body during tibialis anterior vibration in the standing subject has been interpreted in the following way. The vertical reference value is provided by a set of graviceptors. The artificial Ia input induced by the tibialis muscle tendon vibration is interpreted by the central nervous system as indicating a stretching of that muscle and a backward body sway with respect to the vertical. The forward body sway is viewed as a correction of posture in response to the artificial Ia afferent inputs indicating backward sway.

One possible use of redundant sensory information in the regulation of posture is that different set of sensors are put into action according to the source or the velocity of the postural disturbance. The sensitivity range of each category of sensors is different. For example, visual input gives sensitive information related to low-velocity displacements of the body, whereas labyrinthine inputs are sensitive to high rates of acceleration.

Two modes of interaction between these inputs have been identified by manipulating one category of inputs, the other being unchanged, or by depriving the subject of one or several sources of sensory information.

Additive effect

Usually, each input adds its effect to the effect of the other inputs. Thus, visual vection, by itself, will produce postural changes when the other inputs are unchanged. In addition, the body orientation will be biased with respect to vertical when the visual reference frame is inclined, even though the labyrinthine and proprioceptive inputs are unchanged. In this case, there is a sensory conflict between the two types of information about verticality and the resulting postural orientation is intermediate with respect to the orientation prescribed by each category of sensors.

The additive effect of the various inputs in posture control may partly explain the compensatory mechanisms involved when one of the inputs is suppressed. As shown by Horak et al.,[61] in patients with labyrinthine lesions, postural control is relatively well preserved, though only visual and somatosensory inputs are available. However, disturbance of one of the remaining inputs (vision or somatosensory) markedly decreases the patient's ability to balance.

Selection

When conflicts between the information from one type of input and the others arise, one way of resolving the conflict is to select one input which becomes dominant. For example, Achilles tendon vibration produces backward body sway with eyes closed because the somatosensory system is signaling stretch to the gastrocnemius/soleus muscles and thus forward sway. However, when vision is available, the vibration has no postural effect. One could regard this as indicating that the retinal input is dominant and the erroneous input is disregarded. An alternative explanation is that, with eyes open, both vision and vestibular inputs are signaling that no movement is taking place, and somatosensory inputs are thus the only inputs signaling movement. In this case the single conflicting input is disregarded.[34]

It should be stressed that there are individual differences in the dominance patterns of the three sensory inputs. Some subjects rely more on vision, while others rely more on somatosensory inputs.

POSTURAL CONTROL IN RESPONSE TO BALANCE DISTURBANCES

In the last section we reviewed research pertaining to balance control during quiet stance. In many ways this is the simplest form of balance control, since the individual is simply maintaining quiet stance. We will now move on to discuss research on balance control in conditions where there are external threats to balance, such as balancing while standing on a bus which is starting and stopping unexpectedly. This is somewhat more difficult than simply controlling background sway and requires the ability to respond to perturbations to balance differing in direction, amplitude and velocity.

Strategies and synergies

A researcher who has influenced research in postural and movement control considerably is Nicholai Bernstein, a Russian investigator, who argued on theoretical grounds that it would be difficult for the brain to regulate independently the incredible number of motions of the many mechanical linkages of the body and the activities of the associated muscle groups.[29] He thus hypothesized that the nervous system organizes movement in a hierarchical manner, with higher levels of the nervous system activating lower level synergies, which are groups of muscles constrained to act together as a unit. This would thus free up the higher levels of the nervous system for other roles, such as adapting responses to changing task conditions. He hypothesized that such actions as breathing, walking and postural control would use synergies to coordinate the activation of muscles as a unit.

In order to test this hypothesis, researchers have explored the characteristics of muscle responses activated when a subject is exposed to external threats to balance. Gurfinkel and his colleagues performed the first extensive experiments on the contributions of the peripheral and central neural control mechanisms to posture during quiet stance.[62,63] They showed that the excitability levels of the monosynaptic stretch reflex decrease during stance compared with less demanding postural tasks such as lying down, sitting or standing with support. Why would this be the case? They suggested that this would allow postural control to be dominated by longer latency responses (latencies of 70–125 ms, which may be spinally or supraspinally mediated), which are more adaptable and thus more useful in dealing with stance balance control under a wide range of conditions. Gurfinkel and his colleagues proposed that this reorganization in neural control of posture was the result of the functioning of central programs which coordinate the activity of different muscle groups during postural control.

Other research by Nashner[21] and Nashner and Woollacott[64] has further explored Bernstein's hypothesis by examining whether the responses activated in muscles of the leg and trunk in response to perturbations to balance are part of a pre-programmed neural response or synergy or are the result of independent stretch and activation of individual muscles, owing to a simple mechanical coupling of ankle and hip motion during the perturbation.

Subjects were asked to stand on a platform which could be moved unexpectedly in the forward or backward direction or rotated, to cause ankle dorsiflexion or plantarflexion (Fig. 1.3). The different types of platform motions destabilized balance in different ways, requiring the activation of different muscle groups in order to regain balance. The activity of muscles which contribute to the control of the movements of the ankle, knee and hip was monitored.[21,64]

The results showed that, in response to backward platform translations causing anterior sway, gastrocnemius, the stretched ankle muscle was activated approximately 90 ms after platform movement onset, followed sequentially by the hamstrings muscle and the paraspinal muscles at approximately 20-ms intervals. Note that the gastrocnemius response is about 50 ms later than monosynaptic stretch reflex latencies, suggesting that it involves more complex neural pathways. Forward translations caused backward sway and activation of the stretched tibialis anterior muscle, followed by the quadriceps and abdominals (Fig. 1.4).

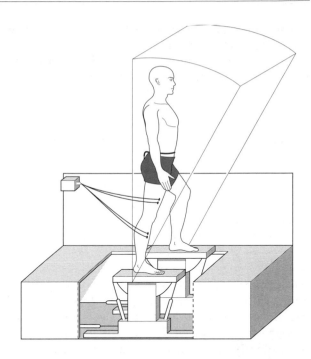

Figure 1.3 *Diagram of the hydraulically activated platform used to perturb the balance of standing subjects. The platform may be translated in the antero-posterior direction or rotated about an axis collinear with the ankle joints (reproduced from ref. 109 with permission from The American Physiological Society).*

Was this response the result of a synergic coupling of these muscles or, alternatively, the result of independent stretch of the individual muscles? In order to answer this question the authors changed the mechanical coupling of the ankle and hip motions by giving the subjects platform rotations, which directly rotated the ankles without causing movements at the other joints. These platform rotations caused activation of the same groups of leg muscles, thus suggesting that it was movement in a single joint, the ankle joint, that was activating the responses in multiple muscles.[21,64]

Experiments were also performed to test whether ankle joint rotation is required to activate the response. In these experiments the platform was moved forward, but during the movement it was rotated in order to keep the ankle joints at a constant 90°, thus eliminating ankle rotation. Under this condition, the muscle responses were delayed. Because the response was delayed it was concluded that the early response was elicited primarily by ankle joint inputs, while a later response possibly activated by vestibular and/or visual inputs, served to stabilize balance. This evidence supported the hypothesis that balance is controlled by neurally programmed synergies, and since the coupling of the muscles served the function of stabilizing ankle sway, the response was termed the 'sway synergy'.[1,21]

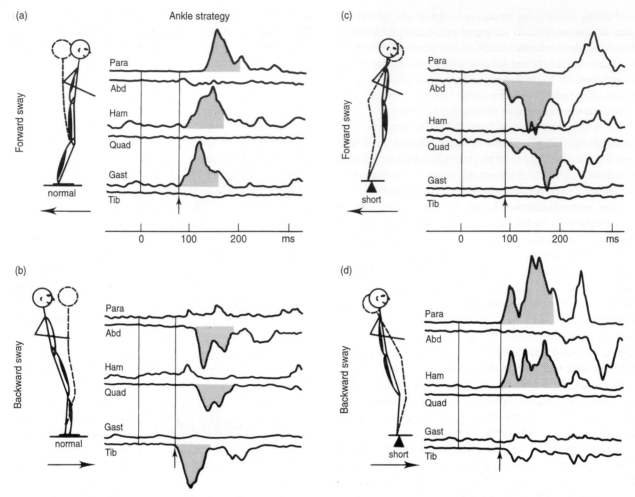

Figure 1.4 *Examples of the muscle activation patterns observed in response to (a) backward platform movements causing forward sway; (b) forward platform movements causing backward sway. These activate the ankle synergy, with responses starting in the stretched ankle muscle, followed by the leg and trunk muscles. (c,d) Muscle response patterns observed when subjects are balanced on a short support surface (restraining the use of ankle torque) while the platform moved backward (c) or forward (d), and activated the hip synergy (adapted from ref. 65).*

Are strategies versus synergies invariant?

In further research, Horak and Nashner[65] found that under conditions in which it was difficult to use ankle torque to balance (standing on a surface that was much shorter than the foot), subjects mainly used motion at the hip to compensate for threats to balance. Under this condition, forward and backward platform movements were compensated for by activating the thigh and trunk muscles on the unstretched aspect of the leg (see Fig. 1.4c,d).[65] This muscle response pattern or synergy restored balance primarily through movement at the hip and was termed the 'hip strategy' as opposed to the 'ankle strategy' by which balance is restored primarily through movement at the ankle.

Although the responses of select muscles and body movement patterns associated with balance recovery give some information on motor control strategies underlying balance, the calculation of joint torques used in postural recovery gives information on the sum of forces provided by all the muscles acting at a given joint. Thus, one can observe the work of additional muscles beyond those recorded through electromyographs (EMGs).

Researchers[66,67] have used this technique to explore the conditions under which subjects use ankle vs. hip strategies when recovering balance on a normal surface. They tested the hypothesis that ankle strategies are used primarily for low velocity (center of mass stays well within the stability limits) threats to balance while hip strategies are used for higher velocity threats (center of mass moves closer to the limits of stability). It has been shown that, as platform movement velocities gradually increase from 10 cm/s up to as much as 55–80 cm/s, subjects increase muscle forces at the ankle, and then begin to add in forces at the hip at a certain critical threshold point. This point varies across subjects. Pure hip strategies, previously observed by monitoring EMG patterns when subjects responded to postural perturbations while standing on a narrow support surface[65] were not found.[66,67]

How could strategy be defined with respect to synergy and is this distinction between two concepts justified? During voluntary movement, the strategy is defined as the path that is selected for reaching a goal. For example, during a reaching task designed to pick up an object on a table, the usual trajectory of the hand is a straight line. When an obstacle is present on this straight-line trajectory, a curvilinear trajectory is performed (see, for example, ref. 68). Straight-line and curvilinear trajectories can be defined as strategies. The execution of the strategy is realized by muscle patterns or synergies, which are the implementation of the strategy.

The same distinction between strategy and synergy was introduced in the postural domain by Horak and Nashner.[65] The ankle strategy and the hip strategy are two different ways of reaching the same goal of restoration of balance. These strategies are defined in terms of kinematics (i.e. changes in the body geometry). In order to control the strategy, muscle patterns or synergies are observed which produce the appropriate muscle force. Under the usual environmental conditions, both strategies and synergies are invariant (i.e. the same muscle pattern is associated with a given 'strategy'). This explains why strategy and synergy are often used as equivalent terms in many papers. However, when the external constraints change, then the muscle synergy should change in order to achieve the same 'strategy.'

The experiments of Macpherson[27] provide evidence that by changing the direction of stance disturbance in the cat, the strategy remains invariant whereas the muscle synergies change. In contrast to the ankle and hip strategies reported by Horak and Nashner,[65] which are defined in terms of kinematics, Macpherson described a strategy in terms of ground reaction forces in the cat: the biomechanical strategy used by the cat involved primarily the hindlimbs and showed invariance in the direction of the vector of force they generated. For any of 16 perturbation directions, the system made a simple two-choice response for vector direction: either backward/outward or forward. This behavioral strategy clearly simplifies the control process. However, the muscle synergies associated with this strategy were more variable. Some of the muscles were co-modulated, including the hip and distal muscles such as the gastrocnemius, and thus may have been activated by a central command. However, others, such as the gracilis, were controlled independently. It was thus concluded that in cat postural control, invariances exist for (1) the direction of force generation by the two hindlimbs (i.e. the strategy), and (2) the grouping of certain hindlimb muscles, which were part of the synergy. However, the independent control of other muscles indicates that they may be used to 'tune' the synergy in order to produce the biomechanical goal of the production of specific ground reaction forces.[69]

Investigations of the flexibility of muscle synergies were also performed in humans. The evidence from previous research supports the concept of the existence of fixed postural synergies when subjects are perturbed in the anterior/posterior direction. However, it is also important to determine if using a variety of different angles of platform motion to perturb balance, including those in the lateral direction, would result in the activation of only a small number of fixed synergies, or whether muscle response patterns would show a continuous variation, as the angle of perturbation was moved from anterior/posterior to lateral. If synergies vary continuously with angle of perturbation, it weakens the hypothesis that balance is controlled by fixed muscle response patterns. In order to answer this question further experiments were performed,[70] in which the balance of subjects was perturbed as in the above experiments, but subjects were asked to pivot at 15° increments between blocks of trials.

It was noted that the pattern of responses in directions near the sagittal plane (300–15°) showed a relatively constant onset latency relationship between muscles, with responses in the gastrocnemius, hamstrings and trunk extensors, as predicted, along with an early response in the abdominals (probably because of the high velocity of perturbation: 25 cm/s versus 13 cm/s used in prior experiments). Muscle patterns were similar for tibialis anterior, quadriceps and abdominals (with an early trunk extensor response) for directions of 165–225°. For other perturbation angles, however, latency relationships varied continuously and sharp transitions in latency and/or amplitude were not seen.

The authors mention that a limitation of the study was that EMG recordings were taken primarily from muscles involved in flexion and extension of the leg and hip, and not muscles that would be responsive to perturbations in the lateral direction, so they could not describe a 'lateral synergy.'[70] Thus, as a whole, the strategy represents the invariant aspect of the postural reactions related to equilibrium control, whereas the muscle synergies are partly fixed, partly flexible.

What makes the muscle synergies flexible? By comparing the respective contribution of mono- and biarticular muscles in postural control and in other tasks, van Ingen Schenau et al.[71] indicated that the biarticular muscles are sensitive to a large variety of peripheral input and might tune the force vector provided by the monoarticular muscles in order to adapt it to the external constraints.

Adaptation of postural synergies

The above evidence suggests that the postural response synergies may be fine-tuned according to the task. Is there also evidence for fine-tuning of postural response synergies in other situations? Research on humans indicates that there are changes in the muscle response parameters within a synergy across successive trials, suggesting that the neuromuscular response synergies may be fine-tuned.[1,72] It has been found, for example, that the amplitude of ankle synergy movements activated by platform rotations (described above) is progressively reduced over 10 trials because under these conditions the sway synergy is destabilizing, causing more sway than the perturbation itself. This change in amplitude has been termed adaptation, since the response is fine-tuned to fit a new task context.[73]

Additional research has indicated that with repeated exposure to horizontal platform displacements, subjects show a reduction in the amplitude of antagonist ankle muscle responses, corresponding to smaller displacements of the body,[72] as if the subjects were changing their postural set during the course of the experiment.

Sensory inputs contributing to the control of perturbed stance

What are the relative contributions of the somatosensory, visual and vestibular systems to postural responses to support surface perturbations? Research performed by Dietz and colleagues suggests that the contribution of the somatosensory system is much greater than that of the vestibular system.[74] In this study, muscle response amplitudes and onset latencies were compared for stance perturbations of two types. The first perturbation consisted of forward and backward support surface movements, while the second perturbation consisted of a forward or backward displacement of a load (2 kg) attached to the head, stimulating the vestibular system (the response was not present in patients with vestibular deficits), but not ankle joint somatosensory inputs. For comparable accelerations, leg muscle responses elicited by the head perturbations were about 10 times smaller than the responses induced by the displacement of the feet. Since comparable accelerations were used for the two perturbations, Dietz et al.[74] concluded that vestibular inputs play only a minor role in recovery of postural control when the support surface is displaced horizontally.

Although vestibular inputs play a minor role in compensation for horizontal support surface displacements, they appear to be more important in compensating for perturbations in which the support surface is rotated toes-upward. This perturbation stretches and activates the gastrocnemius muscle, which destabilizes the subject, and a compensatory response in the tibialis anterior serves to restore stability. It has been shown that the compensatory response in the tibialis anterior muscle, used to restore balance, is activated by the visual and vestibular systems when the eyes are open. When the eyes are closed it is primarily (80 per cent) activated by the vestibular semicircular canals.[75]

The above studies, examining postural control in response to transient horizontal perturbations to stance, suggest that neurologically intact adults tend to rely on somatosensory inputs for the control of horizontal perturbations to balance.

POSTURE CONTROL AND MOVEMENT

One of the main tasks in motor control is to orient the body with respect to the external world. This orientation is necessary for the appropriate coding of the information collected by the sensory organs on the state of the environment. In this respect, the orientation of individual segments and especially of head and trunk (see ref. 9) is critical.

Anticipatory postural adjustments

Anticipatory postural adjustments were first described by Belen'kii and colleagues[76] in association with arm movements, and since then many investigations in both humans and in cats have been devoted to exploring their function, their central organization and their acquisition.[9,77] In their initial work, Belen'kii et al.[76] showed that when standing adults make rapid arm-raising movements, shorter latency postural responses are also activated in the muscles of the legs. For example, responses in the biceps femoris of the leg were activated 80–100 ms after the onset of the signal to start the movement compared with those for the prime mover of the arm (150–200 ms) and thus preceded the onset of the primary mover muscle response by about 50 ms. These postural adjustments act to compensate in advance for changes in posture and equilibrium caused by the movement. This view on the function of the anticipatory postural adjustments was also proposed by Cordo and Nashner[39] and by Bouisset and Zattara.[78,79]

Are the muscle synergies observed in postural reactions also 'utilized' for anticipatory postural adjustments? In one set of experiments by Cordo and Nashner[39] standing subjects were asked to make a rapid arm flexion movement. As in the studies of Gurfinkel and his colleagues, it was found that postural responses occurred in the muscles of the leg in advance of the prime mover muscles of the arm. It is of interest that the same muscle response organization which was previously found to stabilize posture after an external threat to balance (gastrocnemius, hamstrings and trunk extensors) was used to stabilize posture before activation of the prime mover muscle (biceps) in the arm flexion task.[39]

An important characteristic of postural adjustments associated with movement is their adaptability to task conditions.[80] For example, in the experiments described above,[39] when the subjects leaned forward against a horizontal bar at chest height, thus stabilizing the trunk and eliminating the need for postural adjustments in the legs, the leg postural adjustments were reduced or disappeared. This suggests that there is a preselection of the postural muscles to be used in anticipatory adjustments, as a function of their ability to contribute appropriate support.[39]

GOAL OF THE ANTICIPATORY POSTURAL ADJUSTMENTS

Is the goal of the anticipatory postural adjustment to control balance or posture (i.e. the center of gravity and the center of pressure position during movement, or, alternatively, the position or orientation of given body segments)? One should remember that voluntary movement perturbs posture and/or equilibrium for two reasons. First, the performance of a movement of the arm or the trunk while standing changes the body geometry and thus displaces the center of gravity position, resulting in equilibrium disturbance. The second reason is that the internal muscular forces that are at the origin of the movement are accompanied by reaction forces acting on the supporting body segments and will tend to displace them. This will disturb both the position of these segments and equilibrium.

In many tasks (for example arm raising while standing) the anticipatory postural adjustments serve to control balance and to stabilize posture. However, for other tasks, such as trunk bending or bimanual load-lifting tasks, two types of anticipatory postural adjustments can be identified with respect to their goal, those aimed at stabilizing the center of gravity during movement and those aimed at stabilizing the position of body segments. A third goal of the anticipatory postural adjustments is to provide the dynamic support of the postural chain from the ground to the moving segments in order to improve the performance in terms of force or velocity.

Bouisset and Le Bozec[81] and Bouisset et al.[82] introduced the concept of 'posturokinetic capacity' as an assessment of the capacity of the postural chain to assist the movement. This capacity is related to the control of this chain for counteracting the reaction forces associated with movement performance and also for dynamically contributing to the movement force and velocity using the many degrees of freedom from the ground to the moving segments.[83,84]

AN EXAMPLE OF ANTICIPATORY POSTURAL ADJUSTMENT: THE BIMANUAL LOAD–LIFTING TASK

The stabilization of the position or orientation of body segments[85,86] is exemplified by the bimanual load-lifting task. This type of stabilization can be seen independently from the control of the center of gravity during bimanual tasks, when one arm is used to stabilize or hold an object and the other is used to manipulate or lift the

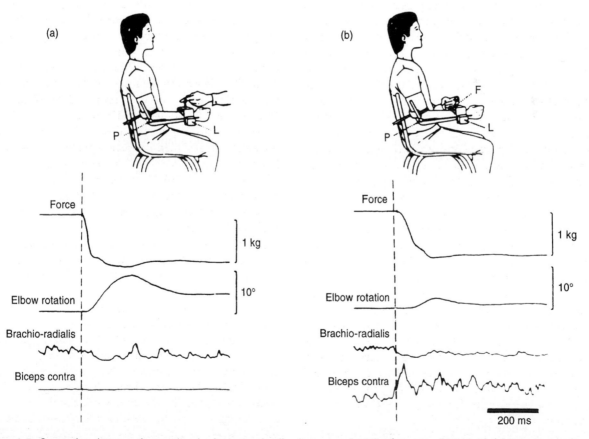

Figure 1.5 *Comparison between imposed and voluntary unloading in a normal subject (average of 20 trials). (a) Force trace recorded from a force platform (F) during unloading of 1 kg weight imposed by the experimenter. Elbow angle was measured by a potentiometer at the elbow joint axis (P). Note the upward rotation. The integrated electromyograph of the brachioradialis showed a reduction of activity after a latency of 30 ms (unloading reflex). (b) Voluntary unloading. Note the reduced elbow rotation, the 'anticipatory' inhibition of the brachioradialis, time locked with the activation of the biceps of the voluntary arm.*

object. For example, during a bimanual load-lifting task, where one forearm was maintained horizontal and supported a 1 kg load, and the other hand lifted the load, the forearm position did not change during unloading (Fig. 1.5). This was because of an inhibition of the elbow flexors of the postural forearm, which preceded the onset of unloading by a short period. This anticipatory postural adjustment was correlated with the onset of the biceps activation of the lifting arm and minimized the forearm disturbance which should normally occur, and is seen when unloading is caused by the experimenter. A similar type of anticipatory postural adjustment is seen to stabilize 'grip force' in advance of a disturbance[87] or to minimize the mechanical impact of a hammer manipulated by the subject to test the tendon reflex of the other arm's triceps.[88]

An insight into the central organization of the anticipatory postural adjustments during bimanual load-lifting tasks was provided by testing the task in patients.[89] It revealed that the anticipatory postural adjustments remained unchanged after callosal section. This suggests that the control of these adjustments did not occur through a direct callosal connection between the cortex controlling the moving side and the cortex controlling the postural side, but by a subcortical connection between the cortex responsible for the movement and the networks responsible for the anticipatory postural adjustment.

Moreover, anticipatory postural adjustments were impaired after a cortical lesion extending to the supplementary area region or to the motor cortex. As the impairment occurred for lesions contralateral to the postural forearm (and not to the moving arm), the authors concluded that the anticipatory postural adjustment networks were under the control of these contralateral cortical areas. It is suggested that the role of these networks is to select the segments utilized as a reference frame for the movement and to gate on the appropriate network for stabilizing the corresponding postural segment during the movement.

Further investigations on the central organization of anticipatory postural adjustments are crucial for the understanding of the neurological deficit specifically related to their dysfunctioning.

How is the control organized?

A main difficulty for understanding postural control is the complexity of the biomechanical constraints underlying human posture. The body is supported by a narrow support base, where the action and reaction forces take place. The body is a multi-joint chain, which includes segments of different mass and inertia, linked by muscles with their visco-elastic characteristics. Each single joint movement is associated with dynamic interaction with other segments of the chain; these movements change the impact of external forces such as gravity on the body segments, thus complicating the regulation of posture.

One main concern for understanding the control is to find out how a reduction of the number of degrees of freedom can be achieved in order to simplify the control.[29] The multi-joint chain is not specific to posture; thus, in this respect, the problems of control are common to that of any multi-joint movement. The specific aspect of posture in this control is related to the need to control balance and/or the body segment orientation during the motor act.

A first concept regarding simplifying control is that of 'reference posture'. This concept is in line with the equilibrium point theory of Bizzi et al.[90] and the lambda model of Feldman and Levin,[91] and related to the spring-mass properties of the musculo-skeletal system.

In the development of the lambda model, it was proposed that the critical threshold length for each muscle (which is the threshold for the myotatic reflex) is set in order to define a given reference postural configuration.[91] The control of a referent posture would consist in setting the critical length for the whole set of body muscles at an appropriate value. This concept is attractive due to its relative simplicity and meets a number of observations. For example, forward and backward trunk bendings are accompanied by opposite displacements of lower body segments and as a result the center of gravity position remains inside the support surface.[92] This kinematic synergy with a strong coupling between segment angles[43,93] remains under microgravity conditions[94] and seems to be a behavioral invariant, independent of external constraints, as would be expected from the referent posture hypothesis. If the kinematic pattern is invariant, the EMG patterns do adapt to the constraint. As proposed by Babinski,[95] the coordination between equilibrium and movement, as revealed by the study of upper trunk movements, seems to be under the control of the cerebellum.[96] It is not yet clear how far this model is able to account for the dynamic interaction between segments which disturbs movement performance and balance.

The inverse dynamic model was proposed by Ito[97] and by Gomi and Kawato;[98,99] it implies that an internal model of the body segments kinematics and dynamics does exist. When performing a goal-directed movement, the dynamical interactions between segments which disturb the trajectory have to be compensated. A feed-forward inverse dynamic model is built up which corrects in advance for these dynamic interactions. The cerebellum would be the site where the inverse model is stored. As the dynamic interactions between segments are a major source of balance disturbance during movement, one might think that the inverse model would accurately control balance during movement performance.

A third possibility for postural control during movement is derived from the observation on hip and ankle strategies for restoring balance.[65] The hip and ankle strategies are considered as basic multi-joint movement units of the biomechanical system which can be scaled both in terms of kinematics and kinetics.[100,101] In a task such as trunk bending, one is used for performing the movement (hip synergy), the other for balance control (ankle synergy) by accelerating the CG forward, in an opposite direction to the CG acceleration resulting from the hip flexion. Thus, two parallel controls would be present, one responsible for the movement, the other for the anticipatory postural adjustment.

LEG MOVEMENTS

Movements of the legs are a source of disturbance of balance because they take part in body support; thus a displacement of the center of gravity is observed preceding leg movement onset to compensate for this disturbance. The center of gravity shift occurs, for example, during the initiation of gait, standing on tip-toes or on the heels, or raising one leg.[8,102–104]

The neural control by which the center of gravity shifts toward a new position compatible with equilibrium during movement, is clearly different from the neural control responsible for the anticipatory position adjustment which prevents center of gravity displacement during movement such as occurs during upper trunk bending. It can be compared to a goal-directed movement except that the goal is expressed not in terms of geometry (object in space) but in terms of forces (new center of gravity position). This type of control is related to equilibrium constraints and disappears under microgravity conditions.[105] Its central organization in humans is still an open question. However, ablation experiments in quadrupeds performing leg-raising tasks suggests that this type of control is highly dependent on motor cortical areas.[106]

Integrating postural responses into the step cycle

Studies on the control of balance during unperturbed gait suggest that this task is very different from the task of balance control during stance.[107] During walking, the center of gravity moves outside the base of support of the feet and thus creates a continuous state of imbalance. Falling is prevented by placing the swinging foot ahead of and lateral to the center of gravity as it moves forward (see Chapter 4).

A key aspect of balance during locomotion is the control of the mass of the head, arms and trunk (the HAT segment) with respect to the hips, since this is a large load to keep upright. It has been hypothesized by Winter and colleagues[108] that the dynamic balance of the head, arms and trunk is controlled by the hip muscles, with almost no involvement of the ankle muscles. They suggest that this type of control is more efficient since the hip has a much smaller inertial load to control (that of the HAT segment) than the ankles, which would have to control the entire body.

Although balance control during unperturbed gait appears to be controlled by hip musculature, compensations for balance perturbations during gait have been shown to be controlled primarily by responses in the ankle and thigh musculature.[109–111] In experiments in which the balance of young adults was disturbed at different points within the stance phase of gait, it was shown that the young adult elegantly modulates postural response organization primarily in the leg and thigh muscles to compensate for disturbances.

Thus, when the foot slipped forward at heel-strike, which slowed forward momentum of the body, a response was elicited in anterior bilateral leg muscles (tibialis anterior) as well as anterior and posterior thigh muscles. These muscles showed early (90–140 ms), high magnitude (four to nine times the activity in normal walking) and relatively long-duration bursts.[111] Although proximal hip muscle activity was often present during the first slip trial in young adults, it tended to adapt away during subsequent trials. As shown previously for recovery of balance during quiet stance, muscle response patterns to balance threats during walking were activated in a distal to proximal sequence.

CONCLUSIONS

Postural or equilibrium control is considered to be the foundation for voluntary skills, because almost every movement that an individual makes is made up of both (1) postural components, which stabilize the body and (2) the prime mover components which relate to a particular movement goal.

The task of postural control involves the maintenance of the alignment of body posture, of stability, or bodily orientation to the environment and also serves as a mechanical support for action.

Postural tone depends on and is modulated through the myotatic reflex loop, tonic labyrinthine reflexes, the tonic neck reflexes, lumbar reflexes and positive supporting reactions. In addition, the tactile, visual and labyrinthine placing reactions adapt the activity of the postural muscles of the limbs to their function of body support.

In humans, where the supporting surface is narrow, there is a direct regulation of the center of gravity by displacement of body segments.

The main substrate that has been proposed as the basis for body orientation is the so-called postural body schema, an internal representation of body posture, which includes a representation of body geometry, of body kinetics and of the body orientation with respect to gravity (vertical).

Information on orientation with respect to verticality comes from the labyrinthine and visual sensors located in the head and possibly from body graviceptors. The use of sensory information from multiple sources, including the visual, vestibular and somatosensory systems, is a key feature of the neural control of both body orientation with respect to vertical and stabilization against external disturbances.

Research on postural compensatory responses to support surface perturbations indicates two levels of control: strategy and synergy. The strategy is invariant and corresponds to the way in which the nervous system restores balance. Examples are the ankle strategy, used to balance in response to small perturbations on a normal surface, and the hip strategy, used to control balance on a short surface or with respect to large, fast perturbations. The neurally programmed synergies provide the muscular forces for achieving the strategy. They are partly fixed and partly flexible. These postural response synergies may be fine-tuned according to the constraints of the task and the individual.

The contribution of the somatosensory system is much greater than that of the vestibular system when compensating for transient horizontal support surface perturbations.

Postural control is not organized as a single unit. Independent control of the position or orientation of segments such as the head, trunk and forearm has been shown to exist. These segments serve as a reference frame for perception and action processes.

The execution of potentially destabilizing voluntary movements is preceded by activation of postural muscles (anticipatory postural adjustments), which serve to compensate in advance for changes in equilibrium or posture caused by the movement. The same muscle response organization that was previously found to stabilize posture after an external threat to balance was used to stabilize posture before an arm flexion task.

Balance control during unperturbed gait appears to be controlled by the hip musculature, while compensations for balance perturbations during gait appear to be controlled by responses in the ankle musculature.

REFERENCES

1. Nashner LM, McCollum G. The organization of human postural movements: a formal basis and experimental synthesis. *Behav Brain Sci* 1985;**8**:135–72.
2. Paï YC, Patton J. Center of mass velocity-position predictions for balance control. *J Biomech* 1997;**30**:347–54.
3. Horak FB, Macpherson JM. Postural orientation and equilibrium. In: Shephard J, Rowell L, eds. *Handbook of physiology section 12, exercise: regulations and integration of multiple systems.* New York: Oxford University Press, 1996; 255–92.
4. Droulez J, Berthoz A. Servo-controlled (conservative) versus topological (projective) mode of sensory motor control. In: Bles W, Brandt T, eds. *Disorders of posture and gait.* Amsterdam: Elsevier, 1986:83–97.
5. Martin JP. *The basal ganglia and posture.* London: Pitman, 1967.
6. Berthoz A, Pozzo T. Intermittent head stabilization during postural and locomotory tasks in humans. In: Amblard B, Berthoz A, Clara C, eds. *Posture and gait.* Amsterdam: Excerpta Medica, 1988:89–98.
7. Gresty M. Stability of the head: studies in normal subjects and in patients with labyrinthine disease, head tremor, and dystonia. *Mov Disord* 1987;**2**:165–85.
8. Guitton D, Kearney RE, Wereley N, Peterson BW. Visual, vestibular and voluntary contributions to human head stabilization. *Exp Brain Res* 1986;**64**:59–69.
9. Massion J. Movement, posture and equilibrium: interaction and coordination. *Prog Neurobiol* 1992;**38**:35–56.
10. Mouchnino L, Aurenty R, Massion J, Pedotti A. Coordination between equilibrium and head–trunk orientation during leg movement: a new strategy built up by training. *J Neurophysiol* 1992;**67**:1587–98.
11. Assaiante C, Thomachot B, Aurenty R. Hip stabilization and lateral balance control in toddlers during the first four months of autonomous walking. *NeuroReport* 1993;**4**:875–78.
12. Gurfinkel VS, Lipshits MI, Popov KE. Stabilization of body position as the main task of postural regulation. *Fiziologya Cheloveka* 1981;**7**:400–10.
13. Berthoz A. Reference frames for the perception and control of movement. In: Paillard J, ed. *Brain and space.* Oxford: Oxford University Press, 1991;81–111.
14. Biguer B, Donaldson IML, Hein A, Jeannerod M. Neck muscle vibration modifies the representation of visual motion and direction in man. *Brain* 1988;**111**:1405–24.
15. Caminiti R, Johnson PB, Galli C, et al. Making arm movement within different parts of space:the premotor and motor cortical representation of a coordinate system for reaching to visual targets. *J Neurosci* 1991;**11**:1182–97.
16. Magnus R. *Körperstellung.* Berlin: Springer, 1924.
17. Rademaker GGJ. *Das stehen: Statische Reaktionen, Gleichwichtsreaktionen und muskeltonus unter besonderer Berucksichtung ihres Verhaltens bei kleinhirnlosen Tieren.* Berlin: Springer, 1931.
18. Paillard J. Motor and representational framing of space. In: Paillard J, ed. *Brain and space.* Oxford: Oxford University Press, 1991;163–82.
19. Sherrington C. *The integrative action of the nervous system,* 2nd edn. New Haven: Yale University Press, 1947.
20. Lloyd DPC. Principles of spinal reflex activity. In: Fulton JF, ed. *A textbook of physiology.* Philadelphia and London: WB Saunders, 1950;78–109.
21. Nashner LM. Fixed patterns of rapid postural responses among leg muscles during stance. *Exp Brain Res* 1977;**30**:13–24.
22. Shumway-Cook A, Woollacott M. *Motor control: theory and practical applications.* Baltimore: Lippincott Williams & Wilkins, 2001.
23. Dietz V. Human neuronal control of automatic functional movements: interaction between central programs and afferent input. *Physiol Rev* 1992;**72**:33–69.
24. Forssberg H, Neural control of human development. *Curr Opin Neurobiol: Motor Systems* 1999;**9**:676–82.
25. Roberts TDM. *Neurophysiology of postural mechanisms.* London: Butterworths, 1979.
26. Tokizane T, Murao M, Ogata T, Kondo T. Electromyographic studies on tonic neck, lumbar and labyrinthine reflexes in normal persons. *Jpn J Physiol* 1951;**2**:130–46.

27. Macpherson JM. How flexible are muscle synergies? In: Humphrey DR, Freund H-J, eds. *Motor control: concepts and issues*. Chichester: John Wiley, 1991:33–47.

28. Massion J. Postural control systems in developmental perspective. *Neurosci Biobehav Rev* 1998;22:465–472.

29. Bernstein, N. *Co-ordination and regulation of movements*. New York: Pergamon Press, 1967.

30. Gurfinkel VS, Levik YS. Perceptual and automatic aspects of the postural body scheme. In: Paillard J, ed. *Brain and space*. Oxford: Oxford University Press 1991;147–62.

31. Clement G, Gurfinkel VS, Lestienne F, et al. Adaptation of postural control to weightlessness. *Exp Brain Res* 1984;57:61–72.

32. Gurfinkel VS, Levik YuS, Popov KE, Smetanin BN. Body scheme in the control of postural activity, In: Gurfinkel VS, Ioffe ME, Massion J, Roll J-P, eds. *Stance and motion: facts and concepts*. New York: Plenum Press, 1988;185–93.

33. Head H. *Studies in neurology*, Vol. 2. London: Hodder & Stoughton, 1920.

34. Roll JP, Roll R. From eye to foot: a proprioceptive chain involved in postural control. In: Amblard B, Berthoz A, Clarac F, eds. *Posture and gait: development adaptation and modulation*. Amsterdam: Elsevier, 1988:155–64.

35. Lackner JR. Some proprioceptive influences on the perceptual representation of body shape and orientation. *Brain* 1988;111:281–97.

36. Roll J-P, Popov K, Gurfinkel V et al. Sensorimotor and perceptual function of muscle proprioception in microgravity. *J Vestib Res* 1993;3:259–73.

37. Lund S, Broberg C. Effects of different head positions in postural sway in man induced by a reproducible vestibular error signal. *Acta Physiol Scand* 1983;117:307–9.

38. Kavounoudias A, Roll R, Roll JP. The plantar sole is a 'dynamometric map' for human balance control. *NeuroReport* 1998;9:3247–52.

39. Cordo PJ, Nashner LM. Properties of postural adjustments associated with rapid arm movements. *J Neurophysiol* 1982;47:287–302.

40. Dietz V, Horstmann GA, Trippel M, Gollhofer A. Human postural reflexes and gravity – an under water simulation. *Neurosci Lett* 1989;106:350–5.

41. Massion J, Mouchnino L, Vernazza S. Do equilibrium constraints determine the center of mass position during movement. In: Mergner T, Hlavacka F, eds Multisensory control of posture. New York: Plenum Press, 1995:103–7.

42. Pagano CC, Turvey MT. Eigenvectors of the inertia tensor and perceiving the orientations of limbs and objects. *J Appl Biomech* 1998;14:331–359.

43. Vernazza-Martin S, Martin N, Massion J. Kinematic synergy adaptation to microgravity during forward trunk movement. *J Neurophysiol* 2000;83:453–464.

44. Mergner T, Rosemeier T. Interaction of vestibular, somatosensory and visual signals for postural control and motion perception under terrestrial and microgravity conditions – a conceptual model. *Brain Res Rev* 1998;28:118–135.

45. Amblard B, Cremieux J, Marchand AR, Carblanc A. Lateral orientation and stabilization of human stance: static versus dynamic visual cues. *Exp Brain Res* 1985;61:21–37.

46. Lestienne F, Soechting J, Berthoz A. Postural readjustment induced by linear motion of visual scenes. *Exp Brain Res* 1977;28:363–84.

47. Dijkstra TMH, Schöner G, Gielen CCAM. Temporal stability of the action-perception cycle for postural control in a moving visual environment. *Exp Brain Res* 1994;97:477–86.

48. Dichgans J, Held R, Young L, Brandt T. Moving visual scenes influence the apparent direction of gravity. *Science* 1972;178:1217–19.

49. Bronstein AM, Guerraz M. Visual-vestibular control of posture and gait: physiological mechanisms and disorders. *Curr Opin Neurol* 1999;12:5–11.

50. Jeka JJ, Lackner JR. The role of haptic cues from rough and slippery surfaces in human postural control. *Exp Brain Res* 1995;103:267–76.

51. Mittelstaedt H. A new solution to the problem of the subjective vertical. *Naturwissenschaften* 1983;70:272–81.

52. Riccio GE, Martin EJ, Stroffregen T. The role of balance dynamics in the active perception of orientation. *J Exp Psychol* 1992;18:624–44.

53. Massion J. Postural control systems in developmental perspective. *Neurosci Behav Rev* 1998;22:465–72.

54. Dietz V. Neuronal basis of stance regulation: interlimb coordination and antigravity receptor function. In: Swinnen S, Heuer H, Massion J, Casaer P, eds. *Interlimb coordination: neural, dynamical and cognitive constraints*. San Diego: Academic Press, 1994:167–78.

55. Dietz V, Gollhofer A, Kleiber M, Trippell M. Regulation of bipedal stance: dependence on 'load' receptors. *Exp Brain Res* 1992;89:229–31.

56. Jami L. Golgi tendon organs in mammalian skeletal muscle; functional properties and central actions. *Physiol Rev* 1992;72:623–66.

57. Asai H, Fujiwara K, Toyama H et al. The influence of foot soles coding on standing postural control. In: Brandt T, Paulus W, Bles W, et al., eds. *Disorders of posture and gait*. Stuttgart: Georg Thieme, 1990:198–201.

58. Magnusson M, Enbom H, Johansson R, Pyykko I. The importance of somatosensory information from the feet of postural control in man. In: Brand T, Paulus W, Bles W, et al., eds *Disorders of posture and gait*. Stuttgart: Georg Thieme, 1990:190–3.

59. Hlavacka F, Kriskova M, Horak FB. Modification of human postural response to leg muscle vibration by electrical vestibular stimulation. *Neurosci Lett* 1995;189:9–12.

60. Karnath HO (1994) Subjective body orientation in neglect and interactive contribution of neck muscle proprioception and vestibular stimulation. *Brain* 1994;117:1001–12

61. Horak FB, Shupert CL, Mirka A. Components of postural dyscontrol in the elderly:a review. *Neurobiol Aging* 1989;10:727–38.

62. Elner AM, Gurfinkel VS, Lipshits MI, et al. Facilitation of stretch reflex by additional support during quiet stance. *Agressologie* 1976;17:15–20.

63. Gurfinkel VS, Lipshits MI, Popov KE. Kinestetic thresholds in the orthograde posture. *Agressologie* 1979;20:133–4.

64. Nashner L, Woollacott M. The organization of rapid postural adjustments of standing humans: an experimental-conceptual model. In: Talbott RE, Humphrey DR, eds. *Posture and movement*. New York: Raven Press, 1979:243–57.

65. Horak F, Nashner L. Central programming of postural movements: Adaptation to altered support surface configurations. *J Neurophysiol* 1986;55:1369–81.

66. Runge CF, Shupert CL, Horak FB, Zajac FE. Postural strategies defined by joint torques. *Gait Posture* 1999;10:161–70.

67. Jensen JL, Bothner KE, Woollacott MH. Balance control: the scaling of the kinetic response to accommodate increasing perturbation magnitudes. *J Sport Exerc Psychol* 1996;**18**:S45.

68. Moll L, Kuypers HGJM. Premotor cortical ablations in monkeys: contralateral changes in visually guided reaching behavior. *Science* 1977;**198**:317–19.

69. Macpherson JM. The neural organization of postural control – do muscle synergies exist? In: Amblard B, Berthoz A, Clarac F, eds. *Posture and gait: development, adaptation and modulation*. Amsterdam: Elsevier, 1988;381–90.

70. Moore SP, Rushmer DS, Windus SL, Nashner LM. Human automatic postural responses: responses to horizontal perturbations of stance in multiple directions. *Exp Brain Res* 1988;**73**:648–58.

71. van Ingen Schenau GJ, Pratt CA, Macpherson JM. Differential use and control of mono- and biarticular muscles. *Hum Mov Sci* 1994;**13**:495–517.

72. Woollacott M, Roseblad B, Hofsten von C. Relation between muscle response onset and body segmental movements during postural perturbations in humans. *Exp Brain Res* 1988;**72**:593–604.

73. Hansen PD, Woollacott MH, Debu B. Postural responses to changing task conditions. *Exp Brain Res* 1988;**73**:627–36.

74. Dietz M, Trippel M. Horstmann GA. Significance of proprioceptive and vestibulospinal reflexes in the control of stance and gait. In: Patla AE, ed. *Adaptability of human gait*. Elsevier: Amsterdam, 1991;37–52.

75. Allum JHJ, Pfaltz JCR. Visual and vestibular contributions to pitch sway stabilization in the ankle muscles of normals and patients with bilateral peripheral vestibular deficits. *Exp Brain Res* 1985;**58**:82–94.

76. Belen'kii VY, Gurfinkel VS, Paltsev YI. On elements of control and voluntary movements. *Biofizika* 1967;**12**:135–41.

77. Massion J. Postural changes accompanying voluntary movements. Normal and pathological aspects. *Hum Neurobiol* 1984;**2**:261–7.

78. Bouisset S, Zattara M. Biomechanical study of programming of anticipatory postural adjustments associated with voluntary movement. *J Biomech* 1987;**20**:735–42.

79. Bouisset S, Zattara M. Segmental movement as a perturbation to balance? Facts and concepts. In: Winters JM, Woo SLY, eds. *Multiple muscle systems: biomechanics and movement organization*. Springer: New York, 1990;498–506.

80. Lee WA, Buchanan TS, Rogers MW. Effects of arm acceleration and behavioural conditions on the organization of postural adjustments during arm flexion. *Exp Brain Res* 1987;**66**:257–70.

81. Bouisset S, Le Bozec S. Body balance stability and postural adjustments associated with voluntary movements. In: Gantchev GN, Mori S, Massion J, eds. *Motor control, today and tomorrow*. Academic Publishing House 'Prof M Drinov' 1999;275–91.

82. Bouisset S, Richardson J, Zattaraa M. Do anticipatory postural adjustments occurring in different segments of the postural chain follow the same organizational rule for different task movement velocities, independently of the inertial load value? *Exp Brain Res* 2000;**132**:79–86.

83. Stapley P, Pozzo T, Grishin A. The role of anticipatory postural adjsutments during whole body forward reaching movements. *Neuroreport* 1998;**9**:395–401.

84. Kingsma I, Toussaint HM, Commissaris DACM, Savelsbergh GJP. Adaptation of center of mass control under microgravity in a whole body lifting task. *Exp Brain Res* 1999;**125**:35–42.

85. Hugon M, Massion J, Wiesendanger M. Anticipatory postural changes included by active unloading and comparison with passive unloading in man. *Pflügers Arch Physiol* 1982;**393**:292–6.

86. Paulignan Y, Dufossé M, Hugon M, Massion J. Acquisition of co-ordination between posture and movement in a bimanual task. *Exp Brain Res* 1989;**77**:337–48.

87. Johansson RS, Westling G. Programmed and triggered actions to rapid load changes during precision grip. *Exp Brain Res* 1988;**71**:72–86.

88. Struppler A, Gerilovsky L, Jakob C. Self-generated rapid taps directed to opposite forearm in man: anticipatory reduction in the muscle activity of the target arm. *Neurosci Lett* 1993:**159**:115–18.

89. Viallet F, Massion J, Massarino R, Khalil R. Coordination between posture and movement in a bimanual load lifting task: putative role of a medial frontal region including the supplementary motor area. *Exp Brain Res* 1992;**88**:674–84.

90. Bizzi E, Hogan N, Mussa-Ivaldi FA, Giszter S. Does the nervous system use equilibrium-point control to guide single and multiple joint movements? *Behav Brain Sci* 1992;**15**:603–13.

91. Feldman AG, Levin MF The origin and use of positional frames of reference in motor control. *Behav Brain Sci* 1995;**18**:723–806.

92. Crenna P, Frigo C, Massion J, Pedotti A. Forward and backward axial synergies in man. *Exp Brain Res* 1987;**65**:538–48.

93. Alexandrov A, Frolov A, Massion J. Axial synergies during human upper trunk bending. *Exp Brain Res* 1998;**118**:210–20.

94. Massion J, Gurfinkel V, Lipshits M, et al. Axial synergies under microgravity conditions. *J Vestib Res* 1993;**3**:275–87.

95. Babinski J. De l'asynergie cerebelleuse. *Rev Neurol* 1899;**7**:806–16.

96. Viallet F, Massion J, Bonnefoi-Kyriacou B, et al. Approche quantitative de l'asynergie posturale en pathologie cerebelleuse. *Rev Neurol* 1994;**150**:55–60.

97. Ito M. *The cerebellum and neural control*. New York: Raven Press, 1984.

98. Gomi H, Kawato M. Equilibrium-point control hypothesis examined by measured arm stiffness during multijoint movement. *Science* 1996;**272**:117–20.

99. Gomi H, Kawato M. Human arm stiffness and equilibrium-point trajectory during multi-joint movement. *Biol Cybern* 1997;**76**:163–71.

100. Alexandrov A, Frolov A, Massion J. Biomechanical analysis of movement strategies in human trunk bending I. Modeling. *Biol Cybern* 2001;**84**:425–34.

101. Alexandrov A, Frolov A, Massion J. Biomechanical analysis of movement strategies in human trunk bending II. Experimental study. *Biol Cybern* 2001;**84**:435–43.

102. Rogers MW, Pai YC. Dynamic transitions in stance support accompanying leg flexion movements in man. *Exp Brain Res* 1990;**81**:398–402.

103. Brenière Y, Do MC. Control of gait initiation. *J Motor Behav* 1991;**23**:235–40.

104. Crenna P, Frigo C. A motor program for the initiation of

forward-oriented movements in man. *J Physiol (Lond)* 1991;**437**:635–53.

105. Mouchnino L, Cincera M, Fabre J-C, et al. Is the regulation of the center of mass maintained during leg movement under microgravity conditions? *J Neurophysiol*, 1996;**76**:1212–23.

106. Birjukova EV, Dufossé M, Frolov AA, et al. Role of the sensorimotor cortex in postural adjustments accompanying a conditioned paw lift in the standing cat. *Exp Brain Res* 1989;**78**:588–96.

107. Winter DA. *Biomechanics and motor control of human movement*. New York: John Wiley, 1990;80–4.

108. Winter DA, McFadyen BJ, Dickey JP. Adaptability of the CNS in human walking. In: Patla AE, ed. *Adaptability of human gait*. Amsterdam: Elsevier, 1991;127–44.

109. Nashner L. Balance adjustments of humans perturbed while walking. *J Neurophysiol* 1980;**44**:650–64.

110. Gollhofer A, Schmidtbleicher D, Quintern J, Dietz V. Compensatory movements following gait perturbations: changes in cinematic and muscular activation patterns. *Int J Sports Med* 1986;**7**:325–9.

111. Tang P-F, Woollacott MH, Chong RKY. Control of reactive balance adjustments in perturbed human walking: roles of proximal and distal postural muscle activity. *Exp Brain Res.* 1998;**119**:141–52.

2

Adaptive human locomotion: influence of neural, biological and mechanical factors on control mechanisms

AFTAB E. PATLA

INTRODUCTION

Life-sustaining and enhancing behavior, such as searching for food and avoiding predators, includes locomotion as an integral component. Nature has evolved a variety of forms of locomotion, such as flying, swimming and walking, suitable for different environments inhabited by the animal and machinery for implementing this important motor act. A common feature of all forms of locomotion is repetition of cyclical activity of appendages to transport the body. Interestingly, except for organisms such as bacteria, the natural kingdom is without wheels, which we hold as the cornerstone for efficient transportation. Lack of physical fusion between the wheels and the body required by design would also stop the transmission of nutrients and neural command signals to the motors driving the wheels.[1] Although wheels involve minimal accelerations and decelerations during a cycle, reducing pitching motion, legged locomotion offers unique advantages. The ability to step over or under obstacles and use isolated footholds allows legged animals to traverse terrains that are virtually inaccessible to wheeled vehicles.[2]

In this chapter we focus on the neural hardware and software and the sensorimotor apparatus that makes human locomotion possible. The chapter is structured around how the central nervous system (CNS) generates and controls various essential requirements for locomotion, and how biological and mechanical factors influence the control mechanisms.

DESIGN AND FUNCTIONAL SPECIFICATIONS OF THE LOCOMOTOR CONTROL SYSTEM

The requirements that the control system has to satisfy to be able to produce adaptive locomotion are:

1. Set up the initial body posture and orientation needed to initiate locomotion.
2. Initiate and terminate locomotion as and when needed.
3. Produce and coordinate the rhythmic activation patterns for the muscles of the limbs and the trunk to propel the body in the intended direction.
4. Maintain dynamic stability of the moving body counteracting the force of gravity and other forces (expected and unexpected) experienced by the moving body.
5. Modulate the patterns to alter the speed of locomotion, to avoid obstacles, select appropriate stable foot placement, accommodate different terrain and change the direction of locomotion.
6. Guide locomotion towards endpoints that are not visible from the start.
7. Use minimal fuel to maximize distance covered before stopping for replenishment of nutrients.
8. Ensure the structural stability of the locomotor apparatus to minimize downtime or permanent damage during the lifespan of the animal.

These are not desirable but necessary features, although, on a short-term basis, the system may be able to function, for example, if the last two requirements are not rigidly satisfied. The focus in this chapter is on normal locomotion, where normal refers to the state of the locomotor machinery. Although the cardio-respiratory system, which provides the fuel to sustain locomotion, is an integral part of the locomotor system, we restrict our discussion to the neuromotor apparatus. The intention is not to provide detailed neurophysiological description but rather highlight the basic principles of operation and organization that allow the system to meet the requirements outlined above.

Initial body posture and orientation needed to initiate locomotion

Initiation of locomotion in both bipeds and quadrupeds requires an initial standing posture (although locomotion in humans can be achieved from a variety of postures, standing posture is the preferred choice). Weight support is achieved through regulation of postural tonus, particularly in the extensors (anti-gravity muscles). Establishing the orientation of the body for locomotion is also essential for purposeful, goal-directed locomotion.

NEURAL SUBSTRATES INVOLVED

The work by Mori and his colleagues (see review by Mori)[3] have identified two midpontine neuronal structures that are responsible for modulating extensor muscle tone. Stimulating the ventral part of the caudal tegmental field (VTF) in the pons increases the level of extensor muscle tone, while stimulation of the dorsal portion of the caudal tegmental field (DTF) reduces the extensor muscle tone. A cat supporting its weight on the limbs can be made to change its posture to sitting and

even lying down when the DTF is stimulated at increasing intensities. In contrast, increasing the level of VTF stimulation results in the cat going from a lying posture to squatting to standing. Mori's work has shown quite clearly that appropriate postural set is a prerequisite for eliciting locomotor behavior. For example, stimulation of the DTF can override stimulation of the mesencephalic locomotor region (cuneiform nucleus) or subthalamic locomotor region (lateral hypothalamic area) which normally would elicit locomotion.

RELEVANT HUMAN STUDIES

The most pertinent studies related to this functional specification are those examining sit-to-stand behavior. Since in western culture, sitting in a chair is a common posture prior to initiation of locomotion, these studies describe the motor changes associated with setting of initial posture. The majority of these studies have described the changes to the muscle activation patterns, joint moments and powers and outcome measures as reflected in center of mass profiles.[4-11] It is clear that the control of the horizontal momentum is the invariant characteristics of sit-to-stand task, and is heavily biased by the final equilibrium posture.[9] Two distinct strategies are used to perform this task; the locus of propulsive power distinguishes between the two strategies and is either the muscles around the knee joint or the hip joint compensating for the amount of trunk flexion before seat-off.[11] The center of mass (COM) and center of pressure (COP) profiles during the execution of such a task clearly provide a useful way of understanding how the control signal captured by the COP regulates the controlled parameter, COM (see Fig. 2.1). As expected,

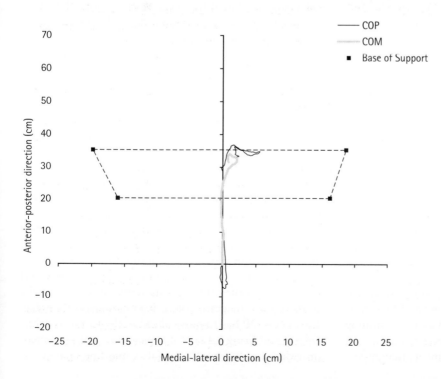

Figure 2.1 *Center of mass (COM) and center of pressure (COP) profiles during a sit-to-stand task.*

COM has to move outside the base of support (BOS) defined by the contact area of the buttocks and the feet (assuming no use of arms). The COP initially moves behind the COM to accelerate the COM forward and quickly moves ahead of COM to bring it to a controlled stop. The difference between the COP and COM determines the magnitude of the COM acceleration.[12] Unlike the patterns observed during gait initiation (see next section), there is no appreciable lateral movement of COP or COM; the profiles show excursions primarily in the forward direction. Setting of orientation during gait initiation has not been investigated.

Initiation and termination of locomotion

Locomotion while involving repetition of cyclical movement patterns is an episodic rhythm and not continuous like the heart or respiratory rhythm. Therefore, we need to be able to turn on the rhythm for gait initiation and turn it off for gait termination.

NEURAL SUBSTRATE AND PATHWAYS INVOLVED

The reticulo-spinal system is the mediating link between the excitatory signals from the higher brain areas and the spinal pattern generator. Research reviewed by Jordan[13] shows the convergence of input to the cells in the medial pontomedullary reticular formation (MRF) region. The latency of the excitatory postsynaptic potentials at the motoneuron level following stimulation of various brainstem regions to initiate locomotion suggests a polysynaptic pathway with a relay in the MRF region. These pathways use glutamate as a transmitter. The input to the spinal network can be characterized as tonic, with the amplitude (intensity) controlling the speed of locomotion.

Identification of these well-defined regions in the midbrain (midbrain locomotor region or MLR) and the lateral hypothalamic area (subthalamic locomotor region, or SLR) was instrumental in the study of locomotion. It is interesting to note that these regions are not hierarchical in the sense that a lesion in the MLR does not abolish locomotion induced by stimulation of the SLR region. The stimulation used to elicit locomotion from these regions is generally electrical. The majority of the studies documenting the behavior of the animal following stimulation of these regions is carried out in a decerebrate preparation (structures rostral to the brainstem and the cerebellum removed). Mori et al.[14] stimulated these regions in an awake cat. It is clear that the stimulation of the two regions elicits quite a different response. The MLR stimulation is accompanied by changes in posture from sitting to standing (mediated through VTF) and results in fast walking and then running movements.[15] The animal behaves as if it is running away from a noxious stimulus. In contrast, stimulation of the SLR results in locomotor movements that appear

very normal and involves 'orienting and searching behavior' before and during locomotion. Although appropriate cardio-respiratory changes accompany locomotion induced in a decerebrate preparation, in an intact animal as studied by Mori et al.,[14] 'behavioral arousal reactions' are also induced (mediated through the ascending activating system from the reticular formation to the higher cortical centers). Termination of locomotion is achieved through removal of the excitatory inputs to these regions.

RELEVANT HUMAN STUDIES

Gait initiation has been studied extensively.[7,16–20] Since the study by Carlsöö,[16] it is realized that the defining feature of gait initiation is the inhibition of activity in postural muscles, specifically the ankle plantarflexors resulting in movement of the COP behind the COM causing the COM to move forward. As shown recently by Couillandre et al.,[21] however, inability to move the COP backward does not limit the ability of the CNS to initiate forward progression. The inhibition of ankle plantarflexors is accompanied by increased activation of the ankle dorsiflexors, which assists in forward displacement of COM. The latency of inhibition and excitations of muscles show a tight linkage and are not influenced by the movement velocity.[7] Gait initiation has been shown to be unaffected by postural instability of the stance limb,[20] cerebellar deficits[22] or vestibular input.[23] This suggests that gait initiation is run in a feed-forward manner with limited on-line control. Winter and colleagues have shown that in addition to backward displacement of COP there is a concomitant lateral displacement of the COP initially towards the limb that is going to be used to take a step.[24] Lateral displacement of COP serves to move the COM towards the stance limb and is achieved by the abductor/adductor muscles about the hip joint. COM and COP profiles during a forward step are shown in Fig. 2.2.

Gait initiation clearly involves purposeful destabilization of a stable upright posture to assist in a forward step. In contrast, gait termination involves the converse; the forward body momentum acquired during steady-state locomotion must be arrested and a stable upright posture must be achieved. While problems in gait initiation are problematic and not desirable, gait termination poses greater threat to balance control. As in a car, ignition failure may be a nuisance, but the failure of the brakes can lead to devastating consequences. Several researchers have studied gait termination and described the interplay between COM and COP,[24] changes in ground reaction force which capture COM acceleration profiles,[25] and electromyographic changes.[26,27] The COM and COP profiles during gait termination essentially show mirror images of the gait initiation profiles (Fig. 2.3). The COP has to move ahead of the COM to decelerate it and bring it to a stable position. Foot placement provides coarse control of COP, while fine changes in

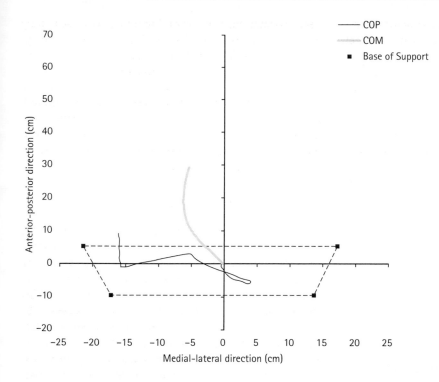

- COP
- COM
- ■ Base of Support

Figure 2.2 *Center of mass (COM) and center of pressure (COP) profiles during gait initiation.*

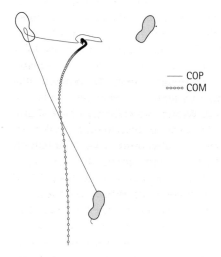

- COP
- ○○○○ COM

Figure 2.3 *Center of mass (COM) and center of pressure (COP) profiles during gait termination.*

COP during the weight-bearing phase are influenced by ankle musculature in the anterior–posterior plane.[24] Hase and Stein[26] identified two distinct strategies based on the electromyograph (EMG) profiles, depending on when the cue to stop is given: extensor synergy when cue is given late stance or early swing and a flexor synergy when the cue arrives in the late swing phase. Crenna et al.[27] found that the weight support limb synergy is dependent on the velocity of locomotion, while the swing limb synergy is relatively robust and immutable. Perry et al.[28] showed that sensory manipulation influenced the interplay between COM and COP during gait termination, suggesting that, unlike gait initiation, gait termination is under feedback control.

Production and coordination of rhythmic muscle activation patterns

Locomotion in all animals involves repetition of cyclical activity of appendages (legs, fins or wings) to transport the body. Without this feature locomotion would not be possible. How this rhythmic activation of the muscles in the appendages is generated has been the subject of much research for over 100 years.

NEURAL SUBSTRATES INVOLVED

The spinal cord represents a large part of the CNS, and on the evolutionary scale is the antecedent for other CNS developments. It is much more than a relay center for commands received from the supraspinal system: it plays a critical role in the generation and control of locomotion. The spinal cord can produce reasonably complex and 'near normal' muscle activation patterns in response to an unpatterned stimuli. The unpatterned stimuli generally consist of injection of pharmacological agents that increase the background excitability of the spinal cord. These patterns of muscular activation are not restricted to muscles within a limb; rather, the spinal cord can provide appropriate interlimb coordination in addition to the intralimb coordination. When the intensity of the unpatterned stimuli is increased, the frequency of the step cycle is also increased along with appropriate interlimb coordination.[29] A spinalized animal is also able to functionally modulate reflex responses[30] and carry out other stereotypic tasks concurrently.[31] Modulation of reflex responses will be discussed later when we focus on the role of the sensory system. The ability to carry out other stereotypic tasks concurrently suggests that the spinal cord is not fully taxed for locomotion: reserves can be used for other tasks.

Although the spinal cord is able to release pre-stored complex motor patterns, these are by no means sufficient for weight support and active propulsion in the intended direction. The ability to propel oneself in the intended direction manifests itself in the generation of appropriate forces exerted on the support surface. For example, to locomote forward the limbs have to produce forces that act downwards and backwards; the reaction forces, as dictated by Newton's third law, will produce forces acting forward and upward on the animal necessary for forward progression. Muscle activity alone cannot provide the necessary information; the anterior–posterior forces, which constitute the resultant action of the activity of many muscles, best reflect this active propulsion. Only one study has examined these forces in the spinalized cat,[32] and their records (see their Fig. 6) show that the animal is not actively pushing itself forward. Others have also observed that spinal stepping lacks the 'vigor' of intact animals, being unable to push the belt of a passive treadmill, and the animal has to be supported in a sling.[33] When one examines the muscle activation patterns along with some kinematic data observed in a spinalized cat for example,[34] two points become clear. First, the burst patterns are primarily restricted to when the muscles are contracting eccentrically and, second, there is an apparent lack of any co-contraction among the muscles. Thus, the spinal cord is necessary but not sufficient for expression of even the most rudimentary stepping behavior.

The demonstration that a simple unpatterned input to the spinal cord can produce complex rhythmic activation patterns led to the principle of central pattern generator (CPG) for the control of locomotion.[35,36] The input plays no role in the generation of basic rhythm; rather, it is necessary to release and sustain the rhythm. The pre-organized rhythmic activation patterns in the spinal cord simplify the control of locomotion by harnessing the large degrees of freedom. It is not clear what 'unit (limb, joint)' of the locomotor apparatus performs this CPG control. Split belt treadmill experiments and other research clearly suggest that there is probably a separate CPG for each limb. Because most animals can walk backwards or sideways, for example, which involve different inter-joint coupling, researchers have suggested that there are CPGs for each joint whose coupling can be changed for different modes of locomotion.[36] There are several aspects mediating against such a proposal. Pattern recognition analyses do not reveal any feature pattern grouping according to a joint. Muscle activity patterns during forward and backward walking show changes that cannot be accounted for by simply changing the sign of coupling.[37] It is more likely that the same spinal circuitry can be reconfigured based on other supraspinal inputs for use in different forms of locomotion.[38]

RELEVANT HUMAN STUDIES

In humans, the evidence for the central pattern generator for locomotion in the spinal cord has been primarily indirect, coming from developmental studies. Young infants produce stepping like behavior (very similar to stepping produced by a spinalized animal), which include appropriate inter- and intra-limb coordination patterns (that are not stable on a cycle to cycle basis, as observed in spinalized animal) when propulsion and balance requirements are eliminated through external support.[39–41] Work on paraplegic patients has provided some direct evidence for a spinal stepping generator in humans.[42] Their work has shown that the pattern of reflexes elicited by flexor reflex afferents (FRAs) is similar to spinal stepping in animals treated with L-DOPA (these FRAs excite the locomotor related interneurons). They have also observed rhythmical activity in one patient that is attributed to the spinal stepping generator.[42] The rhythmic activity was almost synchronous in all the muscle groups and was highly influenced by FRAs. Although the form of locomotor behavior is species specific (e.g. walking vs. flying), the basic framework of the control system is remarkably similar throughout the vertebrate phylum.[35,36] Therefore, there is no reason why this general principle of organizing rhythmic behavior should be different in humans. Recently Duysens and van de Crommert[43] provided a thorough review of the evidence for central pattern generators in humans.

Characterizing output patterns from a central pattern generator in humans has not been very successful. Beginning with the work by pioneers such as Muybridge and Marey in the early 1900s, early researchers used a variety of tools and measures to describe the basic patterns of level, straight-path human locomotion. Many researchers have measured and catalogued the muscle activation patterns, endpoint and joint kinematics, and ground reaction forces during normal human locomotion (for a review see Winter).[44] While muscle activation patterns are useful, it is not easy to determine the net effect of these patterns at the joints and consequent changes in limb/body movement. This lack of unique one-to-one mapping between muscle activation patterns and movement outcome results from the complex effects of muscles on joints they do not span[45] and difficulties with activation of antagonist muscles and muscles spanning more than one joint. Calculation of joint moments and powers using Newton's laws (inverse dynamics) has provided a way around this difficulty. Winter[44] provided an exhaustive catalogue of calculated joint kinetics in the sagittal plane during normal human locomotion.

In Table 2.1 we have described the basic stride cycle and the role that various types of muscle activity play in the control of normal human locomotion. It is clear that

Table 2.1 *Gait phases and definitions*

Overall function	Specific role	Double support IFC to CTO	Single support CTO to CFC	Double support CFC to ITO	Swing ITO to IFC — Early	Late
Balance control	Stability of head and spinal column	Neck extensors, Spinal extensors, Hip extensors		Neck extensors, Spinal extensors, Hip flexors		
	Preventing a forward/backward fall					
	Preventing a fall to the side					
	Preventing collapse		Hip abductors, Hip extensors, Knee extensors, Ankle extensors			
	Control of foot contact to prevent slip					Hip extensors, Knee flexors, Ankle flexors
Movement control	Energy generation for propulsion	Hip extensors		Ankle extensors, Hip flexors	Hip flexors	
	Generation of swing limb trajectory				Hip flexors, Hip abductors/adductors, Knee extensors, Ankle flexors	

CFC, contralateral foot contact; CTO, contralateral toe-off; IFC, ipsilateral foot contact; ITO, ipsilateral toe-off while muscles are used for propulsion and movement (limb trajectory) control, more often their roles are to ensure dynamic stability during different phases of the gait cycle. Thus, to isolate the patterns that constitute essentially output from a putative central pattern generator in humans and the activity that relates to the maintenance of stability is by no means easy. The same muscle activity may serve two functions. One way of determining electromyographic activity related to rhythmic movements of the limb is to study locomotion when individuals are supported in a harness, thereby obviating the need for stability control. Researchers involved in rehabilitation of spinal cord injured patients use harness-supported treadmill walking:[46] monitoring activity in normal individuals in a similar setting can be useful in identifying the rhythmic muscle activation profiles needed to move the limbs cyclically.

Maintaining dynamic stability of the moving body

Maintaining balance is essential to locomotion. The COM of the body is outside the base of support during the single support phase, which constitutes approximately 80 per cent of the stride duration. Therefore, from a static stability perspective, bipedal locomotion is unstable. Falling is avoided by the ability of the nervous system to change the base of support and control the COM that is moving towards the new base of support. This delicate balance is achieved through a combination of reactive (responses elicited after the perturbation is detected by the sensory systems), predictive (responses based on prediction of perturbation generated by changing velocity of on-going movement) and proactive (responses mediated by acquisition of information at a distance primarily through the visual system) control.

REACTIVE CONTROL OF DYNAMIC STABILITY

Mono- and polysynaptic reflexes provide a good first line of active defense against unexpected perturbations (see review by Dietz[47]). The most interesting feature is the functional modulation of these reflexes to provide appropriate phase- and task-specific responses to perturbations in humans (see review by Stein[48]) and other animals.[30] Stein and his colleagues have shown that the gain of the soleus H-reflex (electrical analogue of the monosynaptic stretch reflex) is modulated during the step cycle. It is low in the early stance and swing phases, and high during the mid to late stance. During early stance, when the body is rotating over the foot stretching the soleus muscle, a high reflex gain would impede forward progression and therefore would be undesirable. Similarly, during early swing when the foot is being actively dorsiflexed for ground clearance, a high reflex gain could result in tripping. In contrast, during late stance high reflex gain could assist in the push-off

action and therefore would be desirable. To provide functionally appropriate responses, the incoming sensory information has to be modulated by the supraspinal input and spinal pattern generator output. Presynaptic inhibition has been argued as a mechanism for modulating the stretch reflex during locomotion.[48] While H-reflex studies are useful surrogates for investigating contributions of stretch reflex, there are some differences between H-reflex and stretch reflex modulations during gait, as shown by Sinkjaer et al.,[49] particularly during the swing phase. Polysynaptic reflexes such as the flexor reflex[50–52] are also modulated and gated to provide functionally appropriate responses. The flexor reflex is mediated by skin mechanoreceptors rather than nociceptors (pain receptors). These long latency responses are probably more effective for responding to larger unexpected perturbations applied during locomotion.[47] It is interesting to note that the spinal cord in cats is sufficient for functionally modulating these reflexes.[30] The modulation of mono- and polysynaptic reflexes involves task-, phase- and muscle-specific control of the reflex gain (even the sign), and has been argued to be a basic control strategy.[53]

While the study of specific reflexes using artificial stimuli to specific classes of receptors have been very useful, it is realized that direct perturbations to balance activate many different types of receptors, leading to more complex functional responses. Early work on perturbing balance during locomotion in humans suggested that the recovery strategies are similar in organization to strategies used to maintain upright stance.[54] Later work by Dietz et al.[55,56] suggested that group II and III afferents were responsible for the triggering and organization of the recovery response. Flexor response modulation studies do not adequately predict the complex response seen during an unexpected trip. Responses to an unexpected trip occurring at different times in the swing phase[57] exhibited the following characteristics:

1. They were phase dependent, with perturbations early in the swing phase producing an elevating strategy and perturbation later in the swing phase producing a lowering strategy
2. Muscle response (in ipsilateral and contralateral limb) latencies were in the order of 60–140 ms, suggesting a polysynaptic reflex response
3. Recovery response, particularly for perturbation late in the swing phase, persisted into the subsequent step cycle.

These results demonstrate the complex sensorimotor transformation of essentially similar afferent input, giving rise to a context-dependent reflex response. Similar latency responses have been seen when an unexpected slip is induced during locomotion, both in the perturbed limb and unperturbed limbs.[58–61] Typical responses during an unexpected trip highlighting some of these characteristics are shown in Fig. 2.4.

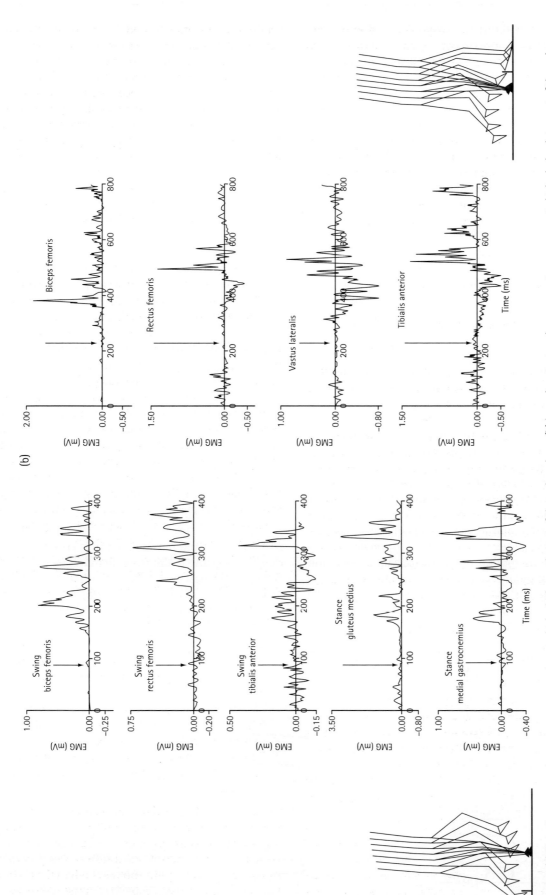

Figure 2.4 (a) Elevating strategy in response to an unexpected trip during early part of the swing phase. (b) Lowering strategy in response to an unexpected trip during later part of the swing phase.

In most cases the perturbation magnitude is sufficiently large such that recovery response takes place over more than one step cycle. Recently, while studying dynamic stability during locomotion in the frontal plane, we have shown that COM recovery takes place over a longer time-frame than typically considered by researchers studying reflexes.[62] Figure 2.5 shows mediolateral COM changes in response to a push from the right side during treadmill locomotion, illustrating the complex recovery response that is needed to return the system to its normal walking pattern.

Two important attributes about recovery responses emerge from many studies on gait perturbation. First, a truly reactive response is most often seen in the first trial.[58,64] Subsequent responses to repeated perturbations often show proactive adjustments based on prior experience with the perturbation.[58] Prior knowledge about a slippery surface, for example, can also influence the recovery response.[58]

PREDICTIVE CONTROL OF DYNAMIC STABILITY

Feed-forward control is also essential for compensating for movement-generated perturbations. Every movement, even the normal locomotor movements, perturbs the body by virtue of displacement of the COM and reactive moments. A pioneering study by Belenkii et al.[65] demonstrated that postural muscles were recruited prior to those required for intended movement. Since then numerous studies have documented the role of anticipatory or proactive control in responding to perturbations applied to upright posture (see Chapter 1). Winter[44] has documented the joint moments that counteract the perturbations produced by the normal locomotor movements. Pitching motion of the trunk with acceleration and deceleration in each step cycle is controlled primarily by the moments about the hip joint. Tipping of the upper body towards the unsupported side is primarily regulated by the hip abductors: the magnitude of destabilization is controlled by the foot placement with respect to body COM. Collapse in the vertical direction is prevented by controlling the moments about the knee joint, which have been shown by Winter[44] to co-vary with the hip joint moments. By using the hamstrings to decelerate the limb extension during the swing phase, gentle foot contact (a horizontal velocity of about 0.4 m/s) is achieved and chances of slipping are minimized. During normal level locomotion, as simulations have shown, tripping is avoided primarily through active dorsiflexion.[66] Studies examining postural responses to additional movement generated perturbations applied during locomotion are relatively few.[54,67,68] These studies have shown that proactive responses to perturbations initiated by arm movements are functional, ensuring stability and forward progression. This mode of proactive control of balance suggests the presence of a movement and body schema within the nervous system.

PROACTIVE CONTROL OF DYNAMIC STABILITY

The most powerful means of ensuring stability is to actively avoid the perturbation. Identification and avoidance of potential threats to stability are made possible by the visual system. Whereas sensory modalities such as the kinesthetic system need physical contact with the external world to transduce and supply relevant information, vision can provide us with information from a distance. Much of our knowledge about the external world is derived from vision, which plays an essential role in guiding movements. Information about the static and dynamic features about the environment in which an animal lives and moves about in is critical. Although receptors sensitive to diffusing chemicals (sense of smell) and to mechanical energy (kinesthesis and auditory system) can provide considerable information about the environment, nothing surpasses the ability of receptors

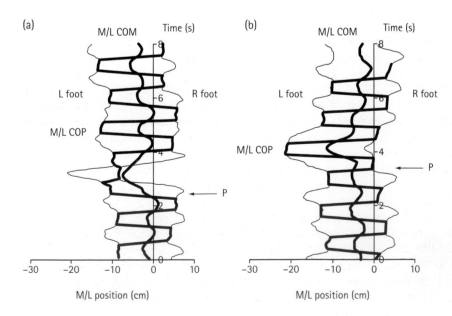

Figure 2.5 *Center of mass (COM) and center of pressure (COP) profiles before and following perturbation from the right side during (a) left and (b) right single support. (Reproduced from ref. 63.)*

detecting light energy to provide information about inanimate features or animate beings that are silent or far away in the environment.[69] Most animals obtain information from the intensity, direction, frequency and polarization of reflected lights. Dusenbery[69] has provided estimates of the large rates of information transmitted in the human visual system (10^6–10^8 bits/s). It is not surprising that the Bible's first imperative is 'Let there be light', and vision is accorded primacy and dubbed the queen of the senses. Vision allows us to interpret and take appropriate action before reaching the site of potential perturbation. These actions are classified as avoidance strategies[70] and include: selection of alternate foot placement by modulating step length and width; increased ground clearance to avoid hitting an obstacle; changing the direction of locomotion (steering) when the obstacles cannot be cleared; and stopping. Clearly, avoidance strategies represent locomotor adaptations that are primarily implemented to ensure dynamic equilibrium of the moving body.

The work done in my laboratory has provided insights into the basis for selection of alternate foot placement,[71] minimum time (expressed in terms of the step cycle metric) required for implementing these avoidance strategies[71–74] and the characteristics of locomotor pattern changes.[70,72,73,75–79]

The major findings from our studies on avoidance strategies are as follows. (1) Most avoidance strategies can be successfully implemented within a step cycle; only steering has to be planned one step cycle ahead. (2) Selection of alternate foot placement is guided by simple rules. Minimum foot displacement from its normal landing spot is a critical determinant of alternate foot placement position. When two or more choices meet the above criteria, modifications in the plane of progression are preferred. Given a choice between shortening or lengthening step length, subjects choose increased step length; inside foot placement is preferred over stepping to the outside provided the foot does not cross the midline of the body. As discussed by Patla et al.,[71] these rules for alternate foot placement selection ensure that avoidance strategies are implemented with minimal changes while maintaining the dynamic equilibrium and allowing the person to travel forwards safely. (3) The modifications made to the locomotor pattern to implement avoidance strategies are complex and task specific. They are not simple amplitude scaling of the normal locomotor patterns: Rather, both ipsilateral and intralimb muscle activation patterns show phase- (of the step cycle) and muscle-specific modulations.[70] (4) Both visually observable and visually inferred properties of the environment influence the avoidance strategy selection and implementation.[70] We have shown, for example, that perceived fragility of the obstacle modulates limb elevation.[77] When obstacle avoidance response has to be initiated quickly, subjects show a two-stage modulation of limb trajectory; initial large change in response to an obstacle is followed by adjustments related to the height of the obstacle.[80]

Different terrains have to be accommodated as we travel from one place to another. These terrains may have different geometric characteristics, such as sloped surfaces or stairs, and/or may have different surface properties, such as compliance (a soggy field), and frictional characteristics (e.g. icy surface) that can influence the body–ground interaction.[70] Unlike avoidance strategies that normally would influence one or two steps, accommodation strategies usually involve modifications sustained over several steps. The types of changes made to the normal locomotor rhythm may include those discussed under avoidance strategies. For example, while walking on a icy surface step length is often reduced. Other changes include a change in locus of propulsive power, as found in stair climbing (propulsive power from the muscles around the hip and knee joint) compared with level walking (major propulsive power from muscles around the ankle joint).[44]

Although the sense of touch (cutaneous afferents) has other roles besides control of movement, the resources of the kinesthetic and vestibular systems are primarily dedicated during the control of locomotion. Visual system resources on the other hand cannot be dedicated completely to the guidance of locomotor task. Intermittent sampling of the environment is adequate.[81–83] This is not surprising considering evolutionary pressures which required the predator or the prey to attend to other things while walking. Our work[83] has shown that when the terrain is even and no specific foot placement is required, subjects visually sample the environment for less than 10 per cent of the travel time (not including the initiation and termination phase). When foot placement is constrained (by requiring the subjects to step on specific locations) the sampling time increases to slightly over 30 per cent. Gaze patterns during adaptive locomotion, whether it involves avoiding an obstacle, landing on specific targets or steering, also show intermittent sampling of environmental features.[84–86]

Kinesthetic and visual systems, unlike the vestibular system, may be subjected to sensory errors. When the support surface moves (for example while standing on a compliant surface) the kinesthetic output can be in error because its output is referenced to the support surface. Similarly, since the visual system detects relative motion between the body and environment, environment motion can be perceived as self-motion. The three sensory modalities, with their different frames of reference,[87] help to resolve conflict when one of the sensory system outputs is in error. The information from the visual system, however, can dominate the movement response, as demonstrated by the elegant studies of Lee and his colleagues (see review by Lee and Young[88]). For example, rotation of the room in which a person is running, leads to compensatory rotation of the trunk to stabilize the visual surround.[88] Recent work by Lackner and DiZio[89] in a rotating room and by Pailhous et al.[90] and Prokop et al.[91] using projected visual flow, also demonstrate the influence and dominance of visual input on the control of locomotion.

Modulation of basic patterns of locomotion

The basic patterns of locomotion discussed in the section 'Production and coordination of rhythmic muscle activation patterns' (page 23), are adequate for walking over a straight level path at a constant speed. Clearly, such constraints on the locomotor control system would not be very useful for us: we need to be able to modify these basic patterns to satisfy internal and external environmental demands. The modulations of basic stepping patterns include changes in speed of locomotion, steering control, selection of foot placement, avoidance of obstacles on and above ground, and accommodating surfaces of different geometry (slopes or stairs) and/or physical properties (icy path or soggy field). The changes can be sensory driven based on external environmental information or internally driven by desired objective. For example, to reach a desired destination sooner we would like to speed up. Modulations in speed of walking can also be externally driven: such as when crossing a street to avoid collision with a moving car. Similarly, steering control can be internally driven to reach a particular end goal or externally driven to avoid collision with a large immovable object, such as a tree. It is the ability of the locomotor control system to meet this requirement that makes legged locomotion so versatile.

NEURAL SUBSTRATES, PATHWAYS AND SENSORY SYSTEMS INVOLVED

While the basic patterns of stepping are generated in the spinal cord as discussed in the section 'Production and coordination of rhythmic muscle activation patterns' (page 23), most other structures of the nervous system and the sensory apparatus are involved in adapting these basic patterns to meet internal and external environmental demands. We begin with discussion of the various neural substrates and pathways involved and bring in the contributions of various sensory systems. Although in other animals sensory modalities such as olfaction and auditory systems play an important role in the modulation of basic locomotor patterns, in humans, as in most mammals, the three sensory systems – kinesthetic, vestibular and visual – are critical for mobility. When vision is compromised in humans, olfaction, haptic and auditory systems can help in guiding locomotor movements.[92] While we have been able to measure activity patterns in various descending and ascending tracts, how sensory input is mapped onto these patterns and eventually the motor output is not well understood.

The major motor tracts that provide phasic modulation to the spinal circuitry are the vestibulospinal tract (VeST) originating in the vestibular nuclei, the rubrospinal tract (RuST) originating in the red nucleus, the reticulospinal tract (ReST) from the reticular formation, the tectospinal tract (TeST) originating in the superior colliculus) and corticospinal tract (CST) originating in the motor cortex. Phasic modulation implies that the activity in these tracts is rhythmically active, with their activity related to specific phase of the step cycle. Generally, ReST and RuST provide excitatory inputs during the swing phase of the step cycle while the VeST primarily provides excitatory input during the stance phase of the step cycle.[93] The cerebellum receives information about the output of the spinal pattern generator called efference copy or corollary discharge [via the ventral spino-cerebellar tract (VSCT) and spino-reticulo-cerebellar tract (SRCT)], afferent inputs generated by the locomotor movements, both active and passive [via the dorsal spino-cerebellar tract (DSCT)], and the vestibular and visual inputs; it modulates the basic locomotor patterns by regulating the activity in all descending pathways. Neurons in the DSCT have been shown to code global parameters such as limb length and orientation.[94] This information would be very useful in planning for changes in activity patterns in the various descending tracts. Cerebellar ablation results in tonic rather than phasic activities in all but the corticospinal tract. The rhythmic modulation of activity in the corticospinal is considerably reduced when the cerebellar input to the sensory motor cortex is eliminated.[93] When the afferent inputs generated by the locomotor movements are abolished, as in a fictive preparation, the phasic modulation of the descending tracts still persists, emphasizing the importance of the activity in the VSCT and SRCT. The functional outcome of the cerebellar input is improved inter- and intralimb coordination of the locomotor movements. In humans, cerebellar deficits (most commonly associated with lesions of the vermis or flocculonodular lobe of the cerebellum) lead to irregular stepping, both spatially and temporally, and poor balance.[95]

The TeST is involved in orienting and attending to novel stimuli. The superior colliculus is an integral part of the visual system different from the geniculostriate system (discussed later) and is involved in visual attention and orienting behaviors (for review see Stein and Meredith).[96] It receives not only visual input from the retina but also from other sensory modalities, and controls the eye and head movements through the tectoreticular tract, and the other musculature through the TeST. Although the superior colliculus is separate from the geniculostriate system, it is influenced by the cortical input.[96] Lesions of the superior colliculus lead to specific behavioral deficits: the animal neglects visual stimuli in the field even though the animal is not blind and can avoid obstacles in the path. The visual stimuli that are most effective in eliciting a response in neurons in the superior colliculus are slow-moving rather than stationary, and novel as opposed to repeated presentation of the same stimulus.[96] It is also clear that input from other sensory modalities, such as the auditory system, is integrated with the visual stimuli to generate an appropriate response. Therefore, steering action during locomotion to attend to novel and moving environmental stimuli is controlled by this structure in the roof of the brainstem.

The corticospinal tract is actively involved in visually mediated obstacle avoidance, foot placement and accommodating different support surfaces in the travel path during locomotion. Animals with lesions of the corticospinal tract are able to travel over smooth surfaces at different speeds quite well. When the animal is required to go over barriers in the travel path or is constrained to place its paws on a specific location (such as the rungs of a ladder), the intensity (but not the phase) of the activity in the corticospinal tract increases dramatically. The neurons in the corticospinal tract are active during the swing phase, as expected; the outputs from these neurons have been shown to precisely encode not only limb elevation to clear the obstacle, but also foot placement.[97] Depending on the intensity of the cortical volley, the ongoing locomotor rhythm may be modified or reset (i.e. initiate transition from stance to swing phase).

RESEARCH ON ADAPTIVE HUMAN LOCOMOTION

There is a wealth of literature on adaptive locomotion patterns in humans. Various avoidance and accommodation behaviors have been studied, although the most commonly studied behavior is obstacle avoidance. Systematic manipulation of sensory inputs and environmental characteristics coupled with detailed measurement of motor strategies has led to some general observations. These are summarized below.

1. Vision provides unique, accurate and precise information at the right time and location that cannot be matched by other sensory modalities.[70,74] The visual system provides three categories of information. Environmental information both visually observable and inferred is available at a distance. Postural and movement information about body/body segments and self-motion information is gathered in the peripheral visual field and is available on-line. Visual information is acquired in a sampled mode and is used both in a feed-forward and on-line manner to modulate locomotion pattern. Because information is sampled, it is subject to top-down processing and distractions. If the sampling is not consistent and predictable, accuracy and precision of control can be adversely affected. Patient study has shown that visual information is processed in the dorsal stream (occipito-parietal cortex).[98]
2. Kinesthetic information has been shown to play a critical role in adapting movement patterns to unexpected disturbances as discussed in the section 'Maintaining dynamic stability of the moving body'

(page 26). The dynamic temporal stability margin (time it would take the body COM to fall outside the projected base of support) during adaptive locomotion is constrained within narrow limits, necessitating a fast backup reactive system (reflexes) to ensure stability in case of error in visual–motor transformation. Kinesthetic input is also essential for implementing successful adaptive strategies. Swing limb knee joint proprioceptive input, for example, is used to monitor limb elevation during obstacle avoidance. Prediction of spatial location of foot landing during locomotion derived from kinesthetic input is critical for selecting alternate foot placement to avoid dangers such as potholes and puddles.
3. Recent research has shown that vestibular information during locomotion has a more pronounced effect on locomotor patterns during walking than in running.[99,100] This suggests that vestibular influence on descending tracts can be selectively gated.
4. Proactive adaptive gait strategies involve global modifications to movement patterns; the changes are not restricted to a joint or even a limb, but involve coordination of whole body.
5. Cognitive factors play an important role in both selection of adaptive strategies and modulation of locomotion patterns.

Guiding locomotion to endpoints

Since locomotion is essential for survival, it is not surprising that animals rarely move around aimlessly: locomotion is goal directed. When the route or path is visible from a single viewpoint, no spatial knowledge of the terrain is necessary. For example, when going from one part of the room to another that is visible from the point of origin, visual input alone can guide the selection of path (even around obstacles if present). When moving in a large-scale spatial area such as a city block or town, route planning generally depends on some mental representation of the area.[101–103] Cognitive spatial maps are the mental representation of large-scale areas. This ability to store and retrieve information about their living environment affords animals tremendous advantage: it confers greater flexibility in locomotor behavior and greatly extends the range of travel than would be possible if locomotion were simply triggered and guided by stimuli available in the field of perception.

NATURE OF COGNITIVE SPATIAL MAPS

The stored spatial information is allocentric, that is, independent of the subject's location and contains both topological (absolute location of objects and landmarks and their various spatial relationship) and metric representation (for review see Poucet[104]). When obstacles in the travel path constrain movements, topological knowledge becomes critical. In contrast, results showing that animals are capable of taking direct shortcuts between two locations, demonstrate the importance of metric representation of space (for true vectorial summation).[104] It is clear that representation of space is not homogeneous: some places may have more value than others. Thus, these maps are not like the cartographic maps used by travelers for navigation in a large-scale environment, but contain relevant information that allows us to select novel paths and guide our locomotion to goals not visible from the start. In addition, the maps have to be associated with specific temporal events (episodic memory). For example, scrubjays time their retrieval of stored foods: foods that decay faster are retrieved earlier.[105]

NEURAL SUBSTRATES INVOLVED

Clinical studies of patients with lesions and electrophysiological and lesion studies in animals have identified several neural substrates in the cerebral hemispheres that store these cognitive spatial maps. Electrophysiological studies have identified neurons in the hippocampus that fire when the animal is in a particular location (place cells), and others that fire when the animal is orientated in a particular direction irrespective of the animal location (direction cells).[102–104,106] This led to the proposition that the hippocampus is a major site for storing these cognitive spatial maps. Lesions of the hippocampus in animals leads to a variety of spatial problems. Although acquisition of new spatial information is adversely affected, well-learned spatial information is spared, suggesting that the hippocampus is critical for acquisition but not long-term storage of spatial maps. Exploratory activity in hippocampal-lesioned animals is greatly reduced. In humans, hippocampal damage does lead to memory deficits, but the information affected is declarative (explicit and accessible to conscious awareness) and not procedural (implicit and accessible through performance).[107]

Damage to the parietal cortex also results in loss of spatial abilities in humans and animals, affecting both the acquisition and retention of spatial information. Egocentric (body referenced) spatial information about objects in the extrapersonal space is unaffected. In contrast, damage to the frontal lobe affects egocentric spatial information and spares the allocentric information. Electrophysiological studies on the parietal or frontal cortex similar to those carried out on the hippocampal neurons are few, although recent work has shown cells in the posterior parietal cortex that fire when the animal looks in a particular direction.[108]

Poucet[104] has proposed in his review article that the parietal cortex and the hippocampus play dual and critical roles in the storage of cognitive spatial maps. The hippocampus is responsible for coding topological information, while the posterior parietal cortex, which receives both visual information (from the occipitoparietal pathway from the visual cortex) and locomotor related information (from the somatosensory cortex), provides metric representation of the allocentric space. The fronto-striatal system is then responsible for converting this allocentric spatial information into appropriate spatially directed locomotor movements in the egocentric frame.[109]

RESEARCH ON HUMAN NAVIGATION

While considerable work has been done on animal navigation, work on human navigation is still in its infancy. The most studied aspect of human navigation is non-visual guidance of locomotion. Typical paradigms involve guiding individuals to a location via varied and circuitous routes and requiring them to return to the start location via the shortest path. Sensory information from the vestibular and kinesthetic systems gathered during the outgoing phase can be used to guide the return journey. Successful charting of a return journey that does not simply involve retracing the outward journey suggests that subjects are able to use sensory signals effectively. Creatures such as desert ants rely on this navigational ability, called dead reckoning, to forage for food and return to their nests. Research has shown that vestibular information is used to gather directional cues while kinesthetic information provides distance cues. Reliance on vestibular information to also code distance by double integrating acceleration signals detected is, like all integration, subject to cumulative errors. This non-visual but sensory-based ability to navigate in humans has only limited spatial range: travel over wider areas is made possible by use of vision and stored spatial memory. Researchers have shown that priming with a visual target improves performance in a purely vestibular navigational task.[110]

Research on the use of visual landmarks and stored spatial memory has been limited by lack of appropriate methods and instruments. Table-top spatial memory tests on navigational ability have major limitations. The perspective is aerial versus viewer centered; information is acquired in the egocentric frame (since the body is stationary) versus allocentric and is available in one field of view as opposed to the multiple fields of view acquired during normal navigation.[106] Virtual reality technology has been a tremendous boon to this field of work. Modern technology can immerse the individual in the visual environment giving a realistic perception of, for example, navigating through a city block. Nevertheless, in most studies using virtual reality the individual does not get other relevant sensory cues from vestibular and kinesthetic systems since they are tethered to a fixed location. Also, the field of view, while improving, is still narrow and limited.[106] Training in a virtual reality environment does transfer to real life and can be used to explore the strategies used by individuals to code and store spatial maps.

Minimizing energy needed during locomotion

Moving the body through an environment requires energy. Minimizing these locomotor-related energy costs can increase an animal's endurance, allowing it to travel farther and longer, provide more energy for reproduction, and reduce time spent on hazardous foraging to replenish the energy sources.[111] These benefits would clearly increase the chances of survival and therefore selection pressures would have favored locomotor structure and patterns that require less energy.

BODY MORPHOLOGY AND MUSCLE CHARACTERISTICS

To achieve lower energy costs, the body morphology is matched to the environment that the animal travels through. Movement of fish through water is energy efficient because of the shape; at cruising speed the flow is laminar, resulting in lower energy costs. In long-legged animals such as humans, the relative mass distribution assists in reducing energy costs. Large-mass muscle is concentrated around the proximal joints, reducing inertia and resulting in lower energy requirements. Elasticity in various tissues has been argued to provide storage capabilities in one phase which can be used later in another phase of the step cycle, thereby reducing energy costs.[111] However, in kangaroo rats, the large hindlimb muscles are designed not for storage and recovery of elastic strain energy but to withstand large forces associated with acceleration to avoid predation.[112] It is well recognized that muscles provide a unique power-to-weight ratio unmatched by any motor that humans have created.

PATTERN OF MUSCLE ACTIVATION

Researchers have shown that terrestrial animals minimize limb extensor muscle strain (<6 per cent) during stance phase of locomotion when the muscles are active. This allows better recovery of elastic energy stored in the muscle tendon actuator and efficient muscle force generation to minimize metabolic costs during locomotion.[113] Similarly, leg stiffness is regulated to exploit recovery of energy from travel surface compliance and minimize energy costs:[114] leg stiffness regulation must involve changes in muscle activation, although these have not been documented.

CONTRIBUTION OF INTERSEGMENTAL DYNAMICS TO MINIMIZING ENERGY COST OF LOCOMOTION

During the swing phase of locomotion, the gravity- and motion-dependent torques can contribute substantially to the motion of the limb, minimizing the need for active muscle involvement.[115] In fact, many researchers have argued that during normal locomotion, the swing phase trajectory is primarily dictated by the pendular dynamics of the swinging limb;[66,116] the initial conditions set at the end of the stance phase coupled with the compound pendulum dynamics produce major aspects of the limb trajectory. Minimal active muscular effort is required; when muscular effort is used, such as at the end of the swing phase, it serves to control rather than generate the limb movement. Intersegmental dynamics are also important in the control of adaptive locomotion. Limb elevation over an obstacle exploits the intersegmental dynamics to minimize energy consumption.[117] Even though swing limb elevation is achieved through flexion of all three joints, only the knee joint is actively flexed. Hip and ankle joint flexion occurs due to motion-dependent torques.[117] The movements generated by muscle action are not as simple as those predicted by the literature on functional anatomy. In order to understand the mechanisms behind the use of intersegmental dynamics to facilitate movement control, we need to re-examine the relationship between muscle action and movement. Modeling the muscle action in multi-articular movement[45] has demonstrated that muscles act to accelerate all joints, even those not spanned by the muscles. The complex action created by active muscle involvement arises from inertial dynamics, which introduce non-linear coupling between limb segments due to Coriolis and centrifugal effects. For example, during a feedforward simulation of the leg movement, it is possible to show that flexor torque applied at the knee joint during the swing phase not only flexes the knee joint, but also the hip joint.[118] These strategies are not immutable: lower limb amputees with intact knee joint musculature choose to use active control about the hip joint rather than the knee joint, thereby minimizing knee joint instability.[119]

PREFERRED SPEED AND FORM OF LOCOMOTION REDUCE ENERGY COST

Humans, like all terrestrial animals, have a preferred speed of locomotion and change their form of locomotion from walking to running as speed requirement increases. In their classic study, Hoyt and Taylor[120] showed that for a given form of locomotion, the energetics of locomotion in horses demonstrate a U-shaped curve as a function of speed: speed selected by the horses coincides with the minima in the U-shaped curves. In humans the relationship between metabolic cost and speed for a given form of locomotion is only U-shaped for walking and not running. Even for horses, energy costs during gallop show a much flatter curve than for walk and trot.[120] Thus, there is not a clear speed of galloping that corresponds with minimum energy cost. While preferred speed for walking in humans does fall around the minimum cost value of the U-shaped curve, this is not the case for running (Fig. 2.6).[121]

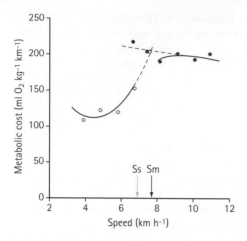

Figure 2.6 *Energy cost during walking and running at various speeds in humans. (Reproduced from ref. 121.) Sm, speed where the metabolic cost for walking and running is similar; Ss, speed of spontaneous gait switch from walking to running.*

Many researchers have examined the transition from a walk to a run in humans to determine whether increased energy cost is the trigger for change in the form of locomotion from walking to running. The results to date have been equivocal. While it is true that energy cost can be reduced if there is a change in form of locomotion (different gait patterns), increased energy costs are not the trigger for such a transition. This is partly because humans are not sensitive to small changes in energy demands over short duration. Others have argued that bone strain is the determinant of gait and speed.[122] This does not preclude energy minimization, rather, as researchers have pointed out, that at preferred speeds the peak level of muscle stress is similar, thereby linking energetics and mechanics.[123]

Ensuring the structural stability of the locomotor apparatus

The locomotor apparatus, however functional, would not be useful if it has a high probability of mechanical failure under normal operating conditions. Structures made by humans are designed with high safety factors: the ratio of failure stress (force per unit area) to those stresses normally experienced by the structure ranges from 4 to 10. Evolutionary pressures have engineered biological structures of the locomotor apparatus (bones, muscles, tendons and ligaments) to minimize their failure during the animal's lifetime.

POSTURAL CHANGES TO MINIMIZE STRESS

Biewener[124] has reviewed how the changes in form, material properties and mass of the biological structure in animals of varying sizes have evolved to minimize failure during locomotor activities. This review shows that the organization and composition of skeletal bones, muscles

and tendons are generally similar across species. To maintain stress within the biological range during locomotion, selection has preferred instead to modify muscle mechanical advantage and limb posture as the size of the animal increases. The upright posture in bipedal locomotion affords a greater effective mechanical advantage, defined as the ratio of propulsive muscle moment arm to the moment arm of the ground reaction forces,[124] thus reducing the muscle force and hence skeletal stress. Postural changes in larger animals have minimized stress at the expense of maneuverability and accelerative capability.

STRUCTURAL CHARACTERISTICS MATCH THE NEED OF THE ANIMAL

Pigeon flight feather shafts are designed for better flexural stiffness than strength. The limb bone safety factor in bending and shear are different for species that sprawl (alligator or iguana) compared with species that have an upright posture (birds and mammals) because the loading patterns are different. For example, bones during sprawling gait experience greater torsion, therefore, alligator bones have a higher bending (and shear) safety factor compared with those of horses. Bone curvature improves load predictability at the expense of strength,[125] and it changes with size of the animal to ensure similar peak bone stress.[126]

PATTERN OF MUSCLE ACTIVATION DURING LOCOMOTION TO MINIMIZE HARMFUL STRESS

Most long bones fracture as a result of bending and/or torsional loading. During human locomotion, Scott and Winter[127] have shown that co-contraction serves to minimize bending load at the expense of compressive load.[128] Bones are designed to tolerate compressive loads much better than torsional loads.

SUMMARY

The deceptively simple task of locomotion so critical for survival and well-being continues to challenge researchers. One way of understanding this area of research is to examine how each functional subtask of successful adaptive human locomotion is generated and controlled. All parts of the central nervous system from the spinal cord to the cortex and the major sensory systems are involved in the control of locomotion. The control system, which has to operate in the gravito-inertial environment, exploits the mechanics to simplify control and save energy. Evolutionary forces have shaped both the structure and form of locomotion to ensure that energy costs are held to a minimum and the structure lasts a lifetime. The review highlights two important points. First, our knowledge is by no means complete: many aspects of locomotor control remain to be discovered. Second, this area of research has attracted workers from different fields, as indicated by the variety of journals where one finds articles related to locomotion. The nature of questions has demanded involvement of neurophysiologists, neurologists, kinesiologists, engineers, roboticists, rehabilitation personnel and biologists. Hopefully, we have posed the right questions, which is the most important aspect of any scientific endeavor. Answers should follow.

ACKNOWLEDGEMENT

The support from NSERC, Canada is gratefully acknowledged.

REFERENCES

1. Gould SJ. *Hen's teeth and horse's toes: further reflections in natural history*. London: WW Norton and Co, 1984.
2. Raibert MH. *Legged robots that balance*. Cambridge: MIT Press, 1986.
3. Mori S. Integration of posture and locomotion in acute decerebrate cats and in awake freely moving cats. *Prog Neurobiol* 1987;**28**:161–95.
4. Kelley DL, Dainis A, Wood GK. Mechanics and muscular dynamics of rising from a seated position. In: Komi PV, ed. *Biomechanics V-B*. Baltimore: University Park Press, 1976;127–34.
5. Pai YC, Rogers MW. Control of body mass transfer as a function of speed of ascent in sit-to-stand. *Med Sci Sports Exerc* 1990;**22**:378–84.
6. Pai YC, Rogers MW. Segmental contributions to total body momentum in sit-to-stand. *Med Sci Sports Exerc* 1991;**23**(2):225–30.
7. Crenna P, Frigo C. A motor programme for the initiation of forward-oriented movements in humans. *J Physiol* 1991;**437**:635–53.
8. Riley PO, Schenkman ML, Mann RW, Hodge WA. Mechanics of a constrained chair-rise. *J Biomech* 1991;**24**(1):77–85.
9. Pai YC, Lee WA. Effect of a terminal constraint on control of balance during sit-to-stand. *J Motor Behav* 1994;**26**:247–56.
10. Doorenbosch CA, Harlaar J, Roebroeck ME, Lankhorst GJ. Two strategies of transferring from sit-to-stand: the activation of monoarticular and biarticular muscles. *J Biomech* 1994;**27**(11):1299–307.
11. Coghlin SS, McFadyen BJ. Transfer strategies used to rise from a chair in normal and low back pain subjects. *Clin Biomech* 1994;**9**:85–92.
12. Winter DA, Patla AE, Prince F, et al. Stiffness control of balance during quiet standing. *J Neurophysiol* 1998;**80**:1211–21.
13. Jordan LM. Brainstem and spinal cord mechanisms for the initiation of locomotion. In: Shimamura M, Grillner S, Edgerton VT, eds. *Neurobiological basis of human locomotion*. Tokyo: Japan Scientific Societies Press, 1991;3–20.
14. Mori S, Sakamoto T, Takakusaki K. Interaction of posture and locomotion in cats: its automatic and volitional control aspects. In: Shimamura M, Grillner S, Edgerton VT, eds. *Neurobiological basis of human locomotion*. Tokyo: Japan Scientific Societies Press, 1991;21–32.
15. Barnes GR. Visual–vestibular interaction in the control of head and eye movement:the role of visual feedback and predictive mechanisms. *Prog Neurobiol* 1993;**41**:435–72.
16. Carlsöö S. The initiation of walking. *Acta Anat* 1966;**65**:1–9.
17. Herman R, Cook T, Cozzens B, Freedman W. Control of postural reactions in man:the initiation of gait. In: Stein RB, Pearson KG, Smith RS, Redford JB, eds. *Control of posture and locomotion*. New York: Plenum Press, 1973;363–88.
18. Cook T, Cozzens B. Human solution for locomotion III: the initiation of gait. In: Herman RM, Grillner S, Stein PSG, Stuart DG, eds. *Neural control of locomotion*. New York: Plenum Press, 1976;65–76.
19. Brenière Y, Do MC, Bouisset S. Are dynamic phenomena prior to stepping essential to walking? *J Motor Behav* 1987;**19**(1):62–76.
20. Fiolkowski P, Brunt D, Bishop M, Woo R. Does postural instability affect the initiation of human gait? *Neurosci Lett* 2002;**323**(3):167–70.
21. Couillandre A, Brenier Y, Maton B. Is human gait initiation program affected by a reduction of the postural basis? *Neurosci Lett* 2000;**285**(2):150–4.
22. Timmann D, Horak FB. Perturbed step initiation in cerebellar subjects: 2. Modification of anticipatory postural adjustments. *Exp Brain Res* 2001;**141**(1):110–20.
23. Bent LR, Inglis JT, McFadyen BJ. Vestibular contributions across the execution of a voluntary forward step. *Exp Brain Res* 2002;**143**:100–5.
24. Jian Y Winter DA Ishac MG Gilchrist L. Trajectory of the body COG and COP during initiation and termination of gait. *Gait Posture* 1993; **1**:9–22.
25. Jaeger RJ, Vanitchatchavan P. Ground reaction forces during termination of human gait. *J Biomech* 1992;**15**:1233–6.
26. Hase K, Stein RB. Analysis of rapid stopping during walking. *J Neurophysiol* 1998;**80**:255–61.
27. Crenna P, Cuong DM, Breniere Y. Motor Programmes for the termination of gait in humans: organisation and velocity-dependent adaptation. *J Physiol* 2001;**537**:1059–72.
28. Perry SD, Santos SD, Patla AE. Contribution of vision and cutaneous sensation to the control of center of mass (COM) during gait termination. *Brain Res* 2001;**913**(1):27–34.
29. Rossignol S, Saltiel P, Perreault M-C, et al. Intralimb and interlimb coordination in the cat during real and fictive rhythmic motor programs. *The Neurosciences* 1993;**5**:67–75.
30. Forssberg H. Spinal locomotor functions and descending control. In: Sjolund B, Bjorklund A, eds. *Brain stem control of spinal mechanisms*. Amsterdam: Elsevier Biomedical Press, 1982;253–71.
31. Carter MC, Smith JL. Simultaneous control of two rhythmical behaviours. II. Hindlimb walking with paw shake response in spinal cat. *J Neurophysiol* 1986;**56**:184–95.
32. Forssberg H, Grillner S, Halbertsma J. The locomotion of the low spinal cat. I. Coordination within a hindlimb. *Acta Physiol Scand* 1980;**108**(3):269–81.
33. Armstrong DM. The supraspinal control of mammalian locomotion. *J Physiol* 1988;**405**:1–37.
34. Barbeau H, Rossignol S. Recovery of locomotion after chronic spinalization in the adult cat. *Brain Res* 1987;**412**:84–95.

35. Delcomyn F. Neural basis of rhythmic behaviour in animals. *Science* 1980;**210**(31):492–8.

36. Grillner S. Neurobiological bases of rhythmic motor acts in vertebrates. *Science* 1985;**228**:143–9.

37. Burford JA, Smith JL. Adaptive control for backward quadrupedal walking. H. Hindlimb muscle synergies. *J Neurophysiol* 1990;**64**:756–66.

38. Pearson KG. Common principles of motor control in vertebrates and invertebrates. *Annu Rev Neurosci* 1993;**16**:265–97.

39. Thelen E, Ulrich BD, Niles D. Bilateral coordination in human infants: stepping on a split-belt treadmill. *J Exp Psychol Hum Percept Perform* 1987;**13**:405–10.

40. Forssberg H. Ontogeny of human locomotor control I. Infant stepping supported locomotion and transition to independent locomotion. *Exp Brain Res* 1985;**57**:480–93.

41. Pang MY, Yang JF. Interlimb co-ordination in human infant stepping. *J Physiol* 2001;**533**:617–25.

42. Bussel B, Roby-Brami A, Yakovleff A, Bennis N. Late flexion reflex in paraplegic patients. Evidence for a spinal stepping generator. *Brain Res Bull* 1989;**22**:53–6.

43. Duysens J, van de Crommert HWAA. Neural control of locomotion; Part I: the central pattern generator from cats to humans. *Gait Posture* 1998;**7**:131–41.

44. Winter DA. *The biomechanics and motor control of human gait: normal elderly and pathological.* Waterloo: University of Waterloo Press, 1991.

45. Zajac FE, Gordon ME. Determining muscle force and action in multi-articular movement. *Exerc Sport Sci Rev* 1989;**17**:187–230.

46. Barbeau H, Norman K, Fung J, et al. Does neurorehabilitation play a role in the recovery of walking in neurological populations? *Ann N Y Acad Sci* 2001;**860**:377–92.

47. Dietz V. Human neuronal control of automatic functional movements: interaction between central programs and afferent input. *Physiol Rev* 1992;**72**(1):33–69.

48. Stein RB. Reflex modulation during locomotion. In: Patla AE, ed. *Adaptability of human gait: implications for the control of locomotion.* Amsterdam: Elsevier, 1991;21–36.

49. Sinkjaer T, Andersen JB, Larsen B. Soleus stretch reflex modulation during gait in humans. *J Neurophysiol* 1996;**76**:1112–20.

50. Belanger M, Patla AE. Corrective responses to perturbations applied during walking in humans. *Neurosci Lett* 1984;**49**:291–5.

51. Duysens J, Trippel M, Horstmann GA, Dietz V. Gating and reversal of reflexes in ankle muscles during human walking. *Exp Brain Res* 1990;**82**(2):351–8.

52. Yang JF, Stein RB. Phase-dependent reflex reversal in human leg muscles during walking. *J Neurophysiol* 1990;**63**:1109–17.

53. Prochazka A. Sensorimotor gain control: a basic strategy of motor systems? *Prog Neurobiol* 1989;**33**:281–307.

54. Nashner LM, Forssberg H. Phase-dependent organization of postural adjustments associated with arm movements while walking. *J Neurophysiol* 1986;**55**:1382–94.

55. Dietz V, Quintern J, Berger W. Afferent control of human stance and gait: evidence for blocking of group I afferents during gait. *Exp Brain Res* 1985;**61**:153–63.

56. Dietz V, Horstmann GA, Berger W. Interlimb coordination of leg-muscle activation during perturbation of stance in humans. *J Neurophysiol* 1989;**62**:680–93.

57. Eng JJ, Winter DA, Patla AE. Strategies for recovery from a trip in early and late swing during human walking. *Exp Brain Res* 1994;**102**(2):339–49.

58. Marigold DS, Patla AE. Strategies for dynamic stability during locomotion on a slippery surface: effects of prior experience and knowledge. *J Neurophysiol* 2002;**88**:339–53.

59. Tang P-F Woollacott MH Chong RKY. Control of reactive balance adjustments in perturbed human walking: roles of proximal and distal postural muscle activity. *Exp Brain Res* 1998;**119**:141–52.

60. Tang P-F Woollacott MH. Inefficient postural responses to unexpected slips during walking in older adults. *J Gerontol Med Sci* 1998;**53A**:M471–80.

61. Tang P-F, Woollacott MH. Phase-dependent modulation of proximal and distal postural responses to slips in young and older adults. *J Gerontol Med Sci* 1999;**54A**:M89–102.

62. Hill S, Patla AE, Perry SD, et al. Base of support changes ensure a constant stability margin following unexpected lateral trunk perturbations during overground walking. In: Duysens J, et al. eds. *Control of posture and gait.* Maastricht, Netherlands, 2001;436–9.

63. Patla AE. Strategies for dynamic stability during adaptive human locomotion. *IEEE Engineering in Medicine and Biology* 2003;**22**(2):48–52.

64. Grabiner MD, Koh TJ, Lundin TM, Jahnigen DW. Kinematics of recovery from a stumble. *J Gerontol* 1993;**48**(3):M97–102.

65. Belenkii YY, Gurfinkel VS, Paltsev YI. Element of control of voluntary movements. *Biofizika* 1967;**12**:135–41.

66. Mena D, Mansour JM, Simon SR. Analysis and synthesis of human swing leg motion during gait and its clinical applications. *J Biomech* 1981;**141**(2):823–32.

67. Patla AE. Adaptation of postural responses to voluntary arm raises during locomotion in humans. *Neurosci Lett* 1986;**68**:334–8.

68. Hirschfeld H, Forssberg H. Phase-dependent modulations of anticipatory postural activity during human locomotion. *J Neurophysiol* 1991;**66**(1):12–19.

69. Dusenbery DB. *Sensory ecology.* New York: WH Freeman, 1992.

70. Patla AE. Understanding the roles of vision in the control of human locomotion *Gait Posture* 1997;**5**:54–69.

71. Patla AE, Prentice SD, Rietdyk S, et al. What guides the selection of alternate foot placement during locomotion in humans? *Exp Brain Res* 1999a;**128**:441–50.

72. Patla AE, Robinson C, Samways M, Armstrong CJ. Visual control of step length during overground locomotion:task-specific modulation of the locomotion synergy. *J Exp Psychol Hum Percept Perform* 1989a;**25**(3):603–17.

73. Patla AE, Prentice S, Robinson C, Neufeld J. Visual control of locomotion: strategies for changing direction and for going over obstacles. *J Exp Psychol Hum Percept Perform* 1991a;**17**(3):603–34.

74. Patla AE. How is human gait controlled by vision? *Ecol Psychol* 1999;**10**(3–4):287–302.

75. Hollands MA, Sorensen KL, Patla AE. Effects of head immobilization on the coordination and control of head and body reorientation and translation during steering. *Exp Brain Res* 2002a;**140**(2):223–33.

76. Patla AE, Armstrong CJ, Silveira JM. Adaptation of the muscle activation patterns to transitory increase in stride length during treadmill locomotion in humans. *Hum Mov Sci* 1989b;**8**:45–66.

77. Patla AE, Rietdyk S, Martin C, Prentice S. Locomotor patterns of the leading and trailing limb while going over solid and fragile obstacles: some insights into the role of vision during locomotion. *J Motor Behav* 1996a;**28**(1):35–47.

78. Patla AE, Adkin A, Ballard T. On-line steering: coordination and control of body centre of mass head and body re-orientation. *Exp Brain Res* 1999b;**129**:629–34.

79. Vallis LA, Patla AE, Adkin AL. Control of steering in the presence of unexpected head yaw movements: influence on sequencing of subtasks. *Exp Brain Res* 2001;**138**(1):128–34.

80. Patla AE, Beuter A, Prentice S. A two stage correction of limb trajectory to avoid obstacles during stepping. *Neurosci Res Commun* 1991b;**81**(3):153–9.

81. Thomson JA. Is continuous visual control necessary in visually guided locomotion? *J Exp Psychol Hum Percept Perform* 1983;**9**:427–43.

82. Assaiante C, Marchand AR, Amblard B. Decrete visual samples may control locomotor equilibrium and foot positioning in man. *J Motor Behav* 1989;**21**:72–91.

83. Patla AE, Adkin A, Martin C, et al. Characteristics of voluntary visual sampling of the environment during locomotion over different terrains. *Exp Brain Res* 1996b;**112**:513–22.

84. Patla AE, Vickers JN. Where and when do we look as we approach and step over an obstacle in the travel path. *NeuroReport* 1997;**8**:3661–5.

85. Patla AE, Vickers J. How far ahead do we look when required to step on specific locations in the travel path during locomotion. *Exp Brain Res* 2003;**148**:133–8.

86. Hollands MA, Patla AE, Vickers JN. 'Look where you're going!': gaze behaviour associated with maintaining and changing the direction of locomotion. *Exp Brain Res* 2002b;**143**:221–30.

87. Gibson JJ. *The senses considered as perceptual systems.* Boston: Houghton Mifflin, 1966.

88. Lee DN, Young DS. Gearing action to the environment. *Exp Brain Res Ser* 1986;**15**:217–30.

89. Lackner JR, DiZio P. Visual stimulation affects the perception of voluntary leg movements during walking. *Perception* 1988;**17**:71–80.

90. Pailhous J, Ferrendez AM, Fluckiger M, Baumberger B. Unintentional modulations of human gait by optical flow. *Behav Brain Res* 1990;**38**:275–81.

91. Prokop T, Schubert M, Berger W. Visual influence on human locomotion: modulation to changes in optic flow. *Exp Brain Res* 1997;**114**:63–70.

92. Strelow ER. What is needed for a theory of mobility: direct perception and cognitive maps – lessons from the blind. *Psychol Rev* 1985;**92**(2):226–48.

93. Orlovsky GN. Cerebellum and locomotion. In: Shimamura M, Grillner S, Edgerton VT, eds. *Neurobiological basis of human locomotion.* Tokyo: Japan Scientific Societies Press, 1991;187–199.

94. Bosco G, Poppele RE. Proprioception from a spinocerebellar perspective. *Physiol Rev* 2001;**81**(2):539–68.

95. Hallett M, Stanhope SJ, Thomas SL, Massaquoi S. Pathophysiology of posture and gait in cerebellar ataxia. In: Shimamura M, Grillner S, Edgerton VR, eds. *Neurobiological basis of human locomotion.* Tokyo: Japan Scientific Societies Press, 1991;2756–830.

96. Stein BE, Meredith A. *The merging of the senses. A Bradford Book.* Boston: MIT Press, 1993.

97. Drew T. Visumotor coordination in locomotion. *Curr Opin Neurobiol* 1991;**91**(4):652–7.

98. Patla AE, Goodale MA. Obstacle avoidance during locomotion is unaffected in a patient with visual form agnosia. *NeuroReport* 1996;**8**:165–8.

99. Brandt T, Strupp M, Benson J. You are better off running than walking with acute vestibulopathy. *Lancet* 1999;**354**:746.

100. Jahn K, Strupp M, Schneider E, et al. Differential effects of vestibular stimulation on walking and running. *NeuroReport* 2000;**11**(5):1745–8.

101. Bryne RW. Geographical knowledge and orientation. In: Ellis AW, ed. *Normality and pathology in cognitive functions.* London: Academic Press, 1982;239–64.

102. O'Keefe J, Nadel L. *The hippocampus as a cognitive map.* Oxford: Clarendon Press, 1978.

103. Schacter DL, Nadel L. Varieties of spatial memory: a problem for cognitive neuroscience. In: Lister RG, Weingartner HJ, eds. *Perspectives on cognitive neuroscience.* Oxford: Oxford University Press, 1991;164–85.

104. Poucet B. Spatial cognitive maps in animals: new hypotheses on their structure and neural mechanisms. *Psychol Rev 100* 1993;**2**:163–82.

105. Claydon NS, Dickinson A. Episodic-like memory during cache recovery by scrub jays. *Nature* 1998;**395**:272–4.

106. Maguire EA, Burgess N, O'Keefe J. Human spatial navigation: cognitive maps sexual dimorphism and neural substrates. *Cogn Neurosci* 1999;**9**:171–7.

107. Squire LR, Zola-Morgan S. Memory: brain systems and behaviour. *Trends Neurosci* 1988;**11**(4):170–5.

108. Zeki S. *A vision of the brain.* London: Blackwell Scientific Publications, 1993.

109. Paillard J. Cognitive versus sensorimotor encoding of spatial information. In: Ellen P, Thinus-Blanc C, eds. *Cognitive processes and spatial orientation in animal and man: neurophysiology and developmental aspects. NATO ASI series no. 37.* Dordrecht: Martinus Nijhoff, 1987;43–77.

110. Israel I, Bronstein AM, Kanayama R, et al. Visual and vestibular factors influencing vestibular 'navigation'. *Exp Brain Res* 1996;**112**(3):411–19.

111. Alexander RMcN. Optimization and gaits in the locomotion of vertebrates. *Physiol Rev* 1989;**69**(4):1199–227.

112. Biewener AA, Blickhan R. Kangaroo rat locomotion: design for elastic energy storage or acceleration. *J Exp Biol* 1988;**140**:243–55.

113. Gillis GB, Biewener AA. Hind limb muscle function in relation to speed and gait: *in vivo* patterns of strain and activation in a hip and knee extensor of the rat, *Rattus norvegicus. J Exp Biol* 2001;**204**(15):2717–31.

114. Kerdok AE, Biewener AA, McMohan TA, et al. Energetics and mechanisms of human running on surfaces of different stiffnesses. *J Appl Physiol* 2002;**92**(2):469–78.

115. Smith JL, Zernicke RF. Predictions for neural control based on limb dynamics. *Trends Neurosci* 1987;**10**:123–8.

116. Mochon S, McMahon TA. Ballistic walking. *J Biomech* 1980;**13**:49–57.

117. Patla AE, Prentice SD. The role of active forces and intersegmental dynamics in the control of limb trajectory over obstacles during locomotion in humans. *Exp Brain Res* 1995;**106**:499–504.

118. Patla AE, Prentice SD, Armand M, Huissoon JP. The role of effector system dynamics in the control of limb trajectory

over obstacles during locomotion: empirical and modeling approaches. In: Taguchi K, Igarashi M, Mori S, eds. *Vestibular and neural front*. Amsterdam: Elsevier Science, 1994;333-6.

119. Hill SW, Patla AE, Ishac ME, et al. Altered kinetic strategy for the control of swing limb elevation over obstacles in unilateral below-knee amputee gait. *J Biomech* 1999;**32**:545-9.

120. Hoyt DF, Taylor CR. Gait and the energetics of locomotion in horses. *Nature* 1981;**292**:232-40.

121. Minetti AE, Ardigo LP, Saibene F. The transition between walking and running in humans: metabolic and mechanical aspects at different gradients. *Acta Physiol Scand* 1994;**150**:315-23.

122. Biewener AA, Taylor CR. Bone strain: a determinant of gait and speed. *J Exp Biol* 1986;**123**:383-400.

123. Perry AK, Blickhan R, Biewener AA, et al. Preferred speeds in terrestrial vertebrates: are they equivalent? *J Exp Biol* 1988;**137**:207-19.

124   Biewener AA. Biomechanics of mammalian terrestrial locomotion. *Science* 1990;**250**:1097-103.

125. Bertman JE, Biewener AA. Bone curvature: sacrificing strength for load predictability? *J Theor Biol* 1988;**131**:75-92.

126. Biewener AA. Allometry of quadrupedal locomotion: the scaling of duty factor bone curvature and limb orientation to body size. *J Exp Biol* 1983;**105**:147-71.

127. Scott SH, Winter DA. Internal forces of chronic running injury sites. *Med Sci Sports Exerc* 1990;**22**(3):357-69.

128. Munih M, Kralj A, Bajd T. Calculation of bending moments unloading femur and tibia bones. In: Popovic DB, ed. *Advances in External Control of Human Extremities* X. Belgrade: NAUKA, 1990;67-79.

3

Development of balance and gait control

MARJORIE H. WOOLLACOTT, CHRISTINE ASSAIANTE AND BERNARD AMBLARD

INTRODUCTION

Children normally develop a wide range of motor skills during the early years of life, including sitting, standing, walking and running, and finally combine these skills into intricate repertoires in such performance areas as dance and gymnastics. The basis for their ability to move in these intricate and refined ways lies in their having learned and mastered foundational postural and loco-motor skills early in life. For example, it has been shown that whenever children make even a simple voluntary movement, such as reaching for a toy, they activate postural muscles in advance of the movement to prepare the body for the destabilizing effect of the movement itself and the added weight of the toy to be lifted.

In the same way, delays or abnormalities in postural development could potentially constrain a child's ability to develop walking and reaching skills. In addition, the ability of the clinician to effectively assess walking and manipulatory skills is tied to the ability to assess the systems contributing to posture and balance control.

When children arrive in the clinic with a motor problem, it is thus essential for the clinician not only to assess and improve their performance in the more refined motor skills, including locomotion, but also in basic postural skills that are the foundation of these movements.

In this chapter we will first discuss various approaches to studying balance and locomotion, and explain why we think the 'systems' approach is not only the most practical for research on postural and locomotor control, but also for assessment and treatment. We will then review the research on the development of balance and locomotion in normal children and in children with motor dysfunction, and finally, we will discuss ways this research might be applied to clinical management of postural and locomotor disorders.

NEW APPROACHES FOR RESEARCH ON BALANCE AND LOCOMOTION

Early studies on the development of motor skills in children described specific 'motor milestones' that children would normally master in a given sequence and within a specific period of developmental time.[1] These included crawling, creeping, sitting, pull-to-stand behavior, cruising (walking, holding on to furniture), independent stance and independent walking. Most of the traditional assessment scales used to assess motor development come from developmental norms established by Gesell and McGraw.[1,2]

There are several theories of neural development which attempt to correlate the development of neural structures with the emergence of behaviors. Early theories of child development attempted to correlate the progressive development and disappearance of a variety of reflexes with the emergence of specific behavioral milestones. For example, the asymmetric tonic neck reflex is estimated to emerge between birth and 2 months and is reported to be integrated at approximately 6 months with the emergence of the righting reactions.[3] It is said that this reflex aids in the development of reaching behavior, since the ipsilateral arm extends when the head turns toward the side. However, recent research has found no correlation between reaching behavior and the presence or absence of this reflex in infants 2–4 months old.[4]

In addition, vestibular righting reactions, optical righting reactions and head on body righting reactions are reported to appear at about 2 months of age, as the child begins to control the head in space. The Landau reaction is said to combine the effects of all three head-righting reactions,[5] and is reported to appear at approximately 3–4 months of age, being activated most readily at 5–6 months. As higher-level behaviors emerge, it is said that higher-level reflexes have begun to mature with the concomitant inhibition of lower-level reflexes. Thus, with further development, other balance and protective reflexes are reported to appear, which are controlled by higher levels of the brain, and which inhibit lower-level, more primitive reflexes.

This perspective, often called the 'reflex-hierarchy theory,' thus suggests that it is the development and integration of hierarchically arranged reflexes within the nervous system that are responsible for the appearance and refinement of postural and locomotor skills. A newer perspective on motor development, often called the 'systems perspective,' suggests that postural and locomotor skill development is a much more complex process. According to the systems perspective, the emergence of posture and locomotor behaviors in a child results from complex interactions between (1) the nervous and musculoskeletal systems of the child, (2) the requirements of the task, and (3) the changing environmental conditions.[6]

What does this mean? It means that the emergence or onset of a particular behavior in a child, such as independent stance, may be due to a number of contributing neural or musculoskeletal systems and there may be specific systems that are 'rate-limiting,' that is, until they mature sufficiently the behavior will not appear. Possible systems contributing to motor development include such neural systems as the different sensory systems (visual, vestibular, somatosensory), motor systems, higher-level adaptive systems, and motivational systems and the musculoskeletal systems (e.g. muscular strength, and growth of the limbs and trunk). The difficulty of the task and the environment in which it is performed are also important.

For example, it has been hypothesized that either the maturation of muscle response synergies underlying postural control or the development of sufficient muscle strength is the rate-limiting factor in the development of independent stance and locomotion. However, environmental factors are also important. For example, the child may be willing to stand on a normal support surface, with no visual distractions, but will be unable to stand on a compliant surface, such as a thick carpet, or when visual distractions are disorienting for postural control. Thus, the ability to stand independently might be present in a child in one environmental setting and not another because of complex interactions between the contributing systems of the child and the environment.

In the same way, contributing systems to the emergence of locomotion could include (1) rhythmic pattern generation, (2) postural stability (including all the systems described above), (3) muscle strength, and (4) motivation.

In addition, static balance control might appear earlier than locomotion, because of the different requirements of the two tasks. That is, locomotion also requires the muscle strength and the ability to balance on one leg in a dynamically moving situation.

The use of this systems perspective allows clinicians to broaden their viewpoint of the systems contributing to balance and locomotor control in children, and also to determine more easily the constraints on postural and locomotor control in children with motor disabilities. Using this perspective, assessment would include (1) an evaluation of each of the systems described above, in order to determine the system or systems that constrained the child most heavily, and then (2) the formulation of a treatment strategy designed to improve the function of those systems.

In the rest of this chapter we review the research on balance and locomotor development in infants from the systems perspective, aiming to show the systems most important in contributing to the emergence of major balance and locomotor milestones in normal infants, and the systems most likely to cause constraints on balance abilities in specific populations of infants with motor disabilities.

PRENATAL DEVELOPMENT OF POSTURE AND LOCOMOTION

Postural control

Studies by Prechtl and colleagues have examined fetal position and orientation in the uterus, and also in preterm infants (28–40 weeks).[7,8] They noted that there is no recognizable posture of preference, yet the fetus and the preterm infant show a repertoire of repeated active postures. They thus concluded that the posture of the fetus and preterm infant is variable, but relatively unrelated to the orientation of the force of gravity.

Locomotion

The earliest locomotor-like activity observed prenatally has been recorded with real-time ultrasonography in fetuses at 10 gestational weeks.[9] Using similar techniques, Prechtl and colleagues also showed that prenatal infants make alternating flexion and extension movements of the legs, which result in a somersault if the legs are positioned against the wall of the uterus. It has been suggested that the fetal locomotor-like movements may play a role in positioning the fetus with the head in the birth canal prior to delivery.[10]

NEONATAL CONTROL OF POSTURE AND LOCOMOTION

Postural control

MOTOR COORDINATION

It is well known that infants have poor antigravity function at birth. Many authors have noted that infants show a general dominance of flexor muscle activity during the first 3 months of life. However, it is not clear whether the poor postural control of neonates is due to problems with muscle weakness (peripheral mechanisms) or to the fact that they do not yet possess appropriate antigravity muscle response organization (central mechanisms). In order to determine whether lack of muscle strength was the sole cause of lack of head postural control in the infants, Schloon et al.[8] recorded from neck muscles of full-term infants in the supine and prone position at 5 days of age. They observed that electromyograph (EMG) activity was similar in waking and in sleep. Analysis of EMG patterns did not show any organized activity that would counteract the force of gravity.

They also noted that when an infant is picked up, an active posture is observed. However, this could again be due to either a simple 'en bloc' response or to their actively counteracting the force of gravity. To test this they put neonates on a rocking table that tilted 15° Infants under 8–10 weeks of age did not respond to head downward or upward tilts. However, at 10 weeks of age, at the onset of spontaneous head control, they began to show clear EMG and behavioral responses.

VISION

When do infants start showing visually controlled postural responses? Jouen has performed a study with preterm infants as young as 32–34 weeks of gestation, both with and without visual feedback (goggles were worn).[11] The infant's head was initially maintained in a midline position and then was released. Subsequent movements of the head were measured and it was noted that without vision there was a significant tendency to turn the head to the right, but with vision present this tendency was suppressed and the infant oriented to midline. It was concluded that from 32 to 34 weeks of gestation infants show a simple type of postural control, which keeps the head at midline, and which depends on the presence of vision.

Additional research investigated the neonate's sensitivity to optical flow.[11,12] Three-day-old infants were placed in a darkened room in which an alternating pattern of stripes was activated in either a forward or backward direction. Postural responses were then measured with air-pressure transducers embedded in a pillow behind the infant's head. Infants showed significant compensatory postural adjustments of the head in response to the optical flow patterns. That is, when the visual patterns moved backwards, the infants probably perceived forward head movement, because they moved the head backwards, as if to compensate. The same was true for patterns moving in the opposite direction. This same effect has been clearly observed in standing infants and in adults.[13]

VESTIBULAR

Studies have also been performed by Jouen to study the early development of the vestibular system in infants.[14] In these studies, infants of 2–5 months were placed in an experimental room that allowed the control and modification of both visual information and vestibular information (the chair in which the infant was placed could be tilted to the right or the left 25°). A red wool ball was placed in the visual field, to catch the infant's attention.

The essence of an antigravity response was to keep the head from falling to the side to which the baby was tilted. This reaction showed changes with developmental level, with the older infants dropping the head less than the younger infants did. In addition, when an object (wool ball) was present in the visual field, both age groups tilted the head less, with the effect being strongest in the youngest infants. These results show, first of all, a significant effect of vision on the vestibular otolithic reaction in the infant. They also show a clear improvement in the vestibular response with age. However, in this experiment it is difficult to determine if the improvement is due to improved neck muscle strength or to improved vestibular/motor processing.

INFANT STEPPING

Locomotor movements can be elicited directly after birth if the infant is held under the arms in an upright posture with foot–surface contact and tilted slightly forward.[15] These alternating movements look like walking and are called the stepping reflex. It has been described in premature infants as young as 28 gestational weeks of age,[16] and is most easily elicited during the first two postnatal months.

Infant stepping differs from mature locomotion in several important ways. First, the stepping pattern is not associated with balance control. The newborn is able to produce the stepping pattern on inclined planes, when submerged in water, in the air, and when held upside down.[17] In fact, infants only carry about 40 per cent of their weight on each limb, and the person supporting the infant must carry the remaining weight because of their insufficient muscular strength.[18] Second, the infant makes contact with a flat foot, typically on the lateral aspect of the sole. During the newborn period, there is a significant coactivation of antagonist muscle groups in movements, which contrasts with the reciprocal activation patterns seen in independent walking. In addition, newborn steps are highly flexor dominant with coactivation of the flexor muscles, the tibialis anterior and rectus femoris.[19,20] Finally, the vertical and the forward propulsive forces are small or absent during foot lift-off. This is due to an absence of a propulsive burst in the calf muscles.[10]

This stepping reflex normally disappears by 3 or 4 months of age. It has been hypothesized that it must either be inhibited, eliminated or incorporated into normal stepping, to enable the development of more adaptive movement control, such as autonomous walking. Although there is agreement on the presence of locomotor movements at birth, their relationship to later developing mature walking patterns has been interpreted in a variety of ways.

Why would a well-coordinated stepping pattern completely disappear, to reappear many months later? The traditionally accepted explanation for the disappearance of the infant stepping reflex is that maturing cortical centers inhibit subcortically controlled primitive reflexes.[15,17,21,22]

However, there is more recent evidence that makes this explanation appear insufficient to explain the disappearance of stepping. For example, Zelazo and his colleagues showed that when infants received daily practice in stepping, their number of steps per minute increased during the period of the so-called disappearance, contrary to the notion of cortical inhibition.[23,24] In addition, these trained infants walked independently earlier than untrained control infants.[23] On the basis of these results, Zelazo[23] hypothesized that the disappearance of the stepping reflex was attributable to lack of use, rather than cortical inhibition.

How reflexive movements change into adaptive movements presents a challenge for development theories in general. According to Zelazo,[24] with training, the reflex was converted into instrumental behavior, a necessary transition before independent walking. Zelazo hypothesized that the cognitive change that appears around 12 months of age is a necessary but not sufficient condition for bipedal locomotion to occur.[25] Clearly, there are many constraints on the emergence of independent walking, including such neural and musculoskeletal constraints as the presence of appropriate pattern generators, sufficient leg length, muscle strength and postural control.

Using a dynamic systems approach to the development of locomotion, Thelen argues that stepping is not a reflex at all, but rather is a manifestation of a spontaneous pattern generator similar to other rhythmical activities such as kicking.[26,28] On the basis of kinematic and EMG analysis, Thelen and Fisher[29] showed that kicking and stepping were identical movement patterns, probably mediated by the same neural circuits, and that upright posture was not essential for eliciting alternating, steplike movements of the legs. In fact, these authors suggest that kicking is a developmental continuity of the

manifestation of spontaneous pattern generation, during the period where stepping disappears. Thelen simply explains the disappearance of stepping to a change in the infant's body proportions, including an increase in fat, which leads to the inability to lift the weight of their legs while upright.[28] She concludes that the 'locomotor silence' during the first year is mainly due to these constraints and the lack of posture control. This point of view is supported by the fact that when 4-week-old infants are submerged up to their trunk in water, thus making them more buoyant and counteracting the effects of gravity, stepping increases in frequency.

This continuity hypothesis is consistent with Forssberg's studies.[19] Despite the various and important differences observed between newborn stepping, supported walking, independent walking and adult walking, Forssberg suggests that innate pattern generators in the spinal cord contribute to the movement patterns observed in infant stepping as well as the adult locomotor rhythm.

POSTURAL CONTROL OF THE HEAD AND TRUNK – SITTING

Motor coordination

In infants, head control is generally considered as constituting the beginning of body equilibrium development.[30] Head control improves with emergence of reaching.[31] Head and gaze stabilization relative to the target establish a stable reference frame for reaching.[32] In the sitting position, studies by Hadders-Algra et al.[33] reported the priority of head stabilization in postural control. In response to forward translations of the support surface, the youngest infants (5–6 months) preferred to activate their neck muscles first with respect to the trunk and the leg muscles, suggesting a top-down recruitment, which differs from the bottom-up recruitment normally present in standing and sitting adults[34,35] and sitting children.[36] These results suggest an articulated operation of the head–trunk unit associated with a descending temporal organization of postural control during the first year of life, as proposed by Assaiante and Amblard[37] in their ontogenetic model for the sensorimotor organization of balance control in humans.

During the process of learning to sit independently, and thus balance the head and trunk as a unit, the nervous system of the infant must learn to coordinate sensorimotor information from two body segments as an ensemble. This means that the rules that were developed for sensory–motor relationships involving control of the head need to be extended to the additional set of trunk muscles.

The development of muscle coordination underlying balance control during independent sitting has been studied by a number of research groups.[38–40] In a first set of studies,[38,39] infants were placed in an infant seat or sat independently on a moveable platform, and the platform was moved forward or backward to disturb the balance of the infant, causing a postural adjustment. The experimental paradigm is shown in Fig. 3.1. Muscle responses from the muscles of the head and trunk were recorded with surface EMGs.

In this study, the youngest infants tested (2 months old) did not activate consistent, directionally appropriate responses to the platform perturbations. Infants of 3–4 months old activated directionally appropriate responses in only the neck muscles in 40–60 per cent of the trials. However, with the onset of the transition to independent sitting at 5 months old, infants began to activate coordinated responses in the neck and trunk muscles in compensation for platform perturbations in 40 per cent of the trials. And by 8 months infants consistently activated both neck and trunk muscles in a co-ordinated pattern similar to that of adults.

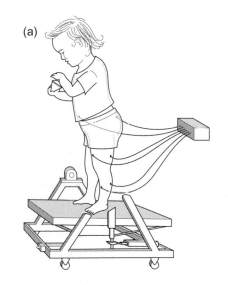

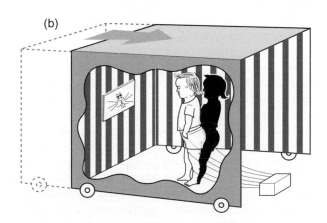

Figure 3.1 *Experimental set-up used to study balance control in infants. (a) Moving platform; infants were either seated or standing; (b) moving room paradigm. (Adapted from ref. 57.)*

A recent study by Hirschfeld and Forssberg[40] using similar support surface perturbations to balance has also indicated that platform movements causing backward sway give much stronger and less variable responses than those causing forward sway. This may be caused by the larger base of postural support in the forward direction.

The developmental principles contributing to these response synergies have been interpreted in alternative ways by different laboratories. They have been described as being selected from a wide variety of response patterns[33] or as being constructed gradually, with a resulting reduction in non-organized tonic background activity in non-participating muscles.[38–39] The above research does not indicate whether it is nervous system maturation or experience that allows neck and trunk muscle responses to emerge. This is because both the maturation and the refinement of synergies through experience are gradual, and occur concomitantly.

Vision

Do seated infants require experience to respond appropriately to visual inputs indicating postural sway? In order to answer this question Bertenthal and Bai[41] placed seated infants in a room with ceilings and walls that moved, but with a floor that was stable. Forward or backward movement of the room caused the illusion of postural sway in the opposite direction, without disturbing the child's balance. One would thus expect that the child would sway in the direction of room movement in order to compensate for the perceived sway. Results showed that (1) 5-month-olds (unable to sit independently) did not show directionally appropriate postural sway of the trunk in response to room movement, while (2) 7-month-olds showed appropriate postural sway if the whole room moved (front and sides), and (3) 9-month-olds showed a response even when only the sides of the room moved. This indicates that seated infants show an increased sensitivity to visual flow, indicating postural sway both with age and with experience in sitting.

Vestibular

In one set of the experiments by Hirschfeld and Forssberg[40] mentioned above, head tilt in response to platform perturbations was systematically varied, while trunk sway remained the same. This allowed the determination of the relative contributions of vestibular signals reporting motion of the head and somatosensory signals reporting body sway to the subsequent muscle response patterns used in compensation for sway. Results showed that the patterns of muscle activity stabilizing the trunk did not change regardless of how the head was oriented. Thus, it appears that it is somatosensory inputs at the hip joints, rather than vestibular inputs that primarily control balance during normal sitting.

The above research on the development of sitting balance indicates that coordinated activity of the neck and trunk muscles develops gradually during the time that the infant is developing the ability to sit independently. We might hypothesize that the nervous system first 'maps' relationships between sensory inputs and the neck muscles for appropriate balance control of the head, and then with the onset of independent sitting, extends these relationships to include the trunk muscles. This gradual development of the head–trunk coordination is illustrated by a recent study by Zedka and Assaiante.[42] These authors reported that infants (6–10 months) sitting on a rocking platform were unable to dampen the oscillations at the trunk level using their lumbar musculature, probably because of the incomplete rostro-caudal maturation of the neuromuscular system. In contrast, older infants with autonomous walking experience (12–18 months) were able to reduce the perturbation at the trunk level using their lumbar musculature.

PRECRAWLING, CRAWLING AND CREEPING

During their first 6 months when infants are placed face-down (prone) or on their back (supine), they will remain in that position with little change in direction or location.[43] Their true mobility begins with the landmark achievement at 6 months of rolling over from supine to prone, as well as in the reverse direction. Infants at this age can also pivot or turn in a prone position. They can change their location somewhat by a series of rolls and turns.

The first true locomotion appears when, at about 7 months, infants can move forward in a prone position. Bayley[44] has called this a prewalking progression. One of the available prelocomotor strategies is crawling, in which the arms are used to pull the body forward and/or the legs used to push.[43] Crawling does not emerge all at once, but rather emerges over a fairly extended period. About 1–2 months occurs between the signs of forward propulsion and skilful crawling, as defined by McGraw.[21] Infants may also move by sitting and scooting on their bottoms across the floor.[45] Creeping is a very frequent mode of forward progression, where palms and knees and/or toes are the only contacts with the ground. When progressing with palms and toes, infants raise their bottom higher than with palms and knees.

In both crawling and creeping, infants may adopt various arm and leg sequences. They can successively pull with the arms and then push with the legs. Keogh and Sugden[43] have described a homolateral pattern, where the leg and arm of one side alternate with the leg and arm of the opposite side, and a contralateral pattern, where the right leg and left arm alternate with left leg and right arm. Many combinations of these elementary patterns may also occur.

Many observations on crawling have mainly focused on psychological consequences of this behavior. Indeed, we can surmise with Gibson and colleagues that, in evolutionary terms, exploratory activity insures cognitive development.[46] Supporting this point of view, Bai and Bertenthal have shown that, in 33-week-old infants, precrawling, crawling and creeping experience clearly influences their search performance.[47] In studies investigating the perception of the affordance for traversing a supporting surface, Gibson et al.[46] have shown that crawling and walking behaviors differentially influence perceived traversability of either a rigid or a waterbed surface. It is interesting that it has been reported that crawling may not be a necessary prerequisite for early ambulation in mentally retarded children.[48]

SUPPORTED LOCOMOTION

Supported locomotion emerges at 7–9 months of age, whether the stepping reflex has been present or not. The movements during supported locomotion seem to be voluntarily elicited and goal directed. During supported locomotion, the child can support the body weight with one leg but still needs assistance to maintain balance. Even with support, infants' muscle activation patterns are highly variable. Individual infants showed both co-contraction (considered less mature but necessary to increase joint stability) and more efficient reciprocal activation in successive step-cycles.[49,50] It is possible to spontaneously change the muscle activation patterns of infants' step-cycles and reduce their variability, when experimenters provide postural support.[50]

The immature non-plantigrade locomotor pattern recurs when children begin to walk with support during the later part of the first year. However, the step frequency is more regular than during neonate stepping. The leg is still hyperflexed and the joints are rotated in phase, although the ankle starts to move more reciprocally with respect to the other joints. Flexor and extensor muscles are co-activated, producing synchronized flexion–extension movements in all joints of the leg. The calf muscles are activated during the end of the swing phase, plantarflexing the foot before ground contact. This produces a digitigrade gait, in which the toes or the fore part of the foot are placed on the ground first.[19]

Traditional accounts of how human upright locomotion develops have, for the most part, taken a maturational perspective according to which, for example, the maturing cerebral cortex or other neural circuits transform early infant stepping into adult-like locomotor patterns.[19,21] An alternative interpretation has been proposed, emphasizing the importance of self-organizing properties of the sensorimotor system to the infant's developing motor competencies.[51–53] In this view, motor skill development is seen not only as prescribed by the growing infant's neuromuscular system, but also emerging from the dynamics of the moving and growing infant.

According to this view, toward the end of the first year of life, there is a maturation of subcortical pattern generating centers and an integration of these centers with developing mechanisms for the maintenance of balance in both static posture and during movement. At the same time, body proportions change to favor erect stance. Muscle strength also increases, to allow muscular control in the assumption of an erect posture. In addition, flexor and extensor muscle tone becomes balanced. Finally, cognitive or voluntary motivation to move forward matures. The synthesis of these central and peripheral influences determines the emergence of independent walking.

INDEPENDENT STANCE

Motor coordination

In the above section on the development of postural control while sitting we proposed the hypothesis that perception–action 'rules' are developed during this period that allow the appropriate mapping of sensory inputs on to motor system centers for balance control of the head and trunk. Do the rules that we have described thus far for the development of head and sitting balance control also extend to the development of stance balance control? Experiments indicate that there are many similarities. However, in learning to stand independently, the infant must learn to coordinate the motions of two new joints, the ankle and knee, with the hip and head.

BALANCE CONTROL DURING QUIET STANCE

As children develop, the amplitude of sway during quiet stance decreases.[54,55] Research including children from 2 to 14 years of age found considerable variability in sway amplitude in young children, with variance systematically decreasing with age and improved balance. Use of the Romberg quotient (eyes-closed sway expressed as a percentage of eyes-open sway), allowed researchers to determine the contributions of vision to balance during quiet stance. They found very low Romberg quotients in the youngest children able to complete the task (4 year olds) with values of less than 100 per cent, showing that they swayed more with eyes open than with eyes closed.[55] By 9–12 years, sway magnitudes reached adult levels for eyes-open and by 12–15 years for eyes-closed conditions.[54]

REACTIVE BALANCE CONTROL

As was described in Chapter 1 on normal postural control, previous research on reactive balance control in standing adults has used an experimental paradigm similar to that described above for neonates and seated infants, in which a platform on which the adult is standing is unexpectedly moved forward or backward, to cause sway (see Fig. 3.1). The muscle responses that the adult uses to compensate for that sway have a characteristic response pattern that is directionally specific. Small movements of the platform (i.e. 2.5 cm) cause sway principally about the ankles and activate muscles in the legs and trunk in a coordinated distal to proximal sequence. For example, if the platform moves backward, causing forward sway, the stretched ankle muscle, the gastrocnemius, is activated first, followed by muscles of the thigh (hamstrings) and hip (abdominals).

In order to determine the manner in which these synergies develop in infants and children longitudinal experiments similar to those described above have been performed during the transition to independent stance.[56,57] The studies examined the gradual development of postural responses in the muscles of the legs and trunk for controlling stance in infants from 2 to 18 months of age (pre-sitting to independent walking). Since the younger children could not stand independently, they were either held by their mother or played with a toy castle placed in front of them while the platform was moved forward or backwards.

The data from this longitudinal study indicate that a sequential process occurs in the development of muscle response synergies controlling balance. For example, infants younger than 7–9 months (the time of acquisition of 'pull-to-stand' behavior, where the infant begins pulling up to a standing position, holding on to furniture) did not show coordinated muscle response organization when balance was disturbed. With the appearance of 'pull-to-stand' behavior they began to show directionally appropriate responses to platform movements, but typically only in the stretched ankle muscles. Shortly afterward, muscles in the thigh segment were added and a consistent distal to proximal sequence began to emerge. Later in 'pull-to-stand' the trunk muscles were also added to the synergy. Thus, by the end of this behavioral period, prior to the onset of independent stance, the infants begin to organize the muscles within the leg and trunk into appropriate synergies, with the ankle muscles being consistently activated first, followed by the upper leg and trunk muscles. Figure 3.2 gives examples of the disorganized muscle response patterns of a child in early pull-to-stand versus the organized patterns of the same child later, when she was able to walk independently.

These experiments showed the approximate time and way in which balance synergies are normally constructed, but can learning or experience affect the characteristics of this process? Experiments aimed to answer this question compared the postural responses of an experimental group of children given extensive experience in balance control in response to platform pertur-

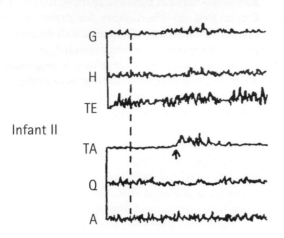
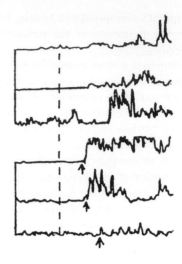

Figure 3.2 *Muscle responses from one child during early pull-to-stand behavior (left) and when the infant was able to independently walk (right) in response to platform perturbations. Platform moves forward, and child sways backward. G, gastrocnemius; H, hamstrings; TE, trunk extensors; TA, tibialis anterior; Q, quadriceps; A, abdominals. Dashed lines show the start of the perturbation. Arrows show start of muscle response. Total time for trial was 1 s. (Adapted from ref. 57.)*

bations (100 perturbations/day for 3 days) and a control group that did not receive this training.[58] Both groups were in the pull-to-stand stage of development, and were thus in the process of acquiring postural response synergies. The muscle responses of the training group showed an increase in the probability of activation. This implies that experience may increase the strength of connections between the sensory and motor pathways controlling balance.

ADAPTATION

A question that has been addressed by a number of laboratories concerns the time at which infants gain the ability to adapt responses to changes in support surface characteristics. Stoffregen et al.[59] tested the ability of children in their first year of walking experience (13–14 months old) to control their balance under altered support surface conditions, including high friction (high friction plastic), low friction (Formica coated with baby oil), and foam surfaces. They also asked them to stand in a crosswise stance on a narrow beam. The children were given two poles to grasp to help with balance, when needed. They found that the infants spent the greatest amount of time in independent stance (minimal hand support) on the high friction surface. When the surfaces were either more compliant (foam) or lower in friction (baby oil), the infants increased pole-holding substantially. The infants were unable to stand crosswise on the beam independently. Since this activity uses active hip control, it appears that the ability to use the hips in balance is not mastered during the first year of walking.

Research on balance control in adults has shown that recovery from large-amplitude balance threats often involves a hip strategy (activated by abdominal muscle

activity), rather than an ankle strategy, as the center of mass nears the margin of the base of support. Researchers have determined when the ability to control the hips during balance recovery emerges[60] by giving children, from new walkers (10–17 months) to hoppers (2–3 years), gallopers (4–6 years) and skippers (7–10 years of age), increasing magnitudes of balance threats in order to attempt to elicit a hip strategy. Hip-dominated responses were occasionally seen during balance recovery in the new walkers with only 3–6 months' walking experience. However, it appeared that these responses were passively activated, using the viscoelastic properties of the muscles and tendons of the joint, since minimal abdominal activity was present. It was only the 7–10 years old age group (skippers) that consistently showed active hip control, with high levels of abdominal muscle activity.

Sensory systems

Are the postural muscle response synergies activated by stimulation of the visual system in the same way as those activated by platform perturbations, and do they develop at the same time for standing infants? Research has shown that these synergies have many characteristics in common. However, those activated by the visual system are available to standing infants as young as 5 months of age, and create significant sway in response to visual flow. Sway responses increase in magnitude through the onset of independent stance, and then, after the first year of walking experience, begin to decrease to the very low levels found in adults (since visual stimulation, in fact, erroneously signals postural sway).

REFINEMENT OF STABILITY

Motor coordination

Maturation of balance control continues to at least 10 years of age.[61–64] It has been shown that postural responses of young children (1 year) were more variable and slower than those of adults, resulting in large sway amplitudes. In addition response amplitudes were consistently greater, and the durations of these responses longer, than those of older children (4–6 years) and adults. Figure 3.3 shows samples of muscle response patterns of 1- to 3-year-olds, 4- to 6-year-olds, 7- to 10-year-olds, and an adult.

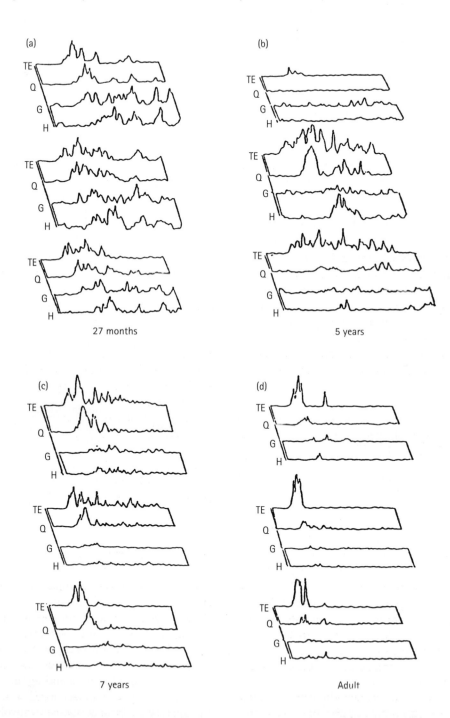

Figure 3.3 *A comparison of muscle activation patterns in leg and trunk muscles in response to forward perturbations in four age groups of normal subjects. G, gastrocnemius; H, hamstrings; TE, trunk extensors; Q, quadriceps. J Motor Behav, The growth of stability: postural control from a developmental perspective, Shumway-Cook A and Woollacott M, 17, 130–47, 1985. Reprinted with permission of the Helen Dwight Reid Educational Foundation. Published by Heldref Publications, 1319 18th Street, NW, Washington, DC 20036–1802. www.heldref.org. Copyright © 1985.*

There is also an unusual change in the muscle response characteristics of the 4- to 6-year-olds, with these children apparently 'regressing' in their postural response organization. For example, postural responses are, in general, more variable and longer in latency than those found in the 1- to 3-year-olds, 7- to 10-year-olds, or adults (see Fig. 3.3). By 7–10 years of age, postural responses are basically like those of the adult.

It has been hypothesized that this temporary regression in postural abilities in the 4- to 6-year-olds is caused by the fact that they are beginning to expand their postural skill repertoire to include intersensory integration abilities. The attempt to master this new skill may cause the temporary increase in variability and slowing of normal postural responses.[62]

Sensory organization abilities

In normal adults, balance control includes the ability to integrate information from multiple senses about the position and movement of the body in space. For a given task and environment the child must determine the validity of a given sensory input for postural control and then select the most appropriate for that context.

Experiments examining the maturation of the ability to integrate sensory information in children have measured postural sway under different conditions that changed the availability and accuracy of visual and somatosensory inputs for postural orientation. Under even normal sensory conditions, 4- to 6-year-olds swayed significantly more than older children or adults (Fig. 3.4). Balance deteriorated somewhat with eyes closed (SnVc), but became significantly worse when ankle joint information was made inaccurate by rotating the surface to keep the ankle joint at 90° (SsVn). When ankle inputs were minimized (as above) and eyes were closed (SsVc), leaving mainly vestibular cues to aid in balance, the majority of 4- to 6-year-olds lost balance while none of the older children or adults needed assistance (see Fig. 3.4). This suggests that (1) 4- to 6-year-olds are just learning sensory-integration abilities and are unable to balance efficiently when both ankle somatosensory and visual cues are removed and (2) by 7 years, children have mature intersensory integration abilities in this postural context.[62]

INITIATION OF GAIT

Gait initiation is an interesting paradigm for studying the control of balance from the perspective of the transition from upright stance posture to locomotion. First, the subject must activate anticipatory postural adjustments in order to shift the weight laterally toward the stance leg and forward. In addition to propelling the body forward and shifting from a bipedal to a single limb

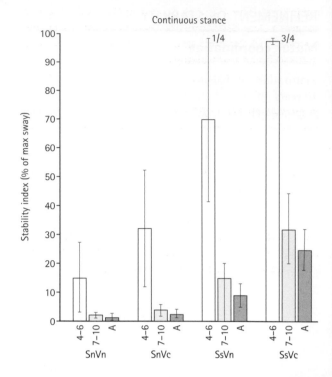

Figure 3.4 *A comparison of body sway in children (4–6 years, 7–10 years) and adults (A) in the four sensory conditions. (Reproduced from ref. 62.)*

support, postural adjustments must be activated in order to stabilize balance during the swing phase of gait, when the body is supported by one leg. This is the most difficult balance problem encountered by infants learning to walk.[28,37,43,65] Developmental research has shown that an anticipatory backward shift in center of pressure is present in children as young as 2.5 years, but becomes systematically used only in 6-year-olds.[66,67] In a recent developmental study,[68] kinematic and EMG analysis indicated that anticipatory postural adjustments were present in toddlers (infants with 1–4 months of walking experience), including a clear anticipatory lateral tilt of the pelvis and of the stance leg in order to unload the opposite leg shortly before its swing phase. There was an anticipatory activation of hip abductor of the leg in stance phase prior to heel-off, suggesting pelvis stabilization.

However, anticipatory postural adjustments did not appear consistently until 4–5 years of age. Indeed, a decrease in segmental oscillations occurred across the ages, indicating a better control of the intersegmental coordination in the frontal and sagittal plane during the postural phase of gait initiation. Young walkers used anticipatory postural adjustments involving movements of both upper and lower parts of the body while 4- to 5-year-olds laterally shifted only the pelvis and the stance leg, similar to adults. Older children (4–5 years of age) and adults also showed lower activation levels of hip and knee muscles, but higher activation of muscles at the ankle level. These kinematic and EMG results together suggest a clear developmental sequence from an '*en bloc*' operation of the body to an articulated operation with maturation and/or walking experience.

INDEPENDENT WALKING

The acquisition of independent bipedal locomotion can be said to be a milestone in the development of balance control. Indeed, the onset of this stage in locomotion involves solving a number of difficult balance problems.[28,65] With the acquisition of upright posture and locomotion, infants have to control their whole body in relation to gravity, so that equilibrium control becomes global rather than segmental. The body is less stable because the center of gravity is higher and the supporting base is smaller than in the previous positions (lying or sitting). Maintaining locomotor balance is a complex task, since it involves achieving a compromise between the forward propulsion of the body, which involves horizontal as well as vertical highly destabilizing forces (Fig. 3.5) and the need to maintain the lateral stability of the body. In bipeds, the difficulty of maintaining equilibrium during locomotion is further accentuated by the fact that the weight of the whole body has to be supported by one leg at a time during the swing phase of gait.

In order to assist in equilibrium control, toddlers show a characteristically wide base of support, arms abducted and elbows flexed. Walking on narrow supports can only be achieved at around the age of 3 years, that is to say, about 2 years after the onset of independent

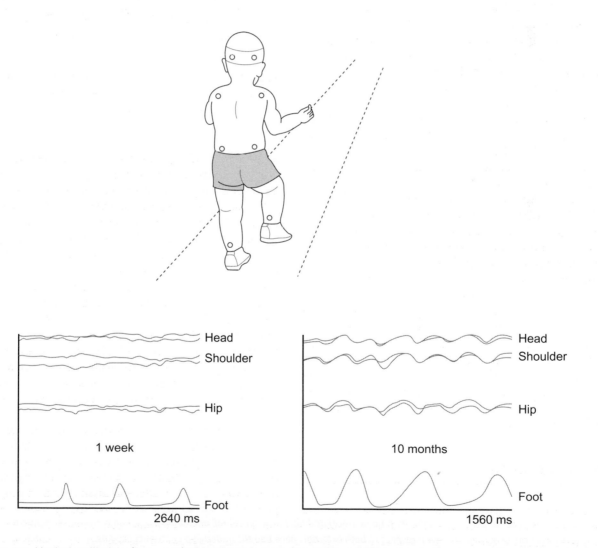

Figure 3.5 *Vertical oscillations (lower part) of various body levels (see position of the markers in the upper part), as measured during locomotion in children having 1 week (left lower trace) and 10 months (right lower trace) of walking experience. In the last case, vertical impulses at foot level were strong enough to induce vertical movements of the whole body at the step frequency, whereas at the very beginning of autonomous walking, children maintained the body level almost constant while walking.*

walking.[69,70] At this age, infants succeed in reducing the gap between their feet while walking,[65,71] thus reducing the supporting base, which indicates that they then become able to maintain balance while walking.

Recently, Assaiante et al.[72,73] have shown that at the onset of autonomous walking, in order to minimize the upper body destabilization induced by foot movements and thus prevent falls, lateral body stabilization is first initiated at the hip level (Fig. 3.6). This hip stabilization in space is probably aimed at controlling the lateral movements of the center of gravity and seems to be a prerequisite for autonomous walking in toddlers. Moreover, hip stabilization clearly helps minimize the vertical foot oscillations, which increase in size with increased walking experience. At about 2 months of walking experience, shoulder stabilization in space improves, indicating an improvement in active control of body balance, since no significant change in either body weight or height occurs over this period. This study shows that hip stabilization clearly occurs before that of the shoulder and the head. This suggests an ascending progression with age of the ability to control lateral balance during locomotion. In addition, in toddlers, the hip movements occur before shoulder and head movements, as well as before foot movements, indicating an anticipatory activity at the hip level. This suggests a hip-centered

temporal organization of balance control while walking, ascending from hip to head and descending from hip to foot.[74] A recent study by Zedka and Assaiante[42] also reported an ascending temporal organization of balance control in response to rhythmical perturbations in sitting toddlers (12–18 months). Young children with walking experience activated their lumbar muscles with a phase advance in relation to the support surface movement cycle, as in adults, but their neck muscle activation occurred too late for an efficient head counter-rotation. It was concluded that the lumbar stabilization strategy using prediction of the periodic surface movement does not emerge before independent walking.

The walking characteristics of the toddler have certain differences and deficiencies compared with fully mature locomotion, including the absence of certain joint angle rotation reversals during stance and swing. Most often, new walkers initiate the stance phase of the step cycle with the toes or flat foot and, correspondingly, show late swing-phase and premature stance phase activity of the ankle plantarflexor muscle groups.[75] New walkers also show a very strong hyperflexion of the hip during the swing phase, similar to that seen in newborn stepping. The persistence of digitigrade locomotion is considered by Forssberg[10] as a remnant of a phylogenetically older quadrupedal form of locomotion. Forssberg

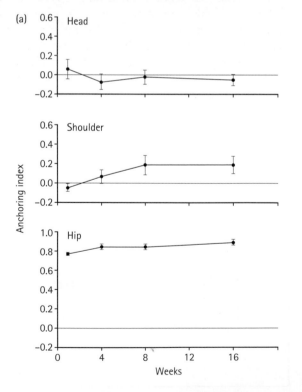
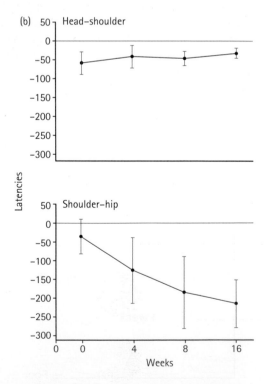

Figure 3.6 *(a) Head (upper trace), shoulder (middle trace) and hip (lower trace) roll anchoring index (index used to compare the stabilization of the given segment with respect to both external space and the underlying anatomical segment) (with standard deviation) while walking on flat ground as a function of weeks of walking experience. A positive value of the anchoring index indicates a better stabilization in space than on the inferior supporting anatomical level, whereas a negative value indicates a better stabilization on the inferior anatomical level than in external space. (b) Latencies (in ms) between head and shoulder (upper trace) and between shoulder and hip (lower trace) correlated movements in roll during locomotion, as a function of walking experience.*

suggests that the neuronal systems responsible for fully efficient plantigrade locomotion do not develop until some 6 months of walking experience. Note that despite all these differences, Clark and Phillips[76] showed that infants who have been walking for 3 months exhibit a step-cycle that is remarkably similar to that of mature walkers, both in terms of overall organization and in method of adjusting to changes in speed. Moreover, with 3 months of walking experience, the infants appear to have found an adult-like coordinative relationship between the two lower limbs.[77]

As soon as upright stance and walking are acquired, mastering motor coordination becomes a priority task. Infants have to develop appropriate postural tonus in their legs and they have to balance the effects of the flexor and extensor muscles by increasing the action of the latter.[78] Coactivation of tibialis anterior and lateral gastrocnemius during the stance phase of walking tends to decrease during the first weeks of independent walking. The lateral gastrocnemius is also activated during swing phase at the beginning of independent walking. The quadriceps and hamstrings activity changes from a pattern of coactivation to reciprocal activation after 2–3 months of autonomous walking.[10,19,79] Reciprocal arm-swing and heel-strike, indicators of gait maturity, are present in most children by the age of 18 months. A mature gait pattern, determined by duration of single limb stance, walking velocity, cadence, step length and the ratio of pelvis span to ankle spread, is well established at the age of 3 years.[75] For example, step length and duration of single-limb support increase almost linearly up to 3 years of age.[75]

Although maturation of the gait pattern is mainly complete by 3–4 years of age, many studies have shown that the final development of locomotion requires many years to be refined. In a study on the normal development of children's gait using an electrophysiological and biomechanical approach, the features typical of the immature state were found to gradually change to the adult pattern at around the age of 5–7 years.[80] In particular, a reciprocal mode of antagonistic leg muscle activation was observed, along with further increases in the gastrocnemius EMG during the stance phase and the disappearance of monosynaptic reflex potentials.[81] Moreover, only the 6- to 10-year-old children showed mature compensatory EMG responses (lacking a monosynaptic reflex component) in response to postural perturbations during gait.[82,83]

Various kinematic studies have also shown that the features typical of the adult locomotor cycle, such as acceleration and braking, are obtained only at around the ages of 5–6 years.[84] Assaiante and Amblard[85] have also emphasized the long maturation of locomotor balance, reporting that the development of head–trunk coordination during locomotion under normal vision can be said to involve at least three main periods (Fig. 3.7).[85] The first period occurs from the age of 3–6 years, when the head stabilization in space strategy is adopted only when walking on the flat ground, a condition with minimal balance difficulty. While walking on a narrow surface, children in this age group tend to increase the head–trunk stiffness, especially at 6 years of age. These data also suggest that under difficult equilibrium conditions, the simplest strategy is likely to consist of blocking the head on the trunk, with an 'en bloc' mode of operation, in order to minimize the number of degrees of free-

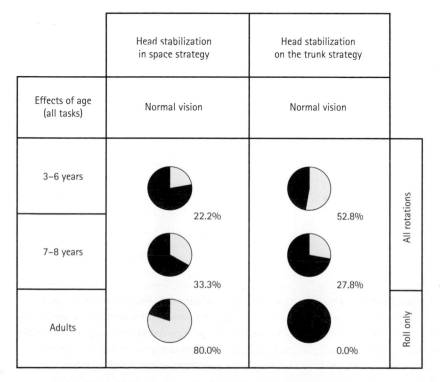

Figure 3.7 *Summary of the age dependence of both frequencies of head stabilization in space strategy and head stabilization on the trunk strategy in 3- to 8-year-old children and adults.*

dom to be controlled simultaneously during the movement.[84-86] In addition, in children, the lateral trunk rotations induced by locomotion occur before lateral head rotations, whereas in adults head and trunk rotations are simultaneous. This suggests an ascending temporal organization of balance control.[85,86]

The second period occurs from the age of 7–8 years. Children of this age become able to adopt the head stabilization in space strategy while walking on a narrow surface. During this period, this strategy is associated with a large decrease in the correlations between head and trunk movements, indicating an articulated operation of the head–trunk unit and is thought to initiate a descending pattern of balance organization, already proposed in adults.[70,85,87,88]

Lastly, in adulthood, the head stabilization in space strategy is commonly adopted, but specifically involves the roll component associated with the lateral body oscillations while walking. This result suggests also a descending temporal organization of balance control associated with an articulated operation of the head–trunk unit and selective control of the degrees of freedom at the neck level, presumably depending upon the task.

The age of 6 years seems to constitute a turning point in both postural[62,89] and locomotor[37,85,90] equilibrium control. In a postural study, Berger et al.[91] have reported that the balance strategy adopted in 2- to 6-year-old children, in response to a horizontal sinusoidal perturbation of the support, consists of blocking the various body joints. The reduced damping in children could represent a strategy that minimizes the number of degrees of freedom that have to be controlled simultaneously during a difficult balance task.[84,85,92] In contrast, in adults the amplitude of the oscillations decreased sharply from the foot to the head, suggesting an articulated operation of the whole body.

VISUAL AND VESTIBULAR CONTRIBUTIONS TO LOCOMOTOR BALANCE CONTROL

The role of vision in the acquisition of the main posturokinetic skills has been thoroughly documented in the literature, particularly during babyhood and childhood. It has been reported moreover, that vision predominates in infants during transitional periods in which they attempt to master new postural challenges.[93] This sensitivity increases again with the onset of upright stance and with the onset of unaided walking.[13,94] However, recent reports on posture and locomotion also suggest that this visual predominance is not restricted to infancy and continues up to about the age of 6 years.[62,69,90] For example, before the age of 4 years, a child is unable to walk on a narrow surface with restricted visual motion cues, such as those available with stroboscopic illumination at a frequency of 5 Hz.[70]

Assaiante and colleagues[69,90] have reported that the influence of peripheral visual cues on locomotor equilibrium did not vary in a simple linear fashion with age (Fig. 3.8). The peripheral visual contribution to dynamic balance control increased from 3 to 6 years of age, with a maximum in 6-year-old children. More precisely, frontal vision limited to 30° induces a maximum decrease in speed in 6-year-old children, whereas this restriction suddenly has no effect at 7 years of age. This age corresponds precisely to the beginning of effective use of the head stabilization in space strategy while walking on narrow surfaces, and this new ability is generally assumed to be mainly of vestibular origin. It is therefore possible to interpret the apparent neglect of peripheral visual cues

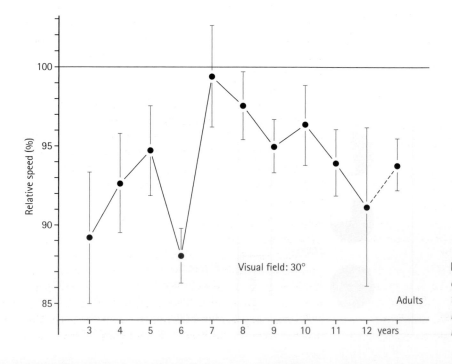

Figure 3.8 *Relative locomotor speed on a narrow beam with frontal vision limited to 30°, calculated in comparison with the locomotor speed recorded without visual restriction, as a function of age.*

associated with the new head stabilization in space skill as being a transient predominance of the vestibular contribution to balance control at 7 years of age. The role played by peripheral vision in locomotor equilibrium control tends to increase again from 8–9 years of age to adulthood.[69,90] In adults, peripheral visual cues as well as visual motion cues have been reported to play an important role in the control of locomotor equilibrium.[70,95]

Visual motion cues as well as peripheral visual cues were found to have little influence on children's ability to stabilize their head in space while walking, whatever their age.[85,96] The complete suppression of visual cues did not affect adults' ability to stabilize their head in space. Moreover, darkness induced an increase in the efficiency of the head stabilization strategy in adults, indicating that head stabilization in space is the most appropriate strategy available for dealing with an increase in the level of equilibrium difficulty and may reflect a top-down planning of postural control while walking. This result also strongly confirms that head stabilization in space while walking does not crucially depend on visual cues and suggests that it may mainly involve vestibular cues. Moreover, Bronstein[97] and Pozzo et al.[98] have reported that patients with vestibular impairments had difficulty in stabilizing their head in space in response to unpredictable body perturbations and while walking. Assaiante and Amblard claim that head stabilization in space may be mainly of vestibular origin and presumably serves to facilitate the visual input processing, particularly that of the motion and peripheral visual cues which are involved in the control of body equilibrium during locomotion.[85] Recent experiments in microgravity in adults[99] confirm that head stabilization in space may be organized on the basis of either dynamic vestibular afferents or a short-term postural body schema stored in memory.

Thus, during the life span, various periods are distinguishable in terms of the relative importance of the visual and vestibular contributions to balance control while walking. During infancy and a part of childhood, visual inputs, particularly peripheral visual cues, play a predominant role, reaching maximum importance at around the age of 6 years. Suddenly, at around the age of 7 years, the peripheral visual contribution becomes minimal, before increasing again from the age of 8–9 years to adulthood. These results, along with the fact that the head stabilization in space strategy begins to be adopted for dynamic balance at around the age of 7 years may indicate that the vestibular inputs become particularly prominent during a transition phase. To date, however, no data have been available as to the visual and vestibular contributions to head stabilization in space between 8 years and adulthood.[70,85] An additional permanent somatosensory contribution may also be at work during all the periods of this model and play a variably important role depending on age.[38,82,83] Lastly, in adults, these three classes of sensory inputs can be coordinated or recruited independently to improve equilibrium control, thanks to their specific efficiency, depending on environmental requirements.

ABNORMAL DEVELOPMENT

Posture

Research on children with neurological impairments indicates that there is a delay in the emergence of behavioral motor milestones. Since normal postural development is important for the performance of voluntary skills, postural abnormalities could contribute to the delays and impairments seen in the child with motor problems. In the following section we discuss the development of balance control in children with motor disabilities, and use the systems perspective to separate the constraints on their motor skills into those involving the musculoskeletal system, the motor system, the sensory systems and adaptational processes.

CEREBRAL PALSY

Musculoskeletal constraints
When normal clinical examinations are made on the child with spastic hemiplegia cerebral palsy in a passive situation, it is clear that the incidence of connective tissue and muscle contractures is high, and that there is increased muscle tone and increased responsiveness to passive stretch in muscles of the involved leg.[100] One would expect that this is an important constraint on the ability to balance normally.

However, surprisingly, in the more dynamic situation of standing balance the passive stiffness of the ankle joint was observed to be the same in both the spastic and more normal leg of the child.[101] In addition, there was almost a complete lack of stretch reflexes in response to platform perturbations, despite the presence of enhanced deep tendon reflexes on the clinical examination. This shows the importance of examining the child with motor disabilities in a variety of task conditions, in addition to the more passive conditions encountered in the clinical examination. It does not necessarily negate the results found in the clinical examination, but it indicates that constraints other than hyperactive reflexes may be more important limitations for standing posture control in the child with hemiplegia.

Neuromuscular constraints
Quiet stance   One of the constraints on balance control in children with cerebral palsy is a restricted range of motion in the ankle, knee and hip joints caused by contractures of the muscles at these joints. In order to determine the extent to which postural alignment itself influences they way in which muscles are activated during balance recovery Burtner and colleagues[102,103] compared

the organization of postural responses during balance recovery in both children with spastic diplegia standing in their normal crouched posture, and in healthy children standing in a similar posture vs. their normal postural alignment. The researchers observed that the children with spastic diplegia showed a high level of coactivation of agonist and antagonist muscles at the ankle, knee and hip joints when responding to loss of balance. Interestingly, healthy children standing in a crouched position used antagonistic muscles more often in response to platform perturbations than in their normal postural alignment. The authors concluded that the musculoskeletal constraints associated with a crouched postural alignment contribute to the atypical postural muscle response patterns observed in children with spastic diplegia.

In experiments similar to those performed on the development of balance control in normal children, it has been shown that in response to balance threats during stance both children with spastic hemiplegia and ataxic cerebral palsy show problems in the timing of postural responses, although there were distinct differences in the types of problems seen in the two groups.[101] For example, children with spastic hemiplegia showed delayed postural response onset latencies in the involved leg, while children with ataxic cerebral palsy showed not only delays in onset latency but also considerable trial to trial variability.

In addition, the spastic hemiplegics showed problems with the organization of muscle responses. Proximal muscles were typically activated before distal muscles in the involved leg. For example, when the platform moved forward and the child swayed backward, the normal distal–proximal gastrocnemius (G)–hamstring (H) synergy was not seen, but instead, H–G was seen. Because of these problems, the leg involved did not generate enough torque to help compensate for the perturbation. Why does one see a late (and low amplitude) G response to stretch caused by postural perturbation despite the indication of spasticity on a clinical examination? This is probably due to their inability to recruit and regulate the firing of motor neurons, a problem also reported by other research. Thus, this may be a primary postural constraint for the child with hemiplegia. In contrast to children with spastic hemiplegia, children with ataxia did not show inter-muscle timing problems.[101]

In experiments analysing balance in the seated position, Brogren and colleagues[104] also reported a disruption in the recruitment order of muscles responding to loss of balance in the seated position in children with the spastic diplegia form of cerebral palsy. Neurologically intact children recruit muscles in response to balance threats during sitting in a distal to proximal sequence, beginning with those muscles closest to the support surface first. In contrast, children with spastic diplegia tended to recruit muscles in a proximal to distal sequence, beginning at the neck and progressing downward. In addition, these children showed coactivation of muscles in the neck and hip, with antagonists being activated before agonists.

Sensory integration

The ability of children with cerebral palsy to balance under changing sensory conditions was examined in a paradigm similar to that discussed above evaluating sensory integration in normal children. Although children with spastic hemiplega showed increases in sway under most sensory conditions compared with normal children, children with ataxic cerebral palsy showed impairments that were significantly greater. The children with ataxia showed sway that was similar to that of adults with cerebellar pathology. Thus, these children appear to have greater problems with sensory organization than with motor coordination, whereas hemiplegic children have greater problems with motor coordination.

Effects of orthoses on balance recovery

Clinicians often use ankle–foot orthoses to control spasticity in children with cerebral palsy to prevent excessive plantarflexion of the ankle. Both solid ankle–foot orthoses (AFOs) (allowing no movement at the ankle) and spiral or hinged AFOs (allowing limited movement at the ankle) have been used. Burtner et al.[105] have attempted to determine the effects of using these AFOs on coordination of muscles underlying postural control by comparing reactive balance response characteristics in both children with spastic diplegia and typically developing children when using no AFO, compared with solid and spiral AFOs. They found that both for children with spastic diplegia and for the control group of children there were significantly fewer trials in which children used the ankle strategy when recovering balance while wearing the solid AFO vs. no AFO and dynamic AFO conditions. When recovering balance in response to balance threats causing forward sway, using a solid AFO also was associated with a significant delay in gastrocnemius onset latency and reduction in the probability of recording a response in the gastrocnemius muscle.

The probability of activation of the normal distal to proximal muscle response sequence was also reduced both in typically developing children and in those with spastic diplegia in the solid AFO condition compared with the no AFO and dynamic AFO conditions. Findings of this type are reminders to clinicians that the orthotic devices used to control position and motion at the ankles can affect the sequencing and timing of muscles used for balance recovery.

In order to explore underlying musculoskeletal problems that might contribute to balance and locomotor dysfunction in children with cerebral palsy, researchers have performed biopsies to examine changes in the structure of skeletal muscle in these children.[106] They found that there was abnormal variation in muscle fiber size and altered distribution of fiber types in children with cerebral palsy with excessive and prolonged muscle contraction. They also found significant differences between type 1 and type 2 fiber mean area. They noted that this was correlated with functional changes in gait, with the extent of muscle pathology being correlated with increased energy expenditure and prolonged EMG activity during gait.[106]

Research also suggests that muscle weakness may contribute to motor control problems in children with cerebral palsy. One study compared strength profiles in lower extremity muscles in children with spastic hemiplegia and spastic diplegia with an age-matched control group.[107] They found that children with cerebral palsy were weaker than age-matched peers in all muscles tested. It is interesting that the children with hemiplegia showed significant weakness not only in the involved limb, but also in the non-involved limb. In addition, the extent of weakness was greater in distal than proximal muscles and in hip flexors and ankle plantar flexors compared with their antagonist muscles. They noted that this weakness was correlated with poor neural control of the muscles, since the children with cerebral palsy typically activated both agonist and antagonist muscles at a joint whenever they were asked to contract just one set of muscles. This was not observed in the control children.

DOWN'S SYNDROME

Shumway-Cook and Woollacott studied 4- to 6-year-old children with Down's syndrome in similar test paradigms.[108] They showed that children with Down's syndrome have normal response organization but show both significant delays in the activation of postural responses to postural perturbations and significant increases in sway, no doubt because of the late onsets of the compensatory responses. The children were also unable to adapt responses to changing task conditions.

In addition, they looked at younger children with Down's syndrome, and found that the youngest one tested (22 months) also showed highly variable responses, with only distal muscles being activated or no response in many trials. This response organization was similar to that seen in the normal 8- to 10-month-old child. Since responses were normally organized in the 4- to 6-year-old child with Down's syndrome, it suggests that a developmental delay contributes to the motor control problems in these children.[108]

Locomotion

In the last 15 years, pathophysiologically oriented analyses of the development of gait in children have considerably increased, especially because of the appearance of some appropriate tools for kinematic, electromyographic and dynamic measurements. Various factors may induce some abnormalities in the development of gait in children, such as central lesions (cerebral palsy), genetic factors (such as Down's syndrome), sensory deficits (visual and vestibular) as well as more diffuse factors (low birth weight, clumsiness). Although studies have often focused on therapeutic considerations, this aspect will not be developed in this chapter.

Many recent quantitative studies of impaired pre-locomotor and locomotor development have been made in children with cerebral palsy. Early motor deficits were described by Yokochi et al.[109] in children with spastic diplegia. In rolling, trunk rotation and elbow support were difficult for the most severely diplegic children. When sitting, most patients had a between-heel sitting pattern in which the thighs were adducted and the knees were flexed. When crawling, the reciprocal thigh movements were insufficient and accompanied by lateral bending of the trunk in many patients. In the more impaired patients, the thighs supported the weight in flexion and did not move reciprocally. Creeping on the elbows without reciprocal leg movements was demonstrated in the most severely affected children after 2 years of age.

During the stage of supported locomotion, children with cerebral palsy (diplegia or hemiplegia) exhibit an immature locomotor pattern similar to that of non-impaired children.[79,110] However, at the age where a plantigrade gait develops in normal children, children with cerebral palsy retain the immature non-plantigrade pattern.[111–114] A prominent dynamic feature is the absence of typical push-off peak in the vertical component of the ground reaction force.[19] Synchronous muscle activity with excessive muscular co-contraction and short-latency reflexes at foot contact are maintained.[79]

Nevertheless, consistent inter- as well as intra-subject variability has been emphasized by Crenna and colleagues.[115,116] These authors have reported that the pathophysiological profile of gait in children with cerebral palsy could be dominated by different factors, including spasticity, co-contraction of agonist and antagonist muscles, or non-neural problems, such as muscle contractures, whereas the paretic component was rarely prominent. Increased co-contraction was apparent on the paretic side, but could also be revealed on the contralateral 'healthy' side, especially at the highest walking speeds. From a kinematic point of view, it has been reported that, in children with neuromuscular impairment (childhood hemiplegia, congenital paraplegia or miscellaneous neuromotor disorders), step length, average maximum foot velocity and walking speed were reduced, while double support time was increased.[117]

Locomotor deficits or delay may also be caused by genetic factors. Ulrich et al.[118] have shown that although Down's syndrome infants begin to walk independently at a much later age than non-disabled infants, 11-month-old infants with Down's syndrome were able to produce alternating steps if supported upright on a motorized treadmill. The authors suggested that the basic neural substrate necessary for upright locomotion is available long before walking occurs in infants with Down's syndrome, just as it is in normally developing infants.

Biomechanical factors such as body weight may also affect the normal development of locomotor proficiency.

According to Molteno et al.,[119] poor head and trunk righting occur at 4 months corrected age in very low birth weight (less than 1500 g) infants. In these children, a delay in maturation is still identifiable on the locomotor subscales at 12 months and 18 months. In addition, Hills and Parker[120] report that obese prepubertal children show the following differences in locomotor characteristics, compared to normal children: longer step-cycle duration, lower cadence, lower relative velocity, and a longer stance period. The obese also displayed asymmetry in step length, with the right limb being favored. Moreover, obese subjects displayed greater instability than normal children at slow walking speeds.

Clumsy children are known to have problems with the control of force, amplitude and tempo of movement.[121] Larkin and Hoare[122] have suggested that in these children, coordination may be impaired as well as control. These authors have described poor running performances in 7-year-old clumsy children, whereas at the same age unimpaired children show a relatively mature movement pattern. The locomotor profile of the clumsy children was characterized by decreased stride length and increased stride time when compared with their well-coordinated peers. In the poor runners, the percentage of cycle time spent in support was greater, whereas the percentage of time in the swing phase was less. During the swing phase, the clumsy runners had limited flexion and extension of the hip and knee and a smaller range of movement. Peak segmental velocities were lower in these poorly coordinated children for the thigh and the leg, and a relatively slower initiation of ankle extension during the support phase was observed.

Sensory deficits may also be an important cause for delaying and/or impairing locomotor development. Although children with visual or vestibular deficits are known to have a delayed and/or abnormal locomotor development, their performances, up to now, have been poorly quantified. Although blind children do not seem to have postural deficits, they seem to encounter more difficulties in mastering dynamic equilibrium.[123] Norris and collaborators[124] have reported that only 50 per cent of blind children displayed autonomous locomotion at the age of 24 months. However, when they are appropriately and regularly trained, autonomous walking emerges at about 19 months.[125] From a biomechanical viewpoint, Sampaio et al.[126] have reported that at the very beginning of autonomous locomotion, blind children walk like non-disabled children of the same age. Nevertheless, it has also been reported that blind children may show asymmetric locomotion, with one foot making a step, and the second one joining the first without passing beyond.[123,127,128] This is presumably a result of the perceptive function of the propelled foot, which analyses the traversability of the supporting surface. Finally, it has been reported that even slight residual vision may markedly improve the speed and quality of locomotion.[128]

It is well known that the development of motor function is frequently retarded in children with congenital deafness, particularly in cases of inner ear anomaly. In particular, Tsuzuku and Kaga[129] have observed that the development of independent walking was delayed in children with inner ear anomalies. To our knowledge, however, there is no recent quantitative study on the impaired development of locomotion in children with vestibular deficits.

ASSESSING POSTURAL DEVELOPMENT FROM A SYSTEMS PERSPECTIVE

Because the systems model of postural control is new, assessment tools based on this perspective are just beginning to be developed. Shumway-Cook and Woollacott[6,130] have described a conceptual framework and preliminary applications of the systems model for assessment. Their systems-based assessment of postural control recommends the assessment of both motor milestones (or the developmental sequences of functional motor behaviors) and the individual subsystems and processes that are required to achieve those motor functions. They also recommend that spontaneous movements and variability of performance of motor skills be evaluated at each developmental level. This is because this spontaneity and variability represents the child's ability to explore and adapt to changing tasks and environments.[6,130]

In assessing motor milestones this approach recommends dividing motor behaviors related to balance control into four sub-areas: (1) the ability to sustain a posture; (2) the ability to regain a posture; (3) the ability to transition between postures; and (4) the ability to integrate posture into movement (walking, manipulation and exploratory behaviors). For example, in assessing stance posture control (see Fig. 3.9) these four categories would be considered as follows: (a) the ability to maintain independent stance (including length of time); (b) the ability to regain stance when perturbed in the anterior–posterior and mediolateral planes; (c) the ability to assume the standing posture from supine, and the pattern used to perform the task; (d) the ability to maintain an upright posture during ongoing movement, such as walking.[130]

In addition to examining postural milestones in this manner, the authors recommend assessing the major subsystems contributing to the acquisition of postural control. These include: (1) the motor systems, including both musculoskeletal (range of motion, strength, alignment of body segments) and neuromuscular components (construction of neuromuscular response synergies); (2) the sensory systems (including the visual, vestibular and somatosensory systems) and the way the child organizes sensory information under changing sensory conditions (e.g. standing in the dark, on thick carpet); and (3) the adaptive and anticipatory mecha-

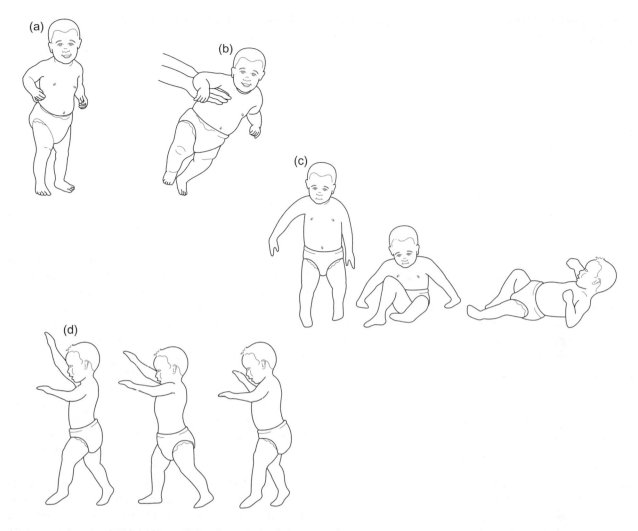

Figure 3.9 *Four categories of postural control abilities which may be used in assessing the control of stance: (a) maintaining a posture, (b) regaining a posture, (c) assuming a posture and (d) using posture in movement. (Adapted from ref. 130.)*

nisms (the ability to predict the postural requirements of a task or environment and balance efficiently in a changing environment).[130]

Table 3.1 shows an example of how these concepts could be used in evaluating head control in an infant of 0–2 months old.[130] Shumway-Cook and Woollacott[130] state that using assessment techniques based on these principles will allow the clinician to gain insight into the following aspects of postural development: 'What is the child's level of function?', 'Is delayed or abnormal postural control a contributing factor to decreased function?', and 'Which systems and processes contributing to postural development are rate-limiting to the emergence of balance and mobility functions?'. Answers to these questions allow the clinician to develop appropriate treatment strategies designed to remediate function in the subsystems contributing to balance dysfunction and to encourage the child to practice balance strategies in a variety of task conditions.

TREATING POSTURAL DYSFUNCTION FROM A SYSTEMS PERSPECTIVE

When treating children with balance dysfunction from a systems perspective the goals of the clinician should include the following therapeutic strategies: (1) to correct impairments that can be changed and to prevent the development of secondary impairments that contribute to balance dysfunction; (2) to train the child in the use of task-specific sensory and motor strategies for maintaining balance; and (3) to retrain functional tasks with different balance control demands (steady state, reactive and proactive) under a variety of environmental contexts.[6]

Interventions aimed at correcting underlying impairments include strengthening exercises focused on the ankle plantarflexors and dorsiflexors, and the hip extensors, flexors and abductors. In addition, flexibility exercises, focused on the Achilles tendon, the hip flexors and

Table 3.1 *Assessment of head control*

A. Functional behaviors observed
1. Ability to sustain head posture
(a) supported vertical position
(b) prone position
(c) supine position
2. Ability to regain head posture
(a) vertical – tip child from vertical
(b) prone – tip child in prone
(c) supine – tip child in supine
3. Ability to maintain head posture during movement
(a) primitive stepping
(b) moving from supine to sit
(c) spontaneous movements
B. Systems tested
1. Motor
(a) musculoskeletal constraints
(1) range of motion – cervical region
(2) strength – neck muscles
(b) motor coordination – neuromuscular synergies involving neck and upper trunk
2. Sensory
(a) capacity of vision to regulate posture
(b) capacity of vestibular and somatosensory inputs to regulate posture
3. Adaptive/anticipation
(a) active exploration
(b) adapting behavior to externally controlled head position
(c) anticipating postural adjustments of head to repeated tips

Adapted from ref. 130.

the neck and trunk will aid in improving postural alignment.

Interventions used to train the child in sensory and motor strategies underlying balance control include focus on sitting and standing postural alignment, and the control of steady state, reactive and proactive balance. Exercises for controlling steady-state balance include asking the child to stand under varying visual conditions (e.g. eyes open, eyes closed, in dim lighting), varying surface conditions (carpet, foam and inclined surface), varying bases of support (normal, narrow, partial tandem, tandem and one foot, when possible) and performing voluntary sway in all directions. These exercises can be practiced both in the clinic and at home. Exercises for developing reactive balance control include giving the child a nudge to the sternum and hip pushes at varying amplitudes and speeds, and asking them to maintain their balance. Tilt boards can also be used for balance practice. These exercises should only be performed in the clinic, under supervision. Anticipatory balance exercises include turns, reaches, leans and stool touches with the two feet alternating when possible.[6]

Intervention at the functional task level includes practice in the maintenance of postural control in a wide variety of tasks and environments, requiring that the child adapt sensory and motor balance strategies to changing conditions.

These therapeutic strategies are used, not sequentially, but in parallel, with the intervention involving an interweaving of exercises to correct impairments, train balance strategies, and practice these strategies in changing conditions and tasks.[6]

CONCLUSIONS

The posture of the fetus and preterm infant is variable, but relatively unrelated to the orientation of the force of gravity, while the earliest locomotor-like activity observed prenatally has been recorded with real-time ultrasonography in fetuses at 10 gestational weeks. From 32 to 34 weeks of gestation, premature infants show a simple type of postural control, which keeps the head at midline, and which depends on the presence of vision. At 10 weeks of age, with the onset of spontaneous head control, infants begin to show clear EMG responses in the neck muscles.

Locomotor movements, called the stepping reflex, can be elicited directly after birth if the infant is held under the arms in an upright posture with foot-surface contact and tilted slightly forward. It has been argued that this is not a reflex at all, but rather a manifestation of a spontaneous pattern generator used for other rhythmical activities such as kicking.

Coordinated activity of the neck and trunk muscles develops gradually during the time that the infant is developing the ability to sit independently. The nervous system may first 'map' relationships between sensory inputs and the neck muscles for appropriate balance control of the head, and then extends these relationships to include the trunk muscles, with the onset of independent sitting. Research indicates that it is somatosensory inputs at the hip joints, rather than vestibular inputs which primarily control balance of infants in response to perturbations while sitting.

Crawling does not emerge all at once, but rather emerges over a fairly extended period (at about 7 months). Supported locomotion emerges at 7–9 months of age when the child can support the body weight with one leg but still needs assistance to maintain balance. The locomotor pattern is immature with the leg still hyperflexed during stepping.

The development of muscle response synergies controlling standing balance occurs gradually beginning at 7–9 months, with the infants gradually organizing the muscles within the leg and trunk into appropriate synergies and with the ankle muscles being consistently activated first, followed by the upper leg and trunk muscles.

Maturation of balance control continues through at least 10 years of age. Maturation brings faster and shorter duration responses and reduced variability, resulting in smaller sway amplitudes.

Although maturation of the gait pattern is mainly complete by 3–4 years of age, many studies have shown that the final development of locomotion requires many years to be refined, with acceleration and braking capabilities developing only at 5–6 years.

The development of head–trunk coordination during locomotion under normal vision can be said to involve three periods in which blocking the head on the trunk, in order to minimize the number of degrees of freedom to be controlled, is gradually reduced. The head stabilization in space strategy is typically observed in older children and adults, even in difficult balance conditions.

Children with cerebral palsy have problems with both postural muscle response organization, slow onset latencies of postural responses, and with sensory organization capabilities.

Children with Down's syndrome show normal response organization but have both significant delays in the activation of postural responses to postural perturbations and significant increases in sway.

The pathophysiological profile of gait in children with cerebral palsy may be dominated by different factors, depending on the child, including spasticity, co-contraction of agonist and antagonist muscles, or non-neural problems, such as muscle contractures, whereas the paretic component is rarely prominent. Increased co-contraction is apparent on the paretic side, but may also be revealed on the contralateral 'healthy' side.

Although Down's syndrome infants begin to walk independently at a much later age than non-disabled infants, infants with Down's syndrome are able to produce alternating steps if supported upright on a treadmill.

The systems perspective is also beginning to be used in the assessment and treatment of balance function.

REFERENCES

1. Gessell A. The ontogenesis of infant behavior. In: Carmichael L, ed. *Manual of child psychology*. New York: Wiley, 1946;335–73.
2. McGraw MB. From reflex to muscular control in the assumption of an erect posture and ambulation in the human infant. *Child Dev* 1932;3:291.
3. Milani-Comparetti A, Gidoni EA. Pattern analysis of motor development and its disorders. *Dev Med Child Neurol* 1967;9:625–30.
4. Larson MA, Lee SL, Vasque DE. Comparison of ATNR presence and developmental activities in 2–4 month old infants. *APTA Conference Proceedings, Alexandria, June, 1990*.
5. Schaltenbrand G. The development of human motility and motor disturbances. *Arch Neurol Psychiatry* 1928;20:720.
6. Shumway-Cook A, Woollacott M. *Motor control:theory and practical applications*, 2nd edn. Baltimore: Lippincott Williams & Wilkins, 2001.
7. Prechtl HFR, Hopkins B. Developmental transformations of spontaneous movements in early infancy. *Early Hum Dev* 1986;14:233–8.
8. Schloon H, O'Brien MJ, Scholten CA, Prechtl HFR. Muscle activity and postural behaviour in newborn infants. *Neuropediatrie* 1976;7:384–415.
9. De Vries JIP, Visser GHA, Prechtl HFR. Fetal motility in the first half of pregnancy. In: Prechtl HFR, ed. *Continuity of neural functions from prenatal to postnatal life. Clinics in developmental medicine*. Oxford: Spastics International Medical Publications, 1984;46–64.
10. Forssberg H. A neural control model for human locomotion development: implications for therapy. In: Forssberg H, Hirschfeld H, eds. *Movement disorders in children*. Basel: Med Sport Sci Karger, 1992;174–81.
11. Jouen F. Head position and posture in newborn infants. In: Berthoz A, Graf W, Vidal PP, eds. *The head–neck sensory–motor system*. New York, Oxford: Oxford University Press, 1992;118–20.
12. Jouen F, Gapenne O. Regulation de la posture encephallique chez le nouveau-ne:L'implication du couplage visuo-postural. *Rev d'Oto-Neuro-Ophthalmol* 1994;28:28–34.
13. Lee D, Aronson E. Visual proprioceptive control of standing in human infants. *Perception Psychophys* 1974;15:529–32.
14. Jouen F. Le role des informations visuelle dans l'elaboration du comportement anti-gravitaire chez le nourrisson. *Cahiers Psychol Cogn* 1982;2:341–56.
15. Peiper A. *Cerebral function in infancy and childhood*. New York: Consultants Bureau, 1963.
16. Heriza C. The organization of spontaneous movements in premature infants. PhD dissertation, Southern Illinois University, USA, 1986.
17. Andre-Thomas AS, Autgaerden S. *Locomotion from pre- to post-natal life*. London: Spastics Society and William Heineman, 1966.
18. Forssberg H, Wallberg H. Infant locomotion: a preliminary movement and electromyographic study. In: Berg K, Eriksson B, eds. *Children and exercise IX*. Baltimore: University Park Press, 1980:32–40.
19. Forssberg H. Ontogeny of human locomotor control infant stepping, supported locomotion and transition to independent locomotion. *Exp Brain Res* 1985;57:480–93.
20. Thelen E, Whitley Cooke D. Relationship between newborn stepping and later walking:a new interpretation. *Dev Med Child Neurol* 1987;29:380–93.
21. McGraw MB. *The neuromuscular maturation of the human infant*. New York: Columbia University Press, 1943.
22. Touwen B. *Neurological development in infancy*. London: Spastics International and Heinemann, 1976.
23. Zelazo PR, Zelazo NA, Kolb S. Walking in the newborn. *Science* 1972;176:314–15.
24. Zelazo PR. From reflexive to instrumental behaviour. In: Lipsitt LP, ed. *Developmental psychobiology: the significance of infancy*. Hillsdale: Lawrence Erlbaum, 1976.
25. Zelazo PR. Learning to walk: recognition of higher order influences? In: Lipsitt LP, ed. *Advances in infancy research*, Vol. 3. Norwood: Ablex, 1984;251–6.
26. Thelen E. Rhythmical stereotypies in normal human infants. *Anim Behav* 1979;27:699–715.
27. Thelen E. Rhythmical behaviour in infancy: an ethological perspective. *Dev Psychol* 1981;17:237–57.
28. Thelen E. Learning to walk: ecological demands and phylogenetic constraints. In: Lipsitt LP, ed. *Advances in infancy research*, Vol. 3. Norwood: Ablex, 1984.

29. Thelen E, Fisher DM. Newborn stepping: an explanation for a 'disappearing reflex'. *Dev Psychol* 1982;**18**:760–75.

30. Jouen F, Lepecq JC. Early perceptuo-motor development: posture and locomotion. In: Hauert CA, ed. *Developmental psychology. Cognitive, perceptuo-motor and neurophysiological perspectives.* Amsterdam: Elsevier 1990;61–83.

31. Thelen E, Spencer JP. Postural control during reaching in young infants:a dynamic systems approach. *Neurosci Biobehav Rev* 1998;**22**:507–14.

32. Berthental B, von Hofsten C. Eye, head and trunk control: the foundation for manual development. *Neurosci Biobehav Rev* 1998;**4**:515–20.

33. Hadders-Algra M, Brogen E, Forssberg H. Ontogeny of postural adjustments during sitting in infancy: variation, selection and modulation. *J Physiol* 1996;**496**:273-288.

34. Forssberg H, Hirschfeld H. Postural adjustments in sitting humans following external perturbations: muscle activity and kinematics. *Exp Brain Res* 1994;**97**:515–27.

35. Horak FB, Nashner LM. Central programming of postural movements: adaptation to altered support configurations. *J Neurophysiol* 1986;**55**:1369–81.

36 Brogan E, Hadders-Algra M, Forssberg H. Postural control in children with spastic diplegia: muscle activity during pertubations in sitting. *Dev Med Child Neurol* 1996; **38**: 379–88.

37. Assaiante C, Amblard B. An ontogenetic model of sensorimotor organization of balance control in humans. *Hum Mov Sci* 1995;**14**:13–43.

38. Woollacott M, Debu B, Mowatt M. Neuromuscular control of posture in the infant and child: is vision dominant? *J Motor Behav* 1987;**19**:167–86.

39. Sveistrup H, Woollacott M. The development of sensori-motor integration underlying posture control in infants during the transition to independent stance. *J Motor Behav* 1996;**28**:58–70.

40. Hirschfeld H, Forssberg, H. Epigenetic development of postural responses for sitting during infancy. *Exp Brain Res* 1994;**97**:528–40.

41. Bertenthal BI, Bai DL. Infants' sensitivity to optical flow for controlling posture. *Dev Psychol* 1989;**25**:936–45.

42. Zedka M, Assaiante C. Different postural strategies in response to rhythmical perturbations in sitting babies and adults. *Society for Neuroscience Abstracts,* 2000.

43. Keogh J, Sugden D. *Movement skill development.* New York: Macmillan, 1985.

44. Bayley N. The development of motor abilities during the first three years. *Monogr Soc Res Child Dev* 1985;1, Ser No 1.

45. Robson P. Shuffling, hitching, scooting or sliding: some observations in 30 otherwise normal children. *Dev Med Child Neurol* 1970;**12**:608–17.

46. Gibson EJ, Riccio G, Schmuckler MA, et al. Detection of the traversability of surfaces by crawling and walking infants. *J Exp Psychol Hum Percept Perform* 1987;**13**:533–44.

47. Bai D, Bertenthal BI. Locomotor status and the development of spatial search skills. *Child Dev* 1992;**63**:215–26.

48. Liao HF, Lee SC, Lien IN, et al. Locomotor strategies before independent walking: prospective study of 50 mentally retarded children. *Taiwan I Hsueh Hui Tsa Chih* 1992;**91**:334–41.

49. Kazai N, Okamoto T, Kumamoto M. Electromyographic study of supported walking of infants in the initial period of learning to walk. In: Komi PV, ed. *Biomechanics V.* Baltimore: University Park Press, 1976;311–18.

50. Okamoto T, Goto Y. Human infant pre-independent and independent walking. In: Kondo S, ed. *Primate morphophysiology, locomotor analyses and human bipedalism.* Tokyo: University of Tokyo Press, 1985.

51. Kugler PN, Kelso JAS, Turvey MT. On the concept of coordinative structures as dissipative structures. I. theoretical lines of convergence. In: Stelmach GE, Requin J, eds. *Tutorials in motor behaviour.* New York: North Holland, 1980.

52. Thelen E. Developmental origins of motor coordination: leg movements in human infants. *Dev Psychobiol* 1985;**18**:1–22.

53. Thelen E, Kelso JAS, Fogel A. Self-organizing systems and infant motor development. *Dev Rev* 1987;**7**:39–65.

54. Taguchi K, Tada C. Change of body sway with growth of children. In: Amblard B, Berthoz A, Clarac F, eds. *Posture and gait: development, adaptation and modulation.* Amsterdam: Elsevier, 1988;59–65.

55. Hayes KC, Riach CL. Preparatory postural adjustments and postural sway in young children. In: Woollacott MH, Shumway-Cook A, eds. *Development of posture and gait across the life span.* Columbia: University of South Carolina Press, 1989:97–127.

56. Woollacott MH, Sveistrup H. Changes in the sequencing and timing of muscle response coordination associated with developmental transitions in balance abilities. *Hum Mov Sci* 1992;**11**:23–36.

57. Sveistrup H, Woollacott MH. Systems contributing to emergence and maturation of stability in postural development. In: Savelsbergh GJP, eds. *The development of coordination in infancy.* Elsevier: Amsterdam, 1993:319–36.

58. Sveistrup H, Woollacott M. Can practice modify the developing automatic postural response? *Exp Brain Res* 1997;**114**:33–43.

59. Stoffregen TA, Adolph K, Thelen T, Gorday KM, Sheng Y-Y. Toddlers' postural adaptations to different support surfaces. *Motor Control* 1997;**1**:119-137.

60. Woollacott M, Burtner P, Jensen J, Jasiewicz J, Roncesvalles N, Sveistrup H. Development of postural responses during standing in healthy children and in children with spastic diplegia. *Neurosci Biobehav Rev* 1998;**22**:583–9.

61. Forssberg H, Nashner L. Ontogenetic development of postural control in man: adaptation to altered support and visual conditions during stance. *J Neurosci* 1982;**2**:545–52.

62. Shumway-Cook A, Woollacott M. The growth of stability: postural control from a developmental perspective. *J Motor Behav* 1985;**17**:130–47.

63. Berger W, Quintern J, Dietz V. Stance and gait perturbations in children: developmental aspects of compensatory mechanisms. *Electroencephalogr Clin Neurophysiol* 1985;**61**:385–95.

64. Hass G, Diener HC, Bacher M, Dichgans J. Development of postural control in children: short-, medium-, and long latency EMG responses of leg muscles after perturbation of stance. *Exp Brain Res* 1986;**64**:127–32.

65. Breniere Y, Bril B, Fontaine R. Analysis of the transition from upright stance to steady state locomotion in children with under 200 days of autonomous walking. *J Motor Behav* 1989;**21**:20–37.

66. Ledebt A, Bril B, Breniere Y. The preparation for movement: acquisition of prospective control in walking. In: *European Conference on Cognitive Science.* INRIA, 1995;145–53.

67. Ledebt A, Bril B, Breniere Y. The build-up of anticipatory behaviour. An analysis of the development of gait initiation in children. *Exp Brain Res* 1998;**120**:9–17.

68. Assaiante C, Woollacott M, Amblard B. The development of postural anticipatory adjustments during initiation of gait: kinematic and EMG Analysis. *J Motor Behav* 2000;**32**:211–26.

69. Assaiante C, Amblard B, Carblanc A. Peripheral vision and dynamic equilibrium control in five to twelve year old children. In: Amblard B, Berthoz A, Clarac F, eds. *Posture and gait: development, adaptation and modulation.* Amsterdam: Elsevier, 1988;75–83.

70. Assaiante C. *Controle visuel de l'equilibre locomoteur chez l'homme:developpement et strategies sensori-motrices.* Aix-Marseille II: CNRS, 1990.

71. Bril B, Breniere Y. Do temporal invariances exist as early as the first six months of independent walking? In: Amblard B, Berthoz A, Clarac F, eds. *Posture and gait: development, adaptation and modulation.* Amsterdam: Elsevier, 1988:23–31.

72. Assaiante C, Thomachot B, Aurenty R. Hip stabilization and lateral balance control in toddlers during the first four months of autonomous walking. *NeuroReport* 1993;**4**:875–8.

73. Assaiante C, Thomachot B, Aurenty R, Amblard B. Organization of lateral balance control in toddlers during the first year of autonomous walking. *J Motor Behav* 1998;**30**:114–29.

74. Assaiante C, Thomachot B, Aurenty R, et al. Hip-centered organization of lateral balance control in toddlers. *Soc Neurosci Abstr* 1993;**19**:556.

75. Sutherland DH, Olshen R, Cooper L, Woo SL-Y. The development of mature gait. *J Bone Joint Surg* 1980;**62**:336–53.

76. Clark JE, Phillips SJ. The step cycle organization of infant walkers. *J Motor Behav* 1987;**19**:421–33.

77. Clark JE, Phillips SJ. A longitudinal study of intralimb coordination in the first year of independent walking: a dynamical systems analysis. *Child Dev* 1993;**64**:1143–57.

78. Thelen E. Treadmill-elicited stepping in seven-month-old infants. *Child Dev* 1986;**57**:1498–506.

79. Leonard CT, Hirschfeld H, Forssberg H. The development of independent walking in children with cerebral palsy. *Dev Med Child Neurol* 1991;**33**:567–77.

80. Berger W, Quintern J, Dietz V. Stance and gait perturbations in children: developmental aspects of compensatory mechanisms. *Electroencephalogr Clin Neurophysiol* 1985;**61**:385–95.

81. Dietz V. Control of natural movements: interaction of various neuronal mechanisms. *Behav Brain Sci* 1992;**15**:732–3.

82. Berger W, Quintern J, Dietz V. Afferent and efferent control of stance and gait: developmental changes in children. *Electroencephalogr Clin Neurophysiol* 1987;**66**:244–52.

83. Berger W, Quintern J, Dietz V. Development of bilateral coordination of stance and gait in children. In: Amblard B, Berthoz A, Clarac F, eds. *Posture and gait: development, adaptation and modulation.* Amsterdam: Elsevier, 1988;67–74.

84. Bernstein, N. *The coordination and regulation of movements.* Oxford: Pergamon Press, 1967.

85. Assaiante C, Amblard B. Ontogenesis of head stabilization in space during locomotion in children: influence of visual cues. *Exp Brain Res* 1993;**93**:499–515.

86. Assaiante C, Amblard B. Organization of balance control in children: an ontogenetic model. In: Woollacott M, Horak F, eds. *Posture and gait:control mechanisms.* Eugene: University of Oregon Books, 1992;338–42.

87. Berthoz A, Pozzo T. Intermittent head stabilization during postural and locomotory tasks in humans. In: Amblard B, Berthoz A, Clarac F eds *Posture and gait: development, adaptation and modulation.* Amsterdam: Elsevier, 1988.

88. Pozzo T, Berthoz A, Lefort L. Head stabilization during various locomotor tasks in humans. I. Normal subjects. *Exp Brain Res* 1990;**82**:97–106.

89. Woollacott MH, Shumway-Cook A. Changes in posture control across life: a systems approach. *Phys Ther* 1990;**70**:799–807.

90. Assaiante C, Amblard B. Peripheral vision and age-related differences in dynamic balance. *Hum Mov Sci* 1992;**11**:533–48.

91. Berger W, Trippel M, Assaiante C, Ibrahim IK, Zijlstra W. Developmental aspects of equilibrium control: a kinematic and EMG study. *Gait Posture,* 1995;**3**:149–55.

92. Gresty MA. Stability of the head in pitch (neck flexion–extension): studies in normal subjects and patients with axial rigidity. *Mov Disord* 1989;**4**(3):233–48.

93. Butterworth G. Some problems in explaining the origins of movement control. In: Wade M, Whiting H, eds. *Motor development in children: aspects of coordination and control.* Dordrecht: Martinus Nijhoff, 1986.

94. Stoffregen TA, Schmuckler MA, Gibson EJ. Use of central and peripheral optical flow in stance and locomotion in young walkers. *Perception* 1987;**16**:113–19.

95. Assaiante C, Marchand AR, Amblard B. Discrete visual samples may control locomotor equilibrium and foot positioning in man. *J Motor Behav* 1989;**21**:72–91.

96. Assaiante C, Amblard B. Head stabilization in space while walking: effect of visual restriction in children and adults. In: Brandt T, Paulus W, Bles W, et al., eds. *Disorders of posture and gait.* Munich: Georg Thieme Verlag, 1990;229–32.

97. Bronstein AM. Evidence for a vestibular input contributing to dynamic head stabilization in man. *Acta Otolaryngol (Stockh)* 1988;**105**:1–6.

98. Pozzo T, Berthoz A, Lefort L, Vitte E. Head stabilization during various locomotor tasks in humans. II. Patients with bilateral peripheral vestibular deficits. *Exp Brain Res* 1991;**85**:208–17.

99. Amblard B, Assaiante C, Fabre J, Mouchnino L, Massion J. Voluntary head stabilization in space during oscillatory trunk movements in the frontal plane performed in weightlessness. *Exp Brain Res* 1997;**114**:214–25.

100. Shumway-Cook A. Equilibrium deficits in children. In: Woollacott M, Shumway-Cook A, eds. *The development of posture and gait across the lifespan.* Columbia: University of South Carolina Press, 1989.

101. Nashner L, Shumway-Cook A, Marin O. Stance posture control in selected groups of children with cerebral palsy: deficits in sensory organization and muscular coordination. *Exp Brain Res* 1983;**49**:393–409.

102. Woollacott M, Burtner P, Jensen J, Jasiewicz J, Roncesvalles N, Sveistrup H. Development of postural responses during standing in healthy children and in children with spastic diplegia. *Neurosci Biobehav Rev* 1998;**22**:583–9.

103. Burtner PA, Qualls C, Woollacott MH. Muscle activation characteristics of stance balance control in children with spastic cerebral palsy. *Gait Posture* 1998;**8**:163–74.

104. Brogren E, Hadders-Algra M, Forssberg H. Postural control in children with spastic diplegia: muscle activity during perturbations in sitting. *Dev Med Child Neurol* 1998;**38**:379–88.

105. Burtner PA, Woollacott MH, Qualls C. Stance balance control with orthoses in a group of children with spastic diplegia. *Dev Med Child Neurol* 1999;**41**:748–57.

106. Rose J, Haskell WL, Gamble JG, Hamilton RL, Brown DA, Rinsky L. Muscle pathology and clinical measures of disability in children with cerebral palsy. *J Orthop Res* 1994;**12**:758–68.

107. Wiley ME, Damiano DL. Lower-extremity strength profiles in spastic cerebral palsy. *Dev Med Child Neurol* 1998;**40**:100–7.

108. Shumway-Cook A, Woollacott M. Dynamics of postural control in the child with Down syndrome. *J Phys Ther* 1985;**65**:1315–22.

109. Yokochi K, Hosoe A, Shimabukuro S, Kodama K. Gross motor patterns in children with cerebral palsy and spastic diplegia. *Pediatr Neurol* 1990;**6**:245–50.

110. Leonard CT, Hirschfeld H, Forssberg H. Gait acquisition and reflex abnormalities in normal children and children with cerebral palsy. In: Amblard B, Berthoz A, Clarac F, eds. *Posture and gait: development, adaptation and modulation.* Amsterdam: Elsevier, 1988;33–45.

111. Thelen E, Bradshaw G, Ward JA. Spontaneous kicking in month-old infants: manifestation of a human central locomotor program. *Behav Neural Biol* 1981;**32**:45–53.

112. Berger W. Normal and impaired development of children's gait. In: Forssberg H, Hirschfeld H, eds. *Movement disorders in children.* Basel: Med Sport Sci Karger, 1992;182–5.

113. Berger W, Quintern J, Dietz V. Pathophysiology of gait in children with cerebral palsy. *Electroencephalogr Clin Neurophysiol* 1982;**53**:538–48.

114. Leonard C. Neural and neurobehavioural changes associated with perinatal brain damage. In: Forssberg H, Hirschfeld H, eds. *Movement disorders in children.* Basel: Med Sport Sci Karger, 1992;51–6.

115. Crenna P, Inverno M, Frigo C, Palmier R, Fedrizzi E. Pathophysiological profile of gait in children with cerebral palsy. In: Forssberg H, Hirschfeld H, eds. *Movement disorders in children.* Basel: Med Sport Sci Karger, 1992;186–98.

116. Crenna P. Spasticity and 'spastic' gait in children with cerebral palsy. *Neurosci Biobehav Rev* 1998;**4**:571–8.

117. Wheelwright EF, Minns RA, Elton RA, Law HT. Temporal and spatial parameters of gait in children. II: pathological gait. *Dev Med Child Neurol* 1993;**35**:114–25.

118. Ulrich BD, Ulrich DA, Collier DH. Alternating stepping patterns: hidden abilities of 11-month-old infants with Down syndrome. *Dev Med Child Neurol* 1992;**34**:233–9.

119. Molteno C, Magasiner V, Sayed R, Karplus M. Postural development in very low birth weight and normal birth weight infants. *Early Hum Dev* 1990;**24**:93–105.

120. Hills AP, Parker AW. Locomotor characteristics of obese children. *Child Care Health Devel* 1992;**18**:29–34.

121. Walton JN, Ellis E, Court SDM. Clumsy children: developmental apraxia and agnosia. *Brain* 1962;**85**:603–12.

122. Larkin D, Hoare D. The movement approach: a window to understanding the clumsy child. In: Summers JJ, ed. *Approaches to the study of motor control and learning.* Amsterdam: Elsevier, 1992;413–39.

123. Mellier D, Jouen F. Remarques a propos des deplacements chez le bebe aveugle. *Psychol Francaise* 1986;**31**:43–7.

124. Norris M, Spaulding PJ, Brodie FH. *Blindness in children.* Chicago: University Chicago Press, 1957.

125. Adelson E, Fraiberg S. Gross motor development in infants blind from birth. *Child Dev* 1974;**45**:114–26.

126. Sampaio E, Bril B, Breniere Y. La vision est-elle necessaire pour apprendre a marcher? Etude preliminaire et approche methodologique. Psychologie Francaise. *Vision Deplacement: Locomotion Passive Locomotion Active* 1989;**34**:71–8.

127. Martinez F. Les informations auditives permettent-elles d'ettablir des rapports spatiaux? *L'Annee Psychol* 1977;**77**:179–204.

128. Portalier S, Vital-Durand F. Locomotion chez les enfants mal-voyants et aveugles. Psychologie Francaise. *Vision Deplacement: Locomotion Passive Locomotion Active* 1989;**34**:79–86.

129. Tsuzuku T, Kaga K. Delayed motor function and results of vestibular function tests in children with inner ear anomalies. *Int J Pediatr Otorhinolaryngol* 1992;**23**:261–8.

130. Shumway-Cook A, Woollacott M. Theoretical issues in assessing postural control. In: Wilhem I, ed. *Physical therapy assessment in early infancy.* New York: Churchill Livingstone, 1993;161–71.

4

Classification of balance and gait disorders

JOHN G. NUTT AND FAY B. HORAK

INTRODUCTION

This chapter presents two classification schemes for balance and gait disorders. The first scheme considers impairments of neurological systems as a means to establish a nosology for balance and gait disorders. The second scheme is based on observed balance and gait patterns that suggest different diagnostic differentials.

BACKGROUND

Postural responses and locomotion are dependent upon all levels of the nervous and musculoskeletal systems. Consequently, gait and balance disorders are common and result from many and diverse diseases.

Independent ambulation requires two capabilities: maintenance of balance (protection of upright stance via anticipatory and reactive postural mechanisms) and movement through the environment via locomotion. Although gait or locomotion can sometimes be separated from balance or postural equilibrium, locomotion and balance are more often inextricably intertwined.[1] Many so-called gait disorders are balance disorders, not disorders in the sequence of foot movements or locomotion. Thus, a nosology needs to include disorders of both gait and balance.

We first consider a classification based on neurological systems required for purposeful ambulation using Hughlings Jackson's hierarchical scheme of lower, middle and higher functions. This classification suggests the range of neurological impairments that can disrupt ambulation and the relationships between various gait and balance disorders.

Patients' walking and balance patterns do not just reflect impairments in neural functioning but also the patient's compensatory strategies for coping with the impairments. Different impairments may elicit the same compensatory strategy, that is, the same abnormal gait or balance pattern. For this reason, classification by neurological impairments may not help the clinician identify the clinical patterns observed in practice. Our second classification scheme considers the common compensatory strategies as clinical patterns or syndromes for which there are differential diagnoses. Problems with ambulation are separated into clinical patterns that are predominantly disorders of balance and those that are predominantly disorders of locomotion, recognizing that in most disorders, both postural responses and locomotion are affected to some extent. Because falls are a common presenting complaint of balance and gait disorders, we also offer a classification for fall patterns.

LOCOMOTION AND EQUILIBRIUM

The temporal and spatial patterns of muscle activation in leg and truncal muscles (synergies) for repetitive stepping or locomotion are programmed at the spinal cord level by central pattern generators (CPGs).[2] Repetitive hind leg stepping can be elicited by movement of a treadmill in cats with total thoracic cord transection[2] and in the legs of humans with paraplegia and quadriplegia.[3] This spinal stepping is activated by sensory stimulation resulting from treadmill motion and by non-specific dorsal root sensory stimulation. The CPGs are also activated by descending pathways from the brainstem.[4] Electrical stimulation of brainstem locomotor centers will produce stepping and, at higher intensity, trotting and running movements of the legs of cats and monkeys.[5] Cerebellum, basal ganglia and primary motor areas appear to refine and adapt the spinal cord generated synergies to varying conditions.[6] Other cortical areas appear to coordinate locomotion and postural responses with the individual's voluntary actions and the immediate environmental constraints.

The neuroanatomical basis of postural control is less well understood than it is for locomotion. The spinal animal does not have postural responses in the limbs below the lesion. The hind limbs of paraplegic cats can support the weight of the trunk with background muscle tone but cannot respond to a postural perturbation to prevent a fall.[7] Spinal cats walking on a treadmill require support to maintain their upright balance.[2,7] These observations indicate that postural responses arise from centers above the spinal cord. Coordinated postural responses can be elicited from the brainstem as evidenced by studies in intact cats with implanted electrodes in dorsal and ventral tegmental regions of the pons. Stimulation of the ventral tegmental region would make a lying cat stand up and then begin walking. Stimulation of the dorsal tegmental region reversed this effect; a walking cat would first stop and then would lie down.[1,8]

Higher centers are presumed to adapt postural responses to the environment and to the individual's needs. Anticipatory postural adjustments precede and accompany any voluntary movement to protect postural stability. These adaptations require accurate neural maps of the body in relation to the earth's gravitational field, the support surface and the immediate environment as well as the relation of various body segments to each other.[9] These maps are synthesized from information obtained from a variety of sensory modalities.[10] Somatosensory information from proprioceptors in muscles and joints are the most important for coordination of posture and gait, including triggering rapid postural responses. Cutaneous sensors provide information about the contour and characteristics of surfaces, the pressure under the feet in contact with support surfaces and a stable reference for posture. Graviceptors in the trunk, some of which appear to be in the kidneys, contribute to perception of postural verticality.[11] Vestibular information helps control trunk and head orientation in space, as well as stabilize gaze during locomotion. Vision contributes to postural stability and is used in a predictive manner to avoid obstacles and plan trajectories and step placement during gait.[12,13] In addition to online sensory information, postural responses are modified and adapted to behavior goals by context, previous experience and expectation.

Functional imaging is beginning to indicate the anatomical basis of various aspects of balance and walking. Positron-emission tomography (PET) studies indicate that the cerebellar vermis and right visual cortex are activated in quiet stance.[14] During walking, supplementary motor area, striatum, cerebellar vermis and visual cortex were activated as measured by a single photon emission computed tomography (SPECT) blood flow study.[15] Navigation through a complex virtual town activated the right hippocampus, right caudate nucleus, right inferior parietal cortex and bilateral medial parietal cortex.[16]

CLASSIFICATION OF BALANCE AND GAIT DISORDERS BY NEUROLOGICAL IMPAIRMENTS

A hierarchical classification, modeled after Hughlings Jackson's approach, considers three levels of neural function controlling gait and balance: lower, middle and higher levels (Table 4.1). 'Lower' to 'higher' correlates with 'simpler' to 'more complex' neural processing. Lower-level processes are the hard-wired locomotor and balance synergies, the primary sensory modalities, and the nerve and muscle responsible for generating force. The middle level organizes sensory input into representations of body parts and their relation to each other, to gravity and to the environment. It also modifies force for effective and precise postural and locomotor synergies. Higher level gait and balance disorders are defined as clinical disorders that are not explicable by weakness, altered muscle tone, primary sensory loss, incoordination or involuntary movements (i.e. lower level functions). This definition of higher level function is, of course, the definition commonly used for apraxia.[17] It differs from the usual concept of limb apraxia in that in addition to disturbed motor plans thought to underlie limb apraxia, it may include dysfunction that is attributed to abnormal sensory integration, sensory or motor neglect, loss of access to automatic brainstem and spinal motor programs, lack of attention and impaired insight/cognitive functioning.

The pathogenesis of higher level gait and balance disorders is assumed to arise from cortical dysfunction. This assumption does not require that the lesion be located in cortex. Subcortical lesions, particularly those in thalamus, basal ganglia and tracts connecting these subcortical nuclei with the cortex, can disturb cortical function indirectly and thereby produce behavioral effects resembling those from cortical lesions. This formulation also parallels that for apraxia, neglect and agnosia, which may arise from subcortical as well as cortical lesions.[18] It is important to note that a single disorder may produce balance and gait dysfunction by effects at several levels. For example, mild to moderate parkinsonism is envisioned as causing mid-level dysfunction by reducing the force generation for balance and locomotor synergies. The consequence is slower, and sometimes ineffective, postural responses as well as slower locomotion. More severe parkinsonism may also affect higher level functions such as adaptation of balance synergies to environmental conditions and coordination of synergies.

Table 4.1 *Neural systems/anatomical classification*

I. Lower level
    A. Spinal locomotor and brainstem postural synergies
        1. Absence of synergies
        2. Abnormal spatial-temporal organization of synergies
        3. Disinhibition of synergies with higher lesions
            a. Spinal stepping
            b. Decerebrate posturing, tonic neck responses
    B. Sensory input
        1. Veering ataxia of acute peripheral vestibular lesions
        2. Sensory ataxia with loss of proprioception
        3. Veering, careful gait of the newly blind
    C. Motor output (force production)
        1. Steppage gait (foot drop) of distal weakness
        2. Waddling gait of proximal (hip) weakness
II. Middle level
    A. Perception/orientation (organization of primary sensory modalities into spatial maps of body parts in relations to each other, the gravitational field and the environment)
        1. Distorted spatial maps
            a. Central vestibular lesions of brainstem and thalamus
            b. Parietal lesions and 'pusher syndrome'
        2. Neglect of spatial information (or distorted maps)
            a. Thalamic astasia
            b. Putaminal astasia
            c. Progressive supranuclear palsy?
            d. Non-dominant parietal lesions?
    B. Force scaling (modulation of force for adaptation of postural and locomotor synergies to individual's purpose and environment)
        1. Hypokinetic and hyperkinetic disorders of basal ganglia origin
        2. Hypermetric and dysmetric disorders of cerebellar origin
        3. Spasticity and clumsiness from corticospinal system damage
III. Higher level
    A. Selection, coordination and adaptation of locomotor and postural responses (less conscious functions).
        1. Dyscoordination of voluntary movement and postural responses
            a. Reduction or loss of anticipatory responses with frontal lesions
        2. Impaired inhibition or excitation of lower postural and gait synergies
            a. Tonic neck reflexes and decerebrate posturing
            b. Freezing with frontal, subcortical and basal ganglia lesions
        3. Impaired adaptation of postural synergies to conditions
            a. Postural inflexibility of advanced parkinsonism
            b. Inability to use experience in cerebellar disease
        4. Inappropriate postural synergies
            a. Disorganized postural shifts such as from lying to sitting and sitting to standing and supporting reactions (standing)
    B. Attention and insight for adaptation to person's goals and limitations (more conscious functions)
        1. Conscious stepping
        2. Inattention
            a. Falls related to centrally active medications, delirium and dementia
        3. Impaired insight
            a. Falls related to lack of caution in dementia
            b. Psychogenic gait disturbances

Lower level gait and balance disorders that arise from musculoskeletal disorders, weakness, end organ vestibular, somatosensory and visual disturbances, are more readily understood and diagnosed by clinicians. Those disorders arising from cerebellum, corticospinal tracts and basal ganglia are also easily recognized by clinicians. The effects of sensory disorganization and higher level neurological dysfunction on balance and gait are less well defined and more problematic clinically.

Lower level

The lower level has three components. The first component consists of the intrinsic locomotor synergies programed in the spinal gray matter (CPGs) and the postural responses programmed in the brainstem. These locomotor and postural responses are the building blocks of successful ambulation. A patient with complete spinal cord section may have no behavioral evidence of locomotor synergies because they lack the necessary facilitation to elicit them. Spinal lesions may also injure CPGs, disrupting spinal locomotor synergies and thereby timing of muscle contractions required for locomotion although, frequently, other neurological dysfunction from higher spinal and brainstem lesions complicates interpretation. Lower level synergies may be disinhibited or excited by higher lesions so that spinal stepping and decerebrate, tonic neck and grasp responses may emerge.[3,19] Another abnormal, possibly disinhibited, postural response seen in some patients that can stand with assistance, is the involuntary hyperextension or active pushing of the center of mass behind the base of support that precludes standing unaided.

The second component of the lower level is the primary sensory modalities with which the person locates his or herself with respect to the support surface, the gravitational field and the immediate environment, and senses the relative positions of various limb segments and trunk. Under most conditions, the information from the visual, vestibular and proprioceptive sensory systems is redundant so that an accurate spatial sense is possible with input from just one or two of the sensory systems. Only in situations that reduce sensory input from intact systems will deficits in other systems be revealed. The disequilibrium of acute and chronic vestibular dysfunction and the sensory ataxia associated with proprioceptive dysfunction are examples of gait and balance disorders associated with reduced, unbalanced and disordered sensory input.

The third component of the lower level is the musculoskeletal system and peripheral motor nerves. These tissues are responsible for generating forces to preserve balance and to move in space. Damage or disease affecting these structures, the effectors of postural and locomotor synergies, will obviously alter gait and postural responses. For the neurologist, the waddling gait and locked knees of muscular dystrophies and polymyositis and the steppage gait of peripheral neuropathies such as Charcot–Marie–Tooth atrophy are prime examples of this type of dysfunction.

Middle level

At the middle level there are two components. The first component is composed of the neural structures that integrate sensory information into spatial maps. This function probably takes place in many areas of the brain. Spatial maps concerned with motor function have been identified in the putamen and premotor cortex. Maps concerned with visual function exist in frontal eye fields and the superior colliculus. The parietal lobes appear to be important in creating spatial maps which may actually reside elsewhere in the brain.[2] Distorted maps can result in body tilt or lean or inappropriately asymmetrical postural responses. Examples of this type of disorientation are the altered perception of visual and postural verticality that may accompany lesions of central vestibular connections[20,21] and right parietal cortex.[22–24] Other disorders, which may represent dysfunction in orienting in space, are progressive supranuclear palsy, thalamic astasia[25] and putaminal astasia.[26] In these syndromes, patients appear to be either unaware of postural vertical, indifferent to this information or unable to use it for appropriate postural responses. Sensory orientation for postural responses is complex and controversial. Perceived visual and postural verticality, actual postural orientation and postural motor responses do not always correlate (see p.158).

The second component of the middle level function is the precise modulation of force for optimal locomotor and postural control. Basal ganglia, cerebellum and cortical motor areas focus and adapt locomotor and postural coordination but do not create the synergies. The clinical manifestations of dysfunction at this middle level are parkinsonism (hypokinetic and stiff/rigid postural and locomotor synergies), hyperkinetic movement disorders (involuntary movements superimposed on normal strategies), ataxia (hypermetric and dysmetric synergies) and spasticity (slowed, stiff and imprecise synergies). These clinical syndromes are a distortion, not loss, of appropriate postural and locomotor synergies caused by the imprecise execution of appropriate synergies.[27–29] Skilled and precise voluntary stepping may be impaired and walking a line or performing a dance step becomes challenging.

Higher level

At the higher level, two components are hypothesized. The first largely operates at a subconscious level. It is responsible for selecting, accessing and coordinating the appropriate brainstem and spinal synergies for balance and walking. The selection of synergies is based on the information about the body, its location in space and the goals of the individual. Anticipatory postural responses accompany voluntary movements to counteract postural perturbations resulting from the voluntary movements. These responses may be impaired by lesions of premotor or supplementary regions.[30,31]

Improper selection of synergies or failure to inhibit synergies may occur with higher level dysfunction. Decerebrate postures and tonic neck reflexes are examples of disinhibited postural responses. The tendency for some patients to push their center of mass behind their support base while standing may be an example of disinhibition of an inappropriate postural response. It may be seen with frontal lesions, deep white matter lesions and severe parkinsonism (which may induce frontal dysfunction).

'Freezing' appears to be caused by disturbed automatic or subconscious access to locomotor synergies. Freezing is associated with an array of frontal, subcortical white matter and basal ganglia lesions.[32–34]

Sensitivity to context is an important component of higher level function. For example, balance and locomotor synergies should be different for walking on a slippery versus a non-slippery surface and for responding to a postural perturbation when holding onto a support versus when standing without a handhold. This higher function is disturbed in Parkinson's disease; when subjects with this disorder are posturally perturbed while seated, they continue to activate leg muscles used in resisting postural perturbations while standing.[35] Similarly, the ability to learn from experience and to predict appropriate responses is a higher level function. Subjects with cerebellar disease have difficulty adapting postural synergies based on prior experience.[29] A gait pattern that is variously termed senile, elderly or cautious gait, is the slowed, short-stepped gait with *en bloc* turns. However, this gait pattern may be an appropriate response to perceived instability; it is used by a normal person moving about in the dark or on a slippery surface. The cautious gait pattern thus indicates that some higher level adaptation is intact.

Another group of subconscious higher level problems is the totally deranged synergies that may fit the concept of apraxia. Although the term apraxia of gait is in common use, most commonly to designate the short-stepped, wide-based gait accompanied by freezing, its appropriateness and clinical definition are problematic.[36] However, apraxia of balance may be justified for righting and supporting responses that are entirely disrupted and mechanically impossible. Inappropriate righting responses such as trying to arise from a chair without bringing the feet underneath the seated body and bizarre supporting responses, such as crossing the legs, not weighting a leg, and pushing the body's center of mass away from the base of support, may be associated with frontal lobe lesions and deep white matter lesions.[37–41]

The second component of the highest system operates at a more conscious level to modify locomotor synergies. It is responsible for precision stepping such as on stepping-stones or performing unfamiliar dance steps. If there are lower and middle level postural and locomotor difficulties, this higher level compensates as best it can to allow ambulation within the constraints imposed by the lower level dysfunction. Under these circumstances, walking and balance are elevated from operation at the largely subconscious level to operation at a conscious level. The more balance and gait are under conscious control, the more attention is required. In this situation, balance and gait deteriorate when the person attempts simultaneous tasks such as talking or carrying something while walking. Using a walker also has attentional demands.[42] Falls occur in older patients that are not attentive to the demands of walking and balance because of dementia or drug-induced impairments of attention. Further, some patients do not have the insight to avoid posturally challenging situations because of dementia. It is for these reasons that dementia and centrally active drug use in the elderly emerge in epidemiological studies as predisposing factors to falls.[43,44] Psychogenic gait disorders could also be seen as representative of dysfunction at this higher level.[45,46]

CLASSIFICATION OF BALANCE AND GAIT DISORDERS BY PATTERNS

The postural response and locomotor patterns that the clinician observes are the consequence of the neurological impairments modified by the compensatory strategies the patient uses to cope with the impairments. Impairments at different levels may invoke clinically similar compensatory clinical patterns. For example, a hyperextended locked knee to prevent knee buckling in stance may be a compensatory strategy for weak quadriceps muscles, hypermetric synergies from a cerebellar disorder or lack of proprioceptive feedback in an individual with profound somatosensory loss.

The pattern or syndrome classification assumes that there are different gait and balance patterns which suggest a different array of etiologies for the pattern. The balance and gait patterns are not mutually exclusive; a patient may demonstrate elements of more than one abnormal pattern.

Classification is based on the history and observed features of gait and postural responses. History is particularly important for patients with falls, as falls are generally not directly observed. Gait and balance features are observed not only during stance and gait, but also during transitions from sit to stand and turning, when balance is challenged by walking in tandem with a narrow base of support, and responding to postural perturbations such as the pull test. The perceived limits of stability can also be evaluated by examining how far the subject can lean forward and backwards in standing and laterally in sitting. Ability to maintain orientation with limited somatosensory information can be evaluated by standing on compliant foam with eyes open and closed. These features will describe gait and balance syndromes. Other clinical features derived from the neurological examination, imaging and laboratory testing will help differentiate between causes of a given syndrome but are not used to define the syndrome. The proposed syndrome classification has three categories; fall patterns, disequilibrium patterns and gait patterns.

Fall syndromes

Fall patterns (Table 4.2) are generally based on history. The first distinction is between falling because of loss of postural tone and falls with retained tone. 'Collapsing in a heap' is a common description of falls from loss of postural tone. Akinetic seizures, negative myoclonus, syncope, otolithic crises and orthostatic hypotension cause collapsing falls. This category of falls is sometimes referred to as 'drop attacks' (but note that the term drop attack may be used for any unexplained fall).[47] Consciousness is retained or is only fleetingly clouded. There is no post-fall confusion. The recognition of the collapsing fall syndrome is an important distinction as the differential diagnostic tests and treatments are very different from the other falls to be considered below (see Chapters 16 and 22).[48]

Table 4.2 *Fall patterns*

1. Collapsing (loss of muscle tone)
2. Toppling (maintained muscle tone)
   a. Drifting into a fall while standing
   b. Falling while changing position/posture
   c. Weaving from side to side or in all directions until falling
3. Tripping
4. Freezing
5. Sensory falls (falling in specific environments or with concurrent sensory symptoms)
6. Non-patterned

In falls with retained muscle tone, the patient falls in some direction and does not just collapse. These are falls in which the patient 'topples like a falling tree.' It may be helpful to distinguish whether the patient actually falls to the ground or has 'near-falls.' 'Near-falls' suggest that the patient recognizes when they are out of equilibrium and performs a late or inadequate postural response. In contrast, patients that consistently fall to the ground clearly have grossly inadequate postural control or are unaware, until too late, that equilibrium has been compromised. Patients and their caregivers can often provide helpful information on the environmental situation, task attempted and type of fall pattern. It is often useful to re-enact the circumstances that led to a fall during the clinical examination.

Some toppling falls occur when the patient is just standing and seemingly drifts out of equilibrium, as seen in progressive supranuclear palsy or thalamic and putaminal astasia.[25,26] More commonly, toppling falls occur when the patient is changing position (arising or turning while standing), as is characteristic of parkinsonism. In both of these types of falls there is often inadequate or no effort to arrest the fall. Patients with cerebellar disease may weave about when standing and fall in any direction, but retain protective responses (putting out an arm to arrest the fall, etc.).

Tripping falls occur because the feet do not clear the support surface adequately and the toe catches on irregularities or obstruction on the surface. The falls are generally forward. Foot drop, spasticity and parkinsonism are common causes of tripping falls.

Falls caused by 'freezing' occur when the feet seemingly stick to the floor while the center of mass continues moving forward. Similarly, with festination the steps are too short and inadequate to keep the feet under the moving center of mass. The patients typically fall forward on to their knees and outstretched arms.

Falls that occur only when the patient is experiencing vertigo, in the dark or in sensory conflict situations, such as when surrounded by moving objects, suggest a peripheral or central vestibular deficit. Falls when walking on uneven surfaces suggest inadequate sensory information for control of balance, especially somatosensory loss as occurs with peripheral neuropathy and dorsal column disease. In these sensory type falls, patients generally recognize their spatial disorientation and attempt to use their arms to grab unto stable objects or voluntarily sit down to prevent injury.

Finally, non-patterned falls – falls that do not seem to fit a consistent pattern – may represent failure of attention and insight, producing carelessness (as can occur in dementia). The patient cannot give many details about the falls and may seem indifferent to falling and its health implications.

Disequilibrium syndromes

Disequilibrium syndromes (Table 4.3) are characterized by impairments of balance that markedly impede or preclude locomotion. They are identified by inspection of arising, standing with eyes open and closed, standing on foam, walking, tandem walking, turning, response to postural perturbation and limits of stability while standing.

Disequilibrium can result from dyscoordination within postural synergies; the relative timing of postural muscle contractions is inappropriate and the clinical consequence is buckling of limbs or hips. Cortical lesions and partial spinal cord lesions can produce abnormal timing of postural responses. An example of a dyscoordinated pattern is the delayed onset of postural responses in gastrocnemius such that the hamstrings muscle activation that normally follows gastrocnemius comes earlier, resulting in knee buckling.[49]

In dysmetric disequilibrium, the postural responses are appropriately organized but improperly scaled, generally being hypermetric. There is increased postural sway while standing still. Postural perturbation often elicits a postural response that is too large and causes the body to be thrown into another unstable

Table 4.3 *Disequilibrium patterns*

1.	Dyscoordination	Excessive motion, buckling, etc. of limb segments caused by disordered timing of body segment movements
2.	Dysmetric (hypermetric)	Excessive sway and over-reaction to postural disturbance caused by correct timing but inappropriately large movements
3.	Hypometric	Postural responses are too small because force develops slowly
4.	Sensory deprivation	Situation-dependent disequilibrium caused by circumstances that limit sensory input
5.	Sensory disorganization	Distorted perception or disregard of postural verticality leading to drifting off balance or actively moving into unstable postures.
6.	Tremulous	Tremulous leg and trunk postural muscles
7.	Apraxic	Completely abnormal or inappropriate postural responses

position. Dysmetric, particularly hypermetric, postural responses are characteristic of cerebellar disorders,[29] the prototype for dysmetric disequilibrium. However, the involuntary movements of chorea superimposed on the normal postural responses can also produce the dysmetric disequilibrium syndrome. High anxiety, fear of falling and suggestibility can also produce hypermetric postural responses and a Romberg sign. Distraction by another task while the subject is standing with the eyes closed, such as identifying coins placed in their hand, will often reduce postural sway in patients with anxiety and suggestibility as causes of increased postural sway.

Hypokinetic or bradykinetic disequilibrium is characterized by the slow development of muscle force so that the execution of postural responses is slow and may not be sufficiently timely or forceful to maintain upright balance. Recovery from the pull test is noticeably slow, the upper body moving back over the center of support over a few seconds. Sometimes, the patients fall without an apparent effort to resist the perturbation. Despite responses that clinically appear delayed, weak or even absent, postural responses are present and the latency, as measured by surface electromyograph (EMG) electrodes, is not prolonged. However, the force is reduced.[27,35]

Sensory deprivation disequilibrium produces instability in situations that deprive the patient of the sensory input necessary for orientation of the body in relation to the environment and gravitational field. Disequilibrium occurs because there is inadequate sensory information to detect, trigger and modify postural responses. In situations in which other sensory systems can serve for organization of postural responses, the patient has no difficulties. Standing with eyes closed to reduce visual input, or standing on foam to reduce proprioceptive input are common ways to reveal deficits. Vision impairments, vestibular disorders, severe peripheral neuropathies and posterior column lesions are common causes of sensory deprivation disequilibrium.

Disequilibrium from sensory disorganization appears to be the cause of falls in which primary sensory input is intact but the synthesis of the information into spatial maps is disturbed or there is inattention to the spatial

information. Falls are characterized by drifting off balance with no apparent effort to correct balance in thalamic and putaminal astasia,[25,26] progressive supranuclear palsy and advanced parkinsonism. Falls may also be caused by active pushing of the center of mass out of equilibrium as occurs with some non-dominant parietal lobe lesions in which there appears to be a distorted sense of body vertical.[23]

Tremulous disequilibrium patterns are associated with tremor in leg and trunk postural muscles. Titubation associated with cerebellar and cerebellar outflow lesions produces a slow, 3–4 Hz tremor in truncal muscles that may contribute to disequilibrium. A 4–5 Hz tremor in legs and truncal muscles may be present in some people with parkinsonism and reduction of the tremor may increase postural stability.[50] Orthostatic tremor is a 16 Hz tremor in the legs that is associated with instability while standing but disappears upon walking.[51] Myoclonus, particularly post-anoxic action myoclonus, can produce an irregular tremor in legs that can prevent standing.[52]

Apraxic disequilibrium is the disorganization of muscle synergies for changing posture, specifically, rolling over in bed, arising from lying to sitting and sitting to standing. The righting and supporting synergies are completely inappropriate to the task. The most common example is patients that try to arise from sitting without bringing the feet under the chair, but other mechanically impossible strategies for righting and standing may be seen. These types of disequilibrium disorders are commonly associated with frontal lobe dysfunction[36] but may also be seen with advanced parkinsonism[53] and other cortical lesions.[39,54]

Gait syndromes

Gait patterns are based on abnormalities that are apparent while the patient is walking. The lateral distance between the feet (base) may be widened or, less commonly, narrowed while standing and walking. Gait speed and stride length are reduced with almost any gait disorder or perceived risk to upright balance and are therefore of little diagnostic assistance. The cadence or regularity of steps, both length and base, may vary during walking. Deviation or veering from intended direction of travel may be observed. Stiffness or rigidity of the legs or trunk manifests in the loss of the normal fluidity of gait and *en bloc* turns. Weakness is identified by waddling and foot drop gait patterns. Difficulty initiating or maintaining gait (freezing) is one of the more striking abnormalities of gait. Adaptability may be estimated by the patient's ability to modify walking speed, avoid obstacles, perform precision walking or turn about. Adaptability is reduced or lost in most gait patterns described below and impaired adaptability may be the earliest sign of gait dysfunction, appearing before the other patterns described below are apparent.

Nine gait patterns are proposed (Table 4.4). The proposed gait patterns are not exclusive; patients may show elements of more than one pattern. Also, gait patterns are not fixed but may change or progress across time in conjunction with the evolution of the neuro-

Table 4.4 *Gait patterns*

1. Ataxic – irregular cadence and progression
   a. Cerebellar ataxia
   b. Sensory ataxia
   c. Chorea
2. Stiff/rigid – loss of fluidity, stiffness of legs and trunk
   a. Spasticity
   b. Parkinsonism
   c. Dystonia
   d. Diffuse cortical and subcortical diseases, such as multi-infarct state
3. Weakness –waddling and foot drop
   a. Muscle disorders
   b. Peripheral neuropathies
   c. Corticospinal tract lesions
4. Veering – deviation of gait to one side
   a. Vestibular disorders
   b. Cerebellar disorders
5. Freezing – start and turn hesitation
   a. Parkinsonism
   b. Multi-infarct state
   c. Normal pressure hydrocephalus
   d. Frontal lesions
6. Wide-based – widened base with standing and walking
   a. Midline cerebellar disorders
   b. Multi-infarct state
   c. In conjunction with other ataxic syndromes
7. Narrow-based – narrow base with standing and walking
   a. Idiopathic parkinsonism
   b. Spasticity
8. Cautious –slowing, short steps and *en bloc* turns
   a. Non-specific, multifactorial
   b. Subcortical white matter lesions
9. Bizarre –strange gait patterns that fit none of the above
   a. Psychogenic disorders
   b. Dystonia
   c. 'Fear of falling' gaits

logical problems. Many gait syndromes begin as a cautious gait and evolve into other syndromes. Finally, gait pattern classification does not exclude that the patients have no balance disorders; most do, and the abnormal gait pattern may be a response to the balance difficulties.

Ataxic gaits are characterized by irregular progression (locomotion). Typically, there is a widened base and shorter stride. Cadence is disturbed. Ataxic gaits reflect an uncertainty about when and where the feet will make contact with the support surface with each step. This uncertainty can be a consequence of dysmetric leg movements, as in cerebellar disorders, superimposed involuntary movements, as in chorea, impaired proprioception in the feet and legs, as in sensory ataxia, and a moving support surface (e.g. a pitching ship deck).

Stiff/rigid gaits are gaits in which the usual fluidity of walking is lost. Rotation of trunk is reduced or absent. The range of motion at the knees and hips is reduced, and arm swing may be decreased or absent. The base may be abnormally narrow, as in idiopathic Parkinson's disease and spasticity, or wide, as in gaits associated with some parkinsonism plus syndromes, frontal lesions or subcortical white matter lesions. Stride is shortened. The stiffness may be unilateral as in spastic hemiparesis or hemidystonia. A stiff/rigid gait may also be associated with musculoskeletal syndromes such as osteoarthritis. Vestibular disorders can sometimes produce this picture, with the patient trying to reduce motion of the head and trunk because of deficient vestibular ocular reflexes.

Gaits disturbed by proximal or distal weakness are easily recognized. Proximal weakness prevents fixation of the pelvis during single support portions of gait and produce waddling. Myopathies and dystrophies that typically affect proximal muscles more than distal ones commonly produce waddling gaits, although occasionally multiple root and peripheral nerve lesions are responsible. Distal weakness generally affects dorsiflexors of the ankle, requiring the leg to be lifted more for the toe to clear the ground. Peripheral neuropathies are the common cause of this problem. Corticospinal tract lesions affect the distal leg muscles more than proximal muscles but stiffness (spasticity) which forces circumduction of the leg differentiates this pattern from weakness caused by peripheral nerve lesions.

Veering gaits are those in which the patient tends to lean, fall or deviate in one direction while walking. Peripheral and central vestibular disorders are the common cause but other brainstem and thalamic lesions may cause similar patterns.

Freezing gaits are those characterized by difficulty initiating (start hesitation and 'slipping clutch' phenomena) and maintaining locomotion while maneuvering in tight quarters, passing through doorways and turning (turn hesitation). There appear to be at least two distinguishable patterns of the freezing gait. Most commonly freezing is associated with a stiff/rigid gait and a narrow base. These patients may have no or reduced lateral sway when trying to initiate walking. Idiopathic parkinsonism is the classical cause of this pattern, although parkinsonism plus syndromes, normal pressure hydrocephalus and vascular parkinsonism may also be causes.[33] A second form of freezing is associated with widened base and often-exaggerated truncal sway and arm swing to initiate gait. It is this pattern to which 'slipping clutch' is an apt description. It has been associated with multi-infarct state and diffuse white matter disease.[55]

Wide-based gaits indicate problems with lateral stability. Often, they are a component of ataxic gaits. In isolation, that is, without obvious dysmetria of the legs and with relatively normal cadence, wide-based gaits can be seen in midline cerebellar syndromes such as alcoholic cerebellar atrophy and in multi-infarct states.

Narrow-based gaits are associated with idiopathic Parkinson's disease and spasticity. Why narrow-based gaits occur in Parkinson's disease is unclear; perhaps because it offers an advantage in initiating gait. In spasticity, the narrowing is related to hypertonus in hip adductors.

Cautious gait is marked by mild to moderate slowing, shortening of stride and *en bloc* turns with only minimal widening of the base. Other gait abnormalities are absent. It is termed cautious because it is the gait pattern assumed by a normal person concerned about their balance, such as when walking on a slippery surface. Cautious gait is an appropriate response to perceived threats to postural balance. As such, cautious gait is non-specific and may be associated with a variety of problems that impact a person's ability to walk safely. Cautious gait may be of multifactorial etiology or may reflect the early stage of a gait difficulty that will progress into some of the gait patterns described above. This gait pattern has been associated with frontal atrophy and subcortical white matter lesions in elderly patients with no other explanation for their disequilibrium.[56]

A final category is most aptly described as bizarre gait patterns: patterns that fit none of the above descriptions. These patterns are often of psychogenic origin. Distractibility, inconsistencies and other non-physiological signs are common pointers to the diagnosis.[45,46] Because some apraxic disequilibrium syndromes and dystonic gaits may be very bizarre, they can be easily confused with psychogenic gaits. An 'over cautious' pattern sometimes termed space phobia or 'fear of falling' occurs in some older people with mild multisystem impairments. Gait is often wide-based, staggering and the person must hold on to another person, furniture or the wall.[57,58] It may be precipitated by a fall or some other event arousing anxiety about falling. The physician needs to be 'cautious' about diagnosing this syndrome and not make the diagnosis without thorough evaluation, including magnetic resonance imaging (MRI) to look for silent infarcts.

DIAGNOSIS OF BALANCE AND GAIT DISORDERS

Each fall, disequilibrium and gait pattern generates a differential. The remainder of the neurological history and examination will narrow the differential and often make a more specific diagnosis possible (Chapter 6). This narrowed differential or diagnosis will direct the workup for etiology. For balance and gait disorders that are unexplained by history and examination, brain MRI is indicated and may reveal unexpected infarcts, hydrocephalus, atrophy and particularly subcortical white matter ischemic lesions. Vitamin B_{12} deficiency is another rare cause of unexplained balance and gait disorders.

CONCLUSIONS

This chapter proposed two classifications for gait and balance disorders that serve different purposes. The neurological systems oriented balance and gait disorders classification is intended to provide a logical hierarchy and indicate interrelations of balance and gait disorders with other manifestations of neurological dysfunction. This classification scheme is based on Hughlings Jackson's concept of lower, middle and higher level function. It is partly hypothetical because higher level disorders have received less attention in clinical and laboratory investigations and the proper place for some disorders in the classification are unproven. The pattern or syndrome classification is based on balance and gait patterns observed by the clinician. It is intended to help the clinician consider the diagnostic possibilities for different patterns of falls, impaired balance and abnormal gait. Clinical experience should continue to refine this classification.

REFERENCES

1. Mori S. Integration of posture and locomotion in acute decerebrate cats and in awake freely moving cats. *Prog Neurobiol* 1987;**28**:161–95.
2. Grillner S, Wallen P. Central pattern generators for locomotion with special reference to vertebrates. *Annu Rev Neurosci* 1985;**8**:233–61.
3. Dietz V, Colombo G, Jensen L. . Locomotor activity in spinal man. *Lancet* 1994;**344**:1260–3.
4. Orlovsky GN, Shik ML. Control of locomotion: a neurophysiological analysis of the cat locomotor system. *Int Rev Physiol* 1976;**10**:281–317.
5. Eidelberg E, Walden JG, Nguyen LH. Locomotor control in Macaque monkeys. *Brain* 1981;**104**:647–63.
6. Armstrong DM. Supraspinal control of locomotion. *J Physiol* 1988;**405**:1–37.
7. Macpherson JM, Fung JR. Weight support and balance in stance in the chronic spinal cat. *J Neurophysiol* 1999;**82**:3066–81.

8. Mori S, Sakamoto T, Ohta Y, et al. Site-specific postural and locomotor changes evoked in awake, freely moving intact cats by stimulating the brainstem. *Brain Res* 1989;**505**:66–74.

9. Massion J. Postural control system. *Curr Opin Neurobiol* 1994;**4**:877–87.

10. Gross CG, Graziano MSA. Multiple representations of space in the brain. *Neuroscientist* 1995;**1**:43–50.

11. Mittelstaedt H. The role of the otoliths in perception of the vertical and in path integration. *Ann N Y Acad Sci* 1999;**871**:334–43.

12. Paulus WM, Straube A, Brandt, Th. Visual stabilization of posture: Physiological stimulus characteristics and clinical aspects. *Brain* 1984;**107**:1143–63.

13. Rondot P, Odier F, Valade D. Postural disturbances due to homonymous hemianopic visual ataxia. *Brain* 1992;**115**:179–88.

14. Ouslander JG, Okada S, Youdim MBH, et al. Brain activation during maintenance of standing postures in humans. *Brain* 1999;**122**:329–38.

15. Fuller RW, Ouslander JG, Matthysse S, et al. Brain functional activity during gait in normal subjects: a SPECT study. *Neurosci Lett* 1997;**228**:183–6.

16. Mahan L, Burguera JA, Dooneief G, et al. Knowing where and getting there: a human navigation network. *Science* 1998;**280**:921–4.

17. Geschwind N. The apraxias: neural mechanisms of disorders of learned movement. *Am Sci* 1975;**63**:188–95.

18. de Renzi E, Faglioni P, Scarpa M, Crisi G. Limb apraxia in patients with damage confined to the left basal ganglia and thalamus. *J Neurol Neurosurg Psychiatry* 1986;**49**:1030–8.

19. Sato S, Hashimoto T, Nakamura A, Ikeda, S. Stereotyped stepping associated with lesions in the bilateral medial frontoparietal cortices. *Neurology* 2001;**57**:711–13.

20. Brandt T, Dieterich M. Vestibular falls. *J Vestib Res* 1993;**3**:3–14.

21. Dieterich M, Brandt T. Thalamic infarctions: Differential effects on vestibular function in the roll plane (35 patients). *Neurology* 1993;**43**:1732–40.

22. Karnath H-O. Subjective body orientation in neglect and the interactive contribution of neck muscle proprioception and vestibular stimulation. *Brain* 1994;**117**:1001–12.

23. Karnath H-O, Ferber S, Dichgans J. The origin of contraversive pushing: evidence for a second graviceptive system in humans. *Neurology* 2000;**55**:1298–304.

24. Ugur C, Gucuyener D, Uzuner N, et al. Characteristics of falling in patients with stroke. *J Neurol Neurosurg Psychiatry* 2000;**69**:649–51.

25. Masdeu JC, Gorelick PB. Thalamic astasia: inability to stand after unilateral thalamic lesions. *Ann Neurol* 1988;**23**:596–603.

26. Labadie EL, Awerbuch GI, Hamilton RH, Rapesak SZ. Falling and postural deficits due to acute unilateral basal ganglia lesions. *Arch Neurol* 1989;**45**:492–6.

27. Beckley DJ, Panzer VP, Remler MP, et al. Clinical correlates of motor performance during paced postural tasks in Parkinson's disease. *J Neurol Sci* 1995;**132**:133–8.

28. Berger W, Horstmann G, Dietz V. Spastic paresis: impaired spinal reflexes and intact motor programs. *J Neurol Neurosurg Psychiatry* 1988;**51**:568–71.

29. Horak FB, Diener HC. Cerebellar control of postural scaling and central set in stance. *J Neurophysiol* 1994;**72**:479–93.

30. Gurfinkel VS, El'ner AM. Contribution of the frontal lobe secondary motor area to organization of postural components in human voluntary movement. *Neirofiziologiya* 1988;**20**:7–15.

31. Massion J. Movement, posture, and equilibrium: Interaction and coordination. *Prog Neurobiol* 1992;**38**:35–56.

32. Achiron A, Ziv I, Goren M, et al. Primary progressive freezing gait. *Mov Disord* 1993;**8**:293–297.

33. Giladi N, Kao R, Fahn S. Freezing phenomenon in patients with parkinsonian syndromes. *Mov Disord* 1997;**12**:302–5.

34. Yanagisawa N, Ueno E, Takami M. Frozen gait of Parkinson's disease and vascular parkinsonism – a study with floor reaction forces and EMG. In: Shimamura M, Grillner S, Edgerton VR, eds. *Neurobiological basis of human locomotion.* Tokyo: Japan Scientific Societies Press, 1991;291–304.

35. Horak FB, Nutt JG, Nashner LM. Postural inflexibility in parkinsonian subjects. *J Neurol Sci* 1992;**111**:46–58.

36. Nutt JG, Marsden CD, Thompson PD. Human walking and higher level gait disorders, particularly in the elderly. *Neurology* 1993;**43**:268–79.

37. Bruns L. Uber storugen des gleichgewichtes bei stirnhirntumoren. *Dtsch Med Wochenschr* 1892;**18**:138–40.

38. Meyer JS, Barron DW. Apraxia of gait: a clinicophysiological study. *Brain* 1960;**83**:261–84.

39. Petrovici I. Apraxia of gait and of trunk movements. *J Neurol Sci* 1968;**7**:229–243.

40. Thompson PD, Marsden CD. Gait disorder of subcortical arteriosclerotic encephalopathy: Binswanger's disease. *Mov Disord* 1987;**2**:1–8.

41. van Bogart L, Martin P. Sur deux signes du syndrome de desequilibration frontale: l'apraxie de la marche et l'antonie statique. *Encephale* 1929;**24**:11–18.

42. Wright DL, Kemp TL. The dual-task methodology and assessing the attentional demands of ambulation with walking devices. *Phys Ther* 1992;**72**:306–15.

43. Salgado R, Lord SR, Packer J, Ehrlich F. Factors associated with falling in elderly hospital patients. *Gerontology* 1994;**40**:325–31.

44. Tinetti ME, Speechley M, Ginter SF. . Risk factors for falls among elderly persons living in the community. *N Engl J Med* 1988;**319**:1701–7.

45. Keane JR. Hysterical gait disorders: 60 cases. *Neurology* 1989;**39**:586–9.

46. Lempert T, Brandt T, Dieterich M, Huppert D. How to identify psychogenic disorders of stance and gait. *J Neurol* 1991;**238**:140–6.

47. Sheldon JH. On the natural history of falls in old age. *BMJ* 1960;**2**:1685–90.

48. Meissner I, Wiebers DO, Swanson JW, O'Fallon WM. The natural history of drop attacks. *Neurology* 1986;**36**:1029–34.

49. Nashner LM, Shumway-Cook A, Marin O. Stance posture control in select groups of children with cerebral palsy: deficits in sensory organization and muscular coordination. *Exp Brain Res* 1983;**49**:393–409.

50. Burleigh AL, Horak FB, Burchiel KJ, Nutt JG. Affects of thalamic stimulation on tremor, balance, step initiation: a single subject study. *Mov Disord* 1993;**8**:519–24.

51. Walker FO, McCormick GM, Hunt VP. Isometric features of orthostatic tremor: an electromyographic analysis. *Muscle Nerve* 1990;**13**:918–22.

52. Lance JW, Adams RD. The syndrome of intention or action

myoclonus as a sequel to hypoxic encephalopathy. *Brain* 1963;**87**:111–36.

53. Lakke JPWF. Axial apraxia in Parkinson's disease. *J Neurol Sci* 1985;**69**:37–46.

54. Kremer M. Sitting, standing and walking. *BMJ* 1958;**2**:63–8.

55. Elble RJ, Cousins R, Leffler K, Hughes L. Gait initiation by patients with lower-half parkinsonism. *Brain* 1996;**119**:1705–16.

56. Kerber KA, Enrietto JA, Jacobson KM, Baloh RW. Disequilibrium in older people. *Neurology* 1998;**51**:574–80.

57. Marks I. Space 'phobia' a pseudo–agaraphobic syndrome. *J Neurol Neurosurg Psychiatry* 1981;**44**:387–91.

58. Murphy J, Isaacs B. The post-fall syndrome: a study of 36 elderly patients. *Gerontology* 1982;**82**:265–70.

5

Orthopedic assessment of gait disorders

JOHN H. PATRICK AND LOUW VAN NIEKERK

INTRODUCTION

Orthopedic surgeons have changed their treatment of musculoskeletal disease in the last 30 years. Orthopedics has become technical and unstoppable in its new-found joint replacement mode; biomechanics is at every corner and implants for almost every conceivable type of fracture abound. The modern orthopedist requires a dedicated operating-room staff to know every nuance of an operation, particularly for using all the implants now available. Assembly of complex external fixators for fracture and deformity treatment, or bone-transplant procedures, the screws, wires, rods, hooks and clamps for spinal operations – even the strange-looking jigs for some joint reconstructions – all need particular training and skills.

All this brings an aura of novelty, of strangeness, to the reputation of the orthopedic surgeon. Horizons for treatable orthopedic conditions and goalposts for defining disability keep changing. The traction and plaster treatments of yesteryear have been replaced in the developed world by fracture fixation devices and joint replacements that produce excellent functional results. Changes in lifestyle, an aging population and attitudes toward recreation as well as for sport present the challenge of diagnosis and treatment of activity-related musculoskeletal disorders in ever increasing numbers. Orthopedic surgery is now a larger subspecialty than general surgery in the UK, but this brings its own problems.

Dissemination of knowledge about advances in orthopedics is difficult enough among even those who practice orthopedics. The interface between orthopedic surgeons and their neurological colleagues is the subject of this chapter: not to describe the how or why of a particular technique (for example, prosthetic joint replacement), but to enlarge upon areas of mutual interest concerning posture, balance and gait. The central nervous system (CNS) controls an anatomical region where our orthopedic and neurosurgical/neurological interests meet. Both orthopedic and neurology departments see and treat walking problems. Modern clinical and investigative techniques allow us both to manage walking abnormality, emphasizing the similarities and differences between our major specialties.

Many of us now require team-working in the assessment and management of the neurologically impaired. Clinical governance emphasizes this, but orthopedic and neurological specialists tend to live separate lives unless driven together by problems presented by patients that cross the divide between their separate interests. In the pursuance of rehabilitation, both specialist groups now abrogate their rights of continuing care in the general direction of another consultant group – the rehabilitationists. In an ideal world, there would be earlier consultation between us; the same team-working needs to be more exact at the outset to foresee potential problems at the completion of the surgical or other intervention. We need true networking among all who treat musculoskeletal and central nervous system control problems. To explore this idea further, we need to consider normal movement and posture.

Vocabulary is a building block for language. The language of gait needs to be understood by all and it is this that the following chapter discusses.

GENERAL ASSESSMENT OF THE PATIENT BY THE ORTHOPEDIC SURGEON OR SPORTS INJURY SPECIALIST

Clearly, as befits normal medical practice, an accurate and detailed history will be taken from the viewpoint of disability.[1] The line of questioning is likely to be very objective about gait. Can the patient stand or initiate a step, or indeed walk? What is the walking distance? Will they fall or need an aid – a carer's arm, a stick or cane, a walker frame, a tripod stick – to avoid a fall? Can stairs or steps be tackled? Is a handrail needed, or two handrails? Can the patient climb stairs or a kerb normally, one leg over the other, or only manage a laborious one step at a time? Additional questions can be pursued if they suggest themselves, such as: Are transfers from the bed, from the chair, the toilet or to the wheelchair possible? Do bath transfers require help? What professional assessments have been made and what conclusions have been reached about a person's physical abilities, and the level of support that social services or a carer is giving to their client? Is it an impairment, a handicap or a disability?[1] The reader may wish to consider using a more detailed scale[2] that demonstrates an exact score of disability for patients. Further use of these types of scoring system may help in assessing outcomes for other diseases that affect mobility.

At the other end of the spectrum, in sports medicine, risk factors for injury in the activity concerned and intensity of the activity have to be ascertained. Overall musculoskeletal flexibility (or lack of movement) and activity-related difficulties or function are determined. A history of previous injury, such as a significant ankle sprain, will place the patient at considerable risk of sustaining recurrent instability or pain.[3] However, beware: even the emphatic history of previous injury does not rule out an underlying neurological cause for the instability. A 32-year-old man recently presented with a history of ankle ligament rupture at age 18 years, with subsequent recurrent ankle sprains. In addition to previous physical findings, however, a mild drop-foot gait and clonus was noted. A prefrontal cerebral tumor was recorded on magnetic resonance imaging (MRI) the same day.

Unhappily, in the authors' experience, a 'neurological diagnosis' often compartmentalizes a client in a special box, which cannot then be opened easily. Neurological disease, a stroke for example, does not mean that orthopedic or other diseases are absent. Degenerative arthritis is no respecter of neurology, and a non-diagnosed arthritic hip, knee or even severe foot pain, especially in the good leg, can cause considerable loss of walking ability – all the while the physical deterioration is being assumed to be caused by a stroke. Similarly, in a recent case seen, a multiple sclerosis paraplegic with insensate buttocks and large ischial pressure sores had had two hospital admissions for septicemia, without attempts being made to involve plastic and orthopedic surgeons in removing the infected bone and, by using rotational flaps, closing the integument and thus achieving a safer future for that patient.

The neurologist needs to pose constant questions: Why is the patient physically disabled? Are there any contributory factors to the type or even diagnosis of the impairment? The same questions can be asked of the surgeon or rehabilitationist, since we may be slow to appreciate that a neurological problem exists. Many patients have Parkinson's disease diagnosed after the hip fracture has been operated upon, even though the fall was caused by the neurological problem. Treatment with X-rays is all too common, especially in the older patient. Diabetic neuropathy affecting the feet may cause 'simple' metatarsal fractures resulting in rehabilitation havoc as Charcot changes occur unexpectedly.

For sport-injured individuals, observation, palpation and assessment of joint movement follow an understanding of the nature of the physical demands of that patient's particular sport. We should understand that the gait cycle changes dramatically when running, and that few sports do not involve running or jumping, together with the complexity of contact sport requiring cutting, turning and maneuvering during motion. Such positional changes have significant implications on the forces passing through the closed kinetic system connecting foot to spine. Ground reaction forces have been shown to change from 80 per cent to 300 per cent of body weight during running.[4] Unsurprisingly failure occurs.

Orthopedic identification of such problems begins with the history. This coincides with observing the patient while seated, recording the quality of voluntary and involuntary movement. Allowing for any obvious functional loss, the next phase of assessment involves observation of the patient standing and walking from in front and behind. If the history suggests a connection between symptoms and running then this too should be observed, although this is difficult by eye. Finally, couch examination commences with the patient being placed supine and then prone. Palpating the affected limb and then assessing both passive and active joint movement follow this.

Clinical examination

OBSERVATION

Erect

Observation of the patient in the erect position is vital to provide clues to postural abnormality, which may explain abnormal biomechanical forces. These may play a role in the patient's symptoms. This is especially true for patients suffering from sports injuries where the overwhelming majority of extra-articular symptoms are caused by enthesopathies. Enthesopathy is the term used to describe a chronic inflammatory response of the bone/soft tissue junction that has been subject to unusual stresses. If the history suggests no recent increase in use one has to, by exclusion, come to the conclusion that abnormal biomechanical forces are responsible for the trauma at these entheses. In the patient with a history of an activity-related symptom (sports injury), such observation may then concentrate our attention on potential abnormal biomechanical forces being applied to a limb that is deformed in comparison to its fellow.

Overall body posture is assessed with the patient first facing the examiner, then facing away and lastly from the side. In the antero-posterior plane truncal asymmetry may be a clue to structural scoliosis, muscle wastage secondary to injury, or a postural scoliosis secondary to a limb length discrepancy. Limb alignment is described as neutral, varus, valgus or windswept on the basis of the tibia's position relative to the femur. A bilateral 6–7° valgus leg alignment in the adult is generally referred to as neutral posture although anything up to bilateral 10° varus knee alignment is regarded as 'normal'. The spectrum for 'normality' in a child is vast and changes with the age of a child.[5] Bilateral varus or valgus posture of the knees in children and young adults is rarely of pathological significance. In the middle to later years of life, degenerative change is possible: a unilateral varus, valgus or windswept posture (one knee in varus and the other in valgus) is always indicative of underlying musculoskeletal pathology.

Observation and description of hind foot posture initially completes this cursory assessment of potential abnormal biomechanical forces that may have a significant bearing on predisposition to sports injury.[6] With the patient still facing the examiner, the posture of the forefoot is described as pronated (often seen with an 'inroll of the great toe nail'), supinated (the opposite, with weight being taken under the fifth ray more than medially), or neutral. Then, with the patient facing away from the examiner, hind foot posture is described on the basis of heel alignment.

As in the knee, heel alignment is described as neutral, varus or valgus. The angle between an imaginary plumb line dropped from the center of the popliteal fossa and the line of the Achilles tendon at its attachment to the os calcis is used to describe hind foot posture. A neutral to 5° valgus posture of the Achilles tendon relative to the aforementioned plumb line is regarded as normal. A wider spectrum of alignment will still fall within the spectrum of 'normality' providing the hind foot is mobile on examination and the posture is symmetrical when compared with the opposite side. Valgus posture greater than this will result in a pes planus (flat foot) and forefoot pronation. This, if unilaterally painful (and of recent onset), is likely to represent dysfunction or possible rupture of the tibialis posterior tendon.[7] Varus heel alignment on the other hand may direct our attention to a pes cavus (high arched foot) which carries an association with congenital talar coalition (seen particularly at the time the coalition ossifies in later adolescence) and thus affects sportsmen of this age. The causes of hind foot deformity are legion, all cases must be examined for the presence of abnormal neurological stigmata.

Supine and prone

First, the examiner looks for the presence of muscle wasting, fasciculation, abnormal movement, obvious joint swelling or contracture, skin callosities, deformity and color change. We examine the overall posture of the limb – especially when compared with the opposite side, if that is indeed healthy. The sports injury specialist will always look for minimal muscle wasting. The patient is then asked to assume a prone position on the examination couch. Rotational limb alignment can only be accurately assessed in this position when the knees are flexed to 90° (Fig. 5.1). Rotating the thigh at the hip in the prone patient while simultaneously palpating the greater trochanter of the femur allows assessment of femoral anteversion. The position where the trochanter becomes less prominent is noted. The angle of the tibia (shank) relative to the vertical is described as the degree of femoral anteversion. In addition, when the knees are flexed to 90° palpation of the medial and lateral malleolus of the ankle allows the degree of tibial rotation to be measured. Both excessive femoral anteversion and external tibial rotation are significant risk factors in the development of sports injuries.[8,9]

In time-honored fashion during palpation, the presence of pain will guide the examiner to the anatomical site of an injury. Assessing both active and passive range of movement in each joint will give an impression of intrinsic joint pathology or soft tissue flexibility. However, lack of movement is sometimes associated with tight supporting ligaments and tendons, rather than because of pain problems *per se*.

PALPATION

Handling the affected part will reveal the presence or absence of warmth, abnormal anatomical relationships, muscle tone changes, pulsations, tenderness, swelling, induration and fluctuations (in a joint or in a fluid-filled cyst). Joint frictions, or crepitus, may be discovered by combining palpation with passive movement. Their importance is clear if the history suggests problems. Clinical acumen is the 'expert-system' that may already be leading the specialist towards a differential diagnosis.

PASSIVE MOTION

The clinician attempts movement of the affected part to compare this with the range of motion on the normal side. Then the quality and amount of joint motion is measured in degrees. Pain causation is noted, if present, and its source localized if possible.

A decreased range of passive joint movement may be produced by intrinsic joint pathology (e.g. degenerative osteophytes) or abnormally tight supporting muscle/tendon units or ligaments. Although the contribution of the latter may be quite obvious in the spasticity produced by neurological disorders, a lack of soft tissue flexibility in the sports-injured individual may be a more subtle manifestation. Decreased range of motion in joints however, even within the physiological bounds of 'normality', has been associated with an increased risk of

(a)

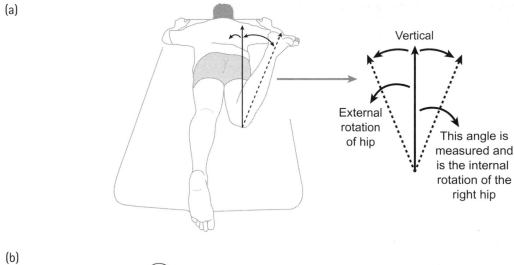

Vertical

External rotation of hip

This angle is measured and is the internal rotation of the right hip

(b)

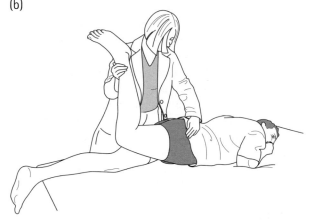

Figure 5.1 *(a) The movement of the shank and foot outwards from the midline measures the amount of internal rotation at the hip joint (and vice versa). (b) The greater trochanter is felt to 'disappear' when the femoral neck lies horizontally in line with the examination couch. The shank angle (from the vertical) at that moment is equivalent to the hip anteversion angle.*

acute injury in sport.[10] Increasing soft tissue flexibility, on the other hand, would appear to decrease the risk of lower extremity overuse injuries.[11]

An abnormal range of motion (to excess rather than restriction) may occur in the normal motion arc of the affected part (hypermobility). Equally, excess motion might be in a new or false direction for a limb segment and this is usually pathological. A Charcot joint is an extreme example of the latter; a recurved or hyperextended knee in a patient with spasticity is an obvious example of the former.

ACTIVE MOTION – EXAMINATION OF LOWER LIMB JOINT FUNCTION STATICALLY

The motion of the affected part that can be moved by the patient without assistance is of great importance, since weakness or paralysis of the muscle groups being tested will commonly allow an explanation as to why there is a gait abnormality. The range of active motion is often less than the passive range. This may be due to pain, but can be aggravated by degrees of spasm or weakness.

It is an interesting point, which is not readily appreciated, that a limp results from a lower limb joint having a decreased or limited range of motion. Any restriction of the normally used range that exists in a lower limb joint

will have an effect on the gait cycle. Obvious, perhaps, in hip osteoarthritis, but not so obvious if the foot or ankle joints, or their muscle levers, are damaged.

Permanent records of active and passive joint ranges in the lower limb can and should be made to assess changing function with time, and a simple joint range goniometer is very helpful for the measurement though not accurate enough for scientific analysis.[12] The examiner lines up the arms of the goniometer with the limb segments on either side of the joint so the angle between their extremes of flexion/extension or abduction/adduction can be directly measured by eye.

LIMB LENGTH

This is sometimes described as the 'height of the joint' when we are considering limb length in the standing functional position. Clinical assessment of leg length begins by looking for asymmetry when the patient is lying with the knees flexed to 90°. This is reliable clinically as a clue for abnormality, but cannot quantify a discrepancy (see below). In children, we have to establish hip location since dislocation or subluxation of a hip can lead to clinical shortening. The commonest cited example is congenital or developmental dysplasia of the hip (DDH) (previously called CDH, or congenital hip dislocation). Imaging may be used by the orthopedists to confirm the amount of shortening, and computed tomography (CT) scanning is now universally used.

FLEXION CONTRACTURES DEMONSTRABLE WHEN SUPINE

Flexion contractures in hip, knee or ankle-foot may be found. The Thomas test (see Fig. 5.2),[13] originally devised to help diagnose tuberculosis of the hip, shows the presence of hip flexion deformity. Much confusion is engendered by the term 'fixed flexion deformity' of the hip joint. Perhaps a better term would be 'hidden flexion', since the distinction is being made between hip disease – commonly causing a limitation of range of hip motion – and the compensations made by the pelvic position which hides the loss of hip range.

In the Thomas test (see Fig. 5.2), the pelvis is fixed by flexing up the opposite thigh and leg towards the abdominal wall. As the lumbar spine straightens from its normal lordotic position, the pelvis can be felt against the hand inserted at the hollow of the back. At this point, the lordosis is eradicated, so the pelvis becomes 'fixed'. If the opposite hip joint is normal, the weight of that leg will keep it flat on the couch. If there is a hip contracture, then as the pelvic position changes, the acetabulae rise, opening towards the ceiling, and the fixed flexed hip cannot extend. Thus, the abnormal thigh rises off the couch and the angle between the couch and the thigh becomes the fixed flexion angle (or hidden flexion angle).

Knee flexion deformity is more obvious since the joint cannot be straightened by the examiner. Occasionally, this is not transparent. The authors suggest placing of the fingers behind the knee joint when the heel and buttocks are on the couch. Normally, the popliteal fossa obstructs the examiner's fingers passing behind the knee. Clearly, a gap for the examiner's hand implies a non-straight knee, and even small (5–10°) flexion contractures can be picked up in this way. This small contracture is often a sign of early and even asymptomatic arthritis.

An equinus at the ankle, or varus/valgus deformity in the subtalar joints will, if present, affect the walk. A Silfverskiöld test[14] will distinguish between gastrocnemius and soleus contracture. It depends upon the spasticity and/or contracture in the three muscles controlling the Achilles tendon, namely, two heads of the gastrocnemii and the soleus muscle. If there is restriction of motion in the ankle joint range then it may be due to inelasticity of the Achilles tendon. If due to a reflex spasticity of the gastrocnemial muscles, then when they are relatively relaxed anatomically (i.e. when the knee is bent) it should be possible to dorsiflex the ankle to a right angle (or above that angle). As the knee is then straightened, the gastrocnemii contribute their effect by recreating the equinus. Conversely, if the soleus is too tight, then knee flexion has no effect on the position of the ankle joint and the equinus persists even when the knee is flexed. An ankle joint dorsiflexion position of more than 10° is used during many sports activities. Normal ankle dorsiflexion has a range from 8° to 26°. During normal gait at least 10° is needed during 1st rocker and toe-off. A dorsiflexion range during ankle loading of at least 20–30° is necessary for most athletes.[15]

It is common for these physical tests to be performed rather haphazardly but this is often foolish in cases of neuromuscular disease or injury, when even slight flexion contractures in the lower limbs can have a grave effect on walking. A careful protocol, used during every examination, will pay long-term dividends in finding these examination changes, even if they are mild. Sutherland et al. drew attention to the flexing moment occurring at the knee joint in Duchenne muscular dystrophy.[16] Such patients cannot counter the flexing moment with an equal and opposite moment of force, giving rise to permanent knee flexion. Such quadriceps weakness/hamstring spasticity is also seen in cases of spasticity from diplegia, mimicking the Duchenne knee position. On other occasions this deformity is dynamic. In the sports environment, a surprising number of 'mild' knee joint contractures are discovered, and recognition of such allows muscle-strengthening treatment to restore the biomechanics of the gait cycle, often significantly. For example 'jumper's knee' has been found to be associated with reduced flexibility of the hamstring and quadriceps muscles, producing the patellar tendinitis often complained of by athletes.

Muscle power

The orthopedist is often reluctant to record the muscle power of individual muscles or groups of muscles that control joint movement. Careful observation and the familiar MRC-based grading system score (from 0 to 5) is presently the most commonly used throughout the world (Table 5.1). These grading scores were developed

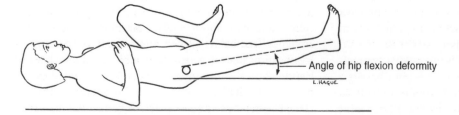

—— Angle of hip flexion deformity

Figure 5.2 *The Thomas hip contraction test. The left hip is flexed up on the trunk to fix the pelvis; the right leg rises to show an angle of fixed (or flexion) deformity.*

Table 5.1 *MRC-based grading system for muscle power*

Grade	Observation
0	No muscle contraction seen or palpable
1	Evidence of muscle contraction but no joint movement
2	Complete range of active motion with gravity absent
3	Complete range of active motion against gravity
4	Complete range of active motion against gravity and some resistance
5	Complete range of active motion against gravity and full resistance

when anterior poliomyelitis was common and lower motor neuron lesions affected muscle groups in a direct fashion. Their adaptation for other conditions is undoubtedly questionable, but has the importance of widespread international use, and is thus very likely to continue. Although suspect as a tool, the alternative in spasticity, for example, is to record only 'Able' or 'Unable'. Normal muscle torque varies with joint position also, an example being the strength of the quadriceps; a loss of 50 per cent strength occurred as the knee was flexed experimentally to 50° from straight (even while the electromyograph (EMG) intensity showed no change).[17] In the MRC grading system we must remember that a finding of Grade 4, rather than 5, is not four-fifths of normal but when scientifically quantified is only equal to 40 per cent of normal strength.

Functionally, for example, we need to measure more exactly how a patient is able to initiate muscle action of the quadriceps in order to straighten the knee in terminal swing phase of the gait-cycle and at that same instant, be able to measure the synergistic contraction of the hamstrings. Such control facility in the normal individual is unsurprisingly subject to change from all manner of disease, disuse or during rehabilitation. Greater understanding of these muscle actions occurs during physiotherapy and exercise targeting maneuvers.[18] Poor integrated control may result in excess hamstring activity and thus knee flexion at initial contact. Experiments on normal individuals have been performed using orthoses to constrain knee flexion in swing, increasing gait energy cost 'significantly'. Thus, therapy must be directed at restoration of integrated muscle action if possible. This is often difficult in disease, but opportunities exist after sports injury.[19]

Dynamic electromyography can distinguish these muscle actions but is a complex and time-consuming investigation. Surface electrodes (or occasionally fine wire electrodes inserted into the targeted muscle) are so placed to allow recordings of muscle activity during the gait cycle. In cases of spasticity, for example, we may find that terminal swing phase flexion of the knee occurs because of abnormal, even constant, hamstring activity. Clearly, a fixed contracture lessens knee exten-

sion but if poor neuromuscular control of the vastii occurs, or they are weak at terminal swing phase, straightening of the knee is lost. If the ankle dorsiflexors are also weak, abnormal forces and moments are applied to all the limb joints, as the fore-foot, not the heel, hits the ground first. Some shock absorption is then lost and stability and progression forwards over the stance foot is compromised. Joint position and limb compensation mechanisms are brought into play but by other muscle actions if this is possible. The resulting patho-mechanics are often wasteful of energy. Lower limb deformity caused by spasticity in the growing child and asymmetrical gait in adults with stroke result from attempts to control these abnormal joint mechanics. These may become insuperable problems during rehabilitation. The vogue for performing EMG on sportsmen has passed: the clinical benefit has been the knowledge of episodic muscle group recruitment during certain sports activities. Knowing normal muscle action allows sports training to be targeted.

Clinical measurement

Careful comparison of the measurements of the affected segment with those of the opposite healthy lower limb will sometimes demonstrate atrophy or hypertrophy. Usually, girth measurements are made at fixed levels above the patella and below. Additionally the length of the limbs – conventionally measured from the anterior superior iliac spine (ASIS) to the level of the knee joint or to the medial malleolus – can be measured. Leg shortening may be apparent or real. To explain the former, think of stance phase *add*uction of the hip. The 'abducted' or normal side will appear longer. The deviation of the abnormal hip towards the midline lessens the leg length measure from the ASIS. Actual shortening is picked up by tape measurement and accurately confirmed using modern imaging techniques.

Other estimations of where shortening occurs around the hip joint were commonly used in the last century before X-ray use became simplified. Nélaton's line or Bryant's triangle can be valuable in discovering the site of clinical shortening of a limb. These lines can assist our understanding of hip pathology.

Nélaton's line extends from the anterior superior iliac spine laterally over the hip, then posteriorly to the tuberosity of the ischium, passing through the upper tip of the greater trochanter in normal people.[20] Sometimes, in cases of hip disease, the trochanter can be palpated above the line so described. If this appears to be the case, then Bryant's triangle[20] should be felt or drawn with a pen. The patient is placed supine and the triangle is formed by drawing a perpendicular line down towards the floor on the upper thigh from the anterior superior iliac spine. The base of the triangle is a line extending from the most proximal tip of the greater trochanter to this perpendicular line and the hypotenuse is represented by the line joining the trochanter and the anterior superior iliac spine. In pathological conditions of the femoral neck or hip (e.g. fracture or degenerative arthritis) the base of the triangle is shortened. In upper femoral subtrochanteric fractures, the shortening of the femur is found not to be in the triangle base and the neck of the hip and normal relations of the triangle are maintained (Fig. 5.3).

A similar, but less well-known line is Schoemaker's line.[20] This is valuable in that its demonstration requires no movement of the patient and may be more appealing to a non-orthopedist. It is drawn from the tip of the greater trochanter through the anterior superior iliac spine and prolonged towards the midline of the abdomen. If the trochanter is displaced upwards, because of disease, the continuation of this line meets the mid line of the body below the umbilicus, whereas in the normal case the line passes above the umbilicus.

These 'lines' are clinically derived and may assist the examiner in noting hip disease, or explaining further the site of some shortening seen in the lower limb. If one leg is shorter as the examiner looks at a patient walking, or lying on a couch, then by flexing the knees and placing the heels together on the couch, estimation of the site of the short bone or segment often becomes obvious. By feeling the top of the tibia (at the joint line) we can appreciate a short below-knee segment, since the 'knee levels' will differ. By looking sideways at the knees (again checking that the heels are together), we may see a longer thigh. A further problem during examination occurs in the presence of knee cruciate ligament injury. The knee may 'sag' backwards when flexed in this fashion. A history of knee injury is inevitable in such cases. Often in hip pathology, no such history or discrepancy is visible, yet a limp is present. Could the pathology be in the spine, pelvis (because of obliquity) or in the hip? Adduction of the hip causes 'apparent shortening', and this deformity is common (being associated with hip osteoarthritis). By feeling for the points described (ASIS and greater trochanter) and drawing these lines, the examiner can deduce clinically what the X-ray will show. Clearly, in a hip dislocation, the lines will be abnormal, but very few patients will unknowingly have spontaneous hip subluxation or dislocation; however early adduction deformity from degenerative arthritis is very common. In high level spinal dysraphism painless dislocation can occur: our clinical diagnosis is confirmed radiologically.

Finally, the orthopedic surgeon is unlikely to use a stethoscope! On occasion, however, it can be used in the neighborhood of joints for locating crepitus or hearing snapping tendons or the friction rubs of tenosynovitis. These can usually be appreciated by sensitive fingers. In sportsman's hip disease, groin strain occurs frequently, with the adductor group muscles and sartorius commonly being subjected to excess load, producing painful bleeds and thus a limp.

Neurological examination

Examination of the CNS will usually have already been performed by the referring neurologist, and the orthopedic surgeon will confirm the salient CNS abnormalities for their own satisfaction, without wishing to challenge a neurological diagnosis (see also Chapter 6). Clearly, any examiner is looking for motor signs that affect gait, such as loss of power or some paralysis of voluntary movement. Similarly, examination of the sensory part of the nervous system to test for pain, numbness, tingling or altered sensation to touch or temperature and loss of position sense is necessary. An orthopedist may be the first to diagnose diabetes while testing two-point discrimination when trying to explain painless major foot deformity or altered gait.

THE MOTOR COMPONENT

In motor disturbance, the signs looked for include atrophy or hypertrophy of muscle bulk, alteration of passive and active ranges of joint motion, the presence of fibrillation or fasciculations in the muscles, spasticity during

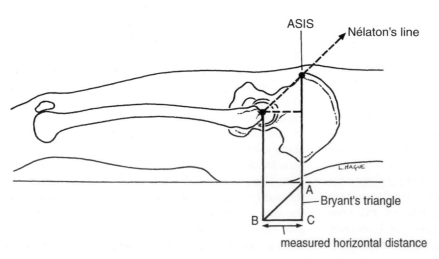

Figure 5.3 *Location of Bryant's triangle. Nélaton's line extends from the anterior superior iliac spine (ASIS) to the tuberosity of the ischium. Schoemaker's line extends upwards from the tip of the greater trochanter, through the ASIS towards the umbilicus.*

attempted movement or irritability in the muscles. Soft tissue contractures producing joint deformities may be present, especially if disease began in childhood. Involuntary movement may be present, either as a regular and spontaneous choreiform movement such as in the athetosis of cerebral palsy. Involuntary but purposeless movement and muscular spasms, tics and tremors arise from many other conditions and extrapyramidal disease. Incomplete paraplegia, multiple sclerosis or cervical disc disease and myelopathy are occasional diagnoses made in the orthopedic department.

Disease of the vestibular system or the connections with the eyes, the spino-cerebellar tracts and connections with the superior corpus quadrigenium of the midbrain and cerebellum, show up as irregular muscle tone and poor coordination of muscle movement. It is to be hoped that early referral to a neurologist for such clinical findings will occur, and patients suffering muscle rigidity, even when minimal, are sent to the appropriate expert. A patient with normal tendon and cutaneous reflexes, but extrapyramidal signs, may present with a disturbed gait pattern, as will cases of ataxia. A high-stepping gait, if present, may be neurologically induced, and diagnosis of the site of the lesion in the upper or the lower motor neuron is required. Rarely, muscle myopathy rather than CNS disease may be discovered by the orthopedist concerned about the gait pattern.

Cervical cord compression or pressure on the exiting nerve roots is a minefield for orthopedic and spinal surgeons, and it is in this area that we believe that a 'call for help' to the neurologist is an imperative. The combination of upper and lower limb signs alert us to exclude cord myelopathy.

THE SENSORY COMPONENT

Touch, pressure, pain, temperature, vibration and proprioceptive sensation are tested. Loss and impairment of superficial and deep sensation is looked for. Although uncommonly found in orthopedic practice, we occasionally see posterior column lesions, showing reduction or absence of the deep senses as well as proprioceptive and vibration sense change. The hemi-spinal Brown–Sequard syndrome is diagnosed in the orthopedic clinics only occasionally but diseases of the sensory cortex itself with contralateral alteration in peripheral sensation, and astereognosis is rarely thought about by the orthopedist. Unfortunately, few of us examine the cranial nerves fully, but alert surgeons will refer their patients to a neurologist.

SPECIFIC TESTS

Orthopedic surgeons use the laboratory to test for full blood count, erythrocyte sedimentation rate, C-reactive protein (CRP) and specifically, serum tests for gout,

rheumatoid arthritis and calcium and phosphate levels and liver function. Cerebrospinal fluid can be obtained from a lumbar puncture with concurrent examination for pressure and tests for complete or partial blocks, if these are indicated from the neurological examination. Both alkaline and acid phosphatase levels may be of importance if indicated by the history or examination.

Electrodiagnostic methods are important, and intensity-duration curves, electromyography and nerve conduction tests can produce accurate diagnoses and pinpoint the site of the lesion in many puzzling cases. The importance of these tests to sports medicine practitioners cannot be underestimated: misdiagnosis in youngsters is always a problem, as mentioned earlier in this text.

All orthopedists need to consider sensory function if they are likely to use plaster or splints (orthoses). Anyone following the healing time of a pressure sore beneath plaster in insensate skin will know sensory abnormality has its price, and is clearly avoidable if we follow simple rules.

Although there are many special tests performed on sportsmen and women, clearly their use will be identified by the site of the problem and the likely cause.

Aspiration of joints or cysts

Aspiration is an all-important therapeutic and diagnostic procedure in the orthopedic outpatients department. Even slight injuries, particularly in the elderly or in the sports-minded child or younger adult, can produce a synovial effusion or hemarthrosis. Aspiration can assist diagnosis if fat globules are found - since this suggests rupture of intra-articular ligaments (e.g. a knee cruciate), implying pull-out from the bone releasing bone marrow fat. Similarly, laboratory examination of the aspirate for infection, rheumatoid factor or crystals can quite often ensure a diagnosis.

Various arthropathies or infection are diagnosable in this way. Bacterial or viral infections remain common. Chronic tuberculous effusions can be aspirated for special stains, though animal inoculation as final proof is always needed. Rheumatoid, osteoarthritic or post-traumatic arthritic effusions are commoner in the elderly. Occasionally, gout and pseudo-gout aspirate needs to be visualized using polarized light microscopy. Clinical suspicion must be high to ask for this but is rewarding if found, since the diagnosis of gout, in particular, can be difficult, with serum levels sometimes obstinately normal.

Effusion examination for luetic infection using the Wassermann test, and in cases of gonococcal arthritis, the gonococcal complement fixation test of the joint fluid, is very specific and, incidentally, is more often positive than testing serum alone.

The importance of performing such aspiration is

often overlooked, even by the trained surgeon. Large effusions stretch the ligaments and joint capsule, thereby interfering with function and irritating nerve endings. Therapeutic aspiration is commonly useful as pain-lessening treatment, at all ages, and diagnosis is assisted by study of the aspirate. Our colleagues in radiology are often keen to assist in such invasive tasks, including the needling of tiny joints or cavities, under ultrasound imaging control.

Particularly following trauma, blood is absorbed very slowly from within a joint and the synovium becomes inflamed. Fibrin can be precipitated and undergo organization, which eventually may form a nucleus for the development of a joint loose body. Early aspiration may avoid this. In cases of infection or rheumatoid and even in degenerative arthritis, the articular cartilage deteriorates. Aspiration (plus joint washout) may slow this process. Because of a natural inclination by the patient to immobilize the joint, atrophy of muscles and bone can develop. Contractures are sometimes caused by muscle spasticity (or imbalance) or within the intramuscular supporting fibrous tissue itself. Current simpler stretching techniques are being superseded by judicious use of orthotics, functional electrical stimulation and the use of botulinum toxin. Rehabilitation treatment may be protracted in such cases, and each of us has a duty to refer early to the physiotherapist to lessen these problems.

Radiographic diagnosis

Although orthopedic surgeons were proud of themselves as being 'the' experts on plain X-rays of the musculoskeletal system, the recent technological advances in imaging techniques have now made them mere courtiers at the court of the 'Grand Vizier'. Both in neurological and orthopedic imaging, the huge expertise and skill of our imaging colleagues has left us ever in their debt. It can be said now that we are unable to ply our trade effectively without their help. Near-perfect images of anatomy of the joints, soft tissues and the central nervous system are available. Further gait study using a mixture of mathematical modeling of joint movement using three-dimensional technology and combining this with imaging techniques is likely to illuminate joint and muscle pathology further in the next few years. This is already occurring in CNS investigation.

EXAMINATION OF GAIT

Development of walking

Although the time of onset of walking has very little significance in itself, late development of walking can often be significant, for example in cases of cerebral palsy hemiplegia or diplegia. In normal development, a baby can partly support the weight of the body and extend the legs, often by week 20, on being lifted to the standing position. They will be able to stand steady for a short while, provided that support is given, at the age of 36 weeks, but do not usually walk alone without support before the age of 1 year. During the following 3–6 months the child will walk without support, but will not run until 18 months old. Stair climbing may start by 18 months but it is not until age 3 years that the child is able to use alternate feet going upstairs and age 4 years before coming downstairs without support.

The width of the walking base does not mature until age 7 years when, as Sutherland has shown, muscle activity and neuromuscular control measurements, and EMGs have adopted an adult form.[21] Asking about these developmental 'milestones' is thus of importance in assessing walking difficulty and its relationship to any earlier difficulty.

Posture

Standing and walking clearly require a postural prerequisite (see Chapter 1). Posture may be defined as the position of the body undergoing gravitational force (which is that force arising from the environment). During standing the line of force (the ground reaction force vector) lies in front of the vertebrae, hip, knee and ankle joint centers in the sagittal plane (see Fig. 5.4). In the coronal plane the 'standing line' joins the mastoid process, the greater trochanter, the tibial tubercle, and reaches the ground at the base of the first metatarsal bone. A state of equilibrium is achieved when a vertical line passing through the center of gravity falls within the boundary of a support base (i.e. between the two feet).

Coordination and integration of many reflex pathways exist and their integrity is vital for the success of gait. These are discussed in detail in Chapters 1, 2 and 8. There is a constant challenge to safe balance in standing, and especially during progression. The center of pressure constantly oscillates several times per second either side of the center of mass to maintain its position within the support area, even in quiet standing. The challenge of movement while maintaining a correct posture requires constant activity of integrated regulatory centers throughout the central nervous system. Normal posture requires multiple input coordination and output activity. There is a great potential for disease processes to change the system, leading to loss of posture, locally or generally.

Assessment of posture requires inspection of the patient walking, standing, sitting and lying to determine the presence or absence of any abnormal movements or response to movement, or any laxity of joint or hypotonia of the muscles and, in the standing patient, whether there are positional spinal deformities.

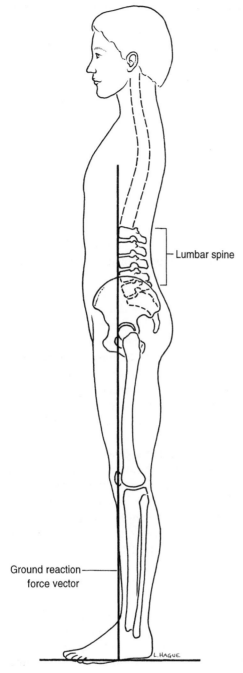

Lumbar spine

Ground reaction
force vector

L.HAGUE

Figure 5.4 *Position of the ground reaction force vector.*

Gait disturbance

NORMAL GAIT

Normal gait has three mandatory requirements, the absence of any one of which prevents walking:[22]

1. Stabilization of a multi-segmented structure – intrinsic and extrinsic.
2. Provision of an energy source (i.e. muscles) which may be manipulated to produce an external reaction.
3. A control system for both 1 and 2.

A definition of intrinsic stabilization involves the concept of the bones of the skeleton being joined at arthrodial joints by capsule and other ligaments which, together with the bony configuration and some muscle activity, keep the joint stable (i.e. mechanically in position). Without these connecting structures, the bones collapse and joint instability results. Free passive motion of joints is fundamental; anything that alters that mobility alters the gait pattern.

Extrinsic stability is a concept of the support area. In normal standing, both feet are used and the support area is encompassed by an oval drawn around each heel and the toes of both feet. Stability is more complex if the person stands on one foot alone, or on the blocks of a ballet dancer's shoe, for example.

Patients with neurological or orthopedic disease often require an extension of their basal support area and add crutch(es), or sticks, to enlarge it. Even with one stick on the ground, the support area inside which the center of mass has to be held extends from between the feet outwards to the reaction point of the aid on the floor. However, less accuracy is required in keeping the center of mass within this much larger support area. 'Control' is less exacting for the impaired patient.

Clearly, muscle activity moves the skeleton, and weakness or absence of muscle contraction will have repercussions for walking. Any disease process of the controlling nervous system will similarly have a major effect.

RECIPROCAL AMBULATION (BIPEDAL GAIT)

Reciprocal ambulation of itself has three basic requirements:[23,24]

- that there is clearance of the swinging foot;
- that there is a forward swing of one leg; and
- that there is forward progression of the trunk.

These need to be discussed in some more detail.

The requirement for clearance of the foot is fundamental to a low-energy-cost walk, since any scuffing of the toe during swing phase results in enormous wastage of energy by the patient. In the normal person, a contraction of the stance side gluteus medius in effect elevates the opposite side hemipelvis (a normal Trendelenburg action). As this is occurring, there is an accelerative activity in the hip flexor muscles of the leg that is about to swing, and hip flexion occurs. This drives the leg forwards by flexing the thigh section towards the abdomen, which in part assists in releasing the foot from the floor, and the second element of reciprocation occurs. Clearly, there has to be some swing leg abduction at this stage to prevent the swinging leg from adducting towards the stance side. This is provided by a smaller gluteus medius contraction on the swing side. Once the swinging leg is accelerating, the main hip flexor – the ilio-psoas – switches off. There is a short prolongation of rectus femoris contraction into initial swing phase, which thus acts to dampen the sometimes massive hip flexion of the psoas, since knee extension results from this rectus activity. By mid-swing phase, the below-knee segment (the shank) has swung, pendulum style, to three-quarters extend the knee without muscle activity occurring. During the following terminal swing phase, the quadriceps become active to straighten the knee and the ankle extensors contract to pull-up the forefoot prior to initial contact under the heel (the pre-tibial muscles also contract in initial swing phase to prevent scuffing of the toes in early swing).

The third element of reciprocal walking demands that the trunk is moved forwards in space. This occurs as the body moves forwards over the 'planted' hind foot in the second rocker of the gait cycle. The trunk moves over the talar dome as the shank moves forwards from behind to in front of the ankle. Just as important is an active contraction performed by the gastrosoleus musculature acting to plantarflex the ankle/foot at 'end stance'. There are some other inertial and other actions which assist this movement. The gastrocnemii actively contract in end stance, pre-swing, lifting the heel off the ground. This pushes the center of mass of the body upwards but also forwards on the 'uphill phase' (Fig. 5.5). Thus, muscle work is performed by the gastrocnemii to raise the center of body mass 2–4 cm upwards and forward. At top dead center, potential energy has been given to the body and this is expended as kinetic energy a little while later, from mid-swing to initial foot contact on the 'downhill phase' of the gait cycle. It will be realized that during this

ankle plantarflexion (called the third ankle rocker or 'push-off'), the trunk advances upwards and forwards and so our third requirement has been achieved.

Normal gait events

Although the reader may be familiar with the definitions of the various sequences of gait, they are described here (and are seen in Fig. 5.6), so that the gait events are broken down into understandable sections. Not only then is the new nomenclature understood, but identification of pathological problems within the gait cycle are more obvious and can be properly communicated to others.

INITIAL CONTACT (IC)

The first event is 'touch down' or initial contact (IC). Most of us know this term of foot contact as a 'heel-strike', but clearly in many diseases the heel never touches the floor or only does so later in the stance phase. This first phase has been redefined in terms of foot contact, to be more realistic.

In normal walking, at the moment of initial contact the specially adapted tissues of the heel dissipate shock energy, and as the first ankle rocker (heel rocker) continues, then the foot comes to lie flat on the ground. The ankle undergoes a plantarflexion during first rocker. Dissipation of the shock continues with the ankle extensor muscles 'lengthening' eccentrically at this stage. Their control of this event allows a smooth 'landing' of the foot on the floor, which is exactly comparable with an

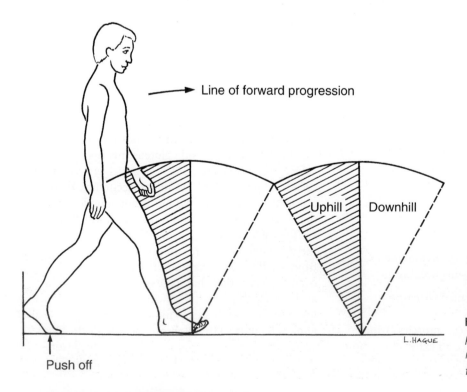

Line of forward progression

Uphill Downhill

Push off

Figure 5.5 *Gastrocnemius activity plantarflexes the ankle in pre-swing, moving the center of the mass forwards and upwards.*

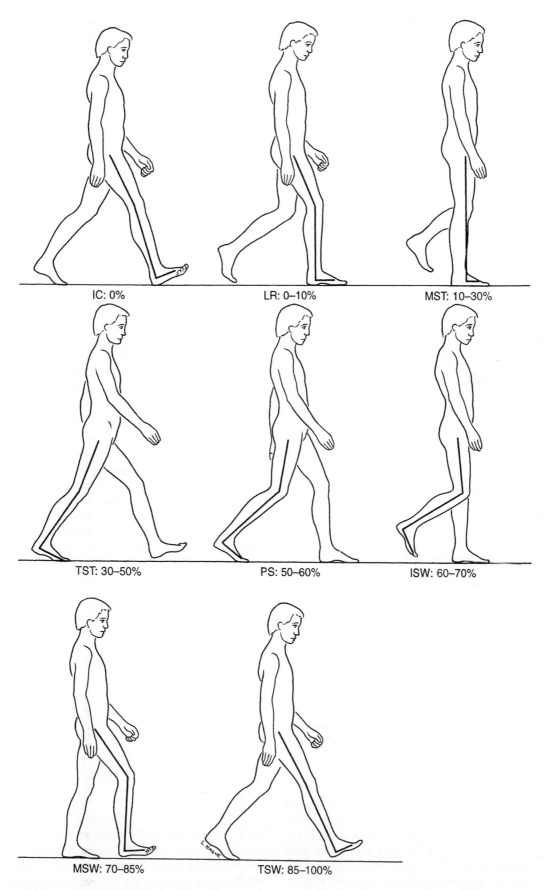

Figure 5.6 *Gait events (for explanation, see text). IC, initial (foot) contact; LR, loading response; MST, mid-stance; TST, terminal stance; PS, pre-swing; ISW, initial swing; MSW, mid-swing; TSW, terminal swing.*

airplane undercarriage absorbing the shock of landing. An audible foot-slap occurs in pathological states where the pre-tibial extensor muscle action is compromised and the foot hurries to the floor.

The second ankle rocker follows (in loading response, see below), when the tibia, or shank, moves forwards at the ankle joint over the talar dome, controlled by an eccentric contraction of the soleus muscle. Both these rockers are energy-absorbing. The third rocker of 'toe-off', or push-off, occurs at the much later pre-swing phase, when stance is nearly over and this leg is preparing to leave the ground once more. This is an accelerative, concentric contraction activity. Clearly, an equinus, varus, valgus or dorsiflexion deformity will all have measurable effects on this sequence of foot rockers. If there is a restriction of normal joint range in the ankle or hindfoot joints, in particular, we can understand the immediate effects on the walk.

LOADING RESPONSE (LR)

This is a novel concept in consideration of understanding gait activity. The human wishes to support body weight on the foot that has newly arrived on the ground, and also wishes to facilitate body advancement over this stance foot. This first 10 per cent of the gait cycle (LR) occurs as the limb is accepting the body weight, and there is clearly a subtle change of body weight moving towards the stance side at the same time as the other leg is leaving the ground. The shock of landing causes the lower limb joints to flex to minimize the upward movement of the pelvis and thus effects a damping of the vertical movement of the center of gravity. If the knee or ankle joint movement range is faulty, the patient will vault over the stance leg or lose these shock-dissipating mechanisms, and extra muscle work is necessary to raise or keep the center of mass higher.

MID-STANCE (MST)

The next phase is mid-stance (MST), occurring at 10–30 per cent of the gait cycle. Here we see weight being fully accepted by the stationary foot as the body progresses forwards over it. The stance hip and knee move into extension and the ankle is vertical, with the whole foot in ground contact.

The center of mass of the body has been raised to its fullest extent at this 'top dead center' position and the weight has shifted towards the stance foot. Reduction of muscle activity is still the primary consideration to conserve energy, but the hip abductors are active on the stance side to prevent the swinging leg hemipelvis from dropping and thus harming swing foot clearance. In many pathologies, the energy-conserving vertical position attained in mid-stance is never achieved (for

example in the crouch gait of diplegia). Excess muscle activity is needed as a consequence – caused by continuing attempts to straighten the hip or knee – and energy is wasted.

TERMINAL STANCE (TS)

The opposite, swinging, leg is now readying itself for 'touchdown', and as it does so, the stance side gastrocnemii fire in terminal stance (TS) or end-stance (EST) phase. This begins when the body moves forward in relation to the support foot. The hip and knee remain extended but the heel rises as the Achilles tendon shortens. This begins knee flexion and truncal movement forwards and upwards, raising the center of mass. Poor control of the gastrosoleus, which is common in neurological conditions, can cause these gastrocnemii to remain quiet or be weak. The result is a lack of body advance, which is so important for walking, as mentioned above.

PRE-SWING (PSW)

Pre-swing (PS) is a transitional phase at 50–60 per cent of the gait cycle, where double support has re-occurred (thus assisting balance), and unloading of the limb occurs rapidly to allow this trailing side to become the new swing leg. The stance hip has now extended, allowing the opposite swing leg its greatest 'reach'. If there is a stance side hip flexion contracture, clearly the swing leg will undergo initial contact much earlier than if the stance hip can extend at the end of terminal stance phase. In PS not only do the gastrocnemii contract hard to push the body forwards (and upwards as has already been explained), but the ilio-psoas and other hip flexors contract strongly in order to lift the limb forwards. The foot dorsiflexors also contract at this stage to prepare for initial swing (ISW) by preventing scuffing.

INITIAL SWING (ISW)

This phase occurs as the foot leaves the ground and is thus dependent upon the integrity of the opposite side gluteus medius to prevent drooping of the swing side hemipelvis, and upon the action of the ipsilateral hip flexors and ankle extensors in order to provide proper foot clearance. Any weakness in these essential muscles will prevent the foot from clearing the ground. Such frictional squandering of energy is very wasteful to the handicapped person, eventually causing tiredness and wasted effort.

MID-SWING (MSW)

Mid-swing occurs at 70–85 per cent of the whole cycle, producing limb advance, under the influence of the inertial forces, continuing the sweep of the leg forwards, together with that motion induced by the hip flexors left-over from the ISW phase. Movement is facilitated by expenditure of kinetic energy as the limb 'falls' forwards on the downhill phase of the curve. Controlling muscle activity at the root of the limb continues the leg and foot advancement in the line of progression. Control problems may significantly worry the patient, who reduces the step length to quickly return to the safer double support where both feet are on the ground.

TERMINAL SWING (TSW)

Terminal swing (TSW) is the last 15 per cent of the cycle, where the limb advances to create a step length, the stance hip on the opposite side extending and the ipsilateral knee and the ankle extensors also contracting to improve this step length. This muscle activity prepares the foot for landing. For completeness, we must state that pelvic rotation plays a part in increasing the step length. As has already been stated, joint range restrictions may mean significant decrease in swing-leg movement affecting those persons suffering major joint disease or deformity.

Temporal and spatial gait definitions

The frequency of succession of left and right steps is called the cadence of the walk, and it is important to know that one walking cycle from a left heel contact to the next left footfall is the stride length; the step length is left foot contact to right foot contact at the next footfall. The combination of cadence and stride length determines speed, and usually we increase our speed of walking by increasing our stride length and increasing the number of steps performed each minute.

Pathological gait

Errors of gait can be identified by the trained eye or by using instruments in the gait laboratory. The orthopedic surgeon will complete the examination by asking the patient to sit and then descend from a couch. Coordination and ability are observed during the maneuver. The standing ability and posture can be judged immediately. Muscle weakness, wasting, tremor or paralysis, and joint contractures are noted (and possibly confirm the couch impression of where the pathology lies). Equally, the stance may still be normal, and the observer none the wiser. Allowing the patient to move and walk may make the diagnosis clear: several differing gait patterns exist and can be spotted at this stage. One of the most dramatic in children's orthopedics is in diagnosis of a very mild congenital hemiplegia, when all seems nearly normal in the examination so far. The instruction to walk fast (or try running) shows up the condition when the classical limb position is seen as the child 'stresses' the CNS.

In some cases the diagnosis remains in doubt. In others, it is not the diagnosis but the further management of a complex case that remains the issue. For example, severe spasticity following head injury may produce a walk that is accepted for assistance with transfers but is so impossible to understand in the context of the conventional sections explained above that observers assume it cannot be altered. With modern gait analysis techniques the demonstration of a muscle group that inappropriately contracts during the gait cycle and blocks the sequence of normal motion may lead to therapeutic decisions that lessen the disability. For example, a dynamic EMG analysis may show inappropriate activity of the hip adductor muscles, making a surgical release effective.

The completion of our orthopedic or neurological examination of a gait difficulty may well require a 'gait assessment'. This is becoming a common request for patients whose problem appears to cross the junction between orthopedic and neurological pathology, or in whom the extraction of a simple plan of the compensations and primary abnormality causing the deformity is well-nigh impossible only on naked-eye examination in a hospital corridor.

MOVEMENT (OR GAIT) ANALYSIS FOR NEUROLOGICAL PATIENTS

Gait or movement analysis (MA) has been said by some to be an investigation looking for a purpose, and thus the more cynical might believe that it is not necessary to submit any neurological patient to a gait analysis. Others may be more generous and wonder if the forces and moments generated about the joints of the lower limbs during locomotion are of importance to the patient. Physicians are naturally concerned about the effect of neuromuscular control difficulties in the widest sense, but the specifics of biomechanics often tug only at the peripheries of their memory. Lack of knowledge about simple mechanics, especially as it relates to human gait, is profound in many specialties of medicine, not least of which is orthopedics and neurology. Technical interest and a growing scientific understanding apply now to the biomechanics of gait. During rehabilitation of neurological or orthopedic gait difficulty patients may need a dynamic medical investigation. Scientific rules and techniques have been 'rolled-up' into a new biomechanical specialty performing measurement. The effects of the forces exerted by muscles can now be measured and calculated. The biomechanical understanding of joint action and pathology encompassed by movement analysis often defines treatment. In cerebral palsy,[24] accurate surgery follows a good analysis (see Fig. 5.7), and children may walk better – cosmetically and functionally.

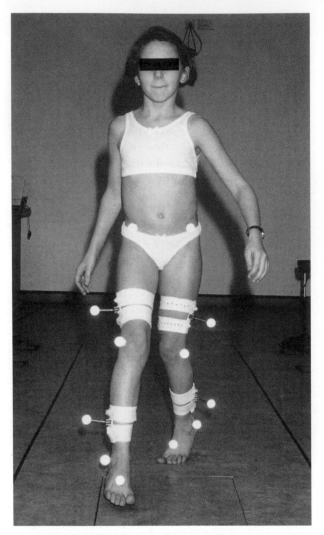

Figure 5.7 *Gait laboratory patient with body markers.*

There is now a positive requirement for gait analysis in cerebral palsy treatment. Why has this come about? Significantly, movement analysis provides distinction between primary causes of deformity and secondary adaptations. The growing child will use cybernetic redundancy during growth: if one or several limb segments will not function effectively, the child will adopt other strategies at an early age, and will continue to adapt and use further compensatory mechanisms as soon as possible. Similarly, the adult with neurological problems will try any mechanism to achieve the objective.

A faulty distinction between compensation and underlying causative problem – by physician, surgeon or physiotherapist – can lead to problems. For example, in the toe-walking child, the cause of the deformity is often gastrosoleus spasticity, but on occasion, for example in Duchenne muscular dystrophy, the mechanics of the walk oblige the boy to stay on tiptoe. By so doing they keep their ground reaction force vector anterior to the knee centers of rotation. In effect, the body weight is

used to augment the weak quadriceps by forcing the knee straight. Lengthen the heel cord to bring the heel down, and the knee sags. Walking and standing cease unless an orthotic (i.e. splinting) augmentation is used to extend the knees.[25]

Numerous examples can be mentioned which, when simple, can be identified by neurologist or orthopedist alike. When complex and involving both legs, the pelvis and truncal movement, say, produces a need to distinguish between primary and secondary disease and compensation. Operations, physiotherapy or splintage applied to the wrong segment or to the compensation will be unsuccessful.[26] This seems obvious, but has only been demonstrable since gait laboratory technology showed the way.[27]

A thorough gait assessment using accurate measurement tools can help to determine where dynamic problems exist and to understand the generation of deformity by inappropriate muscle action, or to see where lower limb muscle power is diminished. We can use instrumented analysis to improve our understanding of the pathology, in order to be able to more certainly suggest good treatment. The adoption of the equinus posture to protect a weak quadriceps is useful for the Duchenne child, and similarly assists some diplegic children also with quadriceps muscle weakness. The same crouch gait is the result for the diplegic walker and for the Duchenne child after Achilles surgery.

Common examples of gait abnormality

Each of us will recognize the redundancy of the musculoskeletal system: if we step on a needle we can continue walking by adjusting our limb support area to avoid putting weight on the injured part of the sole. Similarly, the impaired subject can usually compensate for problems using major or subtle gait changes. I have divided this discussion (which is not exhaustive) into the main segments involved in gait.

FOOT/ANKLE

A permanently everted hind foot produces excess pressures over the medial foot for weight bearing, and the knee moves into slight valgus (knock-knee). This problem can be asymptomatic, for example in flat foot, or may only be indicated by skin thickening or callosity, but sudden loss of posterior tibial tendon integrity causes the internal longitudinal arch to drop and a painful foot and limp result. The opposite varus deformity will produce excess weight bearing under the outer border of the foot and inner compartment of the knee. Skin thickening is found, or shoe wear alteration but no other symptom is common until changing musclo-tendinous functioning produces leg 'tiredness', limping, and some hind foot pain around the outer ankle, sinus tarsi and the heel or mid foot.

If the foot becomes stiff or immobile in any of its many joints – after trauma perhaps, or in inflammatory arthritis – then sufficient redundancy often exists to allow a pain-free gait. Ankle joint fusion, which clearly reduces normal ankle-rocker motions (needful for shock absorption and progression) can be undertaken with impunity, apparently. The resulting walk is achieved with greater energy expenditure and increased foot, knee and hip joint movement as compensation. This can be shown kinematically.

The most obvious ankle deformity is of 'drop-foot', defined as a loss of dorsiflexion in swing phase. Cause may be ascertained by simple clinical testing; the ankle dorsiflexors can be weak, or paralyzed; the gastrosoleus may be spastic or tight. Thus, in initial swing when the foot is first off the ground, the toes lack clearance and a 'scuff' may be seen or heard. Compensatory foot clearance is usual, with excess knee and hip flexion, provided that such motion is possible. This 'high-stepping' may be seen by eye or measured in the gait laboratory if it is subtle. Not so well recognized is the terminal swing phase loss of 'pre-positioning' of the foot in the toe-up position for heel strike contact. In equinus, the step length may be compromised as the plantarflexed foot hits the ground too early. Other causes of drop-foot caused by spasticity or abnormal muscle activity are usually diagnosed clinically. In cases of difficulty, gait laboratory dynamic studies with EMG testing may provide answers. Such analyses guide correct surgical or orthotic treatment. On occasion, clinical examination reveals proximal hip abductor or flexor muscle weakness. This can prevent release of the foot from the floor, masquerading as a foot drop 'scuff' and can only be confirmed in a gait laboratory.

In flaccid paralysis, we can appreciate that a below-knee splint (ankle–foot orthosis, AFO) will restore the possibility for heel strike initial contact; with extensor muscle weakness an AFO will similarly assist. If the gastrosoleus is spastic without ankle joint range impairment (a so-called non-fixed deformity) then AFO treatment is usually effective. Our knowledge of normal gait events and ankle rocker function makes us realize that the orthotist can help with hinged ankle, or fixed orthoses, depending upon the biomechanical deficit and the diagnosis. Too many AFOs are used to attempt ankle control with the splint accommodating only the deformity rather than reducing it anatomically. Thereafter a 'hold' of the foot in the corrected position is essential to restore the ankle rockers. If anatomy is not restored and held, the AFO is ineffective. Discussion between doctor and orthotist is essential in difficult cases. Excess calf spasticity or hamstring tightness are potent causes of continued toe walking during AFO use.

In neurological conditions, spasticity in the gastrosoleus is common, resulting in ankle plantarflexion and the body weight passing directly to the fore foot (even in quiet standing). The ground reaction force vector (engendered by the body weight acting through the limb) is displaced forward – under the metatarsal heads – and then it may lie in front of the knee. If excessive, these forces make the posterior knee capsule painfully stretch into hyperextension. Any rotation of the limb out of plane (for example hip internal rotation in the diplegic) commonly produces pain or excess interface skin force. This results in abandonment of the AFO and callosity, or even skin breakdown if sensory impairment coexists. Untwisting the limb(s) with orthotic twisters attached between waist and the AFO are usually ineffective. Recognition of this rotational (or transverse) plane problem is down to clinical experience or laboratory measurement. Biomechanical derotational corrective surgery may be required, and is often recommended in cases of cerebral palsy diplegia (even for adults).

THE KNEE

The commonest clinical effect of knee arthritis is a limp – often called antalgic – where the patient quickly takes weight off the painful side by reducing the step length on the normal side so that safe double-stance recommences. Some of the body weight is redistributed between the two limbs. Alternatively the subject leans heavily on an ipsilateral stick, allowing the upper limb to take some of the stance-side body weight. Loss of joint range occurring during the walk is a 'limp'. Rarely, a knee is so difficult to flex in swing phase that the compensation occurs at the hip with whole leg circumduction. This movement of the leg into abduction and external rotation, swinging the leg forwards, from the hip, is always performed to clear the foot when the ipsilateral knee is stiff.

Ankle–foot orthoses are also used to control dynamic contractures of the knee. In cases of muscle imbalance between quadriceps and hamstrings the patient may walk in crouch with knee and hip flexed. In cerebral palsy diplegia/quadriplegia this is common. If the knee can be clinically straightened during couch examination and is thus only dynamically in flexion, then the ground reaction force vector of the body weight can be orthotically moved anteriorly to 'extend' the knee. The moments around the knee joint center(s) are altered by adjusting the ankle orthotic angle so that stability in stance is achieved. The polio patient with weak quadriceps presses the anterior thigh in stance phase to achieve the same effect.

Minor knee flexion deformity is often found during careful clinical examination. It cannot be overcome and thus, by definition, it is then a 'fixed' or irreducible deformity. Attempting correction will fail. Even a carefully constructed AFO designed to extend this knee is useless. A rehabilitation aid, contracture correction device (CCD), can stretch muscles, ligaments and the joint capsule to effect extension. Rarely, an above-knee splint (knee–ankle–foot orthosis, KAFO) may be used for partial weight relief, but usually not correction.

THE HIP

Patients with unilateral hip disease (a common example is osteoarthritis) also have a limp, but this is biomechanically different from other limping situations (Fig. 5.8). In order to reduce the time spent on the painful hip, the patient hurries off the painful leg during walking by reducing the step length on the unaffected side. Clearly, as they get back into the double-stance condition they can put more body weight onto the non-painful side. In addition, the osteoarthritic patient adopts a potent mechanism of reducing the force through the painful hip by moving the center of mass of the trunk directly above the left hip (as in Fig. 5.8) by a lateral truncal bend. They eliminate the turning moment produced by the mass of the trunk (length 'l' is reduced to a minimum). With the lever arm (l) shortened, the left hip abductors contract with a lower force since these only have to balance the weight of the right leg. This usually reduces the pain.

In such patients the stick is usually held in the hand opposite the osteoarthritic hip to assist this pelvic elevation on the swing side. Again, force across the osteoarthritic hip is reduced, lessening symptoms.

If the cause of the Trendelenburg is weakness of the hip abductors, then (as in Fig. 5.8b) the left hip musculature is not achieving stabilization of the pelvis in the coronal (frontal) plane. Then, the pelvis dips on the swing side. To assist the weak muscles, the subject will usually use lateral trunk bending to reduce the abnormal hip moments, with the trunk being moved over the affected hip. Sometimes this is called a Duchenne lurch to emphasize its distinction from the force-lowering effect in the arthritic hip. A third abductor lurch, caused by abnormal anatomy, occurs rarely in some orthopedic cases. Local hip joint disease may cause difficulty during walking. If there is a coxa vara or developmental dysplasia of the hip (DDH; formerly called 'congenital' dislocation of the hip), the head and socket are possibly incongruent. In such anatomical abnormality the position of the bony greater trochanter of the femur is changed at the hip, and thus the line of action of the attached hip abductor musculature – to the trochanter - is altered. Usually, the trochanter is moved closer to the pelvis, shortening the muscle overall. It thus cannot contract with its usual force, and the effect again is a limp (see Bryant's triangle earlier).

The 'waddling' gait of the bilateral Trendelenburg is often observed when both hip abductors are paralyzed (e.g. in lumbar-level meningomyelocoele). During movement the trunk is tipped over each stance foot to compensate for the abductor weakness, and the feet are often spread wide

LUMBAR SPINE AND TRUNK POSITIONING

Best observed from the side, lordosis is a common sight in Duchenne muscular dystrophy, but will appear in other cases of hip extensor muscle weakness. The latter muscles, including the hamstrings, should be active at the beginning of stance phase to decelerate the trunk which is flexing forwards in the line of progression. As the heel undertakes initial (ground) contact, the line of action of the body weight passing up the limb (the ground reaction force) will be in front of the hip joint center. This produces a flexing moment, which normally is countered by the gluteus maximus, the hamstrings, and other hip extensors. If these muscles are paralyzed, or weak, the subject compensates by moving the trunk backwards to shift the ground reaction line behind the hip joint axis, and the flexing moment is balanced. To remain upright, a lumbar spine lordosis results. It may be a normal variant associated with tight hamstring muscles, especially in adolescence. It is of importance only if painful or associated with walking difficulty. The commonest cause of flexion deformity of the hip (FFD) is osteoarthritis, but history and physical

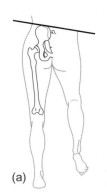 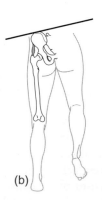 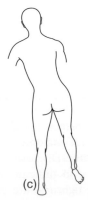

(a)   (b)   (c)

Figure 5.8 *(a) 'Normal' Trendelenburg; the opposite side pelvis rises because of gluteus medius contraction. (b) 'Abnormal' Trendelenburg; the opposite side pelvis droops because of gluteus medius weakness. (c) Osteoarthritic limp with body weight over affected leg. The distance 'l' is reduced by the lean of the trunk; the moment arm is reduced, so the force passing through the hip is lowered. This should lessen pain.*

examination should confirm this diagnosis. Neurological causes of hip FFD are rare except for cerebral palsy. Here, the spasticity of ilio psoas, or weakness of the gluteus and hamstrings, produces an anterior pelvic tilt and lumbar lordosis. Because of lack of hip joint extension on the affected side, the opposite swing-leg step length is reduced. A simple experiment by the reader will confirm this: if the standing posture is adopted, and then both hips are flexed, it is readily appreciated that the step forwards (on either side) is reduced in length. If only one hip is kept flexed, it is similarly appreciated that the step length on the opposite side to the flexed hip remains reduced, while the step on the other side is greater. Neurological disease may affect the hip extensors or the abdominal wall muscles: imbalance causes the lordosis.

The use of clinical gait analysis

The wealth of information from gait laboratories is now becoming more user friendly. Management decisions may be improved after consideration of kinematics, kinetics and electromyographic information as well as more basic clinical input. Although it has been questioned whether such science is useful to patients in an everyday context (rather than being of interest to researchers in gait laboratories), it is now generally agreed that gait analysis is clinically useful. For example, we can now show significant improvements in the energy cost of walking for neurologically impaired children[28] after they had undergone analysis to explain their idiosyncratic gait abnormality. Similarly surgical or other intervention review at repeat gait analysis can be used for audit. Good results of the intervention are obvious, but we all learn from a second analysis of a poor result. Biomechanical lesions identified by gait analysis can now be used to identify similar problems in other neurological diseases.[27] Initially, protocols will need to be derived, and progress will be slow, but repeat gait analysis, months, maybe years, afterwards may allow proper evaluation of chronic interventions and alternative strategies.

CONCLUSIONS

Gait abnormalities defy diagnosis unless three separate sets of information are made available. First, we need to be aware of the functional problems induced by the type of abnormality (muscle weakness, contracture, spasticity or pain). Second, we need to understand normal gait and limb function, and use that as a comparison template in disease states. Third, the observer's eye needs to be very skilled, or we need a gait analysis system that is capable of identifying gait deviations.

Once diagnosis is made, a fourth ideal is to use these findings to set up an appropriate management system for that patient's problem.

REFERENCES

1.   World Health Organization. *International Classification of Impairments, Disabilities and Handicaps (ICIDH)*. Geneva: World Health Organization, 1980;143

2.   Ditunno PL, Ditunno JF. Walking index for spinal cord injury (WISCI II): scale revision. *Spinal Cord* 2001;**39**:654–6.

3.   Verhagen RAW, de Keizer G, van Dijk CN. Long term follow-up of inversion injuries of the ankle. *Arch Orthop Trauma Surg* 1995;**114**:92–6.

4.   Mann RA. Biomechanics of running. In: Mock RP, ed. *Symposium on the Foot and Leg in Running Sport*. St Louis: CV Mosby, 1982;1–29.

5.   Salenius P, Vankka E. The development of the tibiofemoral angle in children. *J Bone Joint Surg* 1975;**57A**:259–61.

6.   Kaufman KR, Brodine SK, Shaffer RA, et al. The effect of foot structure and range of motion on musculoskeletal overuse injuries. *Am J Sports Med* 1999;**27**:285–93.

7.   Meyerson MS. Adult acquired flatfoot deformity: treatment of dysfunction of the posterior tibial tendon. *J Bone Joint Surg* 1996;**78A**:780–92.

8.   Krivickas LS. Anatomical factors associated with overuse sports injuries. *Sports Med* 1997;**24**:132–46.

9.   Turner MS. The association between tibial torsion and knee joint pathology. *Clin Orthop* 1994;**302**:47–51.

10. Tabrizi P, McIntyre WMJ, Quesnel MB, Howard AW. Limited dorsiflexion predisposes to injuries of the ankle in children. *J Bone Joint Surg* 2000;**82B**:1103–06.

11. Hartig DE, Herderson JM. Increasing hamstring flexibility decreases lower extremity overuse injuries in basic military trainees. *Am J Sports Med* 1999;**27**:173–6.

12. Stuherg W, Fuchs R, Miedaner J. Reliability of goniometric measurements of children with cerebral palsy. *Dev Med Child Neurol* 1998;**30**:657–66.

13. Apley AG, Solomon L. *Physical examination in orthopaedics*. Oxford: Reed Elsevier, 1997;7.19, 69.

14. Silfverskiöld N. Reduction of the uncrossed two joint muscles of a one-to-one muscle in spastic conditions. *Acta Chir Scand* 1923;**56**:315–30.

15. Lindsjo U, Danckwardt-Lilliestrom G, Sahlstedt B. Measurement of the motion range in the loaded ankle. *Clin Orthop* 1985;**199**:68–71.

16. Sutherland DH, Olshen R, Cooper L, et al. The pathomechanics of gait in Duchenne muscular dystrophy. *Dev Med Neurol* 1981;**23**:3–22.

17. Haffajee D, Moritz U, Svantesson G. Isometric knee extension strength as a function of joint angle, muscle length and motor unit activity. *Acta Orthop Scand* 1972;**43**:138–47.

18. Dodd KJ, Taylor NF, Damiano DL, et al. A systematic review of strength training programmes for people with cerebral palsy. *Arch Phys Med Rehabil* 2002;**83**(8);1157–64.

19. Yang L, Condie DN, Granat MH, Paul JP, Rowley DI. Effects of joint motion constraints on the gait of normal subjects and their implications on the further development of hybrid FES orthosis for paraplegic persons. *J Biomech* 1996;**29**(2); 217–26.

20. Apley AG, Soloman L. *Apley's system of orthopaedics and fractures*, 7th edn. Oxford: Butterworth Heinemann, 1993.
21. Sutherland DA, Olshen RA, Biden EN, Wyatt MP. *The development of mature walking.* Oxford: Blackwell Scientific Publications, 1988;154–62.
22. Rose GK. *Orthotics. Principles and practice.* London: Heinemann Medical Books, 1986.
23. Perry J. The mechanics of walking: A clinical interpretation. *Phys Ther* 1967;**47**:778–801.
24. Rose GK. Orthoses for the several handicapped – rational or empirical choice? *Physiotherapy* 1980;**66**:76–81.
25. Khodadadeh S, McLelland MR, Patrick JH, et al. Knee moments in Duchenne muscular dystrophy. *Lancet* 1986;**ii**:544–5.
26. Patrick JH. Use of movement analysis in understanding gait abnormalities in cerebral palsy. *Arch Dis Child* 1991;**66**:900–3.
27. Patrick JH. The case for gait analysis as part of the management of incomplete spinal cord injury. *Spinal Cord* 2003; **41**:479–82.
28. Nene AV, Evans GA, Patrick JH. Simultaneous multiple operations for spastic dipelgia: Outcome and functional assessment of walking in 18 patients. *J Bone Joint Surg* 1993;**75B**:488–94.

6

Clinical neurological assessment of balance and gait disorders

PHILIP D. THOMPSON

INTRODUCTION

Walking is a complex action that requires control of trunk posture, balance and stepping. In many instances, the overall pattern of a gait disorder will offer many diagnostic clues. In others, where the abnormality is less obvious, the initial examination should be directed at determining whether the problem lies with one of the three fundamental requirements of locomotion (postural control, balance, and the maintenance and appropriate scaling of stepping) or whether involuntary movements, muscle weakness, sensory loss or other factors such as joint disease or pain are responsible. This chapter discusses a clinical approach to the examination of gait and posture and emphasizes those symptoms and signs that provide clues to the underlying neurological diagnosis.

SYMPTOMS OF GAIT AND BALANCE DISORDERS

Muscle weakness

Walking difficulties caused by leg weakness of peripheral neuromuscular origin are often described in terms of an inability to perform certain movements according to the muscles affected. For example, proximal muscle weakness may lead to difficulty climbing stairs or standing from a seated position, while difficulty walking down stairs may be due to weakness of knee extensors. The circumstances in which the walking problem occur may provide further clues. For example, a tendency to trip when walking over uneven ground or climbing stairs may be due to ankle dorsiflexion weakness and foot drop.

Weakness of upper motor neuron origin in spastic paraparesis or a hemiparesis is often described as stiffness, heaviness or dragging, reflecting loss of the normal freedom and fluidity of movement and an increase in muscle tone. Stiffness is also a common symptom in extrapyramidal disease and is a frequent early complaint in Parkinson's disease. In adults, extrapyramidal disorders of gait are accompanied by slowness of movement, shuffling steps, start hesitation because of difficulty initiating the first steps and freezing on encountering an obstacle or when distracted. Leg stiffness and abnormal posturing of the foot when walking is a common presenting feature of primary torsion dystonia in childhood. Children with dopa-responsive dystonia may develop symptoms only in the afternoon.

Falls

Falls are a common symptom in patients with disorders of posture and gait and an accurate history about them provides much valuable information. It is important to establish whether falls are the result of tripping because of weakness or deafferentation, immobility and poverty of movement, leading to inadequate postural adjustments, or poor balance. Do the falls occur in certain situations, such as after standing up, do falls follow a perturbation, or do they occur spontaneously? Unprovoked falls, forwards or backwards, when standing quietly or in response to a minor perturbation indicate impaired postural reflexes and disequilibrium. A history of falls in the early stages of an akinetic–rigid syndrome is a useful pointer towards symptomatic or secondary parkinsonism, rather than Parkinson's disease. Falls in parkinson's disease may have many causes, including festination, retropulsion and propulsion, tripping or stumbling over rough surfaces and profound start hesitation or freezing. In the late stages of Parkinson's disease, postural reflexes become impaired and falls occur after only minor perturbations. Spontaneous or unprovoked falls are common in sensory ataxia. Falls are uncommon in the early stages of cerebellar ataxia but appear in the later stages of cerebellar degenerations as truncal balance is progressively impaired.

Sudden vestibular or otolith perturbations are a rare cause of drop attacks and falls without alteration of consciousness in which the patient may report a sensation of being thrown to the ground (see Chapter 9).

Fear of falling induces various voluntary maneuvers to minimize the risk of injury. In some patients, a cautious gait pattern dominates the clinical picture and may be the presenting feature. In this situation, it can be difficult to dissect the voluntary compensatory and protective strategies from the underlying neurological syndrome, which is usually a subtle disorder of equilibrium, particularly in the elderly. The cautious gait is often associated with a loss of confidence when walking, especially out of doors, in open spaces where support is not close at hand and in crowded or busy areas where minor perturbations and bumps may occur unexpectedly. Gentle support may dramatically improve the cautious gait.

Unsteadiness

Symptoms of unsteadiness suggest cerebellar disease or proprioceptive sensory loss. Patients with cerebellar gait ataxia stagger and complain of difficulty walking in a straight line and turning suddenly. Patients with sensory ataxia due to impaired proprioceptive sensation complain of uncertainty knowing the exact position of their feet when walking and may be unable to walk in the dark, when visual compensation for the deafferentation is not possible.

Dizziness and vertigo are frequently accompanied by symptoms of unsteadiness. A detailed history is required to ascertain what the patient means by dizziness and to distinguish between the many possible causes, ranging from impending syncope to a vestibular disturbance. Acute peripheral vestibular failure typically produces rotational vertigo, an illusion of body tilt, oscillopsia and nausea or vomiting. The symptoms are induced by head movement and relieved by lying still. In an acute peripheral vestibulopathy, vertigo is severe and disabling, usually forcing the patient to lie quietly in bed. If able to walk, they may veer towards the affected side. Central vestibular lesions are accompanied by symptoms indicating brainstem involvement such as alteration in sensation, especially on the face and weakness. A brief latent period after head movement and before the onset of vertigo is typical of a peripheral vestibulopathy and may also be helpful in distinguishing between central and peripheral vestibular causes of vertigo (see Chapters 7

and 9). Chronic dizziness or disequilibrium is a more difficult problem to analyze and may be associated with only subtle or few symptoms of a gait disturbance. Oscillopsia may accompany head movements when walking and the unsteadiness is more prominent in the dark or on uneven surfaces (see Chapter 7).

Sensory symptoms

Sensory complaints can sometimes help localize the level of the lesion producing walking difficulties. For example, radicular and tract sensory symptoms in a patients with a spastic paraparesis suggest a myelopathy, while distal, symmetrical sensory symptoms suggest a peripheral neuropathy. Exercise-induced weakness of the legs accompanied by pain and radicular sensory disturbances is characteristic of neurogenic intermittent claudication of the cauda equina or spinal cord. Neurogenic claudication can be distinguished from vascular intermittent claudication of calf muscles by the longer time to relief of symptoms after stopping walking, the greater frequency of sensory symptoms such as paresthesia in the affected limbs in addition to pain, and the absence of signs of vascular insufficiency on examination. If doubt remains, the patient should be exercised and examined when symptoms are present. Patients with pain caused by degenerative disease of the hip or knee joints often adopt a variety of motor strategies to avoid bearing weight on the affected joint and to minimize pain when walking (antalgic gait).

CLINICAL EXAMINATION OF POSTURE AND WALKING

A scheme for the examination of posture and walking is summarized in Table 6.1.[1]

Table 6.1 *The examination of gait and posture*

1. Posture	Trunk
	Stance
	Postural reflexes
2. Walking	Initiation
	Stepping
	Associated truncal and upper limb movement
3. Formal motor and sensory examination	
4. Relevant skeletal examination	

Table adapted from Thompson and Marsden.[1]

Posture

TRUNK POSTURE

Normal subjects stand and walk with an upright posture of the trunk. Abnormalities of trunk and neck posture are striking in extrapyramidal diseases.[1] In Parkinson's disease, the trunk becomes stooped and flexed while extension of the neck is typical of Steele–Richardson–Olszewski syndrome. A variety of abnormal truncal postures are seen in torsion dystonia, particularly during walking. Peripheral neuromuscular and musculoskeletal disorders also interfere with truncal posture. Proximal (hip) muscle weakness may cause an exaggerated lumbar lordosis, and is a characteristic sign of a myopathy, particularly muscular dystrophy. Degenerative disease of the hip joint is a common cause of an abnormal truncal posture when standing or walking. Cervical and lumbar spondylosis is also a common cause of mechanical postural abnormality, as is the case in ankylosing spondylitis, where the spine may become immobile and flexed.

STANCE

Stance width, body sway and the ability to balance on two legs are observed during quiet standing and when walking. Wide-based gaits are a feature of cerebellar and sensory ataxias, diffuse cerebral vascular disease and frontal lobe lesions (Table 6.2). Widening the stance base reduces body sway in both lateral and antero-posterior planes and is a strategy employed by those whose balance is insecure for any reason, as in a cautious gait.[2] Subtle imbalance can be unmasked by instructing the patient to adopt a narrow stance width by walking heel-to-toe in a straight line or standing on one leg.

Vision is important in maintaining balance while standing and may be crucial in patients with sensory ataxia due to proprioceptive loss. This is demonstrated by the Romberg test in which the patient is asked to close their eyes during quiet standing. The Romberg test has traditionally been used to distinguish between sensory and cerebellar ataxia. In sensory ataxia, unsteadiness and body sway will increase to the point of falling during eye closure. In contrast, the patient with cerebellar ataxia will, in general, compensate for the increase in body sway brought about by eye closure and not fall. When interpreting the results of a Romberg test it is important to ensure the patient is standing comfortably and securely before the eyes are closed and to bear in mind that body sway increases in normal subjects during eye closure. Vestibular disorders are unlikely to result in an abnormal Romberg test. However, in an acute vestibulopathy the patient may find it difficult to stand with the eyes open or closed and stagger or veer to the affected side, while in chronic bilateral vestibular failure, head movement during eye closure may result in unsteadiness.

A bouncing motion while standing is seen in action myoclonus (as in post-anoxic myoclonus with myoclonic jerks and negative myoclonus or lapses in leg muscle activity) and tremor of the legs (especially orthostatic tremor). A striking finding in orthostatic tremor is the relief of unsteadiness and shaking on starting to walk or merely shifting the stance position. A combination of clonus in spasticity and ataxia can also produce a characteristic bouncing stance and gait, as in multiple sclerosis.

POSTURAL REFLEXES

Postural reflexes maintain a stable upright posture while standing and dynamic equilibrium during walking. These consist of a hierarchy of responses ranging from automatic reflex responses to postural change and perturbations, to voluntary reactions to stop a fall or prevent injury. Postural reflexes are examined by gently pushing the patient backwards or forwards when standing still. An impairment of postural reactions will be evident after each displacement by a few short steps backward (retropulsion) or forward (propulsion). Severe impairment of postural reflexes may render the patient susceptible to falls with even minor perturbations, without any compensatory postural adjustments or rescue reactions to prevent falling, or the protective reaction of an outstretched arm to break a fall and prevent injury. The presence of injuries to the knees, shins, face or back of the head sustained during falls provide a clue to the loss of these postural and protective reactions. Loss of postural reflexes is a common feature of symptomatic or secondary parkinsonism, for example, the Steele–Richardson–Olszewski syndrome.[1]

Table 6.2 *Summary of the major clinical differences between the major causes of unsteadiness and a wide-based gait*

Feature	Cerebellar ataxia	Sensory ataxia	Frontal lobe ataxia
Trunk posture	Stooped/leans forward	Stooped/upright	Upright
Postural reflexes	±	Intact	May be absent
Steps	Stagger/lurching	High stepping	Small/shuffling
Stride length	Irregular	Regular	Short
Speed of movement	Normal/slow	Normal-slow	Very slow
Turning corners	Veers away	Minimal effect	Freezing/shuffling
Heel-toe	Unable	±	Unable
Rombergs test	±	Increased unsteadiness	±
Heel-shin test	Usually abnormal	±	Normal
Falls	Late	Yes	Very common

Table adapted from Thompson and Marsden.[1]

Walking

INITIATION

The initiation of walking involves a complex but stereo-typed pattern of postural adjustments shifting and rotating the body before weight is taken on the stance foot to allow the leading leg to swing forward to take the first step.[3] Because of this complexity, many factors may interfere with gait initiation. Start hesitation with shuffling on the spot ('the slipping clutch' phenomenon) or an inability to lift the feet from the floor ('magnetic feet') are signs of difficulty initiating gait. These are seen in extrapyramidal gait syndromes and may also be prominent in frontal lobe gait disorders (Table 6.3). Occasionally, these signs are seen in relative isolation (gait ignition failure) without other signs of basal ganglia or frontal lobe disease.[4]

A profound disturbance of equilibrium and poor truncal balance may also interfere with the initiation of a step by impairing the ability to balance on one leg and permit the opposite leg to swing forward.

STEPPING

Once walking is underway, the stride length, rhythm of stepping and speed of walking are noted.

Slowness is characteristic of the akinetic–rigid syndromes but also is encountered in ataxic and spastic gaits. In akinetic–rigid syndromes, caused by extrapyramidal disease, the length of each step is short and steps may be slow and shallow although the regular rhythm of normal stepping is preserved (shuffling gait). Shuffling is typically observed on starting to walk and in association with freezing. Freezing may be precipitated by unexpected obstacles or occur spontaneously. The halting progress of Parkinson's disease may be improved by the provision of visual cues for the patient to step over, such as lines on the floor. Rapid small steps (festination) are common in Parkinson's disease but rare in other akinetic–rigid syndromes. In the latter, poor balance and falls are commoner than festination. The differences between the gait of Parkinson's disease and other akinetic–rigid syndromes are summarized in Table 6.3.

In ataxic syndromes, steps are of variable length and irregular in rhythm giving a jerky and lurching quality to the gait, which is exacerbated by turning corners when additional rapid postural adjustments are required. There also may be titubation or rhythmic swaying of the trunk and head in cerebellar ataxic syndromes.

In sensory ataxia, the steps are deliberate and placed carefully under visual guidance, sometimes striking the ground with the heel then the foot, making a slapping sound (slapping gait). In foot drop caused by weakness of ankle and toe dorsiflexors, the legs are lifted abnormally high with each step, descending to strike the floor first with the toe then the heel (steppage gait).

The leg posture and pattern of movement during stepping is abnormal in upper motor neuron syndromes with leg spasticity. There may be slight flexion at the hip and knee when standing but on starting to walk, the affected leg stiffens and extends slightly at the knee. Stepping then involves circumduction of the affected leg during the swing phase of each step, scraping the toe of the shoe on the ground beneath. Slight lateral flexion of the trunk away from the affected side and hyperextension of the hip on that side allow the extended leg to swing through. The characteristic clinical picture of a spastic hemiparesis includes the arm posture of abduction and internal rotation of the shoulder, flexion of the elbow, pronation of the forearm and flexion of the wrist and fingers, with a minimum of associated arm swing on the affected side. The stance may be slightly wide-based and the speed of walking is slow. Balance may be poor because the hemiparesis interferes with corrective postural adjustments on the affected side. In a spastic paraparesis, there is slight flexion at the hips, both legs are extended at the knees and the feet adopt a posture of plantar flexion. The gait is slow and the patient proceeds by dragging the circumducting legs forward one step after the other. There is often a tendency to adduction of the legs (scissor gait).

Table 6.3 *Summary of the clinical features that help differentiate between Parkinson's disease and symptomatic or secondary parkinsonism in patients with an akinetic–rigid gait syndrome*

Feature	Parkinson's disease	Symptomatic parkinsonism
Posture	Stooped (trunk flexion)	Stooped/upright (trunk flexion or extension)
Stance	Narrow	Often wide-based
Postural reflexes	Preserved in early stages	Absent at early stage
Initiation of walking	Start hesitation	Start hesitation/magnetic feet
Steps	Small, shuffling	Small, shuffling
Freezing	Common	Common
Festination	Common	Rare
Arm swing	Reduced/absent	Reduced (may appear exaggerated in frontal lesions)
Heel-toe walking	Normal	Poor (truncal ataxia)
Falls	Late (forwards-tripping)	Early and severe (backwards)

Table adapted from Thompson and Marsden.[1]

Excessive mobility of the hips and lower trunk with an abnormal lumbar posture during quiet stance and walking suggests weakness of proximal leg and hip girdle muscles. These muscles stabilize the trunk on the pelvis and legs during all phases of the gait cycle. Weakness of hip extension leads to an exaggerated lumbar lordosis, flexion of the hips and a failure to stabilize the pelvis during stepping, leading to lowering of the non-weight bearing hip and a tilt of the trunk with each step (waddling gait). Neurogenic weakness of proximal muscles in spinal muscular atrophy and occasionally the Guillain–Barré syndrome, also produce this clinical picture.

Dystonic syndromes may produce bizarre abnormalities of gait. Sustained plantarflexion and inversion of the foot when running is the classical presentation of childhood-onset primary torsion dystonia. Exaggerated hip and knee flexion with each step is another pattern of dystonic stepping. This has been described as a 'peacock' or 'cock-like' gait. An associated sign is tonic extension of the great toe (the striatal toe) when walking. Action dystonia of the leg may not be evident during walking or even running backwards in the early stages.

Patients with chorea frequently incorporate the involuntary movements into their gait, describing an irregular path with a dancing appearance. In patients with Huntington's disease, body sway is increased, stance is wide-based and steps are variable in length and timing.[5] Spontaneous knee flexion and leg raising are common. The disruption of walking by combinations of leg spasticity, ataxia, and dystonia of the trunk and limbs may be the first manifestation of neurodegenerative disease in childhood.

ASSOCIATED MOVEMENTS

Normal subjects walk with flowing synergistic movements of the head, trunk, and arms. Loss of the associated synergistic arm movements when walking is seen in akinetic–rigid syndromes, hemiparesis, and acute cerebellar lesions. Unilateral loss of associated arm swing when walking is often a useful clinical sign in early Parkinson's disease. A loss of truncal mobility will also contribute to loss of normal fluidity of body motion when walking. Truncal mobility is assessed by observing the patient rise from a chair or turn over when supine; it

is often severely affected in frontal lobe gait disorders.[6] While Parkinson's disease and frontal lobe white matter disease may result in similar slow shuffling steps, the preservation of arm and facial mobility in the latter may help distinguish between them. Indeed, the arm swing of patients with frontal lobe disease when walking may appear exaggerated.

FORMAL MOTOR AND SENSORY EXAMINATION

Examination of motor and sensory function of the trunk and legs follows the assessment of gait. In children, particularly those presenting with a limp, limb diameter and length should be measured for any asymmetry in leg size that may accompany congenital malformations of the spinal cord, brain, or leg. The spinal column should be inspected for scoliosis, and the lumbar region for skin defects or hairy patches indicative of spinal dysraphism.

Where pain is a feature, examination of the range of movement at the hip, knee, or ankle joints may be revealing in patients with painful antalgic gaits, or those with short steps and a fixed leg posture. Examination after exercise may be necessary to reveal signs of claudication of the cauda equina.

Examination of muscle bulk and strength is an important step in confirming the presence of muscle weakness and localizing the site of the lesion responsible. Certain patterns of muscle weakness produce characteristic gait abnormalities. Foot drop, caused by weakness or poor activation of the ankle dorsiflexors, has several causes (Table 6.4). These will be identified on clinical examination. Subtle ankle dorsiflexion weakness may be detected by an inability to walk on the heels. A waddling gait suggests proximal leg muscle weakness, particularly hip extension. Proximal leg weakness may be revealed by the use of the arms to push the trunk into an upright posture when attempting to stand from a sitting position, or an inability to stand up from a squatting position (Gower's sign). Myopathic weakness is usually symmetrical and upper limb proximal muscles may be similarly weak. Examination of muscle tone will reveal spasticity in upper motor neuron lesions, rigidity in diseases of the basal ganglia, or gegenhalten (an increase in muscle tone or inability to relax during passive manipulation of the limb) in frontal lobe disease. In the last, other signs such

Table 6.4 *Differential diagnosis of 'foot drop' or equinovarus foot posture while walking*

Upper motor neuron lesion and spasticity	L5 radiculopathy
Dystonia	Lumbar plexopathy
Peroneal muscle weakness	Sciatic nerve palsy
	Peroneal neuropathy
	Peripheral neuropathy (bilateral)
	Myopathy (bilateral-scapuloperoneal syndromes)
Sensory ataxia	

Table adapted from Thompson and Marsden.[1]

as grasp reflexes may also be present. Abnormalities of the tendon reflexes also will yield information about the site of motor disturbance. Brisk reflexes with extensor plantar responses indicate an upper motor neuron syndrome, and absent tendon reflexes suggest a peripheral neuropathy. The sense of joint position should be examined carefully for defects of proprioception in the ataxic patient to look for deafferentation that might give rise to a sensory ataxia.

Heel–shin ataxia will be evident in patients with cerebellar gait ataxia but upper limb ataxia may not be present when lower limb ataxia is caused by restricted cerebellar vermis and anterior lobe cerebellar syndromes. Acute midline cerebellar lesions may produce a profound truncal and gait imbalance, but little in the way of limb ataxia when formally examined in the supine position.

Other discrepancies between the observed walking difficulty and the findings on formal motor and sensory examination include the following examples. Action dystonia of the feet when walking may be the only abnormal physical sign in primary torsion dystonia and the examination when recumbent may be entirely normal. In patients with frontal lobe lesions, hydrocephalus, or diffuse cerebrovascular disease, who are unable to walk, gegenhalten may be the only abnormal sign on examination of the legs when the patient is recumbent. Such patients may be able to perform other leg movements such as the heel–shin test or make bicycling movements of the legs when lying on a bed. Patients with spastic paraplegia caused by hereditary spastic paraplegia, cerebral palsy (Little's disease), or cervical spondylotic myelopathy may exhibit only minor increases in muscle tone when examined supine but have profound leg spasticity when walking.

The remainder of the conventional neurological examination will often provide important clues to the underlying cause of the gait disturbance, for example, a resting tremor in Parkinson's disease. Careful examination of the ocular movements may also reveal a vertical supranuclear gaze palsy in Steele–Richardson–Olszewski syndrome or nystagmus and abnormal pursuit and saccadic movements in cerebellar disease (see Chapters 7 and 11).

Elderly patients with walking difficulties and falls often have signs of multiple deficits. The most common are cervical spondylotic myelopathy with a mild spastic paraparesis and peripheral neuropathy with impaired proprioception.[7] Furthermore, visual and hearing loss also may be evident. The presence of multiple sensory deficits may combine to produce imbalance and an insecure gait.[8]

Finally, the evaluation of the history and physical signs will then guide further investigation to confirm the anatomical basis for the gait syndrome and where possible, the underlying pathology.

REFERENCES

1. Thompson PD, Marsden CD. Walking disorders. In: Bradley WG, Daroff RB, Fenichel GM, Marsden CD, eds. *Neurology in clinical practice*, 3rd edn. Boston: Butterworth Heinemann, 2000;341–54.
2. Day BL, Steiger MJ, Thompson PD, Marsden CD. Influence of vision and stance width on human body movements when standing: implications for afferent control of lateral sway. *J Physiol* 1993;**469**:479–99.
3. Elble RJ, Moody C, Leffler K, Sinha R. The initiation of normal walking. *Mov Disord* 1994;**9**:139–46.
4. Atchison PR, Thompson PD, Frackowiak RSJ, Marsden CD. The syndrome of isolated gait ignition failure: a report of six cases. *Mov Disord* 1993;**8**:285–92.
5. Koller WC, Trimble J. The gait abnormality of Huntington's disease. *Neurology* 1985;**35**:1450–4.
6. Nutt JG, Marsden CD, Thompson PD. Human walking and higher level gait disorders, particularly in the elderly. *Neurology* 1993;**43**:268–79.
7. Sudarsky L, Ronthal M. Gait disorders among elderly patients: a survey of 50 patients. *Arch Neurol* 1983;**40**:740–3.
8. Drachman D, Hart C. An approach to the dizzy patient. *Neurology* 1972:**22**:323–34.

7

Neuro-otological assessment in the patient with balance and gait disorder

ADOLFO M. BRONSTEIN, MICHAEL A. GRESTY AND PETER RUDGE

INTRODUCTION

Symptoms of vertigo/dizziness and related off-balance sensations are some of the commonest in general medical practice and neurology. When a patient reports episodes of frank vertigo in which they feel that they or the world is spinning, a clinician is correct to consider vestibular disease as a likely diagnosis. Patients reporting that they feel unsteady on their feet or afraid of walking outdoors unaided may also suffer from a vestibular disorder. However, even when there is in the background a history of clear cut rotational vertiginous episodes, but even worse when there is no such past history, attaining a certain diagnosis can be difficult. Matters are complicated further by the fact that that patients with long-standing vertiginous symptoms become anxious, a feature that can frequently impede the possibility of achieving a firm diagnosis. An accurate neuro-otological examination can help to identify if the cause of a balance disorder is due to dysfunction of the vestibular system. The problem of falls in vestibular disease is discussed in Chapter 9.

SYMPTOMS OF VESTIBULAR ORIGIN

Dysfunction of the vestibular system causes some of the most distressing symptoms encountered in neurology, yet the signs engendered may be difficult to detect and patients are often considered to have a functional disorder. A careful analysis of the symptoms, especially their evolution, and determination of factors that alter them, is the key to the correct formulation, diagnosis and treatment. Several general points need to be made.

First, the vestibular system comprises components that detect angular (semicircular canal) and linear (otolith organ) acceleration. Further, the former are arranged to detect angular acceleration in the three cardinal planes (sagittal, coronal or torsional, and horizontal) such that derangement of one part can cause symptoms related to that plane. It is important to note the greater development of the vertical canal system compared with the horizontal one in primates that assume a more vertical posture, especially as most of the tests used to detect abnormality of the semicircular canals are concerned with the horizontal pair not with the four vertical ones.[1] It is easy to assume that signaling from the semicircular canals is normal on the basis of tests of the horizontal canal alone when in fact there may be profound dysfunction in the vertical plane. Second, alteration of otolith function can cause profound symptoms yet be dismissed because the patient does not have 'true vertigo'. Third, the patient with vestibular disturbance may complain of visual symptoms, either because of failure of the vestibulo-ocular reflex (VOR), or because of mismatch between the visual and vestibular input. Fourth, dysfunction of the vestibular system may comprise failure of function (e.g. vestibular neuronitis) or excessive activity (e.g. Ménière's syndrome in the acute phase). Since the bilaterally paired vestibular system works in a push–pull fashion these two basic types of pathology cause markedly different signs, namely, the direction of the spontaneous nystagmus. Finally, but certainly not of least importance, in the majority of patients vestibular dysfunction arises peripherally and is therefore commonly associated with auditory symptoms. Assessment of hearing is mandatory in the patient with vestibular symptoms, as is a full history of previous neurological and general disorders. Major errors are made by failing to look at the whole patient and merely dealing with a symptom as if it automatically directed the clinician to, for example, the ear. Vestibular dysfunction can occur anywhere between the otic capsule and the temporal lobe.

Symptoms induced by unilateral loss of vestibular function

Acute unilateral vestibular failure is terrifying. The patient is smitten with severe vertigo, imbalance, nausea and vomiting, prostration, and a fear of impending doom. Initially, the vertigo can be so severe that it is impossible for the patient to determine its direction but, in general, in total unilateral failure the world appears to rotate towards the side opposite from that affected (i.e. right vestibular failure causes rotation of the world to the left). This is because loss of vestibular function on one side leaves the contralateral horizontal canal totally unopposed. The eyes are thus driven slowly towards the damaged side by the remaining intact semicircular canal system (see also Chapter 9). Since vision is suppressed during the fast phase of the nystagmus, the world appears to rotate to the side opposite the affected ear (e.g. right vestibular failure causes rotation of the visual world to the left and of course nystagmus to that side, i.e. fast phase nystagmus to the left). Occasionally, a patient may complain of rotation in some other plane, either vertically, such that the world is scrolling like the failure of the vertical hold on the TV screen or torsionally in the roll or coronal plane like a rotating wheel. Static tilt is less common (e.g. the world seems to lean to one side); this is presumably due to otolith dysfunction (see below). During the initial acute phase of vertigo, some patients say they are unconscious but if questioned carefully they usually say they can hear but cannot see. Why the occasional patient says this is unclear but it is unlikely that patients with acute vestibular failure are truly unconscious for more than a few seconds, perhaps as part of a vestibularly-triggered syncopal episode.

The severe vertigo can last several days and is usually accompanied by nausea, retching and vomiting. The patient is most comfortable lying down and tends to lie on the affected side. Head movement accentuates the symptoms. Initially, the patient may be unable to sit and falls backwards on rising or to one side, usually to that of the affected ear. After 1 or 2 days they can usually stand but need support to walk, often clinging on to furniture and holding their heads absolutely still in an attempt to fixate objects. Removal of fixation may lead to a fall. This can occur in everyday activities such as washing the face, when the patient often falls into the basin and frequently strikes one of the numerous ceramic edifices found in bathrooms, thereby compounding their vestibular problem by a head injury. They tend to veer to the side of the lesion when walking. Over the next few days they gradually recover: the nausea and vomiting settle after a day or two, the vertigo lessens and the gait becomes more confident. At this stage, some patients say that the world no longer spins but may feel that their head does. Finally, the patient recovers but may still complain of not feeling totally normal, often using colloquial expressions to describe these feelings (e.g. 'they feel drunk', 'not with it', 'detached from reality', 'as if they are on a boat', etc.). They may still complain of being very unsteady with their eyes closed.

The above describes the typical symptoms of a patient with an acute vestibular hypofunction. Similar symptoms occur with acute excessive vestibular stimulation but the rotation of the world is of course in the opposite sense. In Ménière's disease there does seem to be some irritative over-stimulation of vestibular apparatus on occasions, hence the direction of the nystagmus is an unreliable indicator of the side involved. In general, however, the duration of vertigo in these cases is short-lived and does not exceed 24 h.

Effect of visual input on vertigo and imbalance

There are complex connections between the retina and the vestibular system, especially in the vestibular nucleus and via the cerebellum, information that updates the vestibular system and enables compensation to occur following vestibular injury or altered input (e.g. during space travel, dancing and ice skating). It should therefore come as no surprise that visual input can cause vertigo or similar symptoms. Many patients with acute vestibular failure prefer to keep their eyes closed to reduce the mismatch between the vestibular and visual systems. Conversely, some patients attempt to increase input from a normal sensory system to compensate for the perceived disturbance. A good example of this is the comfort given to astronauts subjected to gross utricular/semicircular canal mismatch and loss of relevant visual input, by wedging themselves into a seat to attain somatosensory information. Similarly, the motion-sick patient on a boat or in a car will try to remove inappropriate visual input by fixating an earth-bound target; this may be one of the reasons why sailors group on deck if they are sea sick and why drivers of cars are motion sick much less frequently than passengers, especially those in rear seats.

The symptoms of patients with abnormal vestibulo-visual interaction are characteristically related to visual input. The majority find that it is excessive visual motion input that causes most trouble. Thus, optokinetic stimuli make the patient feel disoriented, vertiginous, or unbalanced, a syndrome sometimes called visual vertigo.[2,3] Classic examples of this phenomenon are the patient who cannot walk around a supermarket between the ranks of bottles and cans on either side, a phenomenon certainly worsened by the strobing effect of fluorescent lighting, and the difficulty some people have in ironing striped shirts. Other patients find that cars or people passing by result in a feeling of disorientation and imbalance, and that escalators, especially when passing down a narrow tube, are difficult to negotiate. These symptoms may be so severe that the patients are nauseated with the input. Exceptionally, reading is impossible as it induces the symptom; this phenomenon is more frequent in those using computer screens and word processors, again perhaps due to the strobing effect of the CRT or scrolling of text. Many vestibular patients with such increased sensitivity to visual stimuli have a great deal of anxiety but the physician should not prejudice the diagnosis without appropriate investigations.[3,4]

The converse of this syndrome is occasionally seen. While it is appreciated that removal of visual input in patients with vestibular failure can cause unsteadiness, as described above, some patients complain that they are unable to drive a car in visually impoverished environments as they feel disoriented or even vertiginous. Typically, this occurs in drivers on open motorways and is presumably due to some mismatch between the vestibular and visual inputs in patients using this form of transportation.[5] Some say they are better at certain velocities and others complain of difficulties on broaching a hill or traversing a bend. Oddly, the symptoms usually worsen and the patient tends to drive more and more slowly, finally foregoing the convenience of a vertigo-inducing motorway for the more conventional small roads. Interestingly, a similar hypersensitivity to visual stimuli to that present in patients with visual vertigo can be demonstrated in these 'dizzy' drivers.[3]

Effect of position on vertigo and imbalance

It is most important to determine the effect of position upon vertigo; in particular to see if the vertigo is only induced in certain positions or if existing vertigo and imbalance is altered by such a position. We have already mentioned that head movement worsens vertigo induced by vestibular failure. The Hallpike maneuver in which the patient is placed supine with one or other ear down, can induce vertigo and nystagmus both of benign positional type or of central type (see below and Chapters 9 and 17). From a symptomatic point of view, asking the patient if there is a position of the head that induces the vertigo is extremely valuable. Many patients will say that extension of the neck or looking up (e.g. fixing curtains, or hanging out washing) causes vertigo in its various forms. Further questioning, however, will reveal a subset that have benign positional vertigo; this may be preceded by other forms of vertigo. The symptom recurs in certain circumstances, especially lying down to go to sleep, or on turning in bed. Patients are usually terrified and have often adopted maneuvers to avoid inducing the symp-

tom, such as always lying on the unaffected side – ironically, a practice that tends to perpetuate the problem. Others note that positioning the head while at work may induce an attack (e.g. a car mechanic cannot look under a vehicle). As a general principle the greater the induced vertigo, the less sinister the cause. Certainly, patients with central positional nystagmus rarely complain of vertigo even though their nystagmus is marked. Patients that feel off-balance on looking up are more likely to have a positional vertigo of labyrinthine origin than vertebro-basilar circulatory disorders or cervical vertigo.[6] It is amazing how many patients are given these exotic, more theoretical than practical diagnoses, without having being examined for positional vertigo.

Oscillopsia

'Objective' vertigo in which the patients see the world rotating, is in a sense an example of oscillopsia. However, traditionally, oscillopsia is a term used to indicate apparent to-and-fro movement of the world. It can occur in a variety of conditions including total vestibular failure, abnormality of VOR suppression, and in certain forms of nystagmus.[7]

The VOR may have an abnormally high or abnormally low gain; both of these abnormalities will result in failure of accurate foveation during head movements.[8] In the case of low gain (e.g. loss of vestibular function due to aminoglycoside antibiotics), movement of the head will not cause sufficient corrective movement of the eyes. Conversely, in certain central nervous system (CNS) disorders such as multiple sclerosis (MS) with cerebellar involvement the VOR gain is too high, again resulting in slippage of the image upon the retina. The patients complain of visual blurring or oscillopsia precipitated by head movement. Characteristically, they will say that, on walking, objects either bounce in the vertical plane or, more commonly, they cannot read the numbers on buses or recognize friends until they stand still. Much of the oscillopsia is attributable to loss of canal–ocular reflexes but it has been demonstrated that loss of the otolith–ocular component of compensatory reflexes also contributes in part to the disability.[9] Curiously, nausea does not usually occur during oscillopsia. A patient with gait instability worsened in the dark and oscillopsia on walking or running needs formal vestibular testing. The gait instability in patients with bilateral idiopathic vestibular failure can be slight.[10]

Certain forms of nystagmus can also induce oscillopsia. This particularly applies to vertical upbeat and to a lesser extent downbeat nystagmus and also pendular nystagmus.[11] The patient may find certain positions of the head lessen the oscillopsia. For example, reading can be extremely difficult in these circumstances and patients with vertical nystagmus may find a head position that lessens the oscillopsia, and on examination, the nystagmus. This position may be entirely dependent on eye position or due to alteration of otolith stimulation. For example, some patients with downbeat nystagmus find that their ability to read is improved by lying prone since, in a substantial proportion of these patients, otolith input does alter the nystagmus. Similarly oscillopsia due to downbeat nystagmus is typically worse on looking to one side, a maneuver that increases the nystagmus. Patients with pendular nystagmus, which usually causes intractable oscillopsia and can be more marked in one eye than the other, may find they are better if their temperature is low when the cause is MS or with alcohol ingestion.[12]

Auditory symptoms

Any history obtained from the vertiginous patient is inadequate if it does not include a thorough interrogation for auditory symptoms. Impairment of hearing, its evolution, and associated auditory symptoms are an essential part of the history since there is a close anatomical relationship between the vestibular apparatus and cochlea peripherally, and between the afferent (VIII nerve) fibers. Once the pathways enter the CNS they diverge and are less likely to be simultaneously involved.

In any vertiginous or imbalanced patient it is vital to enquire whether there is an associated hearing impairment, especially if it is unilateral, whether there is tinnitus, and whether there is any alteration in the auditory symptoms with the vertigo and imbalance, especially if the symptoms are episodic. Patients with Ménière's disease and Ménière's syndrome usually have auditory symptoms with fullness in the affected ear, fluctuating tinnitus and hearing loss, with attacks of vertigo lasting up to 24 h. On the other hand patients with cerebello-pontine (CP) angle lesions tend to have progressive impairment of hearing and mild unsteadiness but no true vertigo except in the case of secondary vascular involvement.

A rare but important symptom is the unsteadiness and vertigo induced by sound – the 'Tullio phenomenon'. Patients find that they are pushed to one side by sudden noise in one ear (Chapter 9).[13] This may be frequency specific and can be accompanied by sound-induced eye movements. Exceptionally, such symptoms can be precipitated by pressure on the ear if there is a fistula.

Diplopia and tilt

Some patients with vestibular failure do not complain of rotation of the world or of the head but perceive the world to be tilted. This may be in the roll (frontal) plane or alternatively they may feel that the earth is coming up to meet them or receding from them. The symptom may be continuous or episodic. These symptoms may imply otolith or vertical semicircular canal abnormality.[14,15]

It is important to enquire whether diplopia is present in patients who are unsteady or have vertigo and, if present, whether it is present with just one eye open or not to exclude ocular abnormalities. It is also important to determine whether the diplopia is horizontal or vertical or tilted. Some patients with otolith or brainstem abnormalities do indeed have a skew deviation and this may be symptomatic (skew diplopia). Occasionally, a patient with an internuclear ophthalmoplegia may notice that their diplopia only occurs when they look to one side and that it is transient. This is because of the disconjugate movement of the eyes. This rare phenomenon is an extremely useful point in the history as such patients commonly are imbalanced.

CLINICAL EXAMINATION

Introduction

Despite the progress made in clinical and research vestibular techniques, any sensible clinician should ensure that there are no cranial nerve or long tract or cerebellar signs in a patient with a presumed peripheral vestibular disorder. Involvement of the cranial nerves of the CP angle (V, VI, VII and VIII), or intra-axial brain stem signs should rule out the diagnosis of labyrinthine disease. A full description of the general neurological examination in patients with balance or gait disorders is given in Chapter 6. In the context of a patient with unsteady gait, emphasis on vestibular and ocular examination should be placed in the presence of dizziness, vertigo, lateropulsion, retropulsion, unsteadiness in the dark, head movement induced unsteadiness, oscillopsia, diplopia and auditory dysfunction.

Gait and Romberg test

In the context of vestibular disease, gait and the Romberg test should be systematically examined. As a rule of thumb, a truly positive Romberg (i.e. someone who falls on eye closure) does not have unilateral peripheral vestibular disorder unless observed in the very acute stage of the disease. In this case, they veer or tend to fall towards the side of the lesion, particularly on eye closure. Milder or long-standing cases may show a deviation to the side of the lesion if asked to walk with eyes closed or during the Untenberger test (that is, during marching on the spot with eyes closed). Patients with long-standing bilateral absence of vestibular function can appear fairly normal during a Romberg test unless, in addition to closing their eyes, they stand on a mattress or foam which reduces the accuracy of lower limb proprioception. Acutely (e.g. after a meningitis or ototoxicity) they veer severely in any direction. Postural reflexes, as investigated by pulls or pushes to the trunk for basal ganglia disorders (see Chapter 11) are preserved in vestibular patients but a higher level of unsteadiness can be observed, particularly with the eyes closed. To summarize, unilateral acute vestibular failure will show ipsilateral lateropulsion and probable falls on eye closure. In more compensated stages, patients may show only ipsilateral gait deviation when walking with eyes closed or during the Unterberger test. Patients with acute bilateral vestibular loss will suffer severe difficulty in standing up unaided and may be unable to walk. In compensated stages there may be some unsteadiness on conventional Romberg testing, but the problem will become very severe if standing or attempting to walk on a mattress. In general, heel-to-toe walking will worsen any vestibular gait but not as much as in cerebellar gait ataxia.

Eyes and ears

The eyes and the ears should be carefully examined. Otoscopy should be carried out in all patients with vestibular symptoms, searching for signs of otological disease (suppuration, perforations and cholesteatoma) but also to make sure there is no wax in the external canal which will interfere with investigations such as caloric test or audiometry. (Contrary to what some text books assert, we have never seen a vertiginous syndrome caused by wax in the external canal.)

A clinical examination of ocular motility can be performed in a relatively short time if it is done systematically. A complete examination should include at least the following points which relate to specific ocular motor functions:

- search for spontaneous nystagmus in the vertical and horizontal planes
- convergence;
- smooth pursuit;
- saccades and gaze limitations;
- doll's head (vestibular) eye movements; and
- positional nystagmus.

The ocular-motor system shows well segregated functions subserved by varied anatomical structures (for review see Carpenter).[16] Thus, selective involvement of one system while sparing of others is not a rare occurrence (for a review see Leigh and Zee)[17] Before describing details it should be said that, as a general rule, peripheral vestibular disorders show no abnormality of eye movements unless acute, when spontaneous nystagmus can be observed. In contrast, central vestibular disorders (i.e. brainstem or cerebellar disease) usually show a variety of 'central' eye movement signs including nystagmus, broken pursuit and slow or dysmetric saccades.

Examination of nystagmus

GENERAL CHARACTERISTICS

When assessing a nystagmus it has to be ascertained whether there is a direction of beat. Jerk or saw-tooth nystagmus comprises alternating fast and slow phases in opposing directions. Nystagmus is described in terms of the direction of beat of the fast phase (right/left, up/down) and its intensity (usually described as first degree when visible only with gaze deviation in the beat direction, second degree when present in primary gaze and third degree when it is even visible during gaze deviation in the direction opposite to the beat direction). Pendular nystagmus, an oscillation of the eye without fast phases, and saccadic ocular oscillations, in which there are no slow-phase components, will also be briefly discussed; they are always of central origin.

HORIZONTAL NYSTAGMUS

Clear spontaneous nystagmus in peripheral vestibular disorders is more likely to be seen in general or emergency medicine than in specialized clinics as lesions need to be acute. It can be observed during the first few days in vestibular neuritis or in an acute episode of Ménière's disease. It is mainly horizontal, or with a superimposed torsional component, and it beats away from the hypofunctioning labyrinth (in the irritative phase of Ménière's disease it can beat towards the affected ear, i.e. beats towards the side of the acute tinnitus). After a few days it may be seen as first-degree nystagmus (i.e. nystagmus only present with gaze deviation in the direction of the nystagmus) or with removal of optic fixation (e.g. Frenzel's glasses, infrared viewers or oculography), particularly after vigorous head-shaking. As a general rule, this is the only type of spontaneous nystagmus which can be seen in patients with peripheral vestibular disorders. Large-amplitude nystagmus, particularly in patients with neither acute nor intense vertiginous symptoms, or any nystagmus which is not mainly horizontal must, in principle, be considered as of central origin.

Occasionally, patients with structural brainstem disease, such as Arnold Chiari malformation or small vascular/demyelinating lesions, can show primary gaze horizontal nystagmus; in the acute phase the latter patients feel vertiginous and unsteady, thus mimicking a picture of a vestibular neuritis (Chapter 9). Patients with congenital nystagmus show large horizontal ocular oscillations and do not report vertigo or oscillopsia (see below). Gaze paretic nystagmus, which is due to the inability to maintain eccentric gaze, appears in lesions of the cerebellum or brainstem–cerebellar connections when subjects look in the same direction as the lesion. In extensive or degenerative lesions, gaze paretic nystagmus occurs when looking in any direction. Lesions of the medial longitudinal fasciculus, which connects the abducens (VI) nucleus with the contralateral III cranial nerve nucleus (medial rectus motoneurons), provoke the picture of internuclear ophthalmoplegia.[18,19] This consists of limitation or slowing of the adducting eye on the side of the lesion combined with nystagmus of the abducting eye (dissociated, ataxic or abducting nystagmus). Bilateral internuclear ophthalmoplegia, frequently seen in multiple sclerosis, is often associated with up-beat nystagmus.

VERTICAL NYSTAGMUS

We should distinguish between upwards and downwards directed beating in vertical nystagmus. Downbeat nystagmus, that is primary gaze or second-degree downbeat nystagmus, is a common occurrence in Arnold Chiari malformations and cerebellar atrophy, although in about one-third of patients a clear diagnosis cannot be reached.[20,21] Upbeat nystagmus in primary gaze is less common but it can be seen in various intra-axial, midline brainstem lesions such as tumors or granulomas.[22,23]

TORSIONAL (OR ROTATORY) NYSTAGMUS

This nystagmus is a rotation of the eye, beating around the visual axis. The direction of beat should preferably be specified in right–left terms to avoid confusion: thus 'anticlockwise' nystagmus as seen from the examiner's view, in which the upper pole of the eye beats towards the right shoulder of the patient, should be called right-beating torsional nystagmus. It is usually caused by a lesion in the area of the vestibular nuclei on the opposite side to the beat direction, as in Wallenberg syndrome or demyelinating lesions, in the floor of the fourth ventricle.[24]

PENDULAR NYSTAGMUS

This nystagmus can be seen in association with long-standing or congenital visual defects, in which case it is not necessarily associated with balance or gait disorders, or it can develop weeks to months after structural brainstem disease. The latter case is of interest here as patients usually show cerebellar or pyramidal features or other cranial tremors (e.g. palatal myoclonus) and are considerably disabled.[25–27] These patients describe debilitating oscillopsia which, unlike that seen in peripheral or central vestibular disorders, is largely unchanged (and occasionally improved) by head movements. The nystagmus is frequently in different planes (horizontal, vertical, torsional) and magnitude in the two eyes and complex movement trajectories (ellipses) are common. It would appear that interruption of dentato-rubro-thalamic projections to the inferior olive is the cause of this nystag-

mus. The most common etiologies are demyelinating and vascular lesions of the brainstem.

SACCADIC OCULAR OSCILLATIONS

The commonest of saccadic oscillations is square-wave jerks, in which the eyes jump away from, and immediately come back to, the fixation point provided by the examiner. Generally, square waves are asymptomatic. Unfortunately, they are not a very specific finding and, furthermore, their presence increases in the normal elderly.[28] Abnormally large numbers of square waves are seen in a number of neurological disorders which include gait disorder, such as Steele–Richardson syndrome and cerebellar lesions, particularly in the dorsal vermis.[29] Unlike square-wave jerks, ocular flutter – horizontal back to back saccades without an intersaccadic interval – and opsoclonus ('dancing eyes') – a chaotic combination of back to back saccades in all planes – indicate beyond any doubt the existence of posterior fossa disease. Both can be seen in encephalitis, demyelinating or paraneoplastic brainstem disease.[17] Unfortunately, it is sometimes difficult to distinguish voluntary nystagmus from flutter. Voluntary nystagmus also consists of saccades without an interval but usually occurs during attempting convergence in patients with an otherwise normal neurological examination, is frequently associated with convergence spasm (or other non-organic features), and usually cannot be maintained for more than a few tens of seconds.[30,31]

POSITIONAL NYSTAGMUS

Many forms of nystagmus due to CNS lesions show modulation or even direction reversal when examined in different orientations of the head with respect to the gravitational vertical (Fig. 7.1). This testifies to an otolith component in its mechanism,[32] emphasized in downbeat nystagmus.[20,33] Diagnosis and treatment of peripheral positional vertigo (benign paroxysmal positional nystagmus, BPPV) is discussed in Chapters 9 and 17. The distinction criteria between BPPV and central positional nystagmus can be found in Table 7.1. In general, any nystagmus during the Hallpike maneuver which does not strictly conform to the classical description of BPPV (mainly torsional nystagmus beating to the undermost ear with a latency period, limited duration, and habitua-

Table 7.1 *Distinction criteria between benign paroxysmal positioning vertigo and central positional nystagmus*

	Benign paroxysmal type	Central type
Latent period	2–20 s	None
Adaptation	Disappears in 50 s	Persists
Fatigability	Disappears on repetition	Persists
Vertigo	Always present	Typically absent
Direction of nystagmus	To undermost ear	Variable
Incidence	Relatively common	Relatively uncommon

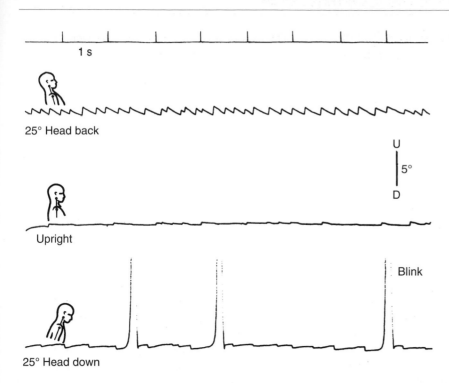

Figure 7.1 *Direction-changing vertical nystagmus in a patient with incipient cerebellar degeneration and slight gait disorder. Note that in the upright position of the head no convincing nystagmus was detected, stressing the importance of looking for positional nystagmus in patients with a disorder of balance or gait.*

tion) should be treated with suspicion that it may be of central origin. Patients should be warned before conducting the Hallpike maneuver that they may experience intense vertigo but that they must not close their eyes, otherwise the diagnostic opportunity may be lost.

OSCILLOPSIA CAUSED BY SACCADIC OSCILLATIONS AND NYSTAGMUS

Not infrequently patients are referred for neuro-otological investigations because of complaints of oscillopsia. This may be caused by involuntary eye movements such as ocular 'flutter', voluntary nystagmus and downbeat nystagmus, as well as being a symptom of vestibular failure. In such cases it is of importance to establish whether the oscillopsia is secondary to the presence of abnormal eye movements (e.g. nystagmus) or occurs only when the head is moved (e.g. while walking), in which case it is likely to be caused by bilateral failure of vestibular function. It is important to be aware that oscillopsia can be caused by minute involuntary eye movements that may only be visible on fundoscopy or high-resolution eye movement recordings.[34,35]

Examination of eye movements

Conjugate eye movements belong to two basic types, slow or fast. Slow-phase eye movements allow continuous fixation of a target that moves (smooth pursuit and slow phase of optokinetic nystagmus) or that remains stationary while the head moves (vestibulo-ocular reflex). Fast eye movements allow shifting gaze from one object to another (refixation saccades or quick phases of vestibular or opto-

kinetic nystagmus). In addition, convergence–divergence complements conjugate eye movements so that images from the two eyes fall on corresponding areas of the two retinas. Eye movement abnormalities in movement disorder patients, most of whom will have balance and gait disorders, have been reviewed.[36,37]

SMOOTH PURSUIT

When examining pursuit eye movements it is vital to obtain patient cooperation and attention. Sometimes unorthodox targets (key rings, cash notes or photographs) can 'normalize' apparently abnormal pursuit movements. The examiner must inspect the eyes in a well-lit room, from a close distance, at not too great a target speed, and be familiar with the fact that pursuit performance decays with age, inattention, alcohol and many neuropharmacological agents. When pursuit mechanisms are insufficient, small saccades catch up with the target so that performance is also evaluated by a more or less saccadic appearance during ocular following ('cog-wheel or broken-up pursuit'). Pursuit pathways are widespread in the CNS, including the parietal lobes, the cerebellum and brainstem; unilateral abnormalities tend to be ipsilateral (i.e. right parietal or cerebellar lesion causes rightwards abnormal pursuit). The link between smooth pursuit and optokinetic (OK) eye movements will be briefly discussed under electro-oculography (EOG) later, but for all practical purposes it suffices to say that, when investigated with a small drum, there usually is good correlation between abnormalities in these two tests; reduced pursuit in one direction is correlated with reduced optokinesis in the same direction. Since OK findings are expressed in terms of the fast phases of the OK nystagmus, hypoactive (broken up) pursuit to the right is normally associated with a directional preponderance of OK nystagmus to the right.

SACCADES

When we shift our eyes from one object to another we are using saccades at speeds frequently greater than 300°/s. The high neural firing rates required to produce such eye motion are generated in the reticular formation of the brainstem and then transmitted to the oculomotor nuclei. Saccades can be examined by providing two targets, for example the examiner's own fingers, and prompting the patient verbally to look right/left or up/down between these two targets (Fig. 7.2). Speed and accuracy should be assessed.

Slow saccades can be seen in involvement of the reticular formation and the oculomotor nuclei, nerves or muscles.[19,38,39] It is clinical context which allows topographical diagnosis: a patient with unilateral slowing of saccades and ipsilateral sensory-motor facial symptoms can only have a pontine lesion whereas another with pan-saccadic slowing, no focal brainstem signs and evidence of muscle disease elsewhere will be diagnosed as ocular myopathy.

Accuracy of saccades is assessed by observing if the patient consistently overshoots or undershoots the target (easily recognizable by the presence of corrective saccades towards the target). A small corrective saccade following a hypometric saccade, particularly if it occurs symmetrically, is normal. Hypometric saccades are a common but not very specific finding in a number of CNS disorders; in hemispheric disease hypometric saccades occur in the direction opposite that of the lesion. In disorders of the frontal lobes and the basal ganglia, difficulty in initiating saccades and hypometria can be seen under specific testing conditions, such as when patients have to move their eyes voluntary, without a target, or repetitively between two targets at will (self-paced saccades) (see Fig. 7.2).[36,37] These findings illustrate that in certain neurological conditions (usually accompanied by gait disorder) the brainstem saccadic generators are in working order but the more complex processes preceding brainstem activation are at fault. Hypermetric saccades are a less common but more valuable sign as these are probably pathognomonic for lesions in the fastigial nuclei or dorsal vermis of the cerebellum (Fig. 7.3).[40]

DOLL'S HEAD MANEUVER AND VOR SUPPRESSION

If a patient is asked to fixate on a target, say the examiner's nose, while their head or whole body is oscillated, they should produce a smooth eye movement in the opposite direction to the head (Fig. 7.4). This 'doll's eyes' response is due to the VOR, which allows the eyes to remain stable in space during head movements. In the clinical context of the patient with balance or gait disor-

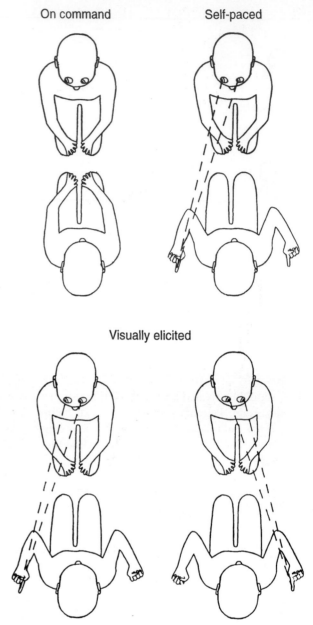

Figure 7.2 *Diagram to illustrate various ways of clinically eliciting saccadic eye movements. Patients with basal ganglia or frontal disorders may show difficulty in initiating saccades and 'multiple step' saccades when the eye movements are in response to a verbal command (e.g. 'just look right or left when I say') or self-paced (e.g. repetitive saccades between the examiner's fingers while they are continuously shown to the patient), but can be normal during saccades to suddenly appearing visual targets (e.g. flicking of the examiner's fingers). When saccades are abnormal because of posterior fossa disease, slowness or dysmetria will be apparent in all modalities.*

der, the doll's head maneuver is conducted with two purposes. First, to investigate the VOR clinically in a patient suspected of having a vestibular disorder. If movements of the head in one direction elicit 'jerky' eye movements, with catch-up saccades, it is likely that the VOR is

(a)

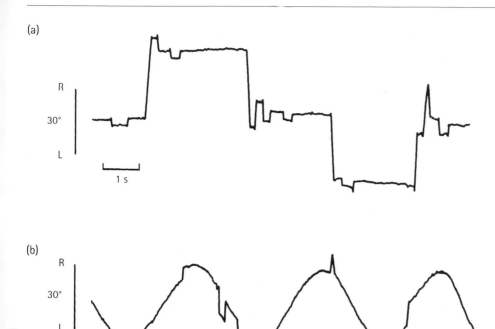

(b)

(b) R 30° L — 1 s

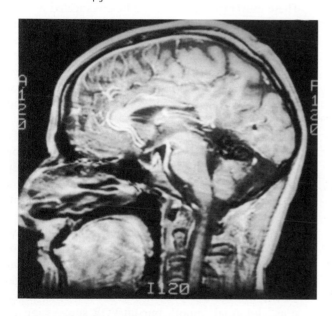

Figure 7.3 *Electro-oculographic recordings in a patient with a dorso-vermal cerebellar lesion (initially thought to be a vascular malformation but later confirmed to be hemosiderosis). Note the hypermetria (overshoots) during saccadic refixations (a). In this particular patient slow-phase eye movements (see sinusoidal pursuit, (b) were not significantly impaired, indicative of relative sparing of floculo-nodular structures. (Slightly modified from ref. 42.)*

hypoactive in the direction of head movement, indicating a vestibular lesion on that same side. Severe bilateral vestibular loss usually produces catch-up saccades with movements in any direction. This procedure can be made more sensitive by moving the patient's head while observing the optic disk by ophthalmoscopy.[41] While observing the disk also note if there is any spontaneous nystagmus but remember that you are examining the back of the eye and, hence, a left-beating nystagmus with the ophthalmoscope is in fact a right-beating nystagmus. If the head movement is very brisk, Halmagyi and Curthoys[43] point out that one can confidently diagnose semicircular canal paresis on the basis of the saccadic compensatory movements observed. In chronic and subtotal vestibular lesions this is not always possible.

Second, the doll's maneuver is applied in patients with certain basal ganglia disease (Steele–Richardson's syndrome and multiple system atrophies; see Chapter 11)[37] or brainstem disorders to establish if a gaze limitation is caused by involvement of the oculomotor nuclei, fasciculi or muscles (nuclear–infranuclear) or supranuclear. Since prenuclear vestibulo-ocular pathways are distinct from voluntary ocular motor pathways, a gaze limitation which is overcome by doll's head maneuver is, by definition, of supranuclear origin.

Normally, the VOR needs to be suppressed in circumstances when we want to keep fixation on objects that move with us (e.g. reading a newspaper we are holding while we walk or travel inside a moving vehicle). If there were no VOR suppression the eyes would hopelessly move

VOR

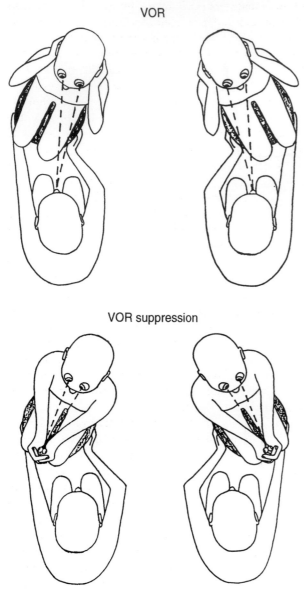

VOR suppression

Figure 7.4 *Clinical examination of the vestibulo-ocular reflex (VOR). Normally this is done by the 'doll's head maneuver' but in patients unable to relax the neck, oscillation of the whole body on a swivel chair should be attempted. Patients are instructed to hold the head fixed to the body and to fixate the examiner's nose. During examination of VOR suppression, patients should fixate their own thumbs.*

away from one's newspaper every time the car in which one was sitting turned. Such suppression is achieved by visuo-motor mechanisms identical or very similar to smooth pursuit. Clinically, VOR suppression can be investigated by asking subjects to fixate on a target held with their teeth (e.g. a ruler or tongue depressor) while their head is oscillated voluntarily or passively by the examiner at a frequency of 0.2–0.3 Hz (1 cycle every 2–3 s).[44] Figure 7.4 shows clinical ways of testing doll's head (VOR) and VOR suppression. The eyes are carefully examined during this oscillation. Normally, the eyes remain fairly still on

the target. In the presence of central lesion VOR suppression is affected and a clear nystagmus beating in the same direction of the head turn can be easily observed. The VOR suppression should be investigated in patients in whom the distinction between a peripheral or central vestibular disorder is not clear. Peripheral patients show normal VOR suppression whereas patients with brainstem–cerebellar lesions usually show clear abnormalities. Such abnormalities are clinically well correlated with pursuit defects (i.e. a right cerebellar lesion will produce abnormal pursuit and abnormal VOR suppression during rightwards motion of the visual stimulus or of the head). This co-directionality is explained by the fact that, during rightwards rotation, the eyes deviate slowly to the left due to the VOR; rightwards pursuit eye movements are therefore used to foveate the target during the rotation. If pursuit is insufficient the VOR cannot be counteracted and the target is re-foveated by saccades, giving rise to a nystagmic pattern.

VERGENCE MOVEMENTS

These movements also need to be investigated with targets able to attract the patient's attention. The patient's own thumb, perhaps because of additional proprioceptive cues, is particularly useful. Reduced convergence is, however, common in subjects over the age of 50–60 years and in patients with minor subclinical squints (exophorias). With these provisos, absent convergence indicates midbrain dysfunction.

In summary, examination of the eye movements is an essential step in the assessment of the patient with a balance or gait disorder. Most patients with a peripheral vestibular disorder will be normal or only show a first-degree nystagmus of low amplitude. The nystagmus may become larger, or be present only on head shaking or when examined with Frenzel's glasses. Patients with brainstem lesions may show slow saccades, abnormal pursuit/VOR suppression and vertical, horizontal or torsional nystagmus. Cerebellar disorder patients may have gaze paretic nystagmus, spontaneous down-beating nystagmus, abnormal smooth pursuit/VOR suppression and hypermetric saccades. Patients with hemispheric lesions may have contralaterally directed hypometric saccades and ipsilaterally abnormal pursuit. In fronto-basal ganglia disease, saccadic abnormalities may have to be investigated with special saccadic paradigms clinically (e.g. self-paced or voluntary 'on command' saccades), or on recordings (anticipatory saccades, remembered saccades).

Clinical assessment of hearing

Hearing must always be assessed in patients with a history suggesting that the cause of a balance disorder may be in the labyrinth, VIII nerve or the brainstem. Conventional techniques included in the general neurological examination can initially be applied, for example ask the patient to repeat muttered words to one ear or to estimate the distance at which the rubbing of fingers can be heard from each ear. Tuning fork tests are useful to distinguish between conductive and sensori-neural hearing loss but neurologists should be aware that false results are common with tuning forks of low frequency (64 or 128 Hz). In a patient with suspected neuro-otological disease, specialized hearing tests should be obtained, as will be described later.

Two further steps should be taken in the aural examination when there is the suspicion that a patient may have a labyrinthine fistula and/or the Tullio phenomenon (vestibular symptoms elicited by loud sounds). The examiner must watch the eyes carefully while pressure is applied to the external auditory canal, either by manual pressure on the tragus or by an insulation pump or the probe of the impedance meter, and during loud sounds either from a tape recorder or from the audiometer. Pressure or tones should last for several seconds otherwise the frequent blink or startle associated with these stimuli may not allow proper description of the eye movements. Abnormal responses are the appearance of nystagmus, usually torsional, beating towards the side of the sound or pressure or, more rarely, a skew eye deviation with hyperdeviation of the eye on the stimulated side and hypodeviation of the contralateral eye (see Chapter 9).

NEUROPHYSIOLOGICAL INVESTIGATIONS

Introduction

The purpose of neuro-otological and related neurophysiological testing in patients with disorders of balance is to detect pathology of structures which have an established role in the organization of posture and movement. More specifically, the procedures examine for the possible involvement of the peripheral vestibular system, its central connections, the oculomotor system and the complex interrelationships between vestibular, visual and oculomotor function.

In order to understand the rationale behind neuro-otological techniques it is worth the reader bearing in mind that *the essential function mediated by visual–vestibular interaction is to signal how the head (and body) is moving in space and in relationship to other static or moving objects in the environment.* Clearly, proprioception also contributes to the assessment of such motions, particularly in relating relative movement of the head with respect to the body.

Oculography

PURPOSE AND METHODS OF OCULOGRAPHY

Eye movement recordings allow one to identify the waveform of an eye movement with precision, to quan-

tify eye movement performance under tasks and to make observations under difficult conditions such as in darkness or with an eye under cover. Oculography also has the educational value that the examiner's ability to recognize types of eye movements can be enhanced by familiarity with their appearance on a chart recorder.

The most commonly available means of recording eye movements are electro-oculography (EOG) and infrared reflection oculography (IRO). Both are best suited to recording eye movements in the horizontal plane; EOG is noisier but transduces over a wider range of eye movement than IRO. Both procedures suffer artifacts from lid movements when applied to vertical eye movements and both are susceptible to artifacts from facial grimacing. Electro-oculography has the advantage that it can be performed within certain limitations on a conventional electroencephalogram (EEG) recorder with solid-state disposable electrodes, as used in neonatal electrophysiological monitoring.

Video-based methods of recording eye movements with computerized analysis of the trajectories of movement are becoming available and offer the advantage of transducing torsional eye movement. At present, their frequency resolution is low, limited by conventional 50 or 60 Hz field rates but rapid development of the technique is to be expected. Cost is high.

The 'scleral coil' technique for transducing lateral, sagittal and torsional eye movements involves placing a silicon contact lens on the eye into which is embedded a 'pick-up coil' of wire which encircles the limbus. The sclera has to be anesthetized and wear time is limited to 30–40 minutes, following which there is edema of the cornea for several hours. Discomfort is experienced and many subjects find the procedure distressing. Transduction is accurate if the lens sticks but slip of the contact lens can be a problem. The signals require corrections for offset and goniometric non-linearity, which require some mathematical expertise. Considering the associated high cost, scleral coil eye movement recording is soon destined to become obsolete.

A comprehensive oculographic screening will include the following.

EXAMINATION FOR SPONTANEOUS NYSTAGMUS IN THE LIGHT AND DARK

The eyes have to be held relatively still in order to have good acuity and the inability to maintain a steady-eye posture signifies disorder.[45] For testing gaze, the subject is instructed to hold their eyes in primary and various eccentric positions of lateral and vertical gaze for durations of 10–20 s. Eye movements may be made on command or in response to fixation targets, which may illuminate in sequence to pace gaze transference. In each gaze position, the stability of the eyes may be observed for tendency to drift, leading to nystagmus, and the occurrence of saccadic instabilities of gaze holding ('square waves')[46] or slow phase oscillations ('pendular nystagmus'). One of the main intentions in gaze testing is to examine for gaze paretic nystagmus which is caused by a disturbance of eye position holding mechanism and which results in the eyes drifting towards their primary position under the elastic forces of orbital tissue. Disturbances of up, down, right or left gaze holding have their respective localizing values.

In each position of gaze the room and target illumination may be turned off so that the subject has to attempt to maintain gaze in darkness. Comparing gaze holding in the light and dark aims to differentiate between nystagmus of central origin and peripheral vestibular nystagmus. As a rule of thumb, a nystagmus that appears minimally in the light and emerges or enhances markedly in darkness and causes the eyes to drift predominately unidirectionally is evidence of a peripheral vestibular imbalance. Nystagmus present significantly in the light, which may enhance further in darkness, points to a disorder of the central nervous system. In the acute or paroxysmal stage of a vestibular disorder, nystagmus may be so intense as to appear significantly in the light, with poor visual suppression. The examiner should also be aware that drug intoxication may also impair the ability to suppress vestibular nystagmus.

SACCADE TRAJECTORIES AND SACCADIC INTRUSIONS

Saccadic eye movements have well-defined parameters for their velocity profile and the accuracy with which targets can be refixated, which can be used to identify abnormalities. The technique used to identify saccade accuracy and velocity is to provoke a number of saccadic refixations to defined target locations. For horizontal eye movements this could, for example, involve refixations to verbal command between targets in center and 30° right and left eccentricity.

The velocity profile of a saccade can be characterized by a simple measurement of peak velocity, which is plotted against amplitude to construct a functional relationship termed the 'main sequence'.[47] Slow saccades can be caused by central disorders of the saccade generating neuronal mechanisms, nerve lesions or muscle disease. Occasionally, one may see a saccade trajectory slow down or fragment into multiple minute steps as in myasthenia in which the steps reflect intermittent quantal release of neuromuscular transmitter.

As a general rule of thumb, saccades to targets at 30° eccentricity should be accurate to within 10 per cent with few corrective steps and centering is usually more accurate then decentering. Excessive inaccuracy manifests as hypometria and/or hypermetria.[48]

Eye movement recordings are useful to quantify saccadic intrusions or 'square waves', which take the eyes away from an intended direction of fixation. Although square waves are present to some extent in normal subjects, excessively large square waves, rapid sequences of square waves and saccadic 'flutter' (to and fro saccades without an intersaccadic interval) can indicate CNS pathology. Flutter occurring simultaneously in sagittal and lateral directions is 'opsoclonus'.[49]

Scanning and surveillance patterns of eye movements involve sequences of refixation saccades which can be abnormal in cortical disorders. Scanning strategies may be impaired and subjects asked to undertake surveillance tasks may be unable to make gaze transference at will or be unable to resist making saccades to distracting targets.[36,37]

PURSUIT AND OPTOKINETIC TESTING

Controversy exists over the relationship between pursuit and optokinetic responses, with some saying that these functions are identical.[50] It is certainly true that both rely on retinal slip signals from the visual cortex and possibly some subcortical structures. Beyond this, a useful operational distinction between pursuit and optokinesis is that the pursuit target is distinguished from background structure and followed preferentially with high accuracy. The target is seen to move independently from background and little sense of subjective vection is induced. In contrast, optokinetic following responses are made typically to movement of large areas of the visual scene, the eyes may follow with only a fraction of the velocity of the target and the subject is susceptible to the illusion that they are moving rather than the visual scene. Accordingly, pursuit is tested with a small target (e.g. a laser spot projected via a mirror galvanometer), whereas optokinesis is tested by confronting the subject with a large field of motion, ideally in the form of a rotating drum which surrounds the subject.

The performance of smooth pursuit in the horizontal plane is a sensitive indicator of the integrity of CNS function.[51] A normal subject should be capable of smooth accurate following of a target at angular velocities of 30–40°/s and with frequencies of rightwards-leftwards sinusoidal oscillation up to circa 0.4–0.6 Hz.[52] At higher velocities and frequencies, saccades are introduced into the pursuit movement to 'catch up' with the target as slow phase following becomes inadequate. Pursuit in the vertical plane has been relatively neglected. It has an intrinsically poorer performance than lateral pursuit, with upwards following worse than downwards and, as such, is not a sensitive indicator of disorder.

Disorders of pursuit most frequently consist of an inability to make adequately quick slow-phase eye movements so that saccades are made to catch up with target position. Thus, the appearance of disordered pursuit is that the target trajectory is followed in a series of steps joined by slow-phase movements with velocities significantly lower than that of the target. Bidirectionally stepped pursuit can be evidence for diffuse brain disease or drug intoxication. Unidirectionally stepped pursuit can be evidence for brainstem–cerebellar disease. The direction in which pursuit is disordered lateralizes the lesion to that side. In brainstem–cerebellar disease the steps tend to be frequent so that the overall envelope of pursuit closely approximates target trajectory. In diseases of the cerebral cortex the steps can be large and poorly controlled. Cortical disorders affecting attention and distractibility can also cause saccadic disruption of pursuit.

Pursuit is invariably deranged when the eyes move into the field of a gaze paretic nystagmus (i.e. the eyes cannot pursue outwards from center as the eyes drift inwards). This arises because pursuit and gaze holding depend upon common brainstem mechanisms in accordance with the lemma that if the eyes could pursue outwards it would cancel the paretic drift inwards.

The presence of a congenital eye movement disorder such as nystagmus associated with infantile strabismus ('latent nystagmus') or idiopathic or familial congenital nystagmus compromises smooth pursuit. The nystagmus interacts with the pursuit movement, producing a distorted trajectory of following, which makes pursuit difficult to assess. In extreme cases the slow phase of the pursuit may appear to be in the opposite direction to that of the target motion; wrongly termed 'inverted pursuit' since the slow phase is caused by the nystagmus. In rare subjects, infantile nystagmus may be brought out only during pursuit eye movements so that disordered pursuit can appear as a specific and isolated abnormality. Frequently, pursuit in subjects with strabismus without nystagmus is interrupted with square waves which take the eyes off-target or frustrate the formation of slow-phase following. This saccadic disruption is attributed, hypothetically, to switching between viewing eyes or uncertainty of visual direction associated with the heterotropia.[32]

Optokinetic following responses are more robust than pursuit in the face of neurological disease. Although they possess high frequency capability, in laboratory testing they are most frequently evoked by prolonged unidirectional motion of large field targets. The response consists of sawtooth-shaped nystagmus (OKN) in which the slow-phase optokinetic response tracks the optic flow, with the saccadic beats of the nystagmus resetting the eyes in anticipation of the oncoming optic flow. Since optokinetic signals project through the vestibular nuclei they give rise to sensations of subjective motion in the same way as vestibular signals. Thus, vestibular and optokinetic signals share the same common path input to oculomotor and perceptual mechanisms.

In the presence of a spontaneous nystagmus arising from peripheral vestibular imbalance and manifesting predominately in the dark, optokinetic slow-phase responses may become asymmetrical and they add or subtract from the nystagmus slow phase according to direction.[53,54] This phenomenon corroborates a vestibular imbalance. Lateralized brainstem lesions affecting the vestibular nuclei can give severe reduction of the slow phase directed towards the side of the lesion. Cerebellar disease has a similar lateralizing effect. In extreme cases of extensive cerebellar disease the optokinetic response may become sluggish and slow, taking 10 or more seconds to build up to even a moderate velocity.[55] This is termed 'slow-onset' OKN, which is the form of OKN occurring in lower mammals; it does not depend upon the integrity of the cerebellum and may be mediated by subcortical pathways.

The velocity of the normal OKN response builds up rapidly, is mediated by the visual cortex and cerebellum and in these respects is very similar to pursuit. The slow build up of slow-onset OKN is due to the retinal slip signals inputting indirect vestibular pathways (the velocity storage mechanism). The low frequency dynamics of the slow onset optokinetic response complement the high frequency capability of the vestibular system in transducing self motion in the environment over a wide dynamic range.

In summary, we think of optokinetic responses as consisting of a quickly responding component which is cortical- and cerebellar-mediated, which superimposes on a phylogenetically older slow response, which is possibly served by subcortical visual pathways that do not route through the cerebellum. Cerebellar lesions affect the fast-onset response whereas brainstem lesions affect both.[12,55,56]

For pursuit, the presence of a congenital oculomotor disorder and particularly latent or congenital nystagmus can interfere with the appearance of optokinetic responses giving asymmetries and slow phases with too-high or too-low velocities. In extreme cases, the OKN can appear inverted in direction, particularly in subjects with congenital nystagmus. The inversion may appear only with certain direction and velocities of stimuli so that testing over a wide range of stimulus parameters may be necessary to identify characteristics typical of congenital disorder.

Vestibulometry

TESTING VESTIBULAR OCULAR 'REFLEXES' – ROTATIONAL STIMULI

Detecting a profound paresis of a horizontal canal using natural head movement is a relatively simple affair and exploits the property that canals signal preferentially in an 'on' direction, with a small velocity range in their 'off' direction. Rapid head movement in the direction of a canal paresis results in a decisively hypoactive VOR with poor compensatory eye movement in the opposite direction to the head, which may be evident on inspection. This is because the remaining canal cannot signal strongly for this direction of rotation. The VOR can be quantified with suitable apparatus to transduce the eye and head movements. The subject can provide the motion stimulus themselves by shaking their head from side to side while fixating a stationary target.[57]

More subtle derangements of canal function rely on establishing the dynamic performance of the vestibular–ocular reflex, which means mapping the frequency response of the VOR and identifying non-linearities, particularly in terms of symmetry.[58,59] This process requires elaborate apparatus in the form of a motorized rotating platform that can carry a subject and recording equipment. The assumption underlying the conventional testing protocols is that the normal VOR dynamic is approximately linear. The test stimuli used are sinusoidal or impulsive.

In sinusoidal testing, say of the horizontal canals, the subject is oriented upright on the turntable, with lateral eye movement recording, and exposed to sinusoidal oscillations across a range of frequencies from around 0.02 Hz to around 1 Hz or more in darkness. The slow-phase eye movement response is also sinusoidal and accordingly is characterized in terms of its gain and phase at each frequency of stimulation in a frequency response or 'Bode' plot. The equation of the Bode plot (an expression in real and imaginary numbers) is the 'transfer function' of the VOR which predicts how much eye movement will be evoked for any head movement.

In the presence of unilateral vestibular dysfunction the VOR becomes non-linear so that the timing relationship between eye velocity and head velocity and/or their peak amplitudes during a cycle of sinusoidal motion are different for rightwards- and leftwards-directed movement. This distortion is apparent on inspection of the raw data records. It may also be plotted conveniently as a Lissajous trajectory with head velocity on the abscissa and eye velocity on the ordinate. A normal response will consist of a narrow ellipse equally balanced about the abscissa. An abnormal response will distort the elliptical trajectory and cause asymmetries about the abscissa.

An enduring problem encountered with vestibular testing is that sinusoidal stimuli are predictable so that a subject with little or no vestibular function may build up a mental picture of how they are moving and generate, through internal signals, a reasonable eye-movement response that is misleading. For this reason, unpredictable rotational stimuli have been used with complex waveforms which may consist of the addition of several sinusoids. The response is complex and has to be decomposed into sinusoidal components by correlation or Fourier analysis. Identification of non-linearities may then be made through calculation of 'coherence' between head and eye movement which quantifies the amount of signal in linear relationship.

The process of analyzing complex waveforms is cumbersome and unsatisfactory, particularly for identifying non-linearities. Alternative stimulus waveforms which reduce predictability and can be analyzed in Lissajous form are 'chirps' or 'swept sines' in which the mode of stimulation is basically sinusoidal but with a rapid frequency change and 'Logons' in which two or three cycles of sinusoidal stimulation are given in an overall crescendo-decrescendo window of amplitude.

At this stage, one can hardly blame the reader for thinking that this is all 'too much' and, indeed, it is common practice to evaluate rotational responses to a brief unidirectional pulse of acceleration, which gives a simple rapid rise of vestibular slow phase followed by an exponential decline – a 'rotational stopping stimulus'. This response is the inverse Fourier transform of the transfer function (i.e. it is the time domain equivalent of the Bode plot) and so embodies the information about linear relationships derivable from sinusoidal testing. It also has the advantage of separating, to some extent, rightwards and leftwards responses. The slow-phase response to an acceleration impulse can be characterized by the peak velocity of slow phase attained just after the impulse has terminated and the time constant of the subsequent decay of the response. From these two values and the magnitude of the acceleration impulse one can calculate the equation of the response. The Fourier transform of this equation is the 'Bode plot'.

In practice, the acceleration impulses are given in the form of steps in rotational velocity (for example, starting from rest, rotating rightwards at 60°/s until the response has died out, and stopping); after the stopping response has died out rotation is repeated but starts in the leftwards direction. This sequence provides two estimates for both peak velocity and time constant to rightwards and leftwards acceleration impulses. The peak velocity of the slow-phase response as a proportion of the step in rotational velocity is the 'high frequency gain' of the VOR which is normally around 0.7 for an alert subject. The time constant for decay is normally around 15 s. This long decay results from prolongation of the time constant by approximately 7 s for decay of the signal in the VIIIth nerve by the central velocity store.

Lateralized disorders of the VOR appear on impulsive rotational testing as asymmetries of peak velocity and time constants or duration for rightwards versus leftwards responses because of hypoactive responses to acceleration directed towards the side of the lesion. In acute vestibular lesions responses to both directions may be diminished in magnitude and foreshortened as part of an initial, global suppressive response to gross vestibular asymmetry. Idealized examples are shown in Fig. 7.5.

Vestibular testing may be generalized by orienting the subject so that vertical canal pairs are stimulated by rotation to test vertical and torsional vestibular-ocular reflexes but, to date, there are few clinical guidelines on interpreting the results obtained from these maneuvers.

Congenital nystagmus (CN) seriously interferes with the structure of vestibular responses so that they may become effectively uninterpretable (see below).[60]

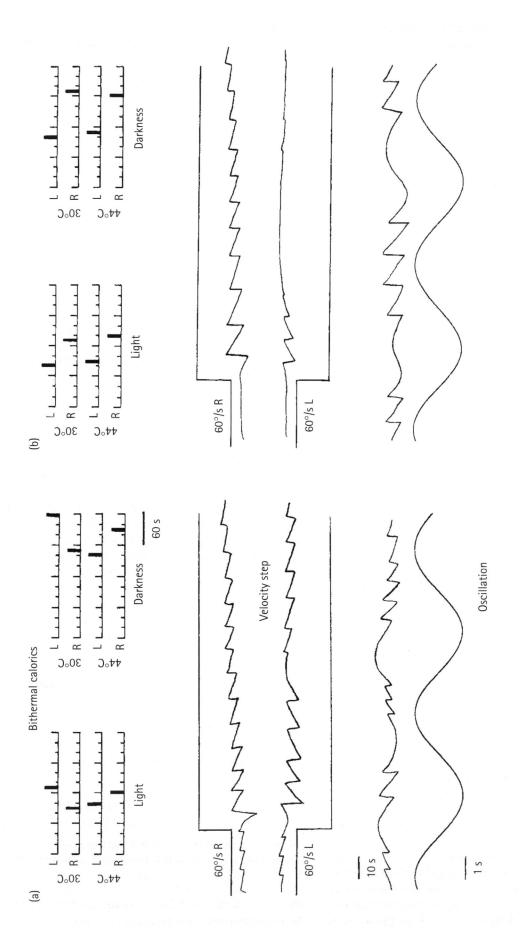

Figure 7.5 Idealized recordings of nystagmus responses to caloric irrigation, steps of rotational velocity and sinusoidal oscillation one might obtain in (a) a directional preponderance of nystagmus to the right and (b) with a partial acute left canal paresis. Note with directional preponderance there is an apparent reversal of response which occurs some time after the initial left beating response for velocity steps to the right. Note the curt response in the case of the left-canal paresis for leftwards rotation. Recordings depict chair velocity and eye displacement; rightwards motion is represented as upwards deflection of the traces and leftwards motion as downwards deflection.

VESTIBULAR–OCULAR REFLEX SUPPRESSION

Tracking a moving target with the head as well as the eyes involves a curious potential antagonism between the vestibular reflex, provoked by the head movement, which is in the opposite direction to the smooth pursuit. For low-velocity head movements, pursuit may simply cancel the VOR whereas for high-velocity head movements the VOR may be inhibited or switched off in some way. Whatever happens the phenomenon is termed vestibular-ocular reflex suppression (VORS) and inability to suppress the VOR results in a nystagmus with slow phases in the wrong direction for target following. Failure of VOR suppression is a sensitive sign of CNS disorder.[44,52,61]

Vestibulo-ocular reflex suppression is tested conveniently as an extension of vestibular sinusoidal rotational testing. The subject fixates a target light which is fixed to the chair and positioned at a reasonable distance from the subject's face; i.e. he is fixing a head stationary target whilst the chair executes sinusoidal oscillation (a similar situation to reading in a moving vehicle). A normal subject will be able to maintain fixation on the target over a frequency range up to c. 0.4–0.6 Hz at peak velocities up to 40°/s; this is a dynamic capability which parallels that of smooth pursuit.[52]

Disorders of VOR suppression appear as nystagmus in the primary position of gaze which is provoked by oscillation and modulates in direction with the velocity of oscillation (i.e. rightwards rotation will induce right-beating nystagmus if the leftwards slow phase of the VOR is unsuppressed). Most often a corresponding reduction in pursuit is to be observed, in this example, rightwards pursuit would be deranged, although there is some evidence that pursuit and VOR suppression can be dissociated. Drug intoxication may lead to failure to suppress the VOR and it is an almost inevitable feature in congenital nystagmus (CN).

CALORIC TEST

Caloric irrigation as a means of testing the function of an individual labyrinth is without equal although the procedure is cumbersome, unpleasant and nauseogenic to many subjects. The rationale of caloric irrigation is that application of a temperature differential across the labyrinth results in endolymphatic flow due to a heat-induced density differential in the endolymph. The flow causes cupular stimulation. There is also a direct effect of the thermal stimulus on the sense organ but this is a relatively small part of the response.

With the subject's head tilted backwards by 60°, the horizontal canals are oriented vertically and appropriately to encourage convection. A thermal stimulus, which may be a stream of water or air, cooler than blood temperature causes endolymphatic flow in the 'off' direction of the horizontal canal and the imbalance in tonus between the labyrinths causes ipsilaterally directed slow-phase eye movement with contralateral nystagmic beats. A stimulus at a temperature higher than that of blood activates the canal, causing contralaterally directed slow-phase eye movement and ipsilateral nystagmic beats. There may be a concomitant vertiginous sensation of rotation in the opposite direction to the nystagmus slow phase.

In practical terms, caloric stimuli are usually delivered under thermostatic control at 30°C and 44°C (within the range of comfortable temperature) for 40 s. The characteristics of the slow phase of the induced nystagmus consist of an initial rise in velocity due to the build up of the thermal stimulus and convection pressure differential followed by a decline in velocity as the stimulus wears off. This profile approximates a linear exponential function for the onset with a linear exponential decay. The overall response can be described conveniently by peak velocity attained and time constant for decay (approximately equal to one-quarter of the total duration). A complete test will comprise cold and hot stimuli delivered to both right and left ears. Several minutes' rest are allowed between individual irrigations to ensure that the thermal stimulus and central adaptation to the unidirectional nystagmus have also declined.

There are two main patterns of disordered response to caloric testing.[62–64] In the case of canal paresis, one ear is unresponsive to hot or cold stimuli, either in terms of relative duration (Fig. 7.5b) or relative peak velocity (right ear compared with left) of the induced nystagmus slow phase. The significance of a canal paresis is clear in that the paretic vestibular apparatus is hypofunctioning but the pathology is not specified with respect to end organ, nerve or nucleus.[65] The second form of distinct response is a directional preponderance in which the nystagmus in the right or left direction is longer in duration or higher in peak velocity than for the opposite direction (Fig. 7.5a). A directional preponderance may be seen, for example, when a patient already has a spontaneous unidirectional nystagmus in the dark. In simple terms one can envisage the spontaneous nystagmus adding to the caloric induced nystagmus to prolong or shorten duration. The directional preponderance is suggestive of vestibular imbalance but does not have localizing value. Profound canal paresis can be evaluated by cold calorics at 20°C or less to give an exceptionally strong stimulus to the canals.

Ratios (Jongkees formulae) may be calculated for canal paresis and directional preponderance which assist comparison with normative data:

canal paresis = (V or D Right side) − (V or D Left side)/(V or D Right side) + (V or D Left side)

directional preponderance = (V or D Right beat nystagmus) − (V or D left beating)/(V or D Right beating) + (V or D Left beating)

where D is duration of response or alternatively V (slow-phase velocity) may be used.

Further evidence for vestibular pathology offered by calorics is markedly asymmetrical subjective sensations and perverted caloric nystagmus in which the eyes execute torsional or vertical trajectories (these are more difficult to quantify and systematize and usually indicate central pathology).

The original technique of Fitzgerald and Hallpike[64] relies on the measurement of the duration of the nystagmic reaction by direct observation, in the presence of optic fixation; such a procedure requires minimal technology and provides much useful clinical information. Caloric responses can be observed in the dark or under Frenzel's lenses or recorded oculographically and be modified to test the ability to suppress caloric nystagmus by switching on room illumination at some defined point during the procedure. Marked failure to suppress caloric nystagmus as for VOR suppression is taken to be a sign of CNS disorder.

Patients may report that the vertiginous sensation they experience during caloric irrigation is similar to their presenting symptoms which may help confirm the suspicion of a vestibular disorder.

GALVANIC STIMULATION OF THE MASTOID

Electrical polarization of the labyrinth, which is normally effected by stimulating the mastoid by means of a DC electric cathodal current of 1 mA typical magnitude for 6 s, induces postural sway and nystagmus or ocular deviations in most normal subjects.[66] Use of the technique in establishing labyrinthine pathology is currently restricted to a few laboratories that have accumulated sufficient experience to establish a comparative data base.

The sway response to cathodal current comprises an initial transient sway to the side of the stimulus lasting approximately 500 ms followed by a sustained postural deviation away from the side of the lesion. At stimulus offset there is a further transient deviation to the stimulated side.

Cathodally induced sway may be reduced or absent in patients with labyrinthine pathology whose canal function is intact, as assessed by rotational and caloric responses. This finding is taken as evidence that the sway is induced via stimulation of the otolith apparatus. Conversely, sway may be intact in some patients that have absent canal responses. It is thought that the electrical stimulus to the nerve ending is responsible for the constant sway offset effect whereas the phasic component of sway is caused by stimulation of the nerve.[67]

HIGH-INTENSITY ACOUSTIC 'CLICK' STIMULATION

Recent years have witnessed a revival or resurgence of attempts to stimulate the vestibular apparatus artificially by high-intensity sound bursts. 'Click' sound stimuli at around 90 dB HL (decibels hearing level) induce periods of silence followed by excitability in neck muscle at short latencies of 8 ms and 20 ms, respectively, which may be detected from background electromyography (EMG) by averaging techniques.[68,69] The equipment needed for setting up this technique is available in most EEG/EMG departments.

Attempts are being made to show that this form of stimulation may have selective effects on subcomponents of the labyrinth which could be exploited for otolith testing; specifically, it is thought that the myogenic potentials may be mediated preferentially by sacculus stimulation. This possibility awaits further study but preliminary communications suggest that the technique is sensitive to abnormalities in certain cochleo-vestibular disorders, including exaggerated responses in patients with Tullio phenomenon.[70]

PSYCHOPHYSICAL ASSESSMENTS

Although by far the oldest methods of evaluating vestibular function, psychophysical estimates of self motion have been neglected for decades in favor of measurements of postural and eye movement responses to vestibular stimulation (perhaps for the reason that these latter methods offer the reassurance that the variables to be quantified are tangible and amenable to neurophysiological study). Although posturographic and vestibular ocular reflex measurements are of relevance to pathophysiology they do not correlate well with patients' symptoms. For this reason there has been a resurgence of interest in psychophysical assessments of how patients with imbalance in general, and vestibular dysfunction in particular, experience self motion. This approach rests on the premise that since inappropriate feelings of self motion are central to their symptoms it is precisely abnormalities of this function that should be addressed.

Testing scenarios aimed at evaluating canal function involve either estimates of how much a subject feels they are rotated, thresholds of sensation of self rotation or estimates of decay of sensation of self rotation. Current emphasis is on estimates of how much a subject feels they are rotated when exposed to passive rotations in rightwards versus leftwards directions.[71,72] At moderate levels of velocity of imposed rotation (c. 60°/s) such assessments are highly successful in indicating unilateral or bilateral canal hypofunction in the more acute phase of loss. Results are simple in that sensitivity is impaired when the subject is rotated towards the lesioned side. As may be expected from such an assessment of 'holistic' function, performance improves with adaptation to the vestibular insult so that the evaluation procedure provides a useful index of disability providing measurements which correlate well with symptom rating scales.[73] Psychophysical assessments may also be useful in patients that have eye movement disorders which impede vestibular ocular reflex testing.[74,75] In its simple form, inquiring if the dizziness obtained from caloric irrigation is approximately the same in the two ears can establish the presence of vestibular function on both sides.

OTOLITH TESTING

Although certain symptoms and signs, including illusory sensations of linear motion and tilt and positional nystagmus, are taken to be suggestive of dysfunction of the otolithic pathways, there are no generally accepted tests of otolith dysfunction in current hospital neuro-physiology departments.[14,76,77] One problem with establishing otolith tests is that we have poorly formed ideas about the functions that otolith signals subserve. A second handicap is that the acceleration stimuli needed to evoke otolith responses also give rise to considerable proprioceptive stimulation, which itself gives responses that can mask presumed otolithic effects.

Current opinion is that otolith signals may have 'oculomotor', 'vestibulo-spinal', and 'perceptual effects'.

Arguably the purest form of otolith response that has been reported is the eye movement generated by sudden-onset linear acceleration of the head. In human subjects a stepwise linear acceleration applied to the skull in the lateral direction along the inter-aural line induces a slow-phase compensatory eye movement in the opposite direction to the head translation, with a latency of approximately 30–50 ms.[78] This response is absent for subjects with bilateral labyrinthine deficiency and its absence contributes to head movement dependent oscillopsia.[9] The response is present in the dark and enhanced with visual fixation. In subjects without labyrinthine function a slow-phase eye movement does occur in the light but at a latency of some 100–150 ms and results from visual guidance of eye movements through pursuit and optokinetic mechanisms. Disorders of the short-latency otolithic slow-phase response are seen as prolongations of latency and reductions in response magnitude and asymmetry.[79–81] Perhaps the most significant finding is that, in the acute phase of unilateral vestibular loss, up to about 4 months the response is consistently hypoactive for linear lateral head motion towards the lesioned side[81] and is thus a clinical sign of unilateral otolith dysfunction. The authors argue that the lateral hair cells of the utricle are responsible for this horizontal otolith reflex because it is these receptors that would be stimulated by motion to the lesioned side if this were intact. The response symmetry is eventually redressed, at least for stimuli of moderate acceleration.

Natural head movements frequently involve linear and angular components and it is thought that the otoliths provide compensatory eye movement reflexes which stabilize vision with respect to the linear components of head movement. The otolith contribution to ocular stabilization may be assessed by performing conventional vestibular rotational tests first with the head centered and then with the head in an eccentric position so there is a significant tangential linear acceleration stimulus. The difference in amplitude in responses between head center and head eccentric can be apportioned to the otolith stimulus.[82,83] Some asymmetries of response in unilateral labyrinthine disease have been reported using this combination of maneuvers. Specifically, the linear components of compensatory eye movements may be diminished in magnitude when rotating towards the lesion side. However, the full potential of combined head eccentric and centered testing has yet to be determined.

The low frequency dynamic and static components of ocular counter-rolling are thought to be, in part, a function of the otolith. Certainly, impoverished ocular counter-rolling in response to slow head tilt is found in bilateral labyrinthine deficiency. It is reported that poor counter-rolling is obtained for head tilt in the direction of the good ear down.[84,85] A drawback to implementing evaluation of counter-rolling as a test of otolith dysfunction is that counter-rolling can be difficult to observe and the abnormalities reported show a high variability with inconsistencies.

Numerous recent studies have addressed the problem of identifying a unilateral otolithic lesion through its effect on static ocular counter-rolling[86,87] and reduced static eye torsion in response to head tilt might point to both a saccular and/or an utricular lesion. It has long been established that following a complete unilateral vestibular lesion there is a static torsional displacement of the eyes towards the lesioned side ('ipsi-cyclo-torsion'), which may be evident on fundoscopy and is manifest as a tilt of the visual vertical.[88–90] The proposed mechanism is that counter-rolling in compensation for head tilt is largely controlled by the medially located hair cells of the utricle and loss of their tonic input to brainstem oculomotor centers leaves an unopposed tonus from the intact utricle which torts the eyes towards the opposite side, as if the head were tilted to the intact side and the otoliths were generating a compensatory eye displacement. Unfortunately, the duration of this effect is highly variable and transitory (up to c. 1 year), probably because compensatory mechanisms redress the asymmetry of vestibular tonus.

In efforts to make the counter-rolling test more sensitive to long-standing lesions, studies have been made on how patients with unilateral vestibular lesions set the visual vertical/horizontal when exposed to strong utricular stimulation by either tilting the head or centrifugation with the head placed eccentrically on a vestibular turntable facing along the tangent to their circumferential trajectory.[91–93] With head tilt to the intact side, the medial utricle is activated by gravity, whereas with tilt to the lesioned side the medial hair cells are deflected in their 'off' direction. Similarly, centrifugation creates an inertial tilt that can be directed to activate or suppress utricular activity according to whether the intact ear is facing out from the axis or facing inwards, respectively. It is argued that greater counter-rolling may be produced by the activation (as with the directional sensitivity of a canal) so that an asymmetry of setting the visual vertical/horizontal may be revealed.

In practice, centrifugation and head tilt can uncover deviations of the visual vertical in chronic patients, however, in short, results are highly variable, compromising the sensitivity and even specificity of the procedure as a clinical test.[94]

Numerous other testing scenarios aimed at eliciting otolith responses have been explored for their clinical utility but (with respect to all investigators that have attempted the difficult task of devising means of identifying otolith dysfunction) one must conclude that, as yet, there are insufficient data about the sensitivity and specificity to identified labyrinthine disorders of the various test tactics that have been deployed to be able to evaluate the ultimate potential of any particular testing scenario.[76]

Posturography

Since one of the symptoms of vestibular disease is unsteadiness while standing and walking it is only natural that, in recent years, there has been a surge of interest in measuring postural stability in patients with vestibular lesions. Posturography is the general term for the recording of postural movements and this can be done with image motion analyzers, accelerometers, goniometers and force platforms. The last of these is the easiest system and the one applied for routine clinical purposes. The problem with force platforms (incorrectly called sway platforms) is that they measure not only the displacement of the center of foot pressure during sway but also the torque actively generated by the ankle. Nevertheless, for most clinical purposes platform signals approximately indicate the degree of stability of the subject being tested.

The terms static and dynamic posturography are often used. In the former, the subject simply stands on the platform, usually with eyes open and closed for periods of approximately 30 s. In this way, posturography is only a quantitative version of the Romberg test and has very little added value if only the overall amount of unsteadiness is measured. If, in addition, the frequency content of the postural movements is measured by fast Fourier techniques, static posturography can contribute to diagnosis more specifically. Normally, most of the power found in sway activity is below 1–2 Hz. Neurological conditions with postural body tremor generate much platform activity above this frequency. In cerebellar disease, particularly involving the anterior lobe such as it seen in alcoholic abuse or degenerative disease, a 3 Hz peak can be distinctly observed (see Chapter 10).[95] Some patients with Parkinson's disease display tremor peaks at 4–6 Hz.[96] A condition called

orthostatic tremor, in which patients experience great discomfort on standing and paradoxically less on walking, can be confidently diagnosed with posturography since it shows an unusually high frequency peak of activity at around 16 Hz.[97] In summary, static posturography can document the degree of unsteadiness in a given patient, or its improvement with time or treatment, but little is gained for specific diagnosis unless tremor activity is looked for.

Dynamic posturography denotes the presence of some kind of sensory stimuli so that information can be gained on the functional status of a particular aspect of the postural control system. The stimulus can be more or less specific for a particular sensory channel (e.g. galvanic stimulation, tendon vibration or moving visual stimuli for vestibular, proprioceptive and visual assessment respectively). This approach has been fruitful in balance research but no clear, simple role can be found for these techniques in the consulting room. A commercial system is available (computerized dynamic posturography, Equitest; see Chapters 8 and 17) which combines a force platform and a visual surround, both of which can be moved by the patient's own sway ('sway referenced' conditions). To some extent, this allows assessment of the separate visuo-vestibular-proprioceptive contributions to balance and for this reason the system is popular among ear, nose and throat (ENT) surgeons and audiologists. Convincing topographic and etiological specificity of this relatively expensive system is, however, lacking and one remains to be convinced of any practical value for the management of an individual patient.

Audiometry

Audiology is an essential adjunct to vestibular testing. Its value lies in providing evidence that may corroborate the presence of a lesion of the cochleo-vestibular end organ or of the VIIIth nerve.[98] The single most important condition to which the audiology must be oriented is the possible presence of an acoustic neurinoma or other space-occupying lesion of the lateral brainstem or CP angle which compresses the VIIIth or facial nerves. This role is being superseded by advancement in imaging techniques.

PURE-TONE AUDIOMETRY

Pure-tone air conduction audiometry combined with masked bone conduction audiometry quantifies hearing thresholds across the range 250 Hz–8 kHz and gives a reasonable estimate of the relative contributions of conductive attenuation due to middle ear disorder and sensorineural components of the overall loss. Threshold is defined as an ascending threshold and is estimated by lowering the intensity of a presented tone in 10 dB HL steps until the listener fails to detect the presentation.

The intensity is then raised in 5 dB HL steps until successfully detected. The estimated is repeated until the same threshold is obtained on two occasions.

A similar procedure is followed to establish bone conduction thresholds,[99] but the ear to be excluded from the test is 'masked' with increasing levels of noise until a stable threshold is found for the ear under test. The difference between air and bone conduction thresholds for an ear is a measure of the conductive attenuation of sound due to middle ear dysfunction.

Middle ear disorders are less likely to be highly correlated with vestibular involvement than sensorineural losses but it is worth bearing in mind that the common condition of otosclerosis, which gives a conductive hearing loss, is also associated with cochlear hearing loss, predominately affecting high tones, and vestibular degeneration, giving symptoms of mild vertigo. Positive identification of otosclerosis may be afforded by the configuration of contraction of the stapedial reflex (see below).

An extension of pure tone audiometry is loudness discomfort levels,[100] which to some extent have been superseded by stapedial reflex thresholds (see below). Loudness discomfort levels (LDLs) are established by increasing the intensity of a 2-s duration pure tone, presented monaurally, in 5 dB HL steps from around 70 dB upwards until the listener expresses reasonable discomfort. Normal LDLs vary from around 75 dB HL to 100 dB HL and are usually similar across frequencies. Hearing 'recruitment' is identified if a subject with a sensorineural hearing loss in certain frequencies has normal LDLs at these frequencies compared with testing at frequencies for which they have normal thresholds. Recruitment is most frequently, but not always, an indication of cochlear hearing loss and thus has differential localizing value between nerve and end organ lesions.

In summary, a unilateral hearing loss may corroborate suspicion of unilateral vestibular dysfunction. Bilateral hearing loss may accompany bilateral vestibular dysfunction. In addition, one should beware that hearing may not always be 'lost'. Diplacusis (as if hearing a metallic echo to sounds) and hyperacusis (extraordinary sensitivity to sounds) may be evidence of cochlear pathology, which may not be reflected in an abnormal audiogram.

Tinnitus may accompany cochlear or sensorineural hearing loss or exist independently. As a rough rule of thumb, tinnitus which masks, meaning that it is suppressed when other sounds are present, is thought of as likely to be cochlear in origin. Unilateral sensorineural hearing loss with tinnitus occurs with cochlear pathology but is also typical of acoustic neurinoma and always indicates appropriate investigations.

TYMPANOMETRY AND STAPEDIAL REFLEXES

Tympanometry provides measures of middle ear pressure and drum compliance (floppiness). High negative pressure is associated with middle ear dysfunction and may accompany conductive hearing loss. Its value in otological studies of balance is in conjunction with evaluation of stapedial reflexes thresholds.

The stapedial reflex is provoked by sound of high intensity and contracts the stapedius muscle thereby stiffening the ossicular chain joining ear drum to oval window in order to attenuate sound transmission to the cochlea. The reflex is evident on the tympanogram as a lowering of drum compliance. The afferent branch of the reflex is the VIIIth nerve, which gives rise to ipsilateral and crossed reflexes that have efferent expression in the VIIth (facial) nerves with a component of lesser significance carried in the trigeminal nerves. Stapedial reflexes are evoked by the monaural presentation of 1-s duration pure tones at increasing intensities until the reflex is evoked and detected as a change in drum compliance, which occurs bilaterally in response to unilateral stimulation. Test frequencies for stapedial reflexes are usually 500 Hz, 1 kHz, 2 kHz and 4 kHz with more weight being given to abnormal responses to the two lowest frequencies. Normal reflexes typically have thresholds similar to loudness discomfort levels and are thus a more objective indicator of hyperacusis.

A stapedial reflex which is sluggish, raised in thresholds or is absent in one ear only indicates a lesion of the facial nerve on that side or a middle ear disorder.[101,102] If on stimulating one ear, ipsilateral reflexes are intact and contralateral reflexes absent, a lesion of the brainstem projection to the opposite side is indicated. Bilateral impairment of contralateral stapedial reflexes probably indicates a midline brainstem lesion. Impaired ipsilateral and contralateral reflexes on stimulation of one ear imply a cochlear or VIIIth nerve lesion on the side of that ear. Impairment of an ipsilateral-evoked reflex in isolation indicates lesion of the ipsilateral brainstem pathways of the reflex.

Stapedial reflex decay is a method of evaluating the integrity of the VIIIth nerve afferent pathway of the reflex. Decay is usually assessed on the contralateral reflex by measuring how well the change in drum compliance sustains throughout a 10-s duration tone (500 Hz and 1 kH) presented 10 dB HL above threshold for the reflex. More than 50 per cent decay in less than 5 s at two frequencies is evidence for the likelihood of a nerve lesion and as such is suggestive of acoustic neurinoma.

Tympanometry and stapedial reflex assessment in combining high-intensity sound tones while manipulating external ear pressure are useful adjunct techniques for investigating Tullio and Henneberg (fistula) phenomena.

BRAINSTEM AUDITORY EVOKED POTENTIALS

The brainstem auditory evoked potentials (BAEP) comprise a series of components, detected with scalp electrodes, that arise from the VIIIth nerve and brainstem in response to auditory stimuli.[103] In general, the stimulus is a short duration click, usually 0.1 ms long, and the record 1000–2000 responses averaged in blocks of 500 obtained from electrodes over the mastoid and vertex. There is evidence that component I arises from activity of the VIIIth nerve while later components, II–V, occur at the time of activation of the cochlear nucleus (II), superior olivary complex (III), and lateral lemniscus and colliculi (IV, V), although there is considerable overlap in the time domain of activity in these structures.[104,105] The response generated bilaterally with components III and V is predominantly contralateral while the earlier components arise from ipsilateral structures.

Brainstem auditory evoked potentials are of use in two situations, namely unilateral hearing loss and neurological disorders affecting the brainstem. In general, a peripheral hearing loss caused by a malfunction of hair cells has little effect upon the BAEP until the deficit at 4 kHz (the frequency at which most of the power is found) reaches 50 or 60 dB. Conversely, in unilateral retrocochlear lesions, there is a marked increase in latency with quite small changes in the pure-tone audiogram.[106–108] If component I can be reliably seen, the I–V interval is a good measure of abnormality and normative data exist which are of use in separating retrocochlear from cochlear lesions. The problem is that component I can be difficult to record reliably and then only a delay of later components is seen, a situation that can also occur in conductive hearing losses (in these, component I is delayed as well as component V and the I–V interval is normal). Selective placement of electrodes can solve this problem; alternatively electrocochleography may help in defining component I.

In neurological practice, BAEP are used to detect and define brainstem lesions.[109] Abnormalities may be of latency or amplitude of the various components. Changes of latency are more robust than those of amplitude, particularly if unilateral stimulation is used; indeed it is necessary to use relative amplitude (ratio of components I/III and V) in the case of unilateral stimulation. While a large number of pathologies have been associated with abnormalities of BAEP, and there is nothing specific about changes seen in terms of etiology, it is in demyelination that the largest changes are observed, particularly in terms of latency.[110,111] As a general rule, if there is good preservation of components but there is a large increase in the I–V interval, demyelination is more likely than a vascular or neoplastic cause. Similarly, total absence of components in a fully conscious patient is most likely to be due to the demyelination. There have been many attempts to site a lesion from the absence of specific components (e.g. absence of component V suggests a lesion in the lateral lemniscus) but this is not always accurate and has now been superseded by magnetic resonance imaging (MRI).

In summary, the BAEP is a useful investigation in the unbalanced or vertiginous patient and would help to separate central from peripheral lesions.

OTOACOUSTIC EMISSIONS

A relatively new technique for studying auditory function and which is of some use in separating central from peripheral causes of vertigo and imbalance is otoacoustic emissions (OAE). If a tone is applied to one ear, energy is emitted from the cochlea at that frequency.[112] This probably arises from activity of the outer hair cells. It is possible to plot the otoacoustic emission over the whole range of audible frequencies. If there is a localized loss of function of hair cells resulting in a dip in the audiogram there is a loss of the OAE at this frequency. The technique is a useful one and, in general, abnormalities of the OAE point to a peripheral cause. There is, however, no agreement over the use of OAE to detect central lesions. It is not clear whether VIIIth nerve tumors, which can cause absence of OAE, do so by interference with the blood supply to the cochlea or due to an effect upon the efferent pathways. Similarly, suppression of the OAE by contralateral stimulation is dependent upon a crossed pathway through the brainstem but absence of suppression has not been shown reliably to detect such lesions. Nevertheless, a normal OAE in the presence of significant pure-tone audiogram abnormality suggests that the problem is of central origin.

IMAGING OF THE VESTIBULAR SYSTEM

Introduction

Imaging of the vestibular system, especially of the VIIIth nerve and central connections, has been revolutionized by the development of MRI. Historically, contrast encephalography using gas or radio-opaque dyes was the only method of outlining the brainstem and its associated nerves; such methods could be used to detect masses, especially extra-axial ones, but were of no value in demonstrating the internal structure of the brainstem. The development of the fast Fourier transform enabled X-ray computed tomograms to be produced in the early 1970s. This technique produced for the first time images of the brain substance as well as its outline, enabling moderately clear definition of hemorrhage and tumor, although the technique was less sensitive in the posterior fossa, the area in which the neuro-otological investigator is primarily interested. Extra-axial tumors in the CP angle were visualized if they were large but it was still necessary to use intrathecal contrast to image small tumors, especially if located in the internal auditory meatus. While computed tomography (CT) X-ray imaging was being developed, parallel experiments using similar transforms to map variations in proton magnetic resonance in tissues were being carried out, culminating in the availability of commercial MRI by the early 1980s. Great improvement in resolution, exploitation of different sequences, and suppression and transfer techniques have culminated in the remarkably high-resolution images of the brain, including those structures within the posterior fossa. Commercial machines routinely enable 1 mm contiguous sections to be obtained, giving good images of the labyrinths and cochlea, VIIIth nerve and many of the major tracts and nuclear clusters (e.g. red nucleus, olivary nucleus, of the neural axis; Figs 7.6

and 7.7). Furthermore pathological changes due to inflammatory lesions, notably those found in multiple sclerosis, (Fig. 7.8) can be visualized with a fair degree of accuracy, a situation that does not apply to CT scanning, while vascular abnormalities and tumors are clearly defined (Fig. 7.9). A further advantage of MRI is the ease with which images can be obtained in any plane, such that foramen magnum abnormalities (e.g. Arnold Chiari malformation), which are so important in neuro-otology, can readily be detected non-invasively.

All the above concerns developments in brain imag-

(a)

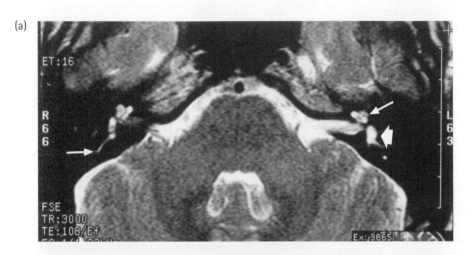

(b)

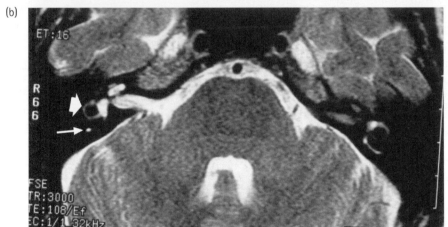

(c)

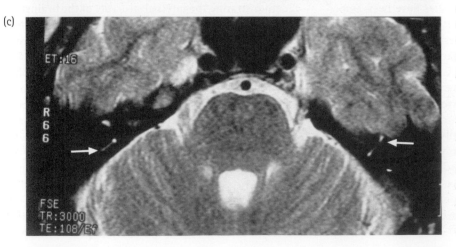

Figure 7.6 *Normal anatomy. Series of magnetic resonance images in the horizontal plane of otic capsule and brainstem. The left side of images are at a slightly lower level than right side. (a) Lowest cut showing cochlea (thin left-pointing arrow), otolith apparatus (open arrow) and posterior semicircular canals (thin right-pointing arrow). (b) Section 1.5 mm higher than previous image showing horizontal canal (open arrow), and vertical part of posterior canal (thin arrow). The superior vestibular nerve is the most posterior component of the VIIIth nerve. (c) Section 1.5 mm above previous image. On the left is upper part of posterior semicircular canal (thin right-pointing arrow), and on the right the anterior semicircular canal (thin left-pointing arrow).*

(a)

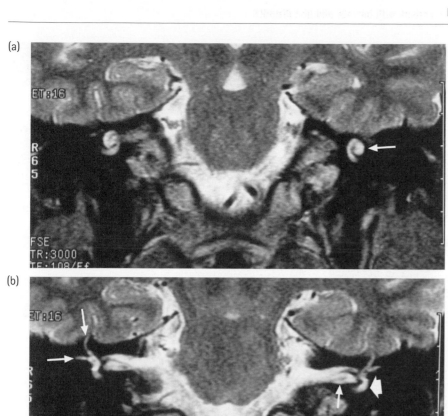

(b)

(c)

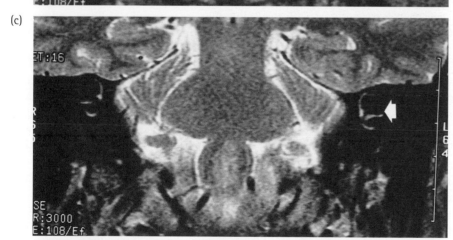

(d)

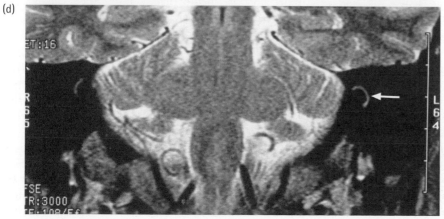

Figure 7.7 *Normal anatomy. Series of magnetic resonance images in the coronal plane of otic capsule and brainstem. Sections are ordered from front to back. (a) Cochlea (thin left-pointing arrow). (b) Superior (thin down-pointing arrow) and horizontal (thin right-pointing arrow) semicircular canals; otolith (open arrow) and VIIIth nerve (thin up-pointing arrow). (c) Superior canal, horizontal canal and anterior part of posterior canal (open arrow). (d) Posterior semicircular canal (thin left-pointing arrow).*

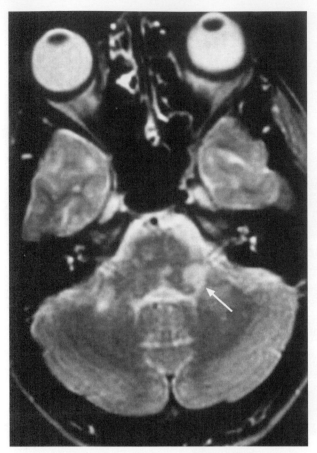

Figure 7.8 *Magnetic resonance images in horizontal plane of VIIIth nerve root entry zone in a patient with multiple sclerosis with left-sided hearing loss and anti-clockwise (right-beating) torsional nystagmus. Note demyelinating plaque in root entry zone (arrow).*

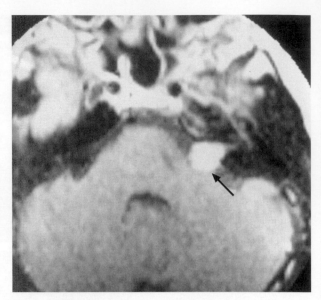

Figure 7.9 *Magnetic resonance image showing acoustic neuroma after gadolinium enhancement (arrow).*

The vestibular end organ

Computed tomography scanning is of great value in determining the integrity of bony structures in the petrous temporal bone (e.g. in detecting erosions caused by tumors) but is of limited value in imaging the vestibular end organ. It has been particularly useful in patients with the Tullio phenomenon (unsteadiness and nystagmus in response to loud sounds). Recently, it has been found that, in many patients with this symptom, the superior semicircular canal is not completely embedded in the petrous bone so that the superior surface is unroofed and covered only by dura (superior canal dehiscence syndrome; Fig. 7.10).[113] This may result in excessive movement of the endolymph in that canal when the subject experiences loud sounds. It is unclear whether this is the only cause of the Tullio phenomenon (see Chapter 9) or what the significance of superior canal dehiscence in asymptomatic subjects is.[114]

There has been some preliminary MRI work on imaging the semicircular canals in patients with acute vertigo especially if hemorrhage into the canals has occurred.[115,116] However, in the vast majority of patients with acute vestibular failure caused by end organ dysfunction, imaging is unrewarding and we still have to rely on physiological tests to site lesions, using imaging only to exclude more sinister central lesions and to encourage us to have faith in our clinical opinion that the lesion is indeed peripheral.

Cerebello–pontine angle lesions

Magnetic resonance imaging is the method of choice for detecting CP angle lesions. Until recently, gadolinium enhancement was necessary to be absolutely sure that

ing. From the 1930s it has been possible to image blood vessels, and excellent pictures of occluded arteries, aneurysms, and vascular malformations have been available to clinicians for 50 years. In addition, displacement of cerebral structures often provided additional information about the distribution and distortion of neural tissue. Intra-arterial injection of contrast was, however, not without risk. The development of digital subtraction techniques enabled low-dose arterial or venous injections to be given, thus reducing morbidity. For the past 5 years magnetic resonance angiography (MRA) has been developed to a degree that is rendering digital subtraction angiography (DSA) obsolete. At present, imaging of patients with neuro-otological symptoms is almost entirely dependent upon magnetic resonance (MRI and MRA) and occasionally temporal bone CT scan.

Of other imaging modalities, isotope scanning is of historical interest, emission computed tomography is of limited use because of the relatively low resolution and expense and impedance tomography has not yet been developed (and may never be developed).

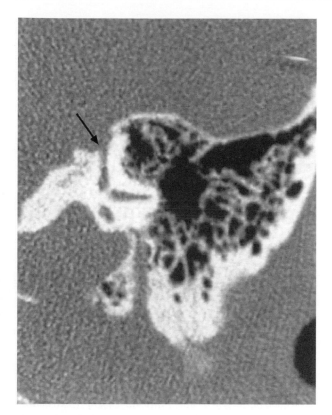

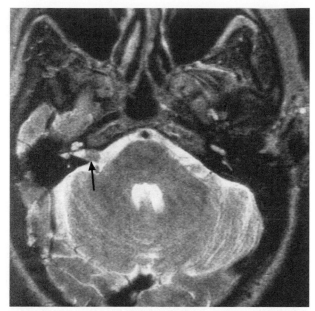

Figure 7.11 *Magnetic resonance image in horizontal plane showing small VIIIth nerve tumor in the internal acoustic meatus (arrow). Section slightly tilted.*

Figure 7.10 *High-resolution bone computed tomography scan of the temporal bone in a patient with Tullio phenomenon. The patient had lateropulsion and torsional nystagmus provoked by loud sounds to the left ear (reported in ref. 13). The Figure shows absence of bony roof of the left superior (or anterior) semicircular canal (arrow).*

small masses adjacent to the VIIIth nerve were detected (Fig. 7.9),[117] but this is no longer the case provided that high-quality MRI pictures using 1-mm slice thickness are obtained in the horizontal and coronal planes (Fig. 7.11). Clearly, such images obtained by using these techniques are expensive and one needs to have a good clinical assessment of the patient to select those requiring such imaging. Acoustic neuromas are common and their presence in some patients with dizziness or unsteady gait may be incidental. Small vascular malformations are also shown and MRI is now of sufficient resolution to render formal intra-arterial injection arteriography obsolete.

Brainstem and cerebellar lesions

It is in the area of central neuro-otological abnormalities that MRI has revolutionized imaging of the patient with a balance disorder.

FORAMEN MAGNUM LESIONS

Lesions of the foramen magnum are not common but are important because the vast majority are benign and are often correctable, at least in part. Prior to MRI, one

had to rely on CT myelography to visualize this difficult area and quite often patients with a clinical picture highly suggestive of Arnold Chiari malformation, pre-pontine epidermoids, or gliomas, or other lesions in this area, were repeatedly studied with invasive methods before a definitive diagnosis was made. Now, a combination of sagittal and horizontal MRI will give a definitive answer in appropriate patients within minutes, since images can be obtained in the required plane, and internal as well as extra-axial areas are visualized.[20]

INTRINSIC BRAINSTEM LESIONS

Lesions of the brainstem may cause unsteadiness, oscillopsia, diplopia, and vertigo and are often demonstrated with MRI (e.g. lateral medullary syndrome; Fig. 7.12). With MRI it has been possible to disentangle the anatomical basis of some of these symptoms.[118] The major problem, however, is to determine in diffuse or multifocal pathology which lesions are responsible for a specific abnormality found on neuro-otological testing. To tackle this difficult problem, averaging techniques using MRI in patients with unequivocal central pathology have been used.[39] In groups of patients it has been clearly shown that canal paresis results from a lesion in the root entry zone of the VIIIth nerve and particularly from involvement of the medial vestibular nucleus.[65] Similarly, unilateral gaze palsies occur with lesions in the nuclei reticulari pontis oralis and caudalis; rather surprisingly, bilateral gaze palsies occur in mid-line ponto-medullary lesions in the nucleus raffe-interpositus, and less surprisingly internuclear ophthalmoplegias (INO) result from high pontine lesions involving the medial

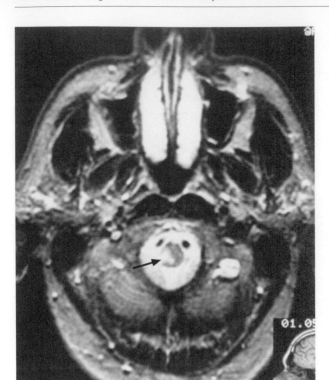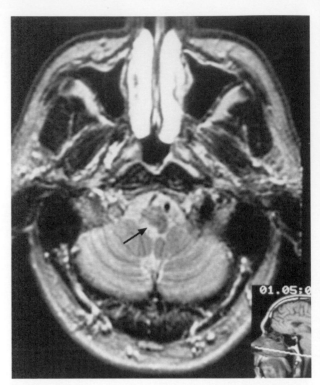

Figure 7.12 *Magnetic resonance images showing area of infarction of medulla (arrows) in a patient with Wallenberg syndrome with lateropulsion and torsional nystagmus. Note patency of vertebral artery and sparing of cerebellum implying occlusion of long projecting branches from the PICA. The left section lies 5 mm lower than right.*

longitudinal fasciculus (MLF).[19] Vertical nystagmus, which is commonly associated with an INO occurs from lesions in the floor of the IV ventricle and just inferior to the aqueduct. More recent studies have shown that pendular nystagmus occurs with lesions in the central tegmental tract and olivary and red nuclei.[27] Torsional nystagmus is caused by lesions in the medial vestibular nucleus.[24] While all these studies are primarily research oriented, they have given clear proof that it is possible to locate specific lesion sites which accompany a given neuro-otological picture and that in patients with that picture MRI will enable anatomical location of the lesion and help unravel its nature.

THALAMIC AND CORTICAL LESIONS

Lesions in the thalamus and neo-cortex are readily demonstrated with combination of CT scanning and MRI. It is uncommon for such lesions to cause vestibular symptoms, with the exception of epileptic activity from the area of the cortex involved in vestibular pathways, namely, the temporal lobe, parietal cortex (area 2v, area 3av), and the posterior insular in monkeys, and presumably, humans. In contrast, lesions in the region of the posterior insular and angular gyrus can cause directional preponderance of optokinetic nystagmus and deviation of visual vertical perception.[119]

DIFFERENTIAL DIAGNOSIS WITH NON-NEURO-OTOLOGICAL CONDITIONS: SYNCOPE, EPILEPSY, CONGENITAL NYSTAGMUS

Syncope

The possibility that the patient with falls or unclearly defined vertiginous symptoms may suffer from syncope is frequently raised. Vaso-vagal syncope, or common faint, can be easily recognized even by an untrained person. It usually manifests in a warm or stuffy room, frequently preceded by a sensation of warmth or nausea that patients with repeated faints recognize well. Slightly more troublesome to diagnose is when the clinician faces the first fainting episode, particularly when this occurs in adult life, or in the elderly when prodromal symptoms may not be prominent. Witnesses of the episodes may report the patients being pale or sweaty or describe muscle twitches or upward deviation of the eyes,[120] which can confuse the picture as they may suggest epilepsy. The recovery of the patient's consciousness is usually quick, less than 1 min or so. The triggers to vaso-vagal syncopes vary, but usually include orthostatic stress, emotional stimuli (the sight of blood being a particularly common one), or painful stimuli. Syncope can also occur triggered by micturition, postural changes or cough, in which case they are called 'situational syncopes'.

Clinical examination in vaso-vagal syncope is entirely normal between episodes and a diagnosis is therefore made on the basis of the clinical history in most cases. Patients referred for cardiological or neurological investigations reach a diagnosis on the basis of exclusion of other conditions. More recently, with the advent of the 'tilt test', confirmation of syncope can be reached as a positive diagnosis rather than by exclusion.[121] In this test, patients usually lie tilted some 30° away from perfect vertical for periods of around 45 min while ECG and blood pressure are continuously monitored. With such techniques well over 50 per cent of patients with syncope will show either a significant drop in blood pressure, bradycardia or both. Reappearance of the patient's spontaneous symptoms by the orthostatic stress, a common occurrence, further reinforces the diagnosis of syncope (see Chapter 22).

The treatment of vaso-vagal syncope is difficult but most patients need only to be reassured and informed about their condition. Specific advice on sitting or lying down when the preliminary symptoms appear should be given and patients likely to injure themselves, such as the elderly, should be carefully instructed on how to rise from bed and avoid the triggering circumstances. A variety of drugs may show some good results including anticholinergic or vaso-active drugs such as sympathomimetic agents, but care should be exercised as aggravation of symptoms can occur with some of these drugs.[122]

The possibility that a loss of consciousness or a fall is due to a structural heart disease, heart arrhythmia, hypoglycemia, vertebro-basilar ischemia or epilepsy should always be borne in mind and appropriate questions should be posed by the clinician. In the specific scope of this chapter dealing with vestibular symptoms – which are so commonly triggered by head movements – it must be borne in mind that syncope can also occur during head/neck movements, in which case carotid sinus hypersensitivity[123] or, exceptionally, vertebral artery blockage by cervical osteoarthritis combined with vascular disease may be the cause. The presence of additional symptoms, such as slurred speech, diplopia, facial or peri-oral numbness should be directly enquired about as they suggest vertebro-basilar ischemia; isolated audio-vestibular or purely vestibular ischemia may occasionally occur in vertebro-basilar insufficiency but, in principle, they should be treated with suspicion. Basal ganglia disorders with orthostatic hypotension syncope and the differential diagnosis of drop attacks are dealt with in Chapters 11, 16 and 22 respectively.

Cardiac syncope

It is vital, in obtaining the history of vertigo, loss of consciousness or falls, to determine if there are features pointing to impaired cardiac output as the cause. Unfortunately, few symptoms can reliably distinguish cardiac dysfunction from vestibular symptoms *per se*, although chest pain does indicate the former. Pallor and sweating occur in both while palpitations are common in patients with peripheral vestibular failure. Nevertheless, palpitations, pallor and sweating consistently and repeatedly occurring in patients with dizziness, especially if they precede the vestibular symptoms, demand full cardiac assessment.

Ictal dizziness

All neuro-otologists are familiar with the occasional misdiagnosis of a simple or complex partial seizure presenting to them. Such patients complain of dizziness (a vague term that can include vertigo, especially if areas of the vestibular cortex are involved). It is vital to obtain a witness account of these cases as so often the patient is unaware of their behavior. This is the only situation where the patient's vestibular symptoms can include unconsciousness. If the attack continues to a major seizure the diagnosis is easy but so often this is not the case, at least initially. A witness may have some valuable information about the appearance of the patient and their movements (e.g. chomping of the jaws, glazed appearance or vacancy). Confusion and incontinence of urine are two useful symptoms to elicit, which point to an epileptic origin of the vertigo. It should be emphasized that diagnostic confusion between such attacks and vestibular failure is rare but it is an important distinction to make.

Congenital oculomotor disorders

Genetic or developmental disorders of eye movements which manifest within a few months after birth pose a problem for the identification of acquired balance disorders.[124] First, since identification of the causes of balance disorders relies greatly on identifying certain patterns of eye movement, the presence of a prior eye movement disorder can mask valuable clinical signs. Second, an early-onset eye movement problem may have previously been overlooked if mild and asymptomatic, so that it may be first detected when a patient presents for neurological examination, under which circumstances it may be taken to suggest acquired disease. Even the patient may not know that they have had a mild oculomotor abnormality throughout their life if it has not given rise to symptoms or of sufficiently florid appearance to provoke social comment.

Undoubtedly, the early-onset eye movement disorders in patients with a more generalized condition, such as fully expressed albinism or retinal–renal abnormalities, will have been identified at an early stage in life. Of more immediate concern are any nystagmus associated with strabismus and 'congenital nystagmus' which may be isolated, idiopathic and pass undetected.

The key identifying feature of nystagmus associated with strabismus is that it may be minimal when both eyes are free to view and enhanced when one eye is covered. This is 'latent nystagmud' and always beats towards the viewing (uncovered) eye.[32] When a latent nystagmus is identified one may expect pursuit to be deranged both monocularly and occasionally binocularly.

Although any early-onset nystagmus is in some sense congenital, the term congenital nystagmus, abbreviated to 'CN', is reserved for a nystagmus in which the slow phases have a bizarre appearance with increasing velocity profiles and pendular distortions of the slow phase waveform. Such nystagmus occurs in association with a number of congenital syndromes, many rare and obscure, of which the most familiar to the reader will probably be albinism. The nystagmus also frequently occurs in isolation and can be proven familial or sporadic. The eye movement is most frequently conjugate in the lateral plane but vertical, torsional and asymmetrical disconjugate forms are seen.

The clinician should be particularly aware that any congenital nystagmus may wax and wane spontaneously or be provoked by illness, when they may become symptomatic, and the less florid forms may have been overlooked in the patient's previous medical examinations.[125]

The compromises that congenital nystagmus can cause in neuro-otological testing and in the assessment of a patient with an acquired balance or gait problem underline the importance of taking a careful history relating to any possible lifelong abnormality of eye movement. In addition, a test for stereoscopic vision, one of which is available in the form of a booklet of pictures viewed through polarized lenses, is a useful adjunct to examination and will identify failure to develop binocular vision. This implies the prior existence of strabismus, even in a patient whose eyes appear 'straight'. In some cases, however, formal eye movement recordings are required to identify the typical CN waveforms.

CONCLUSIONS

Vestibular input is instrumental in the control of balance, in particular in dynamic conditions such as during locomotion. If a balance or gait complaint is or has been associated with vertigo, oscillopsia or hearing disorder, it is likely to be due to a peripheral or central vestibular disorder. The examination must include otoscopy and clinical assessment of hearing, gait with eyes open and closed and eye movements while upright and during the positional maneuver. Clinical examination may be normal in patients with peripheral vestibular lesions outside the acute stage and specialized tests are frequently required. The most useful in practice are the bithermal caloric test and audiological investigations. Central vestibular disorders usually have abnormal eye movements and various types of clinically visible nystagmus but it is important to be aware that a congenital nystagmus may be present in a patient with an unrelated gait disorder. Unexplained falls or dizzy turns of possible syncopal or epileptic origin may require autonomic function or EEG investigations. Magnetic resonance imaging is usually the method of choice for imaging the contents of the posterior fossa and the inner ear when a structural lesion is suspected.

REFERENCES

1. Spoor F, Wood B, Zonneveld F. Implications of early hominid labyrinthine morphology for evolution of human bipedal locomotion. *Nature* 1994;**369**:645–48.
2. Bronstein AM. Visual vertigo syndrome: clinical and posturography findings. *J Neurol Neurosurg Psychiatry* 1995;**59**:472–6.
3. Guerraz M, Yardley L, Bertholon P, et al. Visual vertigo: symptom assessment, spatial orientation and postural control. *Brain* 2001;**124**:1646–56.
4. Redfern MS, Yardley L, Bronstein AM. Visual influences on balance. *J Anxiety Disord* 2001;**15**:81–94.
5. Page NGR, Gresty MA Motorist's vestibular disorientation syndrome. *J Neurol Neurosurg Psychiatry* 1985;**48**:729–35.
6. Brandt T, Bronstein AM. Cervical vertigo. *J Neurol Neurosurg Psychiatry* 2001;**71**:8–12.
7. Bender MB. Oscillopsia. *Arch Neurol* 1965;**13**:204–13.
8. Gresty MA, Hess K, Leech J. Disorders of the vestibulo-ocular reflex producing oscillopsia and mechanisms compensating for loss of labyrinthine function. *Brain* 1977;**100**(4):693–716.
9. Lempert T, Gianna CC, Gresty MA, Bronstein AM. Effect of otolith dysfunction: impairment of visual acuity during linear head motion in labyrinthine defective subjects. *Brain* 1997;**120**:1005–13.
10. Rinne T, Bronstein AM, Rudge P, et al. Bilateral loss of vestibular function: clinical findings in 53 patients. *J Neurol* 1998;**245**:314–21.
11. Rudge P, Bronstein AM. Investigations of disorders of balance. *J Neurol Neurosurg Psychiatry* 1995;**59**(9):568–78.
12. Mossman SS, Bronstein AM, Rudge P, Gresty MA Acquired pendular nystagmus suppressed by alcohol. *Neuro-ophthalmology* 1993;**13**:99–106.
13. Bronstein AM. Faldon M, Rothwell J, et al. Clinical and electrophysiological findings in the Tullio phenomenon. *Acta Otolaryngol* 1995;**520**(Suppl):1209–11.
14. Gresty MA, Bronstein AM, Brandt T, Dieterich M. Neurology of otolith function: peripheral and central disorders. *Brain* 1992;**115**:647–73.
15. Jauregui-Renaud K, Faldon ME, Gresty MA, Bronstein AM. Horizontal ocular vergence and the three-dimensional response to whole-body roll motion. *Exp Brain Res* 2001;**136**:79–92.
16. Carpenter RHS. *Movements of the eyes*, 2nd edn. London: Pion, 1988.
17. Leigh RJ, Zee DS. *The Neurology of eye movements*, 3rd edn. Philadelphia: FA Davis, 1999.

18. Cogan DG, Kubik CS, Smith WL. Unilateral internuclear ophthalmoplegia: report of eight clinical cases with one post-mortem study. *Arch Ophthalmol*. 1950;**44**:783–96.

19. Bronstein AM, Rudge P, Gresty MA, et al. Abnormalities of horizontal gaze. Clinical, oculographic and magnetic resonance imaging findings. II: gaze palsy and internuclear ophthalmoplegia. *J Neurol Neurosurg Psychiatry* 1990;**53**:200–7.

20. Bronstein AM, Miller DH, Rudge P, Kendall BE. Down beating nystagmus: magnetic resonance imaging and neuro-otological findings. *J Neurol Sci* 1987;**81**:173–84.

21. Halmagyi GM, Rudge P, Gresty MA, Sanders MD. Downbeating nystagmus. A review of 62 cases. *Arch Neurol* 1983;**40**:777–84.

22. Fisher A, Gresty MA, Chambers B, Rudge P. Primary position upbeating nystagmus. *Brain* 1983;**106**:949–64.

23. Janssen JC, Larner AJ, Morris H, et al. Upbeat nystagmus: clinicoanatomical correlation. *J Neurol Neurosurg Psychiatry* 1998;**65**:380–1.

24. Lopez L, Bronstein AM, Gresty MA, et al. Torsional nystagmus. A neuro-otological and MRI study of thirty-five cases. *Brain* 1992;**115**:1107–24.

25. Aschoff JC, Conrad B, Kornhuber HH. Acquired pendular nystagmus with oscillopsia in multiple sclerosis: a sign of cerebellar nuclei disease. *J Neurol Neurosurg Psychiatry* 1974;**37**:570–7.

26. Gresty MA, Ell JJ, Findley LJ. Acquired pendular nystagmus: its characteristics, localising value and pathophysiology. *J Neurol Neurosurg Psychiatry* 1982;**45**:431–9.

27. Lopez L, Gresty MA, Bronstein AM, et al. Clinical and MRI correlates in 27 patients with acquired pendular nystagmus. *Brain* 1996;**119**:465–72

28. Shallo-Hoffmann J, Petersen J, Muhlendyck H. How normal are 'normal' square wave jerks? *Invest Ophthalmol Vis Sci* 1989;**30**:225–7.

29. Rascol O, Sabatini U, Simonetta-Moreau M, Montastruc JL, Rascol A, Clanet M. Square wave jerks in Parkinsonian syndromes. *J Neurol Neurosurg Psychiatry* 1991;**54**:599–602.

30. Shults WT, Stark L, Hoyt WF, Ochs AL. Normal saccadic structure of voluntary nystagmus. *Arch Ophthalmol* 1977;**95**:1399–404.

31. Zahn JR. Incidence and characteristics of voluntary nystagmus. *J Neurol Neurosurg Psychiatry* 1978;**41**:617–23.

32. Gresty Ma, Metcalfe T, Timms C, et al. Neurology of latent nystagmus. *Brain* 1992;**115**:1303–21.

33. Chambers BR, Ell JJ, Gresty MA. Case of downbeat nystagmus influenced by otolith stimulation. *Ann Neurol*. 1982;**13**:204–7.

34. Ashe J, Haine TC, Zee DS, Shatz NJ. Microsaccadic flutter. *Brain* 1991;**114**:461–72.

35. Bronstein AM, Gresty MA, Mossman SS. Pendular pseudonystagmus arising as a combination of head tremor and vestibular failure. *Neurology* 1992;**42**:1527–31.

36. Kennard C, Lueck CJ. Oculomotor abnormalities in diseases of the basal ganglia. *Rev Neurol (Paris)* 1989;**145**:587–95.

37. Stell R, Bronstein AM. Eye movement abnormalities in extrapyramidal diseases. In: Marsden CD, Fahn S, eds. *Movement disorders 3*. Oxford: Butterworth Heinemann, 1994:88–113.

38. Zee DS, Optican LM, Cook JD, et al. Slow saccades in spino-cerebellar degeneration. *Arch Neurol* 1979;**5**:405–14.

39. Bronstein AM, Morris J, du Boulay EPGH, et al. Abnormalities of gaze. Clinical, oculographic and magnetic resonance imaging findings. I: Abducens palsy. *J Neurol Neurosurg Psychiatry* 1990;**53**:194–9.

40. Botzel K, Rottach K, Buttner U. Normal and pathological saccadic dysmetria. *Brain* 1993;**116**:337–53.

41. Zee DS. Ophthalmoscopy in examination of patients with vestibular disorders. *Ann Neurol* 1978;**3**:373–74.

42. Kanayama R, Bronstein AM, Shallo-Hoffmann J, et al. Visually and memory guided saccades in a case of cerebellar saccadic dysmetria. *J Neurol Neurosurg Psychiatry* 1994;**57**:1081–4.

43. Halmagyi GM, Curthoys IS. A clinical sign of canal paresis. *Arch Neurol* 1988;**45**:737–9.

44. Halmagyi GM, Gresty MA. Clinical signs of visual-vestibular interaction. *J Neurol Neurosurg Psychiatry* 1979;**42**:934–9.

45. Leech J, Gresty MA, Hess K, Rudge P. Gaze failure, drifting eye movements and centripetal nystagmus in cerebellar disease. *Br J Ophthalmol* 1977;**61**:774–81.

46. Page NGR, Barratt HJ, Gresty MA. Gaze abnormalities with chronic cerebral lesions in man. In: Gale AG, Johnson F, eds. *Theoretical and applied aspects of eye movement research*. Amsterdam: North Holland/Elsevier, 1984;397–402.

47. Behill AT, Clark MR, Stark L. The Main Sequence; a tool for studying human eye movements. *Math Biosci* 1975;**24**:191–204.

48. Barnes GR, Gresty MA. Characteristics of eye movements to targets of short duration. *Aerospace Med* 1973;**44**:1236–40.

49. Gresty MA, Findley LJ, Wade P. The mechanism of rotatory nystagmus in opsoclonus. *Br J Ophthalmol* 1980;**64**:923–25.

50. Barratt HJ, Bronstein AM, Gresty MA. Testing the vestibular-ocular reflexes: abnormalities of the otolith contribution in patients with neuro-otological disease. *J Neurol Neurosurg Psychiatry* 1987;**50**:1029–35.

51. Baloh RW, Honrubia V, Sills A. Eye-tracking and optokinetic nystagmus. Results of quantitative testing in patients with well-defined nervous system lesions. *Ann Otol* 1977;**86**:108–14.

52. Chambers BR, Gresty MA. The relationship between disordered pursuit and vestibulo-ocular reflex suppression. *J Neurol Neurosurg Psychiatry*. 1983;**46**:61–6.

53. Baloh RW, Yee RD, Honrubia V. Clinical abnormalities of optokinetic nystagmus. In: Lennestrand G, Zee DS, Keller EL, eds. *Functional basis of ocular motility disorder. Wenner-Gren Symposium series 37* Oxford: Pergamon Press. 1992;311–20.

54. Baloh RW, Yee RD, Honrubia V. Optokinetic nystagmus and parietal lobe lesions. *Ann Neurol*. 1980;**7**:269–76.

55. Mossman SS, Bronstein AM, Hood JD. Optokinetic nystagmus in response to different stimulus modalities. *Neuro-ophthalmology* 1992;**12**:63–72.

56. Waespe W, Cohen B, Raphan T. Role of the flocculus and para-flocculus in optokinetic nystagmus and visual-vestibular interactions: Effects of lesions. *Exp Brain Res* 1983;**50**:9–33.

57. Halmagyi GM, Curthoys IS, Cremer PD, et al. The human horizontal vestibulo-ocular reflex in response to high-acceleration stimulation before and after unilateral vestibular neurectomy. *Exp Brain Res* 1990;**479**:490.

58. Baloh RW, Hess K, Honrubia V, Yee RD. Low and high frequency sinusoidal rotational testing in patients with peripheral vestibular lesions. *Acta Otolaryngol (Stockh)* 1984;**406**(Suppl):189–93.

59. Waespe W. The physiology and pathophysiology of the vestibulo-ocular system. In: Hofferberth B, Brune GG, Sitzer G, Weger HD, eds. *Vascular brain stem diseases*. Basel: Karger, 1990;37–67.

60. Gresty MA, Barratt HJ, Page NGR, Ell JJ. Assessment of vestibulo-ocular reflexes in congenital nystagmus. *Ann Neurol* 1985;**17**:129–36.

61. Hood JD, Korres S. Vestibular suppression in peripheral and central vestibular disorders. *Brain* 1979;**102**:785–804.

62. Cawthorne TE, Fitzgerald G, Hallpike CS. Observations on the directional preponderance of caloric nystagmus resulting from unilateral labyrinthectomy. *Brain* 1942;**65**:138–60.

63. Cawthorne TE, Fitzgerald G, Hallpike CS. Studies in human vestibular function: observations on the clinical features of Mèniére's disease with especial reference to the results of the caloric tests. *Brain* 1942;**65**:161.

64. Fitzgerald G, Hallpike CS. Studies in human vestibular function: 1. Observations on the directional preponderance ('Nystagmusberietschaft') of caloric nystagmus resulting from cerebral lesions. *Brain* 1942;**65**:115–37.

65. Francis DA, Bronstein AM, Rudge P, du Boulay EPGH. The site of brainstem lesions causing semicircular canal paresis: an MRI study. *J Neurol Neurosurg Psychiatry* 1992;**55**:446–9.

66. Kayan A, Trinder E, Harrison MS. The use of galvanic vestibular nystagmus in clinical otology. *J Laryngol Otol* 1974;**88**:503–13.

67. Tokita T, Takagi K, Ito Y. Analysis of the vestibulo-spinal system with a five-dimensional feedback model. *Acta Laryngol* 1987;**104**(3–4):322–7.

68. Colebatch JG, Halmagyi GM. Vestibular evoked potentials in human neck muscles before and after unilateral vestibular deafferentation. *Neurology* 1992;**42**:1635–6.

69. Colebatch JG, Rothwell JC. Vestibular-evoked EMG responses in human neck muscles. *J Physiol* 1993;**473**:18.

70. Colebatch JG, Rothwell JC, Bronstein A, Ludman H. Click-evoked vestibular activation in the Tullio phenomenon. *J Neurol Neurosurg Psychiatry* 1994;**57**:1538–40.

71. Brookes GB, Gresty MA, Nakamura T, Metcalfe T. Sensing and controlling rotational orientation in normal subjects and patients with loss of labyrinthine function. *Am J Otol* 1993;**14**:349–51.

72. von Brevern M, Faldon ME, Brookes GB, Gresty MA. Evaluating 3D semicircular canal function by perception of rotation. *Am J Otol* 1997;**18**:484–93.

73. Kanayama R, Bronstein AM, Gresty MA, et al. Perceptual studies in patients with vestibular neurectomy. *Acta Otolaryngol* 1995;**520**(Suppl):408–11.

74. Faldon M, Shallo-Hoffmann J, Bronstein AM, Gresty MA. 'Vestibular perception' in subjects with congenital nystagmus. *Neuro-ophthalmology* 1997;**17**:135–47.

75. Okada T, Grunfeld E, Shallo-Hoffmann J, Bronstein AM. Vestibular perception of angular velocity in normal subjects and in patients with congenital nystagmus. *Brain* 1999;**122**:1293–303

76. Gresty MA, Lempert Th. Pathophysiology and clinical testing of otolith dysfunction. *Adv Oto-Rhinol Laryngol* 2001;**58**:15–33.

77. Lempert T, Gresty MA, Bronstein AM. Horizontal linear vestibulo-ocular reflex testing in patients with peripheral vestibular disorders. *Ann N Y Acad Sci* 1999;**871**:232–47.

78. Bronstein AM, Gresty MA. Short latency compensatory eye movement responses to transient linear head acceleration: a specific function of the otolith-ocular reflex. *Exp Brain Res* 1988;**71**:406–10.

79. Bronstein AM, Gresty MA, Brookes GB. Compensatory otolithic slow-phase eye movement responses to abrupt linear head motion in the lateral direction. Findings in patients with labyrinthine and neurological lesions. *Acta Otolaryngol (Stockh)* 1991;**481**(Suppl):42–6.

80. Brookes GB, Bronstein AM, Gresty MA. Otolith-ocular reflexes in patients with unilateral and bilateral loss of labyrinthine function. In: Sacristan T, Alvarex-Vincent JJ, Bartual F, et al., eds. *Otorhinolaryngology, head and neck surgery*. Amsterdam: Kugler and Ghedini, 1990:805–8.

81. Lempert T, Gianna CC, Brookes GB, et al. Horizontal otolith–ocular responses in humans after unilateral vestibular deafferentation. *Exp Brain Res*, 1998;**118**:533–40.

82. Barratt HJ, Gresty MA, Page NGR. Neurological evidence for dissociation of pursuit and optokinetic systems. *Acta Otolaryngol (Stockh)* 1985;**100**:89–97.

83. Koizuka I, Takeda N, Sato S, Matsunaga T. Centric and eccentric VOR tests in patients with Meniere's disease. *Acta Otolaryngol* 1991;**481**(Suppl):55–58.

84. Diamond SG, Markham CH. Binocular counter-rolling in humans with unilateral labyrinthectomy and in normal controls. *Ann N Y Acad Sci*, 1981;**374**:69–79.

85. Diamond SG, Markham CH. Ocular counter-rolling as an indicator of vestibular otolith function. *Neurology* 1983;**3**:1460–9.

86. Kingma H. Clinical testing of the statolith-ocular reflex. *ORL J Otorhinolaryngol Relat Spec* 1997;**59**(4):198–208.

87. Bohmer A, Mast F. Assessing otolith function by the subjective visual vertical. *Ann N Y Acad Sci* 1999;**871**:221–31

88. Friedmann G. The perception of the visual vertical and horizontal with peripheral and central vestibular lesions. *Brain* 1970;**93**:313–28.

89. Dai MJ, Curthoys IS, Halmagyi GM. Linear acceleration perception in the roll plane before and after unilateral vestibular neurectomy. *Exp Brain Res* 1989;**77**: 315–28.

90. Curthoys IS, Dai MJ, Halmagyi GM. Human ocular torsional position before and after unilateral vestibular neurectomy. *Exp Brain Res* 1991;**85**:218–25.

91. Clarke AH, Englehorn A. Unilateral testing of utricular function. *Exp Brain Res* 1998;**121**:457–64.

92. Odkvist LM, Noaksson L, Olsson S, Ledin T. Subjective visual horizontal determination during otolith stimulation by eccentric rotation in conservatively treated Meniere's disease. *Int Tinnitus J* 1998;**4**(1):75–7.

93. Bohmer A, Mast F. Chronic unilateral loss of otolith function revealed by the subjective visual vertical during off center yaw rotation. *J Vestib Res* 1999;**9**(6):413–22

94. Vibert D, Hausler R. Long-term evolution of subjective visual vertical after vestibular neurectomy and labyrinthectomy. *Acta Otolaryngol* 2000;**120**(5):620–2.

95. Diener HC, Dichgans J, Bacher M, Gompf B. Quantification of postural sway in normals and patients with cerebellar diseases. *Electroencephalogr Clin Neurophysiol* 1984;**57**:134–42.

96. Bronstein AM, Hood JD, Gresty MA, Panagi C. Visual control of balance in cerebellar and Parkinsonian syndromes. *Brain* 1990;**113**:767–79.

97. Yarrow K, Brown P, Gresty MA, Bronstein AM. Force platform

recordings in the diagnosis of primary orthostatic tremor. *Gait Posture* 2001;**13**:27–34.

98. Katz J. *Handbook of clinical audiology*, 4th edn. New York: Williams and Wilkins, 1994.

99. Poole JP. Clinical technique in bone conduction tests. *Sound* 1970;**4**:31–34.

100. Dix MR. Loudness recruitment and its measurement with especial reference to the loudness discomfort level test and its value in diagnosis. *Ann Otol Rhinol Laryngol* 1968;**77**:1131–51.

101. Cohen M, Prasher DK. The value of combining auditory brainstem responses and acoustic reflex threshold measurements in neuro-otological diagnosis. *Scand Audiol* 1988;**17**:153–62.

102. Prasher DK, Cohen M. Effectiveness of acoustic reflex threshold criteria in the diagnosis of retrocochlear pathology. *Scand Audiol* 1993;**22**:11–18.

103. Jewett DL, Williston JS. Auditory evoked far fields averaged from the scalp of humans. *Brain* 1971;**94**:681–96.

104. Hashimoto I, Isiyama Y, Yoshimotor T, Nemoto S. Brain stem auditory evoked potentials recorded directly from human brain stem and thalamus. *Brain* 1981;**104**:841–60.

105. Moller AR, Jannetta PJ, Sekhar LN. Contributions from the auditory nerve to the brain stem auditory evoked potentials (BAEP). Results of intracranial recordings in man. *Electroenceph Clin Neurophysiol* 1988;**71**:198–211.

106. Eggermont JJ, Don M, Brackmann DE. Electro-cochleography and auditory brain stem electric responses in patients with pontine angle tumours. *Ann Otol Rhinol Laryngol* 1980 Nov–Dec;**89**(6 Pt 2):1–19.

107. Selters WA, Brackman DE. Acoustic tumor detection with brain stem electric response audiometry. *Arch Oto-laryngol* 1977;**103**:181–7.

108. Robinson K, Rudge P. The differential diagnosis of cerebello-pontine angle lesions. *J Neurol Sci* 1983;**60**:1–21.

109. Robinson K, Rudge P. The use of auditory evoked potentials in the diagnosis of multiple sclerosis. *J Neurol Sci* 1980;**45**:235–44.

110. Robinson K, Rudge P. Auditory evoked responses in multiple sclerosis. *Lancet* 1975;**1**:1164–5.

111. Robinson K, Rudge P. Abnormalities of the auditory evoked potentials in patients with multiple sclerosis. *Brain* 1977;**100**:19–40.

112. Kemp DJ, Ryan S, Bray P. A guide to the effective use of oto-acoustic emissions. *Ear Hearing* 1990;**11**:93–105.

113. Minor LB, Cremer PD, Carey JP, et al. Symptoms and signs in superior canal dehiscence syndrome. *Ann N Y Acad Sci* 2001;**942**:259–73.

114. Carey JP, Minor LB, Nager GT. Dehiscence or thinning of bone overlying the superior semicircular canal in a temporal bone survey. *Arch Otolaryngol Head Neck Surg* 2000;**126**:137–47.

115. Mark AS, Seltzer S, Harnsberger HR. Sensorineural hearing loss: more than meets the eye? *Am J Neuroradiol* 1993;**14**:37–45.

116. Weissman JL, Curtin HD, Hirsch BE, Hirsch WL. High signal from the otic labyrinth on unenhanced magnetic resonance imaging. *Am J Neuroradiol* 1992;**13**:1183–7.

117. The Consensus Development Panel. National Institute of Health consensus development conference statement on acoustic neuroma. December 11–13, 1991. *Arch Neurol* 1994;**51**:201–7.

118. Waespe W, Wichmann. Oculomotor disturbances during visual–vestibular interaction in Wallenberg's lateral medullary syndrome. *Brain* 1990;**113**:821–46

119. Brandt T, Dieterich M, Dnek A. Vestibular cortex lesions affect the perception of verticality. *Ann Neurol* 1994;**35**:403–12.

120. Lempert T, von Brevern M. The eye movements of syncope. *Neurology* 1996;**46**:1086–8.

121. Sneddon JF, Camm AJ. Vasovagal syncope: classification, investigation and treatment. *Br J Hosp Med* 1993;**49**:329–34.

122. Chan WL, Kong CW, Chang MS, Chiang BN. Exacerbation of vasodepressor syncope by beta-adrenergic blockade. *N Engl J Med* 1991;**324**:1219–20.

123. Kenny RA, Traynor G. Carotid sinus syndrome – clinical characteristics in elderly patients. *Age Ageing* 1991;**20**:449–54.

124. Gresty MA, Page NGR, Barratt HJ. The differential diagnosis of congenital nystagmus. *J Neurol Neurosurg Psychiatry.* 1984;**47**:936–42.

125. Gresty MA, Bronstein AM, Page NGR, Rudge P. Congenital-type nystagmus emerging in later life. *Neurology* 1991;**41**:653–6.

8

Objective assessment of posture and gait

KENTON R. KAUFMAN

INTRODUCTION

Every health professional treating patients with clinical disorders of balance, posture and gait must evaluate and treat the patient based on assumptions made about the relative function of the central nervous system, selective motor control, weak or spastic muscles, joint contracture and bony deformities. The usual methods of assessment include physical examination, manual muscle testing and visual observation. Clinical inspection of postural balance and gait are an important part of a routine clinical examination. A treatment plan is formed based on algorithms passed on by others and modified by experience gained from personal observations. However, many centers now have laboratories and skilled personnel to perform objective measurements rather than rely upon intuition and assumptions. These laboratories can provide quantitative information on the abnormal movement pattern. This objective information can then be used as a basis for appropriate therapeutic intervention. Posturography and gait analysis should be used as part of the initial assessment to provide a basis for correct intervention and repeated to aid in the assessment of therapeutic outcome.

The purpose of this chapter is to provide information on the types of instrumentation that are available and to describe how it can be used to measure those aspects of a patient's balance, posture and gait that cannot be assessed quantitatively in a clinical setting.

HISTORICAL PERSPECTIVE

Motion analysis can be described as the objective, systematic analysis of movement. The concept of depicting and recording human motion began during the Renaissance Period. Giovanni Alphonso Borelli, a student of Galileo, was among the first scientists to analyze motion while developing his theory of muscle action based upon mechanical principles.[1] Duchenne conducted the first scientific systematic evaluation of muscle function. His findings were published in the monumental work, *Physiologie des Mouvements*, published in 1867.[2] Edweard Muybridge first performed photographic recording of human motion. Muybridge was asked to settle a bet by Governor Leeland Stanford of California, USA, regarding whether a trotting horse had all four feet off the ground at any instant in time. Muybridge placed cameras at regular intervals along a race track. Thin threads stretched across the track triggered the shutters. The horse's hooves triggered cameras in order and a series of photographs clearly depicted the gait sequence. Muybridge subsequently compiled a detailed photographic account of human and animal locomotion, which was published in 1887, in three volumes.[3]

At the end of the nineteenth century in Germany, Braune and Fischer became interested in measuring the motion of human body segments. They placed Geissler tubes, containing a rarified nitrogen gas, on various limb segments of a human subject dressed in black. Electrical circuits connected to the tubes created incandescence and the illuminated tubes were recorded by cameras as the subject walked. Experiments were carried out at night because there was no means to darken the room in which studies were performed. It took 10–12 hours to put this apparatus on the subject, whereas data collection was completed in minutes using four cameras. The images were digitized using a precision optical device. Coordinate geometry was used to extract three-dimensional coordinates. Equations needed to calculate resultant forces and moments at the joints of a 12-segment rigid body model were formulated. Although their quantitative results were published in 1895, their findings are still valid today.[4]

Inman and colleagues combined rudimentary motion recordings with electromyography (EMG) in the latter part of the last century. Their pioneering work in limb prosthetic research laid the foundation for modern gait analysis. Their text, *Human Walking*, was published in 1981 and represents the seminal text in the field.[5]

Since this pioneering work, much effort has been put into developing the technology needed for human movement analysis. Automated movement tracking systems have replaced hand digitization. Advances in the aerospace industry have been utilized for the development of force plates for kinetic analysis. Computerized electromyography systems have replaced hand palpation. The technology and knowledge for gait analysis has now advanced to a level that permits rapid analysis.

EQUIPMENT AND METHODS

Observation

The simplest form of gait analysis is observational gait analysis. A systematic approach for observational gait analysis was developed at the Rancho Los Amigos Medical Center in Downey, California, USA.[6] An experienced observer can detect many gait deviations during both stance and swing phases. However, an obvious limitation of observation in gait analysis is the difficulty of observing multiple events and multiple body segments interacting concurrently. Further, it is not possible to visualize the location of force vectors in space or electromyographic activity of muscles. Events happening faster than 1/12 of a second (83 ms) cannot be perceived by the human eye.[7] More consistent observations are obtained when motion videotapes are reviewed in slow motion.[8] Three expert observers rated video footage of 15 children that had lower limb disability and wore braces.[8] Pearson's correlation coefficient was 0.6 within observers and less between observers. Thus, observational gait analysis is a convenient, but only moderately reliable technique. Saleh and Murdoch[9] used experienced observers to study the gait of transtibial amputees. The prosthetic limbs of the amputees were intentionally misaligned in the sagittal plane. The agreement of experienced observers with a biomechanical model was 22 per cent. In a similar study, 54 licensed physical therapists with varying amounts of clinical experience rated three patients with rheumatoid arthritis.[10] Generalized kappa coefficients ranged from 0.11 to 0.52, indicating that clinician assessments are only slightly to moderately reliable.

Thus, it is easy to see that limitations in observational gait analysis can lead to misinterpretation of the patient's locomotion capabilities. Hence, it is important to utilize advances in gait analysis techniques to more precisely quantify the patient's functional status. Extensive instrumentation has been developed for recording the various parameters used to describe balance and gait.

Posturography

Upright stance requires multiple sensory inputs with automatic and reflexive motor responses to keep the person's center of mass over the base of support. Once the center of mass deviates from its equilibrium position relative to the force of gravity, the person senses the deviation through a combination of sensory inputs from the balance system, consisting of vision, somatosensation and vestibular sensation. The balance system receives multiple sensory inputs, which provides redundancy and gives a margin of safety for maintenance of postural equilibrium. Therefore, in order to evaluate the balance system, it is necessary to examine critically the integration of these sensory inputs and their ability to handle sensory conflict. In addition, it is important to assess the sensory motor response and coordination of the lower limbs when evaluating balance.

Postural sway has long been recognized as an important indicator of balance function. Stationary force platforms equipped with strain gauges have been used to record postural sway.[11] However, there are no data that suggest measuring balance while standing still predicts or explains functional performance in patients with balance impairments.[12] Alternatively, systems have been built wherein the force platform is mechanized so that it can either translate in a horizontal plane or rotate out of the horizontal plane (i.e. pitch the subject either forward or backward).[13] This type of dynamic system is called computerized dynamic posturography (CDP) and has been combined with other visual stimuli as a means of determining the relative importance of the various sensory inputs critical for balance. It allows some degree of isolation of the visual and somatosensory contributions to balance so that these influences can be analyzed separately from vestibular influences. The CDP system is capable of shifting, tilting, or otherwise perturbing the support surface to challenge the patients with unexpected movements.

Efforts to develop a comprehensive system approach for analyzing postural control have been led by Nashner and Horac.[14,15] A CDP system has been developed with a particular protocol known as a 'sensory organization test'. A summary of the testing conditions available in the sensory organization test part of the CDP system is shown in Fig. 8.1. The sensory organization test consists of six conditions: three on a stable support surface with eyes open, eyes closed and with the visual surround moving with body sway, and the three same conditions with the platform moving with body sway. A second test available is called the 'motor control' test. The motor control test uses a total of nine forward and nine backward translations of three different magnitudes. Also,

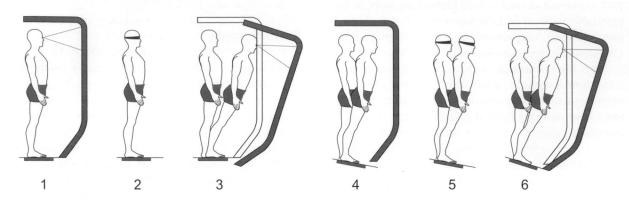

Figure 8.1 *The six conditions tested with the sensory organization portion of dynamic posturography testing. Conditions 1, 2 and 3 provide for accurate foot somatosensory cues with accurate visual cues in condition 1, absent visual cues in condition 2, and stabilized visual input (information that is of no functional use visually for maintaining stance) in condition 3. In conditions 4, 5 and 6, inaccurate foot somatosensory cues are given and the same visual conditions are retested.*

five sequential platform rotations are delivered in a toes-up then a toes-down direction. For both of these tests, patient responses are compared with responses from an age-appropriate control of normal subjects. Nashner and coworkers suggest that postural balance is maintained on the basis of a limited repertoire of centrally generated muscle synergies. During slight balance perturbations, the body rotates around the ankle joints and behaves essentially as an inverted pendulum. Muscle responses are organized in a distal to proximal manner and this is called the 'ankle strategy'. Larger balance perturbations lead to movements around the hip joint and earlier activation of proximal muscles. This is called the 'hip strategy'. A hip strategy is associated with a predominance of shear forces whereas an ankle strategy is characterized by predominance of changes in the reaction forces without much shear.

Computerized dynamic posturography has been shown to be a reliable and valid test of postural stability. It is able to differentiate between subjects with normal and abnormal vestibular function as compared with the clinical standard of reference.[16] Further, CDP appears to provide unique information that quantifies a patient's ability to use vision and somatosensation in maintaining postural stability. Although some of the information provided by CDP can be gained by means of a careful physical examination, much is unique, particularly because the data are quantitative.

Nonetheless, the question remains whether posturography is useful for management of patients that complain of balance problems and dizziness. Proponents of CDP would indicate that it has a clearly identified role in the planning of vestibular rehabilitation therapy and in monitoring treatment progress and outcome.[17]

Further, studies have identified specific clinical indications in which the use of CDP leads to decisions that improve outcome.[18,19] In contrast, other people feel that CDP is of no or very limited value for the patient. Bronstein and coworkers have found that the only disease-specific diagnosis that can be made with posturography is orthostatic tremor.[20,21] Further, there is a lack of correlation between questionnaire data, such as the dizziness handicap inventory and posturography data.[22] Moreover, there is a lack of concurrent validity between balance performance and functional gait measured in the clinic and gait laboratory.[23] A possible explanation for these discrepancies may be the fact that the CDP system uses information from force signals at the feet to reconstruct body sway. The patient's anterior–posterior sway is monitored by measuring vertical force with the force strain gauges that are mounted underneath the two platforms on which the patient stands (i.e. one foot on each platform). A fifth strain gauge is mounted in another direction to measure the shear force that is generated as the hips are thrown forward or backward to maintain balance instead of rotating about the ankles. These force signals are then used to reconstruct a cone of stability for anterior–posterior sway.[24] The cone of stability is assumed to be 12.5°. Thus, it is assumed that a person who sways about 12.5° is at the limits of stability and is likely to fall. This analysis lacks two critical features. First, the force signals might not accurately capture the movement of the center of mass. Second, the CDP analysis does not account for movement in the medial–lateral direction. Therefore, additional tests of a person's full-body mobility and balance are required. These functional tests are available using gait analysis techniques.

Movement measurement

Walking results in cyclic movement patterns at multiple joints. Biomechanical analysis of this motion assumes that the skeletal segments are rigid links moving through space. These rigid links are assumed to be interconnected through a series of frictionless joints. Measurement systems that are aimed at capturing the spatial trajectories of body segments are: a goniometer system, a video-based motion measurement system, an electromagnetic system, or an accelerometer system.

ELECTROGONIOMETRY

Electrogoniometers are electromechanical versions of the standard plastic goniometer frequently used in clinical environments. The simplest form consists of two bars that span the joint to be measured, with one bar attached to the proximal segment and the second bar attached to the distal segment. A rotary potentiometer is attached to the two bars and placed over the axis of rotation for the joint of interest. The potentiometer provides an output voltage proportional to the angular change between the two attachment surfaces. The goniometer operates on the assumption that the attachment bars on the proximal and distal surface move with the midline of the limb segment onto which they are attached and, thereby, measure the actual angular change at the joint. Multi-axial goniometers are more appropriate for human joint motion measurement. These goniometers measure three-dimensional motion by combining at least three potentiometers capable of measuring three rotations between adjacent limb segments (Fig. 8.2).

Electrogoniometers have several advantages:

1. They are relatively simple and easy to use, so they can produce a large quantity of data.
2. They provide direct measurement of joint relative motion instantaneously without a tedious data reduction process.
3. They are reliable and reproducible and have a bandwidth adequate to capture movement dynamics.
4. They are low cost and can be readily interfaced to a standard analog-to-digital converter and a personal computer for data acquisition.

These devices also have some inherent limitations (these limitations can be serious if they are overlooked):

1. When using electrogoniometers, the joint to be measured is assumed to be a ball and socket joint containing three rotational degrees-of-freedom only. This assumption may not always be true, especially in joints with pathological motion where the translational component may be significant.
2. The goniometer linkage system is not located within the joint. Therefore, any combined rotations may cause significant cross-talk in multi-axial goniometers. However, this cross-talk can be corrected theoretically.[25]

3. Care must be exercised in applying the goniometer system to individuals with a high body mass index. Soft tissue interposition between the goniometer linking system and the underlying skeletal system can cause relative movement. The tracking assumption is therefore reasonable for lean individuals but subjects with higher body mass may cause artifacts in measurement.
4. Placement of the goniometer system in relation to the joint axes is very important. Misalignment may result in significant cross-talk. Well-trained personnel are required for equipment application in order to ensure the data are consistent and reliable.
5. Most significantly, a goniometer can only provide relative joint motion. This motion is not referenced to an inertial reference frame. Thus, it is not possible to obtain joint intersegmental force calculations when using electrogoniometry.

VIDEO–BASED STEREOMETRIC SYSTEMS

With a camera, either passively reflective or actively illuminated markers are used (Fig. 8.3). These markers are commonly attached to the subjects as either discrete points or rigid clusters with multiple markers on each cluster. The external markers on the body segments are aligned with particular bony landmarks. Using stereophotogrammetric principles, the planar projections of markers viewed by each camera are used to reconstruct the three-dimensional instantaneous position of the markers relative to an inertially fixed laboratory coordinate system. If the position of at least three non-colinear points fixed to the body segment can be obtained (and the body segment is assumed to be rigid) then the six degrees of freedom associated with the position and orientation of each segment can be obtained. Initially, a body-fixed coordinate system is computed for each body segment (Fig. 8.3b). For example, consider the markers on the shank at an instant in time. A vector, S_{TZ}, can be formed from the lateral malleolus (B) to the lateral knee marker (A). Another vector can be formed from the lateral malleolus to the marker on the shank wand (C). The vector cross-product of these two vectors is a vector, S_{TX}, that is perpendicular to the plane containing all three markers. The unit vector, S_{TY}, may then be determined as the vector cross-product of S_{TZ} and S_{TX}. Thus, the vectors S_{TX}, S_{TY} and S_{TZ} form an orthogonal body fixed coordinate system, called a technical coordinate system. In a similar manner, the marker based, or technical coordinate system may be calculated for the thigh (i.e. T_{TX}, T_{TY} and T_{TZ}).

Once the position of adjacent limb segments has been determined, it is possible to determine the relative angle between adjacent limb segments in three dimensions. This assumes that the technical coordinate systems reasonably approximate the anatomical axes of the body segments (e.g. T_{TZ} approximates the long axis of the thigh

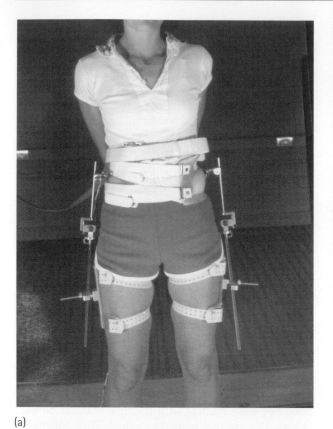

(a)

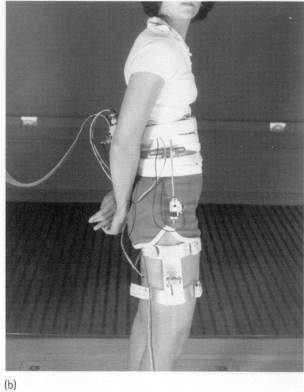

(b)

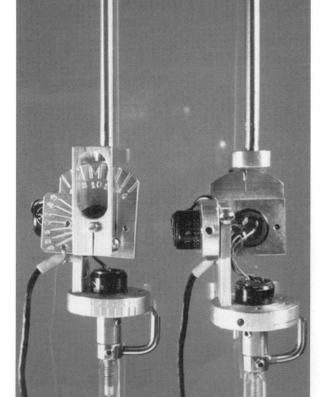

(c)

Figure 8.2 *(a) Frontal, (b) sagittal and (c) close up view of a triaxial electrogoniometer used to measure three-dimensional joint angular motion.*

(a)

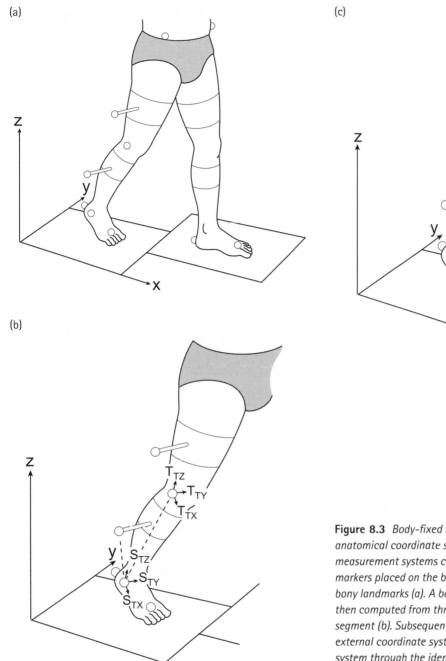

(b)

(c)

Figure 8.3 *Body-fixed reflective markers used for establishing anatomical coordinate systems. Video camera motion measurement systems calculate the location of external markers placed on the body segments and aligned with specific bony landmarks (a). A body-fixed external coordinate system is then computed from three or more markers on each body segment (b). Subsequently, a subject calibration relates the external coordinate system with an anatomical coordinate system through the identification of anatomical landmarks (e.g. the medial and lateral femoral condyles and medial lateral malleoli) (c).*

and S_{TZ} approximates the long axis of the shank). A more rigorous approach adapts a subject calibration procedure to relate the technical coordinate systems with pertinent anatomical landmarks.[26] Additional data can be collected that relates the technical coordinate system to the underlying anatomical coordinate system. The subject calibration is performed as a static trial with the subject standing. Additional markers are typically added to the medial femoral condyle and the medial malleoli during the static calibration trial. These markers serve as anatomical references for the knee axis and ankle axis. The hip center location is estimated from markers placed

on the pelvis.[27] The technical coordinate system is then transformed into alignment with the anatomical coordinate system for each limb segment (e.g. S_{AX}, S_{AY}, S_{AZ}; Fig. 8.3c). The marker system is coupled to a biomechanical model.[28,29] Once the position of adjacent limb segments has been determined (and each body segment is assumed to be rigid), it is possible to determine the relative angle between adjacent limb segments in three dimensions. The Euler system is the most commonly used method for describing three-dimensional motion (Fig. 8.4).[25,30]

The video-camera based systems have several advantages:

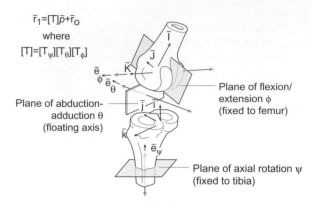

$$\bar{r}_1 = [T]\bar{p} + \bar{r}_O$$
where
$$[T] = [T_\psi][T_\theta][T_\phi]$$

Plane of flexion/
extension ϕ
(fixed to femur)

Plane of abduction-
adduction θ
(floating axis)

Plane of axial rotation ψ
(fixed to tibia)

Figure 8.4 *Description of knee joint motion using Eulerian angle system. An axis fixed to the distal femur defines flexion/extension motion, ϕ. An axis fixed to the proximal tibia along its anatomical axis defines internal external rotation, ψ. A floating axis is orthogonal to the other two axes and used to measure abduction-adduction, θ. (Reproduced with permission from ref. 25.)*

1. The system is capable of providing absolute limb motion data in an inertial reference frame. Thus, it is possible to directly calculate joint forces and moments using Newtonian mechanics.
2. These systems allow measurement of numerous points on multiple limb segments simultaneously. Thus, there is no need to make assumptions about the type of joint being studied and a complete six degrees of freedom motion measurement based on the theory of rigid body motion can be obtained.
3. The markers on each segment are small and have minimal mass so that inertial effects are minimized and motion interference is minimal.
4. Computerized motion analysis systems have been developed that provide marker trajectory data in real time. These systems are now available for applications in biomechanics. The applications make it possible to obtain results of gait analysis studies much faster and will make gait analysis much more clinically available.

The limitations of this method are related to the characteristics of the instruments involved:

1. In order to obtain bilateral, three-dimensional motion, a number of cameras are required. This requires precise alignment and calibration. This process may be time consuming.
2. Synchronization can also be a problem. When multiple cameras are used, the timing of data from each camera must be precisely synchronized. In addition, if data from a force plate are collected, synchronization must also be precisely obtained between the video-based and analog-based signals.
3. The lighting for illuminating markers is typically infrared light. Thus, this prohibits using this system in work environments where outside light sources (i.e. sunlight) may obscure marker positions.
4. Marker positions are identified based on line of sight from the video camera. If a marker is occluded because of an adjacent limb segment passing between the marker and the camera, then the trajectory of the marker may be lost unless there is a redundancy of cameras viewing the marker.
5. Although video data is captured in real time, for many systems the conversion of point-in-space coordinates to joint relative motion and joint kinetics requires additional calculation, which may be time consuming.
6. The cost of video systems is very high.
7. These systems work well in laboratory environments but are seldom applicable for measurements in work environments.

ELECTROMAGNETIC SYSTEMS

The most recent development to be used for quantifying human motion is an electromagnetic tracking system.[31] Electromagnetic systems detect the motion of sensors placed on each segment using an electromagnetic field. A three-axis magnet dipole source and a three-axis magnetic sensor are used (Fig. 8.5).[32] The excitation of the source and

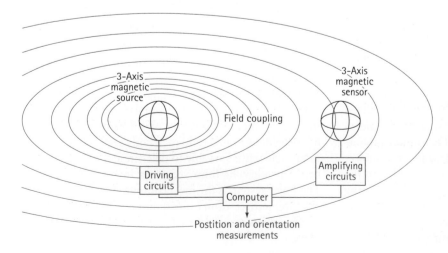

Figure 8.5 *System block diagram of an electromagnetic tracking system. The three-axis magnetic source emits three sequential excitation states that are picked up by the three-axis magnetic sensor. The resultant set of sensor excitation vectors is used to calculate the position and orientation of the sensor relative to the source.*

the resulting sensor output are represented as vectors. The source excitation pattern is composed of three sequential excitation states, each of which produces an excitation vector that is linearly independent of the other two. The sensor is connected to a system controller through a cable. The sensor outputs are preamplified, multiplexed and transmitted to a system electronics unit. The resultant set of three sensor output vectors contains information sufficient to determine both the position and orientation of the sensor relative to the source. Thus, these systems can provide real-time six degree-of-freedom movement data. The use of this equipment is growing in areas of human motion analysis. The advantages are that (1) the instrumentation is simple to use and (2) it is insensitive to limb interference. The limitations are (1) the cabling necessary to connect the sensors, (2) the sampling frequency, which decreases as the number of sensors are increased, and (3) sensitivity to magnetic interference from nearby ferromagnetic metallic structures, such as a total joint replacement. Nonetheless, as electromagnetic system capabilities increase, it is expected that these devices will be used more frequently for movement analysis.

ACCELEROMETRY

Multi-axis accelerometers can be used to measure both linear and angular acceleration. Velocity and position data can then be obtained through numerical integration of the acceleration. Acccelerometry has been used in both clinical and experimental settings to measure human motion. The most general motion of a rigid body segment in space can be determined by properly oriented linear accelerometers.[33] Greater accuracy can be obtained when four non-coplanar triaxial accelerometers are used.[35] However, use of accelerometry has been limited because drift after integration of angular acceleration or angular velocity distorted the results. Recently, however, it has been demonstrated that relative angles can be calculated without integration thereby solving the problem of integration drift.[35]

Although this method is seldom used experimentally, there are several potential advantages:

1. This method is capable of producing complete anatomic joint motion kinematic data without using the potentially erroneous differentiation technique.[36]
2. The instrumentation is not affected by body segment interference. Thus, it can be used for bilateral evaluation of multiple joints.
3. The instrumentation cost is low compared to other methods capable of producing equivalent results.

This technique has limitations both in the analytical techniques and instrumentation required:

1. The theoretical analysis required to calculate joint motion is complex and requires highly trained technical personnel.
2. Instrument noise, drift and other hardware-related errors can cause significant problems in the reliability and resolution of the data.
3. Attachment of accelerometers to skin induces additional noise because of skin movement artifacts.
4. Selection of proper initial conditions for motion calculations is difficult.
5. The cabling necessary to connect the sensors restricts motion.
6. Determination of the orientation of accelerometer system in an inertial frame is difficult and limits application of this technique for calculation of joint kinetics.

Force measurement

Gait analysis is also concerned with the forces that cause the observed movement and the assessment of their effect on locomotion (kinetic analysis). Forces acting on the human body can be divided into internal and external forces. The external forces represent all physical interactions between the body and the environment. These forces include gravitational, ground reaction forces and inertial forces. The internal forces are those transmitted by body tissues, which include muscular forces, ligament forces and forces transmitted through joint contact.

Generally, only the ground reaction forces can be measured using a force plate. Current force plates typically use strain gauge or piezoelectric transducers. Force platforms can be used to define the magnitude and direction of the resultant ground reaction force (GRF) applied to the foot by the ground (Fig. 8.6). The GRF vector is three dimensional and consists of a vertical component plus two shear components acting along the

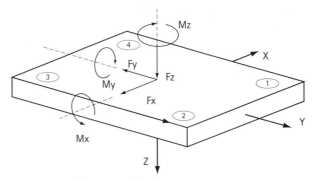

Figure 8.6 *A force plate is used to measure the location and magnitude of the ground reaction force. Transducers are located in the four corners of the plate. The ground reaction force is divided into three force (Fx, Fy and Fz) and three moment (Mx, My and Mz) components. Fx and Fy are shear forces; Fz is the vertical force. Some force plates only measure the moment around the vertical axis (i.e. Mz). This assumes that no tensile forces are imposed on the force plate (i.e. the foot does not stick to the plate). Under this assumption, the other moments are zero.*

force plate surface. The shear forces are applied parallel to the ground and require friction. These shear forces are usually resolved in the anterior–posterior and medial–lateral directions. An additional variable, the center of pressure, is needed to define the location of this GRF vector. The center of pressure, also sometimes called the center of foot pressure, is defined as the point about which the distributed force has zero moment when applied to the foot. It is found by determining the line of action of the forces measured by the platform and calculating where that line intersects the surface of the force platform.

This force data is combined with kinematic data using Newton's Second Law to calculate the intersegmental forces and moments causing motion (Fig. 8.7). The process of proceeding from known kinematic data and external forces to obtain intersegmental joint forces and moments is called the inverse dynamics approach.[37] The gravitational forces acting on each body segment can be determined from the relevant mass and location of the center of mass for each segment. These quantities can be calculated together with the segmental mass moments of inertia using prediction techniques from anthropometric dimensions. The inertial forces can be obtained from calculations of angular and linear position, as well as velocity and acceleration of the body segments with respect to either a fixed laboratory coordinate system or referenced to another body segment using kinematic data. This information can be combined to solve the inverse dynamics problem (Fig. 8.8). Joint power can also be calculated.[38] These data provide understanding of the subtle musculoskeletal adaptations which are used by patients to maintain dynamic balance during gait. Kinetic data is available at the hip, knee and ankle joint. When the position of this force line with respect to joint center has been established by combining force and movement data, the extrinsic joint moment, which is the product of lever arm and the ground reaction force, plus gravity and inertia can be calculated. This moment is of great importance because, in the case of lower extremity

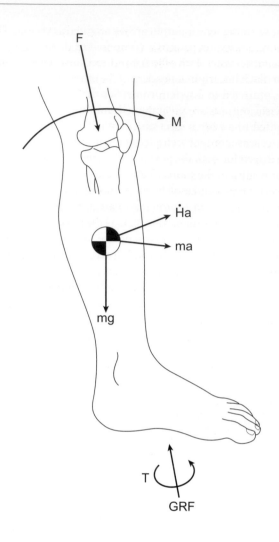

Figure 8.7 *The joint dynamics, which includes the intersegmental forces and moments, is computed through the use of Newtonian mechanics. The computation includes the external loads to the foot; e.g. the ground reaction forces (F) and torque (T), the weight of the limb segments (mg), and the inertial loads (ma and $\dot{H}a$), to calculate the joint intersegmental force (F) and moment (M).*

Inverse dynamic problem

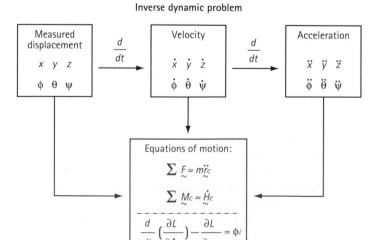

Figure 8.8 *Solution process for inverse dynamics problem. Displacement information must be differentiated twice to yield acceleration. Either Newtonian or Lagrangian formulations can be used to formulate the equations of motion.*

muscles acting during load bearing, it determines the requirements for intrinsic (muscle) force. For example, when the force line falls behind the knee joint center, quadriceps muscle action is required to prevent knee collapse, and when the force line falls in front of the knee, extensor muscle force is not needed.

At each joint, a state of equilibrium exists where the external joint forces are balanced by the internal joint forces. The measurement of internal forces requires sophisticated techniques which are invasive. Analytical procedures have been developed for estimating internal joint forces. These analytical approaches use classical mechanics and mathematical optimization routines.[39] They require the use of simplifying assumptions about the mechanical structure and knowledge of muscle physiology principles. Thus, the accuracy of the analytical predictions depends not only on the quality of the input data but also on the validity of the assumptions. In general, it is necessary to evaluate the estimated quantities by comparing them with experimental observations. Typically, electromyographic data are obtained to provide information regarding muscle activation patterns.

Electromyography

Neuromuscular coordination is required to adjust the varying muscular and ligamentous forces interacting with the abundant degrees of freedom in the joints and other parts of passive locomotive system to obtain dynamic balance during gait. Electromyographic data are useful to provide information about the timing of muscle activity and the relative intensity of muscle activity. Both surface and fine-wire electrodes have been used for gait kinesiological EMG analysis. Each type of electrode has its advantages and disadvantages. Surface electrodes are convenient, easy to apply to the skin and do not cause pain, irritation, or discomfort to the subject. However, they pick up signals from other active muscles in the general area of application. This feature makes surface electrodes the ideal choice for analysis of global activity in superficial muscles or muscle groups. However, surface electrodes are sensitive to movement of the skin under the electrodes and have poor specificity. They are influenced by significant muscle 'cross-talk,' in which the electrode signals of one muscle interfere with the signals from another.[40] Thus, the activity of adjacent muscle groups can interfere and lead to false results. However, a double differential technique has been shown to reduce cross-talk in surface EMGs.[41] The major advantage of fine-wire electrodes is selectivity to measure the activity of specific muscles. The influence of electrical activity of nearby muscles is greatly reduced. Nonetheless, a number of disadvantages are associated with fine-wire electrodes. Pain on insertion, the difficulty of accurate placement, wire movement with muscle contraction and the need for licensure to utilize wire electrodes are some of the drawbacks. Furthermore,

subjects with indwelling electrodes walk more slowly after insertion of the electrodes.[42] Because they are to be inserted transcutaneously, needle electrodes must be sterilized and sufficiently strong to resist breakage. Commonsense considerations, such as time, expense, pain experienced during a long study, the tolerance of the subject to multiple needle insertions and the influence of indwelling electrodes on walking, necessitate a selection of the muscles most relevant to the specific movement abnormalities. Large muscles near the surface can be studied well with surface electrodes, whereas small muscles and those surrounded by other muscles require insertion of fine-wire electrodes. Electrical stimuli are usually given to confirm the accuracy of placement. Electromyography systems are available in either hardwired or telemetry versions. The hardwired versions now send multiple signals on a single cable. These systems are reliable and less expensive than telemetry. Telemetry systems do not encumber the subject with cables but are susceptible to electromagnetic interference.

Once the EMG data are acquired, they must be processed further to provide information about the timing of muscle activity and the relative intensity of the muscle activity. The EMG data are recorded throughout the gait cycle. The gait cycle is indicated either with synchronization of the kinematic data, foot-switch information, or force-plate data to indicate each foot strike and toe-off. Analysis of the EMG is done by a phase–time plot of the activity of the muscle against events of the gait cycle. The raw EMG signal can be analyzed or processed further. The most common methods of EMG signal processing are full-wave rectification, linear envelope and integration of the rectified EMG (Fig. 8.9). Full-wave rectification reverses the sign of all negative voltages and yields the absolute value of the raw EMG. The linear envelope is created by low-pass filtering the full wave-rectified signal. There are many versions of integrated EMGs (IEMGs). The IEMG term is widely used and abused, probably because the first use of the term was by Inman and coworkers[43] when they employed a linear envelope and called this IEMG. The correct interpretation of integration is purely mathematical and means the 'area under the curve'. Thus, the simplest form of integration starts at some preset time and continues during the total time of muscle activity. The IEMG is then the summation of the area under the curve of each muscle activity burst. However, a more common form of integration involves resetting the integrated signal to zero at regular intervals of time (usually 20–200 ms and the time should be specified). This scheme yields a series of peaks which represent the trend of the EMG amplitude with time and gives something close to a moving average. During gait analysis, integrated processing of the rectified signal is usually performed over short duration (i.e. 2 per cent of gait cycle) and then the integration is reset and accumulated again. Normalization schemes may also be used to aid in analysis. Normalization may

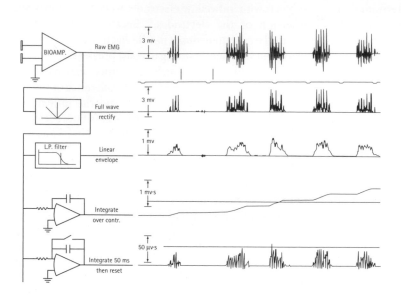

Figure 8.9 *Example of several types of temporal processing of electromyography (EMG) signals. The top trace represents the 'raw' or unaltered EMG signal during five successive contractions. The trace under the 'raw' EMG is the full-wave rectified version of the top trace. The rectification process converts the negative EMG signals to positive signals. The next trace is the rectified and low-pass filtered version of the top trace. This is commonly referred to as a linear envelope. The fourth trace from the top is obtained by integration of the rectified EMG data (i.e. integrated EMG or IEMG). The bottom trace represents the integrated EMG where the integrater is reset every 50 ms. (Reproduced from Winter DA, Rau G, Kedefors R, Broman H and de Luca CJ. Units, terms, and standards in the reporting of EMG research. Ad Hoc Committee of the International Society of Electrophysiology Kinesiology, 1980.*

be based on the maximum manual muscle test or maximum EMG signal obtained during gait. The muscle is considered to be activated when at least 5 per cent of the maximum electrical activity obtained during a manual muscle test is present for 5 per cent of the gait cycle.[44]

The EMG provides a means for studying muscle activity. The signals that result from action potentials and muscle fibers are stochastic and non-stationary, adding to uncertainty in interpretation. While the ultimate source of locomotor activity is muscle force, no study has established that electromyographic signals represent muscle force.[45] The EMG signal is a measure of the bioelectric events that occur in conjunction with contraction of the muscle fibers. Thus, it is a phenomenon related to the initiation of muscle contraction rather than an effect of the muscle's mechanical action. There are many difficulties in correlating the EMG signal amplitude with muscle force magnitude. Both linear and non-linear relationships between the force level of skeletal muscles and the EMG signal have been reported.[46–54] Consequently, the EMG is commonly used in clinical gait analysis to determine phasic patterns for individual muscles or muscle groups. It is possible to examine simple on/off patterns,[55] or the EMG can be processed to find a graduation of signal level, after which EMG patterns are examined as defined by the level of activity over the gait cycle.[56–58] In the latter process, it is common to normalize the signal as a percentage of voluntary maximum muscle contraction. The process of detecting when a muscle is 'turned on or off' is usually one of testing whether the average level of the signal is above some predefined limit. This limit is often defined as a percentage of the maximum voluntary muscle contraction. The determination of on/off time is often done by calculating the EMG level and then testing for occasions when the

level exceeds some threshold value. The EMG on/off times are generally more variable from step to step than either kinematic or kinetic gait measurements.

Problems occur in dynamic situations when using electromyographic activity as a measure of muscle functional capability. A dynamic force produced by a muscle is not proportional to the degree of muscular activity. Other factors may affect the muscle force, such as a change of the muscle length, change of the contraction velocity, the rate and type of muscle contraction, joint position and muscle fatigue. It is desirable to find an alternative measurable mechanical parameter related to muscle force. The electromyographic signal does not assess the tension produced by a muscle because the tension reflects the sum of both the active contraction and the passive stretch. A technique which may provide information about muscle force is measurement of intramuscular pressure. Intramuscular pressure (IMP) is a mechanical variable that is proportional to muscle tension. It is possible to obtain IMP measurements during gait and relate these measurements to the timing and intensity of muscle contraction. Intramuscular pressure has been used to quantify muscle function during dynamic activities.[59] Intramuscular pressure measurements obtained during walking parallel the electromyographic activity and account for passive stretch of the muscle (Fig. 8.10).[59] General types of systems used for measuring intramuscular pressure are either fluid filled or solid state. A comprehensive review of techniques to measure interstitial fluid pressure is provided by Wiig[60] and Aukland and Reed.[61] Fluid-filled methods consist of the needle monometer, wick technique, micropipette technique and perforated implantable colloid osmometer. However, fluid-filled pressure recording systems require infusion to maintain accuracy[62–64] and are sensi-

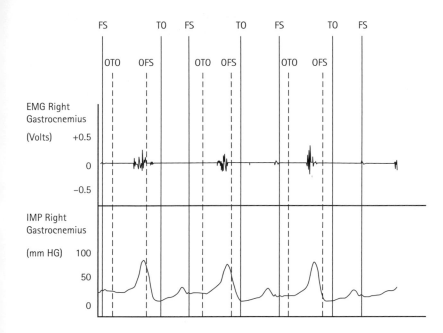

Figure 8.10 *Raw data for a single subject during gait. Both EMG and intramuscular pressure are being recorded from the gastrocnemius muscle. The stance phase of gait occurs from foot strike (FS) to toe-off (TO). The swing phase of gait occurs from TO to FS. Single limb stance occurs from opposite toe-off (OTO) to opposite foot strike (OFS). Peaks in intramuscular pressure during gait can be correlated with peaks of active contraction and passive stretch of the gastrocnemius (Reproduced with permission from ref. 59.)*

tive to hydrostatic artifacts. Thus, fluid-filled systems may be used only with limited movements that do not involve limb position changes relative to the horizontal plane, rendering this technology inappropriate for measuring intramuscular pressure during dynamic activities. In contrast, a fiber optic transducer tipped system is not sensitive to hydrostatic artifact and has been shown to be effective for measuring IMP during exercise.[65] However, commercially available fiber optic pressure transducers are too large for optimum comfort and may themselves induce pressure artifacts based on their extremely large size relative to muscle fibers themselves. In order to address this issue, a new pressure microsensor is being developed for measuring interstitial fluid pressure. This microsensor has a sufficiently small size of 360 μm diameter (Fig. 8.11) that will allow it to be inserted with a small needle, thereby allowing routine clinical use. It has been shown that this microsensor is accurate, repeatable, linear and has low hysteresis.[66]

INTERPRETATION OF GAIT DATA

Once the data which describe the biomechanics of the patient's gait have been collected, the most crucial step of interpreting the data remains to be performed. Based on the clinical examination and measurements performed, the data must be synthesized and integrated in order to supply clinically relevant information. Human locomotion is very complex and multifaceted. The clinical interpretation of pathological gait disorders involves holding in human memory a large number of graphs, numbers,

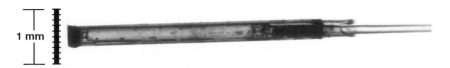

Figure 8.11 *Pressure microsensor for measuring interstitial fluid pressure. This microsensor has a sufficiently small size (360 μm diameter) that it can be inserted with a small needle, thereby allowing routine clinical use.*

and clinical tests from data presented on hard copy, charts, X-rays, video and computer-generated three-dimensional graphics from multiple trials of a subject walking. Further, comparisons must be made to data from an able-bodied normal population in order to identify the potential movement problems for a given individual. The referring clinician, who may not be an expert in gait analysis, is overwhelmed by the magnitude of the number of measurements included in a typical gait report. The person interpreting the data must integrate this information. While data collection techniques for gait analysis have continually evolved over the last 50 years, the method of data presentation has not changed over this time. The data are still reported in two-dimensional charts, with the abscissa usually defined as a percentage of the gait cycle and the ordinate displaying the gait parameter.

Recent developments in computer animation may make it possible to apply advanced methods to visualize human movements. The large volume of variables currently found in a typical clinical report could be replaced with a few graphic images that succinctly provide the needed information. It is difficult to fully appreciate and understand the relationships between motion dynamics and biomechanical variables without scientific graphic visualization. Computer software packages have now advanced to the stage where it is possible to provide a gait analysis report using animation of fully three-dimensional, realistic graphical depictions of human locomotion. The format used for reporting test results is a matter of considerable importance. The data must be presented in an accurate, clear and concise format. If the results are not communicated in an effective format, they will be of little use to the clinician regardless of quality.

TREATMENT PLANNING AND ASSESSMENT

When treatment is being planned, the main objective is to differentiate between the primary causes and compensations for the patient's functional problems. If the treatment is directed at a compensation, the patient will lose their ability to compensate and their movement problems will worsen. The patient will display adaptations in their gait pattern because of their pain, injury, deformity, instability and/or inappropriate muscle activation patterns. The ramifications of these problems cannot be fully assessed without an instrumented gait study. Patients can undergo dynamic adaptation related to the biomechanics of walking which must be factored into the treatment algorithm. For example, it has been shown that when planning corrective osteotomy knee surgery, patients with the same bony deformity will have differing knee loading as a result of dynamic adaptations.[67] These dynamic adaptations will have a direct effect on surgical outcome. The patients that dynamically compensated for their

malalignment had a better long-term outcome.[67,68] For patients with progressive disorders, these dynamic adaptations will also change with time as the disease progresses. It is possible to use motion analysis studies to quantify these dynamic changes in locomotor patterns.

RATIONALE FOR CLINICAL MOVEMENT ANALYSIS

In this era of government reimbursement for medical services, the ability to document the need and effectiveness of a particular treatment will assume an increasingly important role. Managed care will require validation for many types of therapeutic interventions. Pre- and post-treatment measurement will become mandatory. Outcomes will have to be compared. Practitioners and facilities will be rated on their outcomes. Maximizing anticipated outcomes will be required to document that a treatment plan is worthwhile. Objective gait analysis is an essential tool to meet these demands. The technology is at a level where it is both feasible and affordable to provide an objective form of patient assessment.

In all areas of medical care, a need exists for instrumentation and procedures to aid in a differential diagnosis and treatment of patients. Further, information is required to document objectively patient response to treatment. The ability to diagnose, prescribe treatment and document results is common to all areas of medical care. However, the technology available in different medical specialties varies widely. This is particularly evident when the current medical technology for treating patient with cardiovascular conditions is compared with the technology for treating patients with neuromuscular conditions (Table 8.1). For both types of patients the technology can be divided into three levels: static examinations, dynamic examinations and invasive procedures. Typically, the approach is to use the technology available at the lowest level that will meet the requirements for aiding in differential diagnosis and treatment planning. When a patient reports to a physician that they are experiencing chest pain and the risk factors for a myocardial infarction exist, the patient is monitored with an electrocardiogram. In some centers, a computed tomography (CT) scan is obtained to assess the amount of arteriosclerosis in the vessels of the heart muscle. These tests are obtained while the patient is either sitting or lying down. Hence, these constitute static exams. Other static modalities include magnetic resonance imaging (MRI), positron-emission tomography (PET) and ultrasound. If the physician has a high index of suspicion, dynamic tests may be undertaken. These include a stress test or echocardiography. Finally, angiography may be used as an invasive procedure to further examine the heart.

Conversely, for a patient with neuromuscular dysfunction, most of the modalities used are static modalities. Current modalities include X-ray, CT, MRI and

Table 8.1 *Current medical technology*

Level	Examination	Treatment modality Cardiovascular patients	Neuromuscular patients
I	Static	Electrocardiogram Computed tomography Magnetic resonance imaging Positron-emission tomography Ultrasound	X-ray Computed tomography Magnetic resonance imaging
II	Dynamic	Stress test Echocardiography	Motion analysis
III	Invasive	Angiography	Diagnostic electromyography Kinesiological electromyography

nuclear imaging. It is also common to obtain diagnostic EMG to further elucidate the neuromuscular status of the patient. However, during all these examinations, the patient is static and non-weight-bearing. Dynamic assessment of patients with neuromuscular dysfunction can only be obtained using motion analysis techniques along with acquisition of kinesiological EMG.

An objection sometimes raised is that these studies are too costly. However, this objection is unfounded. In terms of cost–benefit ratio, the most compelling consideration is the high cost of inappropriate treatment. It is important to remember that unsuccessful treatment will result in unfavorable changes in function and may require subsequent procedures to deal with the original problem. There is, of course, no assurance that gait studies performed prior to treatment planning will always ensure favorable outcome, but careful planning, based on objective data, will provide a solid foundation for decision making. Post-treatment studies will give the information required for objective evaluation of treatment results. The rate at which gait analysis technologies become more common will depend on the market, the manufacturers and managed care requirements. Objective patient assessment using gait analysis techniques will facilitate the identification of optimal treatment regimens and provide a solid foundation for clinical decision making.

SUMMARY

Human function cannot be fully understood without studies of movement. Balance control is a complex motor skill that involves integration of sensory information and execution of flexible movement patterns in order to maintain upright posture and achieve forward progression. Comprehensive objective assessments of balance and gait are needed in order to provide clinicians with data on the patient's functional status. Balance assessments have evolved to the level where they can provide information on balance strategies with changes in support and sensory conditions, the ability to respond to external perturbations and the ability to anticipate postural demands asso-

ciated with voluntary movements. Current gait analysis systems offer sophisticated methods for tracking limb movements in space, combined with force platforms to provide data on the musculoskeletal responses to the external loading environment. When coupled with a biomechanical model, this equipment is able to provide a complete, three-dimensional, dynamic description of the subject's gait along with information on the timing and intensity of muscle activity. Gait assessments can provide objective information on the ability of the subject to voluntarily and efficiently move the body's center of mass through space while maintaining upright stable posture over the base of support. Interpretation of these data makes it possible to integrate morphology and functional adaptations in order to understand and treat patients with neurological and orthopedic disorders.

ACKNOWLEDGEMENTS

This work was partly supported by NIH Grant R01 HD31476. Appreciation is expressed to Barbara Iverson-Literski for careful manuscript preparation.

REFERENCES

1. Borelli GA. *De motor animalium*. Batavis: Lugduni, 1685.
2. Duchenne GBA. *Physiologie des mouvements démontrée a l'aide de l'expérimentation électrique et de l'observation clinique et applicable à l'étude des paralysies et des déformations.* Paris: J.B. Baillière, 1867.
3. Muybridge E. *Human and animal locomotion.* New York: Dover, 1979.
4. Braune W, Fischer O. *Der Gang des Nenschen [The human gait]*, Leipzig: BG Teubner, 1895.
5. Inman VT, Ralston HJ, Todd F. *Human walking.* Baltimore: Williams and Wilkins, 1981.
6. Perry J. *Gait analysis: normal and pathological function.* Thorofare: Slack, 1992.
7. Gage JR, Ounpuu S. Gait analysis in clinical practice. *Semin Orthopaed* 1989;2:72–87.
8. Krebs DE, Edelstein JE, Fishman S. Reliability of observational kinematic gait analysis. *Phys Ther* 1985;65:1027–2033.

9. Saleh M, Murdoch G. In defense of gait analysis. *J Bone Joint Surg* 1985;**67B**: 237–41.

10. Eastlack ME, Arvidson J, Snyder-Mackler L, et al. Interrater reliability of videotaped observation of gait-analysis assessments. *Phys Ther* 1991;**71**(6):465–72.

11. Terekhov Y. Stabilometry as a diagnostic tool in clinical medicine. *Can Med Assoc J* 1976;**115**:631–33.

12. Dobie RA. Clinical forum: does computerized dynamics posturography help us care for our patients? *Am J Otol* 1997;**18**:108–12.

13. Nashner LM, Black FO, Wall C. Adaptation to altered support and visual conditions during stance: patients with vestibular deficits. *J Neurosci* 1982;**2**(5):536–44.

14. Nashner LM. A model describing vestibular detection of body sway motion. *Acta Oto-Laryngol* 1972;**72**:429–36.

15. Horak FB, Nashner LM. Central programming of postural movements: adaptation to altered surface-support configurations. *J Neurophysiol* 1986;**55**:1369–81.

16. Hamid MA, Hughes GB, Kinney SE. Specificity and sensitivity of dynamic posturography. *Acta Oto-Laryngol Suppl* 1991;**481**:596–600.

17. di Fabio RP. Meta-analysis of sensitivity and specificity of platform posturography. *Arch Otolaryngol Head Neck Surg* 1996;**122**:150–6.

18. Herdman SJ, Clendaniels RA, Mattox DE, et al. Vestibular adaptation exercises and recovery: acute stage after acoustic normal resection. *Arch Otolaryngol Head Neck Surg* 1995;**113**:1056–159.

19. Cass SP, Borellow-France D, Furman J. M. Functional outcome of vestibular rehabilitation in patients with abnormal sensory-organization testing. *Am J Otolol* 1996;**17**: 581–90.

20. Bronstein AM, Guerraz M. Visual–vestibular control of posture and gait: physiological mechanisms and disorders. *Curr Opin Neurol* 1999;**12**(1): 5–11.

21. Yarrow K, Brown P, Gresty MA, Bronstein AM. Force platform recordings in the diagnosis of primary orthostatic tremor. *Gait Posture* 2001;**13**:27–34.

22. Robertson BB, Ireland DJ. Dizziness Handicap Inventory correlates of computerized dynamic posturography. *J Otolaryngol* 1995;**24**:118–24.

23. O'Neill DE, Gill-Body KM, Krebs DE. Posturography changes do not predict functional performance changes. *Am J Otol* 1998;**19**:797–803.

24. Epley JM. New dimensions of benign paroxysmal positional vertigo. *J Otolaryngol Head Neck Surg* 1980;**88**:599–605.

25. Chao EYS. Justification of triaxial goniometer for the measurement of joint rotation. *J Biomech* 1980;**13**:989–1006.

26. Cappozzo A, Catani F, Croce UD, Leardini A. Position and orientation in space of bones during movement: anatomical frame definition and determination. *Clin Biomech* 1995;**10**(4):171–8.

27. Bell AL, Pederson DR, Brand RA. Prediction of hip joint center location from external landmarks. *Hum Mov Sci* 1989;**8**:3–16.

28. Kadaba MP, Ramakrishnan HK, Wootten ME. Measurement of lower extremity kinematics during level walking. *J Orthop Res* 1990;**8**:383–92.

29. Kaufman KR, An KN, Chao EYS. A Comparison of intersegmental joint dynamics to isokinetic dynamometer measurements. *J Biomech* 1995;**28**(10):1243–65.

30. Grood ES, Suntay WJ. A joint coordinate system for the clinical discussion of 3-dimensional motions: applications to the knee. *J Biomech Eng* 983;**105**:136–44.

31. An K-N, Jacobsen MC, Berglund LJ, Chao EY. Application of a magnetic tracking device to kinesiologic studies. *J Biomech* 1988;**21**(7):613–20.

32. Raab FH, Blood EB, Steiner TO, Jones HR. Magnetic position and orientation tracking system. *IEEE Trans Aerospace Electr Syst* 1979;**AES-15**(5): 709–18.

33. Morris JRW. Accelerometry – a technique for the measurement of human body movements. *J Biomech* 1973;**6**:729–36.

34. Hayes WC, Gran JD, Magurka ML, et al. Leg motion analysis during gait by multi-axial accelerometry: theoretical foundations and preliminary validations. *J Biomech Eng* 1983;**105**:283–9.

35. Willemsen ATM, van Alsté RJA, Bloom HBK. Real-time gait assessment utilizing a new way of accelerometry. *J Biomech* 1990;**23**(8):859–63.

36. Chao EY, Rim K. Application of optimization principles in determining the applied movements in human leg joints during gait. *J Biomech* 1973;**6**:497–510.

37. Chao EYS. *Determination of applied forces in linking systems with known displacements: with special application to biomechanics.* Iowa City: University of Iowa, 1971.

38. Winter DA. *Biomechanics and motor control of human movement*, 2nd edn. New York: Wiley and Sons, 1990.

39. Kaufman K, An K, Litchy W, Chao E. Physiological prediction of muscle forces – I. Theoretical formulation. *Neuroscience* 1991;**40**(3):781–92.

40. Zuniga EN, Simons DG. Nonlinear relationship between averaged electromyogram potential and muscle tension in normal subjects. *Arch Phys Med Rehabil* 1969;**50**:613.

41. Koh TJ, Grabiner MD. Cross-talk in surface electromyograms of human hamstring muscles. *J Orthop Res* 1992;**10**:701–9.

42. Young CC, Rose SE, Biden EN, et al. The effect of surface and internal electrodes on the gait of children with cerebral palsy, spastic diplegia type. *J Orthop Res* 1989;**7**(5):732–7.

43. Inman VT, Ralston HJ, Saunders JB, et al. Relationship of human electromyogram to muscular tension. *Electroencephalogr Clin Neurophysiol* 1952;**4**:187–94.

44. Bogey RA, Barnes LA, Perry J. Computer algorithms to characterize individual subject EMG profiles during gait. *Arch Phys Med Rehabil* 1992;**73**: 835–41.

45. Perry J, Bekey GA. EMG-force relationships in skeletal muscle. *Crit Rev Biomed Eng* 1981;**7**(1):1–22.

46. Lippold OCJ. The relation between integrated action potentials in a human muscle and its isometric tension. *J Physiol (Lond)* 1952;**117**:492.

47. Messier RH, Duffy J, Litchman HM, et al. The electromyogram as a measure of tension in the human biceps and triceps muscles. *Int J Mech Sci* 1971;**13**:585–98.

48. Komi PV, Buskirk ER. Effect of eccentric and concentric muscle conditioning on tension and electrical activity of human muscle. *Ergonomics* 1972;**15**:417.

49. Zuniga EN, Leavitt LA, Calvert JC, et al. Gait patterns in the above-knee amputees. *Arch Phys Med Rehabil* 1972;**53**(8):373–82.

50. Maton B, Bouisset S. The distribution of activity among the muscles of a single group during isometric contraction. *Eur J Appl Physiol* 1977;**37**:101–9.

51. Matral S, Casser G. Relationship between force and integrated EMG activity during voluntary isometric and isotonic contraction. *Eur J Appl Physiol* 1977;**46**:185.

52. Moritani T, de Vries HA. Reexamination of the relationship between the surface integrated electromyogram (IEMG) and

force of isometric contraction. *Am J Phys Med* 1978;**57**:263–77.

53. Bigland-Ritchie B, Kukulka CJ, Woods JJ. Surface EMG-force relationships in human muscles of different fibre composition. *J Physiol (Lond)* 1980;**308**:103.

54. Woods JJ, Bigland-Ritchie B. Linear and nonlinear surface EMG/force relationships in human muscles. *Am J Phys Med* 1983;**62**(6): 287–99.

55. Sutherland DH, Olshen RA, Biden EN, Wyatt MP. *The development of mature walking.* Oxford: Mac Keith Press, 1988.

56. Shiavi R, Green N. Ensemble averaging of locomotor electromyographic patterns using interpolation. *Med Biol Eng Comput* 1983;**21**: 573.

57. Limbird TJ, Shiavi R, Frazer M, Borra H. EMG profiles of knee joint musculature during walking: Changes induced by anterior cruciate ligament deficiency. *J Orthop Res* 1988;**6**:630.

58. Wooten ME, Kadaba MP, Cochran GUB. Dynamic electromyography. II. Normal patterns during gait. *J Orthop Res* 1990;**8**:259.

59. Kaufman KR, Sutherland DH. Dynamic intramuscular pressure measurement during gait. *Operat Techn Sports Med* 1995;**3**(4):250–5.

60. Wiig H. Evaluation of methodologies for measurement of interstitial fluid pressure (P_i): physiological implications of recent P_i data. *Crit Rev Biomed Eng* 1990;**18**(1):27–54.

61. Aukland K, Reed RK. Interstitial-lymphatic mechanisms in the control of extracellular fluid volume. *Physiol Rev* 1993;**73**(1):1–78.

62. Matsen FA, Mayo KA, Sheridan GW, Krugmire RB Jr. Monitoring of intramuscular pressure. *Surgery* 1976;**79**:702–9.

63. Rorabeck CH, Castle GSP, Hardie R, Logan J. Compartmental pressure measurements: an experimental investigation using the slit catheter. *J Trauma* 1981;**21**:446–9.

64. Styf JR. Evaluation of injection techniques in recording of intramuscular pressure. *J Orthop Res* 1989;**7**: 812–16.

65. Crenshaw AG, Styf JR, Mubarak SJ, Hargens AR. A new 'transducer tipped' fiber optic catheter for measuring intramuscular pressures. *J Orthop Res* 1990;**8**:464–8.

66. Kaufman KR, Wavering T, Morrow D, et al. Performance characteristics of a pressure microsensor. *J Biomech* 2003;**36**:283–7.

67. Prodromos CC, Andriacchi TP, Galante JO. A relationship between gait and clinical changes following high tibial osteotomy. *J Bone Joint Surg Am* 1985;**67A**: 1188–94.

68. Wang JW, Kuo NN, Andriacchi TP, Galante JO. The influence of walking mechanics and time on the results of proximal tibial osteotomy. *J Bone Joint Surg* 1990;**6**:905–9.

9

Postural imbalance in peripheral and central vestibular disorders

THOMAS BRANDT AND MARIANNE DIETERICH

INTRODUCTION

Vestibular dysfunction is a significant differential diagnosis in patients presenting with irresistible or unexpected falls. This is not adequately recognized by clinicians outside the field of neuro-otology. Peripheral and central vestibular pathways run from the labyrinths via vestibular and ocular motor nuclei to the thalamus and vestibular cortex. Vestibular syndromes – which are commonly characterized by a combination of phenomena involving perceptual, postural, ocular motor and vegetative manifestations – therefore comprise disorders of the labyrinths, vestibular nerves, brainstem and archicerebellum, thalamus and vestibular cortex.[1] They are caused in the majority of cases by dysfunction induced by a lesion, but a considerable proportion result from pathological excitation of various structures. Examples are otolith Tullio phenomenon, vestibular (nerve) paroxysmia, paroxysmal dysarthria and ataxia in multiple sclerosis or vestibular epilepsy. The particular pathological mechanisms that provoke postural instability and may cause vestibular falls differ considerably since they may result from changes in otolith or in horizontal or vertical semicircular canal function. In the following text, examples will be given of peripheral and central vestibular imbalance and falls, with particular emphasis on our current knowledge of how and why the patients fall (Table 9.1 and see Table 9.3).[2] Typically, an imbalance or gait disorder of vestibular origin is characterized by directed deviations or falls: fore–aft, lateral or diagonal.

PERIPHERAL VESTIBULAR FALLS

Vestibular neuritis

Acute unilateral vestibular paralysis causes a vestibular tone imbalance. In vestibular neuritis, the fast phase of the spontaneous rotational nystagmus and the initial

Table 9.1 *Postural imbalance in peripheral vestibular disorders*

Disorder	Direction	Mechanism
Vestibular neuritis	Lateral ipsiversive (diagonal)	Vestibular tone imbalance (yaw, roll) due to horizontal and anterior canal paresis
Benign paroxysmal positioning vertigo (BPPV)	Forward ipsiversive	Ampullofugal stimulation of posterior canal by canalolithiasis and a heavy clot-induced endolymph flow
Ménière's drop attacks (Tumarkin's otolithic crisis)	Vertical (down?)	Loss of postural tone due to abnormal otolith stimulation in sudden endolymphatic fluid pressure changes
Otolith Tullio phenomenon	Backward contraversive (diagonal)	Sound-induced mechanical stimulation of utricle by luxated stapes footplate
Vestibular paroxysmia	Forward contraversive (?) (multidirectional?)	Neurovascular cross-compression causing ephaptic stimulation of vestibular nerve
Bilateral vestibulopathy	Multidirectional, fore–aft	Impaired postural reflexes particularly in darkness

perception of apparent body motion are directed away from the side of the lesion, and the postural reactions initiated by vestibulospinal reflexes are usually in a direction opposite to the direction of vertigo. These result both in the Romberg fall and in past-pointing towards the side of the lesion. Patients with this type of vertigo often make confusing and contradictory statements about the direction of their symptoms. There are, in fact, two sensations, opposite in direction and the patient may be describing either one (Fig. 9.1). The first is the purely subjective sense of self-motion in the direction of the nystagmus fast phases, which is not associated with any measurable body sway. The second is the compensatory vestibulospinal reaction resulting in objective, measurable destabilization and a possible Romberg fall in the direction opposite to the fast phases.[3]

Vestibular neuritis causes a partial loss of labyrinthine function. It affects only part of the vestibular nerve trunk, usually the superior division (horizontal and anterior semicircular canal paresis), which travels separately and has its own ganglion, whereas the inferior part (posterior semicircular canal) is spared.[4] This hypothesis of partial involvement of the vestibular nerve is supported by three-dimensional eye movement analysis,[5] the temporal

bone pathology[6] and also by the histopathology of a case of herpes zoster oticus.[7] The ipsiversive falls described above reflect a horizontal and anterior semicircular canal paresis, but are indistinguishable from unilateral loss of vestibular function produced by acute conditions other than neuritis.

Management of vestibular neuritis involves medical treatment and physical therapy. During the first 1–3 days when nausea is pronounced, benzodiazepines or vestibular sedatives such as antihistamine dimenhydrate (50–100 mg every 6 h) or scopolamine (0.6 mg) can be administered parenterally for symptomatic relief. Their major side-effect is general sedation. These drugs should not be given after nausea disappears because they prolong the time required to achieve central compensation. As soon as the patient is no longer vomiting, this therapy should be replaced by a graduated vestibular exercise program supervised by a physiotherapist. Vestibular exercise programs are based on a combination of voluntary eye movements and fixations (improvement of visual stabilization), active head movements (recalibration of the vestibulo-ocular reflex) and active body movements (improvement of vestibulospinal regulation). A few studies have shown that glucocorticoids facilitate central vestibular compensation and have a beneficial effect on the course of the disease. Antiviral substances, such as acyclovir, have not yet been systematically studied. A double-blind study conducted by Adour et al.[8] found that acyclovir–prednisone is superior to prednisone alone for treating Bell's palsy, which most probably has the same pathogenesis.

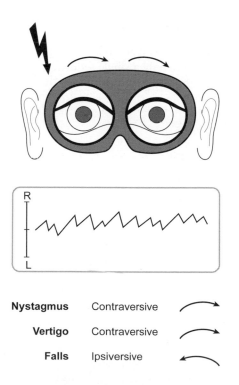

Figure 9.1 *Ocular signs, perception and posture in the acute stage of right-sided vestibular neuritis. Spontaneous vestibular nystagmus is always horizontal-rotatory away from the side of the lesion (best observed with Frenzel's glasses). The initial perception of apparent body motion (vertigo) is also directed away from the side of the lesion, whereas measurable destabilization (Romberg fall) is always towards the side of the lesion. The latter is the compensatory vestibulospinal reaction to the apparent tilt.*

Benign paroxysmal positioning vertigo

Posturographic measurements have been performed in patients with benign paroxysmal positioning vertigo (BPPV), in whom attacks were elicited by head tilt while standing on a force-measuring platform.[4] These measurements revealed a characteristic pattern of postural instability. After a short latency, patients exhibit large sway amplitudes, predominantly in the fore–aft direction (Fig. 9.2) with a mean sway frequency range < 3 Hz. Instability decreases over 10–30 s parallel to the reduction of the nystagmus and sensation of vertigo. When subjects close their eyes, the acute destabilization may lead to an almost irresistible tendency to fall. Posturographic data show a shift of the mean position of the center of gravity forwards and towards the direction of the head tilt (Fig. 9.2) with a concurrent increase in sway amplitude. The measurable shift of the center of gravity in the forward direction and ipsiversive to the tilted head can be interpreted as the motor compensation for the initial subjective vertigo in the opposite direction, the diagonal plane corresponding to the spatial plane and working range of the ipsilateral posterior canal.

Schuknecht[9] postulated a mechanical pathogenesis termed 'cupulolithiasis' because basophilic deposits were found on the cupula of the precipitating posterior

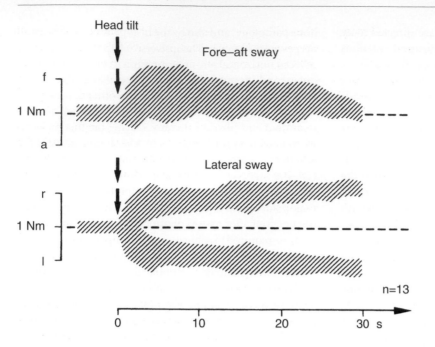

Head tilt

Figure 9.2 *Benign paroxysmal positioning vertigo. Mean amplitudes of body sway with an approximation of the deviation of the center of gravity in 13 patients in whom an attack could be elicited while standing upright on a force-measuring platform. The center of gravity of the body shifts forward and ipsilateral to the affected ear with a reduction of increased sway amplitudes concomitant with a decrease of nystagmus and vertigo.*

semicircular canal in individual patients that manifested unilateral BPPV prior to death from unrelated disease. There is now general acceptance that the debris floats freely within the endolymph of the canal; 'canalolithiasis' rather than 'cupulolithiasis' is the significant causative factor.[10–12] The debris, comprising particles possibly detached from the otoliths, congeal to form a free-floating clot (plug). Since the clot is heavier than endolymph, it will always gravitate to the most dependent part of the canal during head position changes that alter the angle of the canal's plane relative to gravity (Fig. 9.3). Analogous

to a plunger, the clot induces bidirectional (push and pull) forces on the cupula, thereby triggering the BPPV attack.[12,13] Canalolithiasis explains all the features of BPPV: latency, short duration, fatigability, changes in direction of nystagmus with changes in head position and the efficacy of physical therapy.

Positional exercises are an effective physical therapy for BPPV (Fig. 9.3). The Semont[14] and Epley[11] liberatory maneuvers require only a single sequence, making them preferable to the multiple repetitions over many days required by the Brandt–Daroff exercises.[1]

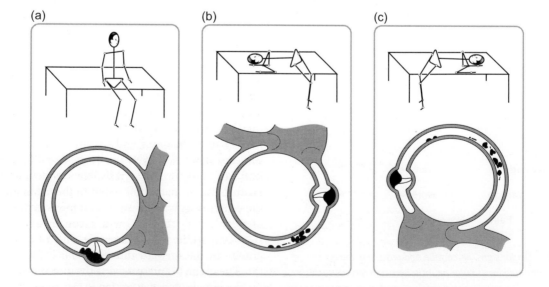

Figure 9.3 *Schematic drawing of the clot of otoconial debris dispersed and sluiced by positioning maneuvers from the upright (a) to the challenging (b) position and to the opposite side (c). According to the change of the head position relative to the gravitational vector, the clot sediments to the lowermost part of the canal and by transition from position (b) to (c), leaves the canal in order to enter other labyrinthine recesses.*

Ménière's drop attacks (Tumarkin's otolithic crisis)

In Ménière's disease periodic endolymphatic membrane ruptures with subsequent transient potassium palsy of vestibular nerve fibers cause vertigo attacks and postural instability with characteristics similar to those in vestibular neuritis. The direction of nystagmus and vertigo depends on the location of the membranous leakage in relation to either the posterior or horizontal ampullary nerve. Rarely, vestibular drop attacks (Tumarkin's otolithic crisis)[15] occur in early and late stages of endolymphatic hydrops[16] when sudden changes in endolymphatic fluid pressure cause non-physiological end-organ stimulation (deformation of utricle of saccule membrane?) with a reflex-like vestibulospinal loss of postural tone. Patients fall without warning; they remain conscious but lose voluntary control of balance. Sometimes during a vestibular drop attack patients have the feeling that they are being pushed or thrown to the ground. However, slower sensations involving apparent tilts of the surroundings also occur, possibly resulting in forward, backward or lateral body tilt.

Pharmacologically, administration of fentanyl and droperidol (Innovar) has been tried with questionable success. Drop attacks disappeared completely after gentamicin treatment.[17] All reported experience with this kind of treatment indicates that one injection per week (1–2 ml with concentrations less than 30 mg/ml) on an outpatient basis could be recommended in order to better monitor the delayed ototoxic effects. The final, rarely used but effective form of treatment is surgery,[18] involving either ipsilateral labyrinthectomy or selective section of the vestibular nerve to preserve useful hearing in the affected ear. On the whole, however, prognosis is relatively benign and attacks often remit spontaneously.

Fistula of the anterior semicircular canal

A new syndrome has been described by Minor and coworkers:[19,20] dehiscence of the bone overlying the anterior semicircular canal. The clinical manifestation is sound- and/or pressure-induced attacks of dizziness and postural instability with vertical and rotatory oscillopsia or diplopia associated with vertical-torsional eye movements typical for excitation or inhibition of the anterior semicircular canal of the affected ear. The bony dehiscence can be identified on high-resolution temporal bone computed tomography (CT) scan. The symptoms improve when the affected canal is patched or plugged.

Otolith Tullio phenomenon

Sound-induced vestibular symptoms such as vertigo, nystagmus, oscillopsia and postural imbalance in patients with perilymph fistulas are commonly known as the Tullio phenomenon.[21] Evidence was presented, based on otoneurological examination of a typical patient as well as re-evaluation of cases described in the literature, that an otolith Tullio phenomenon due to hypermobile stapes footplate typically manifests with the pattern of sound-induced paroxysms of ocular tilt reaction (OTR).[22] The patients complain of distressing attacks of vertical oblique and rotatory oscillopsia (apparent tilt of the visual scene) and of falls towards the unaffected ear and backward elicited by loud sounds (Fig. 9.4). This arises from non-physiological mechanical otolith stimulation; surgical exploration of the middle ear of our patient revealed a subluxated stapes footplate with the hypertrophic stapedius muscle causing pathologically large amplitude movements during the stapedius reflex. The otoliths lie directly adjacent to the stapes footplate.

With the patient standing, a vestibulospinal reflex can be recorded electromyographically at a surprisingly short latency, with an electromyograph (EMG) response after 47 ms in the tibialis anterior muscle and after 52 ms in the gastrocnemius muscle (Fig. 9.4).

Vestibulospinal effects are modulated to a great degree by body position and are abolished with the eyes open (Fig. 9.5) or with the patient in the supine position.[23] The latencies are different for agonists and antagonists, despite a regular co-activation. Increased amplitude and different patterns of activation of leg, arm and neck muscles cannot be interpreted as arising solely from three-neuron reflex arcs, but obviously involve preprogrammed motor patterns intended to maintain postural stability. There is an influence of neck proprioceptive input: turning the head about the vertical Z-axis to the left or right and maintaining it in that position does not alter the position of utriculus and sacculus with respect to the gravitational field. Nevertheless, there are marked and reproducible differences in the latencies of lower leg muscle activation. Turning the head to the right (i.e. towards induced head tilt) results consistently in an activation of the tibialis anterior muscle from about 50–60 ms, whereas voluntary turning of the head to the left (i.e. against induced head tilt) increases latencies to 80–87 ms (Fig. 9.6). Not only the onset of muscle activity but also its peak in the rectified EMG response occurs about 20–30 ms later under head turned left conditions. It appears, therefore, that efference copy signals or the somatosensory input from neck muscles can modify the timing of muscular activation in the lower leg following otolithic stimulation. Both somatosensory and static otolithic inputs are altered when the patient rests on hands and knees (crawling position). The pattern of activation is slightly decreased in amplitude, yet the latencies do not differ significantly from those in the upright stance. Extension or retroflexion of the head does not alter the pattern of activation in a patient with typical otolith Tullio phenomenon. Functional inactivation of vestibulospinal reflexes is dependent on assumed posture.[23] The effect of otolithic stimulation was studied under several conditions in

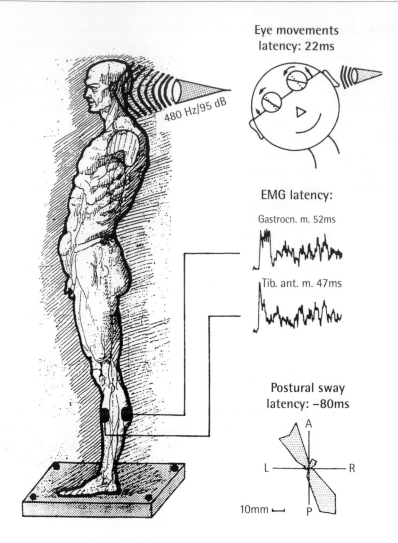

Eye movements
latency: 22ms

480 Hz/95 dB

EMG latency:

Gastrocn. m. 52ms

Tib. ant. m. 47ms

Postural sway
latency: −80ms

10mm

Figure 9.4 *An otolith Tullio phenomenon (left ear) is characterized by a sound-induced ocular tilt reaction (skew deviation with ipsilateral over contralateral hypertropia, ocular torsion counter-clockwise and head tilt with ipsilateral ear up; top) and increased body sway predominantly from right-backward to left-forward (bottom). Latencies of eye movements are 22 ms. Latencies of the vestibulospinal reflex during upright stance are 47 ms in the left tibialis anterior muscle and 55 ms in the left gastrocnemius muscle. Measurable postural sway has a minimum latency of about 80 ms.*

which the lower leg muscles were voluntarily contracted but not used in maintaining upright posture. It was common to all these conditions that, despite the continuous voluntary discharge in the EMG, no increase (or decrease) of activity time locked to the sound stimulation could be detected. When the patient balances on one foot (eyes closed) activation in the tibialis anterior muscle occurs at short latency on the supporting leg, with a slightly more pronounced response in the left, ipsilateral leg than in the right one (Fig. 9.7). In the elevated leg the EMG remains unmodulated with a sustained discharge because of voluntary contraction of the muscles. When sitting or supine, no specific response can be recorded from the lower leg muscles.

Otolithic stimulation, therefore, does not release a rigid vestibulospinal reflex but triggers different patterns

of antigravity muscle activation, dependent on the current posture or intended task. This flexibility is required to maintain balance in situations with combined voluntary-active and involuntary-passive stimulation, for example, walking on a rolling ship.

Bilateral vestibulopathy with predominant forward and backward falls

Bilateral loss of vestibular function causes unsteadiness of gait, particularly in the dark, and – because of the insufficiency of the vestibulo-ocular reflex – oscillopsia associated with head movements or when walking. These patients complain of oscillopsia and imbalance, and the condition can be identified by decreased ocular motor responses to caloric irrigation and angular acceleration.[24]

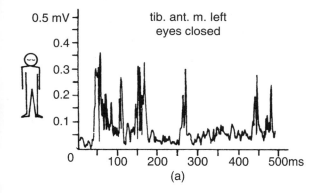

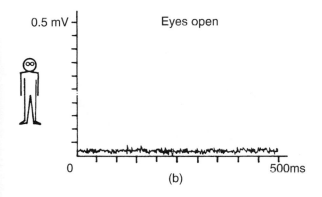

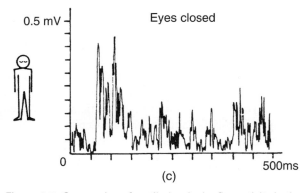

Figure 9.5 *Suppression of vestibulospinal reflex activity in the ipsilateral tibialis anterior muscle when the patient fixated a stationary visual scene (b). In (a) and (c) the muscular response with eyes closed immediately before and afterwards is shown.*

Measurements of postural instability show the largest amplitude in the fore–aft direction (Fig. 9.8), corresponding to the predominant direction of fall. In cases of body perturbations, falls may also occur sideways, particularly in darkness when vision cannot compensate sufficiently for the vestibular deficit. The lack of one channel of sensory input – important as it is for demanding balancing tasks in sport – rarely manifests itself as clinically significant instability.[1] In the absence of sensory information from two of the stabilizing systems, postural control may be severely impaired as, for example, in a patient with sensory polyneuropathy or with bilateral vestibulopathy under restricted visual conditions (darkness).

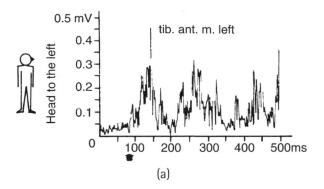

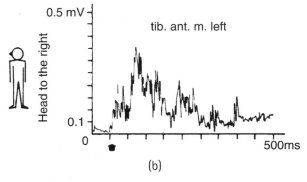

Figure 9.6 *Influence of neck proprioceptions on latency of vestibulospinal reflex recorded in the ipsilateral tibialis anterior muscle following otolith stimulation. Turning the head to the left (a) results in an activation of muscle from 50 to 60 ms, whereas turning the head to the right increases latencies to 80–87 ms.*

Vestibular paroxysmia

Neurovascular cross-compression of the root entry zone of the Vth, VIIth and IXth cranial nerves can elicit distressing attacks of trigeminal neuralgia, hemifacial spasm and glossopharyngeal neuralgia. Ephaptic transmission between bare axons and/or central hyperactivity initiated and maintained by the peripheral compression are discussed as pathophysiological mechanisms by Moller.[25] The syndrome of neurovascular compression of the VIIIth cranial nerve was first described by Jannetta et al.[26] and later termed 'disabling positional vertigo' by the same authors; it is a description for a heterogeneous collection of signs and symptoms.

The lack of a well-defined syndrome and of a pathognomonic test hitherto prevented reliable diagnosis and made it difficult for the non-surgical clinician to accept the existence of this interesting disease.[1] In a study, 11 patients were described as suffering from brief and frequent attacks of rotational or to-and-fro vertigo for months to years, with prompt and significant response to carbamazepine.[27] Typical features were the association with peripheral auditory and vestibular deficits and the dependence of the attacks on changes in head position. The diagnosis was based on four characteristic features:

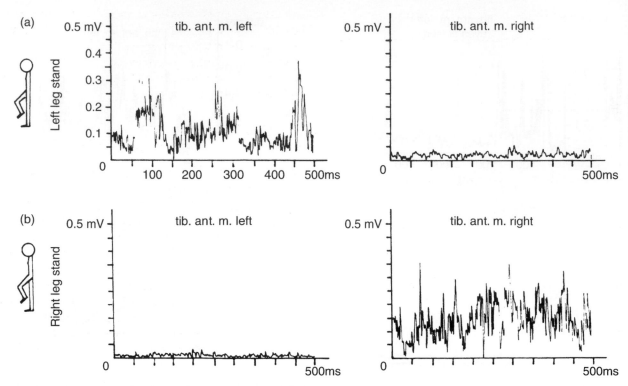

Figure 9.7 *Suppression of vestibulospinal reflex activity in the tibialis anterior muscle of both sides when not used for support of upright stance while the patient balanced on one foot. In the elevated leg the electromyogram remained unmodulated. (a) Balancing on left foot, (b) balancing on right foot.*

1. Short attacks of rotational ($n = 8$) or to-and-fro vertigo ($n = 3$) lasting from seconds to minutes;
2. Attacks frequently dependent on particular head positions ($n = 8$) and modification of the duration of the attack by changing head position ($n = 5$);
3. Hypacusis ($n = 5$) or tinnitus ($n = 7$) permanently or during the attack; and
4. Measurable auditory or vestibular deficits by neurophysiological methods ($n = 10$).

Only those patients that presented with at least three of the four features and that responded convincingly to carbamazepine were diagnosed as having 'vestibular paroxysmia'.[27] The latter criterion seemed essential since earlier studies on 'disabling positional vertigo' emphasized the ineffectiveness of vestibular suppressant medications[26] without evidence that anti-epileptic drugs (first choice for trigeminal neuralgia) were systematically employed in these patients.

Neurophysiological documentation in a typical patient may serve to demonstrate subtle but measurable ocular motor and postural effects during the attacks. This patient complained of oscillopsia, postural imbalance and unilateral tinnitus within the right ear during the attacks, which lasted 26–72 s. The effects were dependent on head position, with a combination of auditory (high-frequency hearing loss, tinnitus at 2000 Hz) and vestibular symptoms. Involvement of vertical canal and otolith input was suggested because of upward spontaneous nystagmus of both eyes, ocular torsion of both eyes and pathological tilt of subjective visual vertical (Fig. 9.9).

Taken together, in audio-vestibular testing most of the patients (10 of 11) exhibited unilateral dysfunction in the symptom-free interval. All patients responded promptly and significantly to carbamazepine (Tegretol), even to a low initial dosage. One or two wash-out phases were performed in four patients, all of whom relapsed within 2 days to 2 weeks.

The strongest argument for a peripheral nerve origin of these attacks of vertigo and imbalance is based on the documented unilateral peripheral audio-vestibular deficits in the symptom-free interval in most of the patients. This is supported by the long duration of monosymptomatic attacks over several years, which makes a central brainstem disorder less likely while multiple sclerosis and vestibular epilepsy have to be ruled out by careful diagnostics [magnetic resonance imaging (MRI) scan, cerebrospinal fluid (CSF) and evoked potentials, electroencephalogram]. A pathological contact of the nerve with a loop of the anterior inferior cerebellar artery can be found by means of special MRI sequences. The dependence of vestibular and auditory symptoms on head position is further indicative for a peripheral disorder. On the basis of our experience we recommend carbamazepine as first-choice therapy and gabapentin as second-choice therapy in suspected neurovascular cross-compression of the VIIIth nerve before an operation is contemplated.[27]

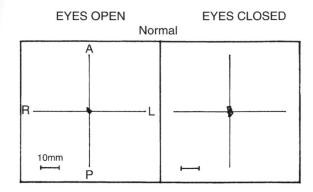

EYES OPEN   EYES CLOSED
Normal

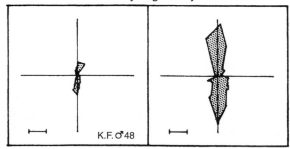

Bilateral vestibulopathy

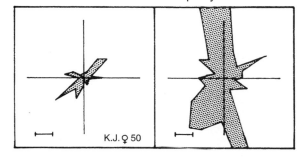

Downbeat nystagmus syndrome

Figure 9.8 *Postural instability in bilateral vestibulopathy and downbeat nystagmus syndrome. Histograms for fore–aft (A, P) and lateral (R, L) postural sway during upright stance with eyes open (left) and eyes closed (right) obtained with a force-measuring platform. For comparison see registration of body sway in a normal subject (top). Preferred direction of postural instability and body sway is in the fore–aft direction for bilateral vestibulopathy (bottom). Body sway increases significantly with eyes closed when visual stabilization cannot compensate for the peripheral vestibular deficit. Force-plates do not measure body displacement, instead they measure the position of the center of foot pressure (CFP). The movement of this point is influenced both by displacement of the center of gravity and by body acceleration (produced by muscle activity). If body displacements are slow the CFP will indicate approximately the position of the center of gravity, but with active postural correction CFP displacements can be considerably larger. The histograms shown here probably contain both components, which does not alter the clinical interpretation much but one should be cautious about describing them as sway histograms and discussing them purely in the context of body displacement.*

Another vertigo syndrome that depends on head position is the rotational vertebral artery occlusion syndrome. Head rotations may elicit recurrent uniform attacks of severe rotatory vertigo and postural imbalance caused by labyrinthine ischemia due to a complete occlusion of the vertebral artery at the C2-level.[28]

VESTIBULOPATHIC GAIT

You're better off running than walking with acute vestibulopathy

The recent finding that patients with acute vestibular disorders balance better when running than when walking slowly led us to suggest that the automatic spinal locomotor program suppresses destabilizing vestibular input.[29]

If an acute unilateral peripheral vestibular failure causes a distressing vestibular tone imbalance, the afflicted subjects move slowly, grasp searchingly for support, or must be guided in order to correct for their deviating gait and lateral falls. Slow motion is commonly believed to be much safer for these patients than fast motion. When walking slowly, the area of foot support is larger (both feet on the ground) than when running (one foot on the ground at a time). Thus, one would expect balance control to rely more on the actual vestibular input during running.

A chance observation of a dog with acute left unilateral vestibular failure showed that running is safer.[29] After awakening one day, the dog suddenly showed a severe postural imbalance and repeatedly fell to the left. When she stood still, head movements caused the falls. When walking slowly, she veered to the left, staggered about in counterclockwise circles and repeatedly fell. Surprisingly, once the dog was outside and began to trot, she was suddenly able to move without deviating from her course and obviously felt better and more confident as her raised, wagging tail indicated. However, as soon as she stopped trotting and began to slowly walk, she again showed the severe tendency to deviate from her intended path and fell to the left.

Neurological examination of the dog revealed a spontaneous nystagmus to the right and an ocular tilt reaction to the left.[30] The high-frequency head rotation test[31] revealed a defective vestibulo-ocular reflex, best explained by an acute unilateral vestibular failure.

This observation prompted video recording of the balance during walking and running of patients with acute unilateral vestibulopathy and healthy volunteers with a post-rotatory transient vestibular tone imbalance.[29] Four patients (all women, aged 57–67 years) had a confirmed diagnosis of vestibular neuritis. Three to 5 days after the onset of the condition, they were requested to close their eyes and slowly walk or run 10 m through a 2.5-m wide corridor. All touched the wall for support two to four times during the 10-m stretch. In

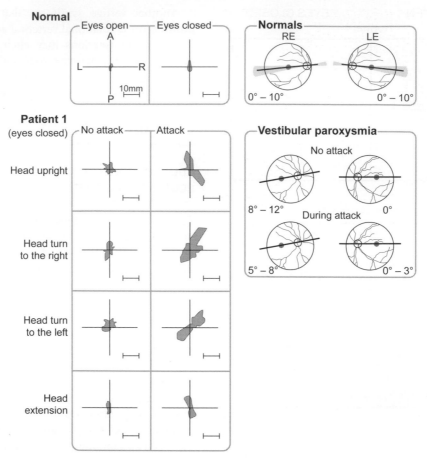

Figure 9.9 *Patients with vestibular paroxysmia may complain of oscillopsia, postural imbalance and unilateral tinnitus during the attacks. (a) Histograms for fore–aft (A, P) and lateral (R, L) postural sway obtained with a force-measuring platform (Kistler, Ostfildern) in a normal subject (top) and a patient suffering from neurovascular cross-compression of the right VIIIth nerve. The patient exhibited a slightly increased body sway with eyes closed (bottom left), which increased during the attack for 26–72 s (bottom right), usually in a diagonal fore-aft direction. The direction of the preferred body sway changed by 90° if the head was turned to the right or to the left. The effects were dependent on head position and a combination of auditory symptoms (high-frequency hearing loss, tinnitus at 2000 Hz) with involvement of vertical canal and otolith input was suggested because of upward spontaneous nystagmus and ocular torsion of both eyes and tilt of perceived vertical. (b) Schematic representation of the fundus indicating normal position of the eyes in the roll plane (straight line through papilla-macula). Normal position in roll is an excyclotropia of 0° to 10°. In the patient, eye position was slightly abnormal in both eyes (as seen by the observer). During the attack a slight clockwise rotation of 2–3° could be repeatedly measured by laser-scanning ophthalmoscope.*

contrast, when running slowly, they maintained their direction for over 10 m and felt much more secure (Fig. 9.10). Increased walking speed also had a clearly stabilizing influence on their balance.

Ten blindfolded, healthy physical therapists (five women; mean age 26.5 years, SD 3.7) were suddenly stopped after 10 rotations in a chair at a constant angular velocity of 360 degrees/s. They were then asked to either walk slowly or run straight ahead for 10 m. There was a mean deviation when they walked of 52.6 (SD 12.4) degrees over 10 m (Fig. 9.11). In contrast, the mean deviation was 14.6 (SD 9.2) degrees when they ran. All volunteers also felt it was easier to maintain their balance while running. Similar data were found when blindfolded subjects were asked to walk or run during galvanic vestibular stimulation.[32] There was, however, no difference in mean

deviations for walking or running when the patients or subjects walked or ran in place without locomotion.

Automatic spinal locomotor pattern largely independent of actual vestibular input

All three observations of dog, patients and volunteers after body rotation demonstrate that an acute vestibular tone imbalance has less effect on balance and the direction of locomotion if the individual runs rather than walks slowly. This apparent paradox is unlikely to have a simple explanation such as increased speed causes a mechanical stabilization of balance ('gyrocompass phenomenon'). Moreover, the same difference in balance and direction during walking or running was observed regardless of whether the subjects swung their arms

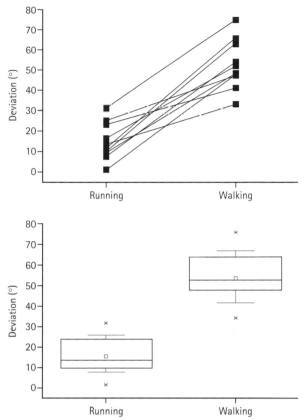

Figure 9.11 *Deviation of gait during running vs. walking in volunteers with a transient physiological vestibular tone imbalance. Ten healthy blindfolded subjects were asked to either slowly walk or run 10 m straight ahead after being suddenly stopped out of a constant velocity body rotation of 360°/s. Individual deviation in degrees was consistently less when running (top); mean deviation when running was 14.6 ± 9.2° and when walking 52.6 ± 2.4° (paired t-test, P <0.001). Open square, mean; horizontal lines of the box, 25th, 50th and 75th percentiles; error bars above and below the boxes, 5th and 95th percentiles; cross, range.*[29]

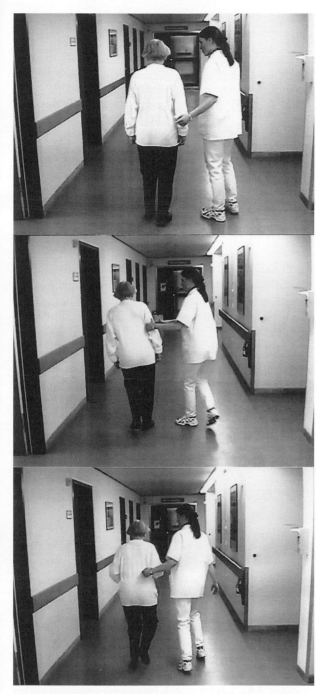

Figure 9.10 *Posture and gait of a 66-year-old patient on day 4 after an acute vestibular neuritis of the left ear (taken from a video sequence). With her eyes closed, she was able to maintain balance by increasing her body sway (top). If she tried to walk in a straight line, her gait showed a marked deviation toward the affected ear and there were lateral falls (middle). She found it easier to run straight ahead with eyes closed without touching the wall on the left (bottom).*

spontaneously, which should aid balance, or held them close to the body. All three examples also show that locomotion is largely independent of the actual control of the vestibular system, especially active linear path integration.

Earlier reports in the literature also demonstrate that the actual control of the vestibular system can be bypassed. For example, blindfolded patients with bilateral vestibular failure are able to perform linear goal-directed locomotion toward memorized targets.[33] Automatic locomotor patterns have been found in the chronic spinal cat (for review, see Grillner[34]) and in paraplegic patients whose body weight was partly unloaded during suspension from a parachute harness connected to an overhead crane while walking on a moving treadmill.[35] This spinal locomotor activity was induced only after signs of spinal shock had disappeared, and it was distinct from spinal stretch reflex activity.[36]

A functional interpretation of the observation that you're better off running than walking with acute vestibulopathy would argue that an automatic spinal program of locomotion triggers the inhibition of descending vestibular sensory inflow. This explanation would agree with the recently proposed concept of sensory down- and up-channeling for multisensory postural control. According to this theory, the vestibular organ is the body's sensor of position (i.e. it receives the 'body-in-space' signals – down-channeling) and the somatosensory system measures the joint angles (i.e. it receives the 'support-in-space-tilt' signals – up-channeling).[37] In our examples, the ascending rather than the descending signals would define the desired value for the joints to control posture. A misleading vestibular signal could thus be suppressed via down-and-up channeling.

Further evidence in the literature supports this functional interpretation. Like the vestibular system, the somatosensory system can also be inhibited. Monosynaptic stretch reflex responses in the human leg, for example, are suppressed and spinal pathways of group I afferents are blocked during gait.[38] Moreover, muscular sense was reported to be attenuated when humans move.[39] This finding is consistent with a general attenuation of sensory feedback which occurs during movement and locomotion.

The multisensory-sensorimotor interaction necessary for postural control is, thus, not a simple fusion, but rather a complex of different processes that are fine-tuned by repetition and learning. How they interact is influenced not only by the pattern of actual motion stimulation, but also by the particular postural and locomotor tasks. This is reflected by the differential effects of an actual vestibular tone imbalance on slow walking and running as well as on walking and running in place without locomotion. Control of slow walking obviously depends on afferent and re-afferent sensory input to a larger extent than does fast walking or running. It makes sense to suppress the vestibular (or somatosensory) input once a highly automatic motor pattern of fast walking or running has been initiated, otherwise the re-afferent sensory stimulations caused by head and joint motion during locomotion would interfere, acting like adverse feedback and modify an already optimized automatic program.

These findings on the differential effects of an acute vestibulopathy on walking or running may have important consequences for the physical therapy and rehabilitation of patients with vestibulopathic gait.

CENTRAL VESTIBULAR FALLS

The acute central vestibular tone is built up by the tonic bilateral vestibular input. It stabilizes the eyes and head in the normal upright position in the yaw, pitch and the roll planes, and dominates our perception of verticality. A lesional vestibular tone imbalance may affect either one of the three major planes of action of the vestibulo-ocular reflex (VOR) – horizontal 'yaw', vertical 'pitch' or 'roll' (Table 9.2).[1,40] It is well established that several ocular motor disorders are secondary to distinct and separate lesions of central vestibular pathways from the

Table 9.2 *Classification of some central vestibular syndromes of the brainstem according to the three major planes of action of the vestibulo-ocular reflex (VOR)*

Disorders of the VOR in horizontal (yaw) plane	Horizontal nystagmus Pseudo 'vestibular neuritis' (lacunar AICA/PICA infarctions; MS plaques)
Disorders of the VOR in sagittal (pitch) plane	Vertical nystagmus Downbeat nystagmus/vertigo, upbeat nystagmus/vertigo
Disorders of the VOR in frontal (roll) plane	Ocular tilt reaction and its components (skew deviation; cyclorotation of the eyes; head tilt; body lateropulsion)

vestibular nuclei to ocular motor nuclei. A first attempt is proposed to classify vestibular brainstem disorders according to a lesional tone imbalance in one of the three major planes of action of the VOR (Tables 9.2 and 9.3).

Vestibular epilepsy with contraversive vertigo and falls

Vestibular epilepsy is a cortical vertigo syndrome secondary to focal discharges from either the temporal lobe or the parietal association cortex[41,42] and the parieto-insular vestibular cortex,[43,44] all of which receive bilateral vestibular projections from the ipsilateral thalamus. Several distinct and separate areas of the parietal and temporal cortex have been identified in animal studies as receiving vestibular afferents, such as area 2v at the tip of the intraparietal sulcus[42,45,46] area 3aV (neck, trunk and vestibular region of area 3a) in the central sulcus,[47] the parieto-insular vestibular cortex (PIVC) at the posterior end of the insula[43,44] and area 7 in the inferior parietal lobule.[48] Our knowledge about vestibular cortex function in humans is less precise, derived mainly from stimulation experiments reported anecdotally in the older literature. It is not always possible to extrapolate from monkey species to human cortex, as Anderson and Gnadt[49] have demonstrated for Brodmann's area 7 in the rhesus monkey and humans. Area V corresponds best to the vestibular cortex as described by Foerster in 1936.[41] The PIVC corresponds best to a region from which Penfield and Jasper[50] were able to induce vestibular sensations by electrical stimulation with a depth electrode within the Sylvian fissure, medial to the primary acoustic cortex. This region was found to be activated during vestibular stimulation, as assessed by focal increase of cortical blood flow[51] or in brain activation studies.[52,53] In a study of 52 patients with infarctions in the middle cerebral artery territory a region could be identified deep in the posterior part of the insula in humans, ischemia of which regularly caused significant (mostly contraversive) tilts of perceived visual vertical.[54] In this study, the overlapping infarcted area of the 23 patients with tilts of the perceived vertical centered on the long

Table 9.3 *Postural imbalance in central vestibular disorders*

Disorder	Direction	Mechanism
Vestibular epilepsy	Contraversive (?)	Simple or complex partial seizures due to epileptic discharges of vestibular cortex
Thalamic astasia	Contraversive or ipsiversive	Vestibular tone imbalance (yaw, roll?) in posterolateral vestibular thalamic lesions
Ocular tilt reaction	Contraversive in pontomesencephalic lesions Ipsiversive in pontomedullary lesions	Tone imbalance of VOR in roll due to lesions of otolith and vertical canal pathways
Paroxysmal ocular tilt reaction	Ipsiversive with pontomesencephalic stimulation Contraversive with peripheral vestibular stimulation	Pathological excitation of otolith and vertical canal pathways mediating VOR in roll
Lateropulsion (Wallenberg's syndrome)	Ipsiversive, diagonal	Lesion-induced tone imbalance of VOR in roll and yaw with concurrent deviation of the subjective vertical
Downbeat nystagmus/vertigo	Backward	Lesional vestibular tone imbalance of the VOR in pitch

insular gyrus, the adjacent superior temporal gyrus and the transverse temporal gyrus, a region probably homologous to the PIVC in monkey.

Vestibular seizures are simple or complex partial sensory seizures with vertigo as the predominant symptom. Patients experience sudden disequilibrium with rotational or linear vertigo, accompanied in most cases by body or head and eye rotation. From the few detailed reports on the direction of apparent self- and surround motion, it is most likely that the direction of perceived self-motion, measurable body motion and eye deviation is contraversive to the epileptic focus, whereas simultaneously perceived surround motion may be ipsiversive.[41] The different effects on the perception of self- and object-motion correspond to the effects of normal locomotion, in which body motion in one direction causes relative surround motion in the opposite direction. That the directions of nystagamus and of measurable body displacement are the same differs significantly from the case of vestibular neuritis (Fig. 9.1), in which the directions of nystagmus and body displacement are always opposite. Thus, in vestibular epilepsy, actual body movements do not represent a vestibulospinal compensation of perceived vertigo but an epileptic postural response. Vestibular seizures can manifest without any objective eye and body movements, as described by Foerster[41] in his stimulation experiments. In the case described by Penfield and Jasper,[50] the direction of eye deviation, nystagmus and perceived surround motion was the same, but this case appears to represent visual rather than vestibular epilepsy.[1]

Anticonvulsive therapy is the same as that for other focal or partial complex seizures (e.g. carbamazepine, gabapentin, valproic acid, or phenytoin).

Thalamic astasia with contraversive or ipsiversive falls?

There are a few instances of presumed central vestibular dysfunction in which patients without paresis, or sensory or cerebellar deficit, are unable to maintain an unsupported, upright posture. The conditions are thalamic astasia,[55] lateropulsion in Wallenberg's syndrome[56,57] and OTR.[58] Postural imbalance with a transient tendency to fall has been noted following therapeutic thalamotomy and thalamic hemorrhages.[59] Thalamic astasia, as described by Masdeu and Gorelick,[55] occurred in the absence of motor weakness, sensory loss or cerebellar signs, as a result of lesions with different causes, all primarily involving super-posterolateral portions of the thalamus but sparing the rubral region. Their patients seemed to fall in a direction contraversive to the lesion or backwards. A critical review of their patients (mostly cases of hemorrhages and tumors), based on current knowledge of the differential effects of thalamic infarctions on vestibular function, reveals that a clear distinction between posterolateral and paramedian thalamic infarctions involving rostral mesencephalic tegmentum is lacking. It is our own experience in some 30 patients with thalamic infarctions that the posterolateral type may cause both contraversive or ipsiversive postural instability (Fig. 9.12), whereas the paramedian type always causes contraversive OTR and falls.[60,61]

Graduated vestibular exercise programs should be started as soon as possible to promote central compensation of the vestibular tone imbalance.

Ocular tilt reaction

Ocular tilt reaction is a central vestibular disorder involving the vertical vestibulo-ocular reflex in the roll plane. It represents a fundamental pattern of coordinated eye-head-roll motion and body tilt. It is based on both otolithic and vertical semicircular canal input, and is mediated by the graviceptive pathways from the labyrinths via the rostral medial and superior vestibular nuclei and the contralateral medial longitudinal fascicle to the rostral midbrain tegmentum (Fig. 9.13). It consists of lateral head tilt and skew deviation of the eyes:

Normal

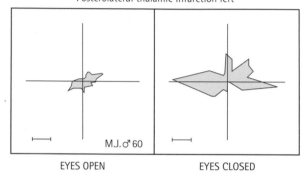

Posterolateral thalamic infarction left

M.J.♂60

EYES OPEN   EYES CLOSED

Figure 9.12 *Postural instability in a patient with a left posterolateral thalamic infarction. Preferred direction of postural instability and body sway is in the lateral direction.*

clockwise with head tilt left, counter-clockwise with head tilt right (viewpoint of the observer). It was first clearly delineated during electrical stimulation of the interstitial nucleus of Cajal.[30]

Ocular tilt reaction is not a rare condition. In acute unilateral brainstem infarctions it can be detected in about 20 per cent of cases if a careful investigation for cyclorotation of the eyes (fundus photographs), subtle skew deviation and subjective visual vertical[62] is carried out. Ocular tilt reaction and concurrent body tilt are always ipsiversive in ponto-medullary lesions,[58,63] whereas OTR and concurrent body tilt are always con-traversive in ponto-mesencephalic lesions.[60,62,63] This can be best explained by a crossing of graviceptive pathways (which is supported by animal experiments) at the pontine level.[64] If OTR is induced by electrical stimulation of the pathways rather than by lesional destruction, then the direction is reversed.[65]

The natural course and management of OTR depend on its etiology. Deviations of eyes and perceived vertical are usually transient, because of the unilateral lesion and the central compensation via the unaffected side. In cases of infarction or hemorrhage recovery occurs within a few days to 6 weeks. Physical therapy may facilitate this central compensation.

The syndrome of OTR in the acute phase of an infarction presenting with deviations of the subjective visual vertical as well as cyclorotation and skew deviation of the eyes has to be differentiated from the syndrome of 'con-

traversive pushing' (Pusher syndrome). Stroke patients in the chronic phase may exhibit a behavior of actively pushing away from the non-hemiparetic side, leading to lateral postural imbalance and a tendency to fall toward the paralyzed side. Measurements of the subjective postural vertical (SPV) and the subjective visual vertical (SVV) revealed that the deficit leading to contraversive pushing is an altered perception of the body's orientation in relation to gravity.[66] Pusher patients experienced their body as oriented 'upright' when it was actually tilted 18 degrees to the non-hemiparetic, ipsilesional side (SPV tilted), while the SVV was within normal range. There seem to be two graviceptive systems which may rely on different input sources, at least in part. The orientation of the visual world and the head to the vertical is perceived through our visual, vestibular and proprioceptive sense organs in the head and the neck, while the posture of the trunk is mainly perceived through sense organs in the trunk.[67]

Lateropulsion in Wallenberg's syndrome

Lateropulsion of the body is a well-known transient feature of lateral medullary infarction in which patients cannot prevent ipsiversive lateral falls. We believe that subjective vertigo is usually absent in these patients because there is no sensory mismatch. The lesion causes a deviation of the perceived vertical. Individual multi-sensory regulation of posture is then adjusted not to the true vertical but to the pathologically deviated internal representation of verticality produced by the lesion. Thus, these patients fall without realizing that it is their active shift of the center of gravity (lateropulsion) that causes the imbalance. It is the incorrect central computation of verticality (despite correct peripheral sensory signals from the otoliths) that is responsible for postural imbalance. Posturographic measurements in thirty-six patients with Wallenberg's syndrome[57] revealed that with minor lateropulsion the preferred body-sway direction is diagonal and becomes more lateral in severe cases, particularly with the eyes closed (Fig. 9.14). All patients exhibited significant tilts of the internal representation of the gravity vector, as indicated by deviations of the subjective visual vertical ipsiversive to the lesion. If one correlates the grade of lateropulsion with net tilt angles of the subjective visual vertical, it is evident that the more pronounced the lateropulsion, the greater the spatial disorientation with respect to verticality.

Downbeat nystagmus syndrome with backward falls

Downbeat nystagmus in the primary gaze position, in particular on lateral gaze, is often accompanied by oscillopsia and postural instability[68] and a tendency to fall

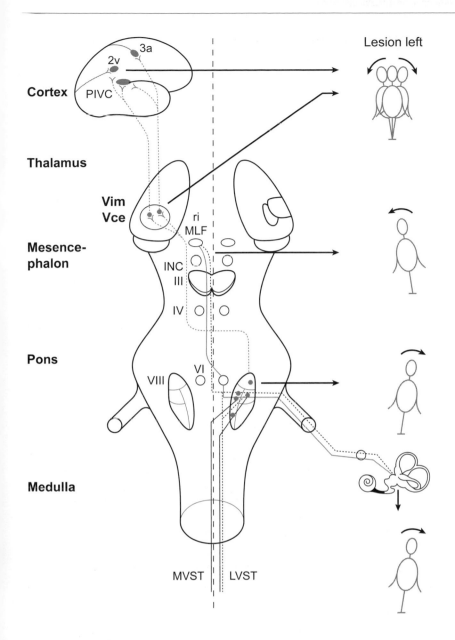

Lesion left

Figure 9.13 *Schematic drawing of graviceptive pathways mediating vestibular reactions in the roll plane. The projections from the otolith and vertical semicircular canals to the ocular motor nuclei (nucleus trochlearis IV, nucleus oculomotorius III, nucleus abducens VI) and the supranuclear centers of the interstitial nucleus of Cajal (INC), and the rostral interstitial nucleus of the fasciculus longitudinalis medialis (riMLF) are shown. They subserve the vestibulo-ocular reflex (VOR) in three planes. The VOR is part of a more complex vestibular response which also involves vestibulospinal connections via the medial and lateral vestibulospinal tracts (MVST and LVST, respectively) for head and body posture control. Furthermore, connections to the vestibular cortex (areas 2v and 3a and the parieto-insular vestibular cortex) via the vestibular nuclei of the thalamus (Vim, Vcc) are depicted. Graviceptive vestibular pathways for the roll plane cross at the pontine level. Vestibular falls are depicted schematically on the right in relation to the site of the lesion: ipsiversive falls with peripheral and pontomedullary lesions, contraversive falls with pontomesencephalic lesions. In vestibular thalamus and cortex lesions the tendency to fall may be contraversive or ipsiversive.*

backward (Fig. 9.8). This fore–aft postural instability can be interpreted as a direction-specific tone imbalance of the vestibular ocular reflex in pitch, due either to a lesion in the floor of the fourth ventricle or to bilateral dysfunction of the flocculus. It can be interpreted as a direction-specific vestibulocerebellar imbalance since it can be observed when the eyes are closed. We believe that the objective measurable backward tilt represents a vestibulospinal compensation in the direction opposite to the perceived lesional 'forward vertigo', which corresponds to the downbeat nystagmus.[69] With the eyes open, a measurable visual stabilization of body sway is preserved but does not sufficiently compensate for the visual ataxia. In the downbeat nystagmus syndrome the patient's pathological postural sway with the eyes open

is dependent on the direction of gaze; it increases with increasing nystagmus amplitude and pathophysiologically it is secondary to a combination both of a vestibulocerebellar ataxia and of reduced visual stabilization owing to the nystagmus.[70] Thus, downbeat nystagmus is not simply an ocular motor syndrome but a central vestibular syndrome comprising ocular motor, postural and perceptual effects.

In some patients with downbeat nystagmus syndrome as well as ataxia treatment with the γ-aminobutyric acid (GABA)-A agonist baclofen (3 × 10 mg p.o. daily) or gabapentin (3 × 400 mg p.o. daily) are helpful and reduce nystagmus amplitude. A beneficial effect was also seen using the GABA-A agonist clonazepam (3 × 0.5 mg p.o. daily).

Table 9.4 *Typical signs and symptoms suggesting vestibular unsteadiness or falls in disorders of the peripheral or central vestibular system*

Signs/symptoms	Lesion site/disorder
Peripheral vestibular system	
Unsteadiness of gait, particularly in the dark or on unlevel ground and oscillopsia associated with head movements or when walking	Both labyrinths or vestibular nerves (bilateral vestibular failure)
Ipsiversive falls with contraversive spontaneous nystagmus, rotational vertigo, and nausea	Acute unilateral peripheral vestibular loss (vestibular neuritis; MS-plaque or lacunar infarctions at root entry zone of eighth nerve)
Paroxysmal loss of postural tone with unexpected falls without impaired consciousness	Labyrinths (vestibular drop attacks and Ménière's disease)
Paroxysmal lateral and forward falls with rotational vertigo and nystagmus elicited by head extension or lateral head tilt	Posterior semicircular canal ipsilateral to the direction of fall (benign paroxysmal positional vertigo)
Episodic vertigo with postural imbalance, nystagmus, nausea, tinnitus, and fluctuating hearing loss	Labyrinth (Ménière's disease)
Frequent spells of postural instability, dizziness, tinnitus, and hearing loss elicited or modulated by changes in head position	Neuro-vascular cross-compression of the eighth nerve (vestibular paroxysmia; disabling positional vertigo)
Central vestibular system	
Paroxysmal vertigo and/or ataxia with ocular motor deficiencies (also in the attack-free interval) and associated headache	Brainstem, cerebellum, labyrinth? (basilar migraine)
Paroxysmal ataxia and dysarthria	Brainstem (paroxysmal attacks in MS)
Paroxysmal lateral or rotational falls with vertigo (nystagmus) and impaired consciousness	Parieto-insular vestibular cortex (vestibular epilepsy)
Episodic familial ataxia (with or without vertigo) with nystagmus or myokymia	Brainstem, cerebellum (familial episodic ataxias)
Fore–aft instability with vertical nystagmus	Ponto-medullary or ponto-mesencephalic-brainstem, or bilateral floccular lesions (downbeat/upbeat nystagmus)
Lateral instability or falls with tilts of perceived vertical and ocular skew deviation (without vertigo, paresis, or cerebellar ataxia)	Ponto-medullary or ponto-mesencephalic brainstem, mid-brain tegmentum, vestibular thalamus, vestibular cortex (lateropulsion in Wallenberg's syndrome, or in vestibular cortex lesions, thalamic astasia)

CONCLUSIONS

Vestibular dysfunction is a significant differential diagnosis in patients who have unexpected falls without loss of consciousness, paresis, sensory loss or cerebellar deficit (Table 9.4).

Peripheral or central vestibular disorders cause postural instability with preferred directions of falling (Tables 9.1 and 9.3), some of which can be attributed to either the particular plane of the affected semicircular canal or a central pathway mediating the three-dimensional VOR in yaw, pitch and roll. Ipsiversive falls occur in vestibular neuritis or in Wallenberg's syndrome, where they are known as lateropulsion. Contraversive falls are typical for the otolith Tullio phenomenon, vestibular epilepsy and thalamic astasia. Predominant fore–aft instability is observed in bilateral vestibulopathy, benign paroxysmal positioning vertigo as well as in downbeat or upbeat nystagmus syndrome. Falls can be diagonally forward (or backward) and toward or away from the side of the lesion depending on the site of the lesion (the ocular tilt reaction is ipsiversive in medullary lesions, but contraversive in mesencephalic lesions) and on whether vestibular structures are excited or inhibited. The observation that patients with acute vestibular disorders keep their intended path better when running than when walking slowly suggests that the automatic spinal locomotor program suppresses destabilizing vestibular input.

A preliminary classification of central vestibular disorders of the brainstem according to the yaw, pitch and roll planes predicts the dominant direction of instability. It is not sufficient to state that the VOR merely subserves stabilization of gaze. Its neuronal pathways also include ascending input to the thalamocortical projections of perception as well as descending input to the vestibulospinal projections for adjustment of head and body posture (Fig. 9.13). This means that both physiological stimulation and pathological dysfunction of the semicircular canal input and the otoliths not only provoke nystagmus but inevitably cause a direction-specific concurrent vertigo and postural imbalance (Table 9.2).

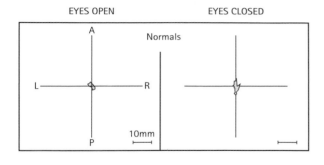

EYES OPEN   EYES CLOSED

Normals

10mm

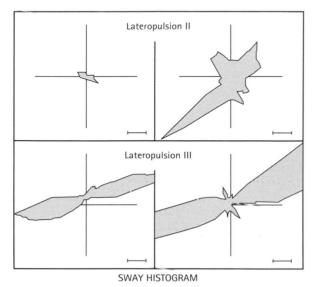

Lateropulsion II

Lateropulsion III

SWAY HISTOGRAM

Figure 9.14 *Typical body sway histograms in two patients with Wallenberg's syndrome during upright stance with the eyes open and closed. Grade II lateropulsion indicates considerable imbalance without falls; grade III lateropulsion represents falls with eyes closed. Body sway increases considerably in patients with Wallenberg's syndrome and the normal dominance of the anterior–posterior (fore–aft) sway component shifts to an abnormal dominance of the lateral sway component which is diagonal in grade II lateropulsion and becomes more lateral in grade III lateropulsion.*

ACKNOWLEDGEMENT

We thank Judy Benson for editing the manuscript.

REFERENCES

1. Brandt T. *Vertigo: its multisensory syndromes*, 2nd edn. London: Springer, 1999.
2. Brandt T, Dieterich M. Vestibular falls. *J Vestib Res* 1993;**3**:3–14.
3. Brandt Th, Daroff RB. The multisensory physiological and pathological vertigo syndromes. *Ann Neurol* 1980;**7**:195–203.
4. Büchele W, Brandt Th. Vestibular neuritis, a horizontal semicircular canal paresis? *Adv Oto-Rhino-Laryngol* 1988;**42**:157–61.
5. Fetter M, Dichgans J. Vestibular neuritis spares the inferior division of the vestibular nerve. *Brain* 1996;**119**:755–63.
6. Schuknecht HF, Kitamura H. Vestibular neuritis. *Ann Otol Rhinol Laryngol* 1980;**90**(Suppl 78):1–19.
7. Proctor L, Perlman H, Lindsay J, Matz G. Acute vestibular paralysis in herpes zoster oticus. *Ann Otol Rhinol Laryngol* 1979;**88**:303–10.
8. Adour KK, Ruboyianes JM, von Doersten PG, et al. Bell's palsy treatment with acyclovir and prednisone compared with prednisone alone: a double-blind randomized, controlled trial. *Ann Otol Rhinol Laryngol* 1996;**105**:371–8.
9. Schuknecht HF. Cupulolithiasis. *Arch Otolaryngol* 1969;**80**:765–87.
10. Parnes LS, McClure JA. Posterior semicircular canal occlusion in the normal ear. *Otolaryngol Head Neck Surg* 1991;**104**:52–7.
11. Epley JM. The canalith repositioning procedure: for treatment of benign paroxysmal positioning vertigo. *Otolaryngol Head Neck Surg* 1992;**107**:399–404.
12. Brandt Th, Steddin S. Current view of the mechanism of benign paroxysmal positioning vertigo: cupulolithiasis or canalolithiasis? *J Vestib Res* 1993;**3**:373–82.
13. Brandt Th, Steddin S, Daroff RB. Therapy for benign paroxysmal positioning vertigo, revisited. *Neurology* 1994;**44**:796–800.
14. Semont A, Freyss G, Vitte E. Curing the BPPV with a liberatory manoeuvre. *Adv Otorhinolaryngol* 1988;**42**:290–3.
15. Tumarkin A. The otolithic catastrophe: a new syndrome. *BMJ* 1936;**I**:175–7.
16. Baloh RW, Jacobson K, Winder T. Drop attacks with Ménière's syndrome. *Ann Neurol* 1990;**28**:384–7.
17. Ödkvist LM, Bergenius O. Drop attacks in Ménière's disease. *Acta Otolaryngol (Stockh)* 1988;**455**(Suppl):82–5.
18. Black FO, Efron MZ, Burns DS. Diagnosis and management of drop attacks of vestibular origin: Tumarkin's otolithic crisis. *Otolaryngol Head Neck Surg* 1982;**90**:256–62.
19. Minor LB, Solomon D, Zinreich JS, Zee DS. Sound and/or pressure-induced vertigo due to bone dehiscence of the superior semicircular canal. *Arch Otolaryngol Head Neck Surg* 1998;**124**:249–58.
20. Minor LB. Superior canal dehiscence syndrome. *Am J Otol* 2000;**21**:9–19.
21. Tullio P. *Das Ohr und die Entstehung der Sprache und Schrift.* Munich: Urban & Schwarzenberg, 1929.
22. Dieterich M, Brandt Th, Fries W. Otolith function in man: results from a case of otolith Tullio phenomenon. *Brain* 1989;**112**:1377–92.
23. Fries W, Dieterich M, Brandt Th. Otolith contributions to postural control in man: short latency motor responses following sound stimulation in a case of otolithic Tullio phenomenon. *Gait Posture* 1993;**1**:145–53.
24. Baloh RW, Jacobson K, Honrubia V. Idiopathic bilateral vestibulopathy. *Neurology* 1989;**39**:272–5.
25. Moller AR. The cranial nerve vascular compression syndrome: I. A review of treatment *Acta Neurochir (Wien)* 1991;**113**:18–23.
26. Jannetta PJ, Moller AR, Janetta PJ, et al. Diagnosis and surgical treatment of disabling positional vertigo. *J Neurosurg* 1986;**64**:21–8.
27. Brandt Th, Dieterich M., Vascular compression of the eighth nerve. Vestibular paroxysmia. *Lancet* 1994;**343**:798–9.
28. Strupp M, Planck JH, Arbusow V, et al. Rotational vertebral artery occlusion syndrome with vertigo due to 'labyrinthine excitation'. *Neurology* 2000;**54**:1376–9.

29. Brandt T, Strupp M, Benson J. You are better off running than walking with acute vestibulopathy. *Lancet* 1999;354:746.

30. Westheimer G, Blair SM. The ocular tilt reaction: a brainstem oculomotor routine. *Invest Ophthalmol* 1975;14:833-9.

31. Halmagyi GM, Curthoys IS. A clinical sign of canal paresis. *Arch Neurol* 1988;45:737-9.

32. Jahn K, Strupp M, Schneider E, et al. Differential effects of vestibular stimulation on walking and running. *NeuroReport* 2000;II:1745-8.

33. Glasauer S, Amorim M-A, Vitte E, Berthoz A. Goal-directed linear locomotion in normal and labyrinthine-defective subjects. *Exp Brain Res* 1994;8:323-35.

34. Grillner S. Control of locomotion in bipeds, tetrapeds, and fish. In: Brookhart M, Mountcastle M, eds. *Handbook of physiology. The nervous system* II. Washington, DC: American Physiology Society, 1981;1179-235.

35. Dietz V, Colombo G, Jensen L. Locomotor activity in spinal man. *Lancet* 1994;344:1260-3.

36. Dietz V, Wirz M, Curt A, Colombo G. Locomotor pattern in paraplegic patients: training effects and recovery of spinal cord function. *Spinal Cord* 1998;36:380-90.

37. Mergner T, Rosemeier T. Interaction of vestibular, somatosensory and visual signals for postural control and motion perception under terrestrial and microgravity conditions – a conceptual model. *Brain Res Rev* 1998;28:118-35.

38. Dietz V. Afferent and efferent control of posture and gait. In: Bles W, Brandt Th, eds. *Disorders of posture and gait*. Amsterdam: Elsevier, 1986;69-81.

39. Collins DF, Cameron T, Gillard DM, Prochazka A. Muscular sense is attenuated when humans move. *J Physiol (Lond)* 1998;508:635-43.

40. Leigh RJ, Brandt Th. A re-evaluation of the vestibulo-ocular reflex: new ideas of its purpose, properties, neural substrate, and disorders. *Neurology* 1993;43:1288-95.

41. Foerster O. Sensible corticale Felder. In: Bumke O, Foerster O, eds. *Handbuch der Neurologie*, Vol VI. Berlin: Springer, 1936:358-448.

42. Fredrickson Z, Figge U, Scheid P, Kornhuber HH. Vestibular nerve projection to the cerebral cortex of the rhesus monkey. *Exp Brain Res* 1966;2:318-27.

43. Grüsser O-J, Pause M, Schreiter U. Localisation and responses of neurones in the parieto-insular vestibular cortex of awake monkeys. *J Physiol* 1990;430:537-57.

44. Grüsser O-J, Pause M, Schreiter U. Vestibular neurones in the parieto-insular cortex of monkeys (*Macaca fascicularis*): visual and neck receptor responses. *J Physiol* 1990;430:559-83.

45. Schwarz DWF, Fredrickson JM. Rhesus monkey vestibular cortex: a bimodal primary projection field. *Science* 1971;172:280-1.

46. Büttner U, Büttner UW. Parietal cortex area 2 V neuronal activity in the alert monkey during natural vestibular and optokinetic stimulation. *Brain Res* 1978;153:392-7.

47. Ödkvist LM, Schwarz DWF, Fredrickson JM, Hassler R. Projection of the vestibular nerve to the area 3a arm field in the squirrel monkey (*Saimiri sciureus*). *Exp Brain Res* 1974;21:97-105.

48. Faugier-Grimand S, Ventre J. Anatomic connections of inferior parietal cortex (Area 7) with subcortical structures related to vestibulo-ocular function in monkey (*Macaca fascicularis*). *J Comp Neurol* 1989;280:12-14.

49. Anderson RA, Gnadt JW. Posterior parietal cortex. In: Wurtz RH, Goldberg ME, eds. *Reviews in oculomotor research. Vol 3, the neurobiology of saccadic eye movements*. Amsterdam: Elsevier, 1989;315-35.

50. Penfield W, Jasper H. *Epilepsy and the functional anatomy of the human brain*. Boston: Little Brown, 1954.

51. Friberg L, Olsen TS, Roland PE, et al. Focal increase of blood flow in the cerebral cortex of men during vestibular stimulation, *Brain* 1985;108:609-23.

52. Bottini G, Sterzi R, Panlesu E, et al. Identification of the central vestibular projections in man: a positron emission tomography activation study. *Exp Brain Res* 1994;99:164-9.

53. Bense S, Stefan T, Yousry T, Brandt T, Dieterich M. Multisensory cortical signal increases and decreases during vestibular galvanic stimulation (fMRI). *J Neurophysiol* 2001;85:886-99.

54. Brandt Th, Dieterich M, Danek A. Vestibular cortex lesions affect the perception of verticality. *Ann Neurol* 1994;35:403-12.

55. Masdeu JC, Gorelick PB. Thalamic astasia: inability to stand after unilateral thalamic lesions. *Ann Neurol* 1988;23:586-603.

56. Bjerver K, Silfverskiöld BP. Lateropulsion and imbalance in Wallenberg's syndrome. *Acta Neurol Scand* 1968;44:91-100.

57. Dieterich M, Brandt Th. Wallenberg's Syndrome: lateropulsion, cyclorotation and subjective visual vertical in thirty-six patients. *Ann Neurol* 1992;31:399-408.

58. Brandt Th, Dieterich M. Pathological eye-head coordination in roll: tonic ocular tilt reaction in mesencephalic and medullary lesions. *Brain* 1987;110:649-66.

59. Verma AK, Maheshwari MC. Hyperesthetic-ataxic hemiparesis in thalamic haemorrhage. *Stroke* 1986;17:49-51.

60. Halmagyi GM, Brandt Th, Dieterich M, et al. Tonic contraversive ocular tilt reaction due to unilateral mesodiencephalic lesion. *Neurology* 1990;40:1503-9.

61. Dieterich M, Brandt Th. Thalamic infarctions: differential effects on vestibular function in the roll plane (35 patients). *Neurology* 1993;43:1732-40.

62. Dieterich M, Brandt Th. Ocular torsion and tilt of subjective visual vertical are sensitive brainstem signs. *Ann Neurol* 1993;33:292-9.

63. Brandt Th, Dieterich M. Vestibular syndromes in the roll plane: topographic diagnosis from brainstem to cortex. *Ann Neurol* 1994;36:337-47.

64. Brandt Th, Dieterich M. Skew deviation with ocular torsion: a vestibular sign of topographic diagnostic value. *Ann Neurol* 1993;33:528-34.

65. Lueck CJ, Halmagyi P, Crawford TJ, et al. A case of ocular tilt reaction and torsional nystagmus due to direct stimulation of the midbrain in man. *Brain* 1991;114:2069-79.

66. Karnath H-O, Ferber S, Dichgans J. The origin of contraversive pushing. Evidence for a second graviceptive system in humans. *Neurology* 2000;55:1298-304.

67. Mittelstaedt H. Origin and processing of postural information. *Neurosci Behav Rev* 1998;22:473-8.

68. Cogan DG. Downbeat nystagmus. *Arch Ophthalmol* 1968;80:757-68.

69. Büchele W, Brandt Th. Vestibulo-spinal ataxia in benign paroxysmal positional vertigo. *Aggressologie* 1979;20:221-2.

70. Büchele W, Brandt Th, Degner D. Ataxia and oscillopsia in downbeat nystagmus/vertigo syndrome. *Adv Oto-Rhino-Laryngol* 1983;30:291-7

10

Cerebellar gait and sensory ataxia

LEWIS SUDARSKY

INTRODUCTION AND HISTORICAL COMMENT

Ataxia means irregularity, disorderliness or incoordination. The term is from the ancient Greek, and can be found in the writings of Hippocrates. Since the late nineteenth century, ataxia has been used more narrowly to describe an incoordination of movement of cerebellar or proprioceptive origin. An important problem of that era was to distinguish the locomotor ataxia of tabes dorsalis (neurosyphilis) from the various forms of hereditary ataxia and spinocerebellar degeneration described by Friedreich[1] and Marie.[2] The classic descriptions of cerebellar ataxia come from studies done by Holmes[3] at the beginning of the twentieth century on patients with gunshot injuries to the posterior fossa. He described the gait in these patients as irregular, slow and halting. There is a wide base of support and a tendency to stumble off to the affected side. Patients are unable to balance when attempting to walk tandem, heel to toe.[3]

We now recognize ataxia as one of the most common and distinctive locomotor disorders. Every good stage actor can mimic the speech and gait of acute intoxication (in many cases, informed by personal experience). A variety of chronic neurological diseases produce cerebellar ataxic gait. While tabetic neurosyphilis is infrequent in contemporary practice, a number of peripheral and spinal disorders produce injury to cerebellar and proprioceptive afferents sufficient to compromise walking. In our studies of elderly outpatients, sensory deficits (18.3 per cent) and cerebellar degeneration (6.7 per cent) are common causes of gait disturbance.[4,5] Sensory deficits in older people most typically produce a cautious gait or a form of sensory ataxia. This chapter considers the physiology and clinical details of cerebellar gait and sensory ataxia.

FUNCTIONAL ANATOMY OF THE CEREBELLUM

The cerebellum is divided into two paired cerebellar hemispheres and a narrow midline portion, the vermis. A detailed review of the anatomy is outside the scope of this chapter, but, briefly, the cerebellum can be divided into functional zones based on its input and output connections (Fig. 10.1). The vestibulocerebellum (the flocculus, nodulus, uvula and midline vermis) projects to the brainstem via the fastigial nucleus. There are also direct projections to the vestibular nucleus in the medulla. The intermediate zone (spinocerebellum) receives afferent projections from the spinocerebellar tracts and projects to the red nucleus in the midbrain via the interposed nuclei. The red nucleus in turn projects back to the spinal cord through the rubrospinal tract. The lateral zone (neocerebellum) receives the bulk of afferent projections from the pontine gray and inferior olive. The cerebellar hemispheres process this information, which is sent to the motor system in the forebrain through the dentate nuclei and superior cerebellar peduncle.

Pathology restricted to the flocculonodular lobe is unusual, but the effects on truncal control may be profound. Lesions of the paravermal zone in the anterior lobe and spinocerebellum produce principally a disorder of postural control and cerebellar gait. Lesions restricted to one cerebellar hemisphere primarily affect motor control of the ipsilateral limbs. There may be a tendency to fall toward the side of the lesion. Clinical correlation with neuropathology and imaging is imperfect, particularly in patients with longstanding or developmental disorders. Patients with near-total aplasia of the cerebellum, for example, may be capable of good standing balance and stable locomotion.

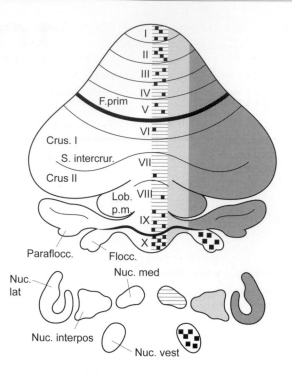

Figure 10.1 *Zonal organization of the cerebellum, based on the pattern of corticonuclear projections. The midline zone (vestibulocerebellum) projects to the brainstem via the fastigial nuclei. There are also direct projections to the vestibular nucleus in the medulla. The intermediate zone (spinocerebellum) projects via the interposed nuclei. The lateral zone (neocerebellum) projects to the forebrain through the dentate nuclei. (Reproduced from Brodal A, Neurological Anatomy 3rd edn, Oxford University Press 1981, p. 299, copyright Springer-Verlag, with permission.)*

MODELING GAIT ATAXIA IN ANIMALS

Human bipedal gait presents a unique challenge integrating locomotion with postural control, but some insights can be derived from animal studies. Well characterized mutations affect the developmental anatomy of the cerebellum in mice and in dogs.[6–8] These animals display many of the qualities of cerebellar gait in humans: irregular step generation, reduced truncal stability, difficulty turning and changing direction (Fig. 10.2). Physiology studies of cats after removal of the cerebellum reveal loss of interlimb (and intralimb) synergy, unevenness of stride and occasional loss of equilibrium.[9] Recordings from awake, behaving cats suggest that the fastigial nucleus may be of particular importance in controlling reticulospinal and vestibulospinal pathways important for locomotion.[10]

The neurodegenerative ataxias differ in the degree to which cerebellar cortical neurons, afferent and efferent connections are lost. Purkinje cell and granule cell loss are a major feature of the SCA-2 mutation. In contrast, patients with Machado-Joseph disease/SCA-3 suffer loss of spinocerebellar and vestibulocerebellar connections, and are particularly prone to stumbling and tripping falls. Single gene mutations responsible for the SCA-1, SCA-2 and SCA-3 mutations have been expressed in animals.[11–13] Studies reveal differences among these diseases in pathological anatomy and cellular mechanism. Such studies allow both a dissection of molecular mechanism and a pathophysiological deconstruction of the hereditary ataxias.

CEREBELLAR ATAXIA IN HUMANS: PHYSIOLOGICAL STUDIES

Holmes[3] described changes in gait and balance stability in patients with traumatic injury to the cerebellum.

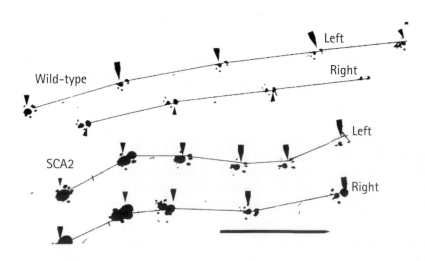

Figure 10.2 *Paw prints indicate the presence of gait ataxia in a transgenic mouse expressing the SCA-2 mutation (bottom track). Note irregular stride and deviation from a straight path, features also observed in bipedal gait of ataxic humans. (Reproduced with permission from Stefan Pulst, MD, Department of Neurology, Cedars Sinai Medical Center, Los Angeles, CA, USA.)*

Lesions of the anterior lobe produce truncal ataxia that is exaggerated when the base of stance is narrowed. Lesions of the lateral parts of the cerebellum produce a deficit in standing balance, with a tendency to fall towards the affected side.[3] Most contemporary physiological studies involve heterogeneous patient groups, subjects with alcoholic cerebellar degeneration and mixed neurodegenerative ataxias. As noted above, these diseases differ in their pathological anatomy and in how the diseases prune the cerebellar circuit. It would be instructive to see focused physiological investigation on genetically defined subgroups drawn from the hereditary ataxias.

Physiology of postural control

The cerebellum is involved in the maintenance of postural control in quiet stance. Positron-emission tomography (PET) studies of healthy normal subjects demonstrate activation of the anterior lobe of the cerebellum when standing with the feet together.[14] Chronic alcoholics with atrophy of the anterior vermis display a 3 Hz sway in the anterior–posterior plane, which can be observed at the bedside.[15] This tremor can be recorded in studies using platform posturography. Truncal tremor is aggravated by eye closure. Gatev et al.[16] studied postural control in 25 patients with cerebellar cortical atrophy and nine with olivopontocerebellar atrophy. Increased sway during quiet stance was correlated with gait and balance impairment on a clinical ataxia rating scale. Patients with structural pathology of the flocculonodular lobe experience an omnidirectional sway with frequency at or below 1 Hz.[17]

Measures of dynamic equilibrium may be more sensitive than studies of static balance in discriminating cerebellar deficits. Cueman-Hudson and Krebs[18] measured lateral excursions of the center of gravity during a repetitive stepping task and found that the cerebellar patients exhibited instability particularly in the lateral (roll) plane. A classic paradigm for investigation of postural control responses places the subject on a platform which has a sudden movement. The electromyograph (EMG) response in the leg muscles to a 4° toe-up perturbation has been studied in cerebellar patients by Diener and others.[19,20] The latency of the immediate and late responses in the leg muscles was normal in cerebellar patients, but the long latency response (beginning around 110 ms) was prolonged and inappropriately scaled, producing an exaggerated force. Studies involving translational movements of the support surface also evoke inappropriately scaled responses in postural muscles.[21] This increased gain in postural responses may be the basis of some of the dysmetria in postural reaction to platform perturbation, and may be a factor in truncal sway or titubation.

Interesting studies have been done to assess the abil-ity of ataxic patients to deal with conflicting and/or inappropriate sensory information. In studies involving a platform sway referenced to neutralize proprioceptive feedback, cerebellar patients did much worse than controls in maintaining their balance when visual information was also absent or distorted.[21] Patients with cerebellar disease are able to respond appropriately to the motion of a visual surround that creates a false illusion of movement.[22] These experiments indicate that cerebellar patients are able to shift from visual to proprioceptive control of postural sway, but have difficulty when the information from more than one modality is compromised.

Physiology of cerebellar gait

Laboratory gait analysis in cerebellar patients tends to confirm features described by observation. Palliyath et al.[23] noted a reduced velocity and stride length in 10 patients with cerebellar degeneration. All components of the gait cycle showed increased variability, and stepping was irregular in direction and distance. Irregularity of step generation can be considered one of the defining features of cerebellar gait. Interestingly, the gait was not wide-based in these patients, although other laboratories have confirmed a wide base of support.[18] There was reduced dorsiflexion of the ankle at the onset of the swing phase, which might predispose to tripping. Analysis of moments about the knee and ankle joints revealed poor intralimb coordination. Kinetic studies of ground reaction forces demonstrated a reduced peak at weight acceptance, reflecting a difficulty planting the foot soundly.

CEREBELLAR GAIT ATAXIA: CLINICAL FEATURES

Cerebellar gait ataxia is distinctive and recognizable. The patient with ataxia walks as if drunk. The gait is typically slow and halting, with a widened base of support. Stepping is irregular in timing and foot placement, as noted above. Progression deviates from a straight path. Erratic stride results in a lurching quality as the upper body segments struggle to maintain alignment. Patients may stumble or veer off to the more severely affected side. Many cerebellar gaits are wide-based, which may in part be a biomechanical adaptation to improve stability; instability is more evident in narrow-based stance. Most patients are unable to walk tandem, heel to toe, and have difficulty maintaining balance when they turn rapidly or change direction. Truncal tremor or titubation are observed in more severely affected patients. Usually, there are additional features to point to a problem of cerebellar origin, such as dysarthria and oculomotor disorder, or dysmetria in the limbs. Occasional patients with cerebellar degeneration (particularly alcoholics with anterior vermis atrophy) may have truncal imbalance and gait ataxia as the principal manifestation of their illness.

Early features of cerebellar gait disorder include a tentative stride and a degree of imbalance in turns. Irregular foot placement can be observed when walking a straight path and imbalance can be brought out by tandem gait. These deficits are often masked if the patient walks briskly and may be more evident walking at a slower pace. Other gaits are affected in addition to walking, and ataxia patients may complain of difficulty jogging (slow running) or cycling.

Differential diagnosis

Many diseases of the nervous system affect the cerebellum, but a full review is outside the scope of this chapter. The intent is to outline an approach. A starting point is the distinction of cases with static injury to the cerebellum from those that reflect an intrinsically progressive disorder. This distinction is not always easy, as many patients with a fixed injury to the cerebellum report a gradual decline in gait as they get older. Serial observations are sometimes needed to establish whether the ataxia is progressive. In addition to trauma and vascular disease, hyperthermia can produce persistent ataxia, as cerebellar Purkinje cells are vulnerable to heat injury.

Table 10.1 summarizes the various causes of progressive ataxia. In some cases there is an exogenous toxin or metabolic disorder which causes pathology in the cerebellum. Patients with multiple sclerosis and other immune-mediated diseases can have ataxia as the principal manifestation. In most of cases of progressive ataxia there is neurodegeneration within the cerebellum and its connections. This point is underscored by a recent report of neuropathology on the playwright Eugene O'Neill, who suffered from a form of cerebellar degeneration.[24] He had a severe tremor and gait disturbance, and ataxia compromised his ability to write in his later years. His

Table 10.1 *Progressive ataxia*

Structural causes	Chiari malformation
	Dandy Walker cyst
	Posterior fossa tumor with or without hydrocephalus
Toxic	Alcohol
	Phenytoin
	Cytosine arabinoside (ara-C)
	Amiodarone
	Lithium
	Metals (methylmercury, lead, thallium, bismuth, manganese)
	Toluene
Common and rare metabolic disorders	Hypothyroidism
	Ataxia with vitamin E deficiency
	Abetalipoproteinemia
	Refsum's disease
	Organic acidurias
	Urea cycle disorders
	Cerebrotendinous xanthomatosis
	Storage disease (late-onset GM2 gangliosidosis, Niemann-Pick C)
Inflammatory and immune mediated	Multiple sclerosis
	Post infectious ataxia of childhood
	Miller–Fisher syndrome
	Gluten ataxia
	Paraneoplastic cerebellar degeneration
	Ataxia with anti-GAD antibodies
Autosomal dominant hereditary ataxia	SCA-1, SCA-2, SCA-3 (Machado–Joseph disease), SCA-4, SCA-5, SCA-6, SCA-8, SCA-10
	Autosomal dominant ataxia with retinal degeneration (SCA-7)
	Dentatorubropallidoluysian atrophy (DRPLA)
	Episodic ataxia, types 1 and 2
Autosomal recessive	Friedreich's ataxia
	Ataxia telangectasia
	Autosomal recessive Friedreich like ataxias (ARSACS)
Mitochondrial disorders	
Sporadic neurodegenerative ataxia	Multiple system atrophy
	Pure cerebellar cortical degeneration

problem was attributed to alcohol abuse by his doctors, although it progressed for years after he had stopped drinking. Post mortem examination identified a form of neurodegenerative ataxia.[24]

The next step in the evaluation of the patient with progressive ataxia is to establish whether there is a family history. Cerebellar degenerations are classified into two major groups: hereditary or sporadic. Estimates suggest that hereditary ataxia has a prevalence of five per 100 000 population, roughly comparable to that of Huntington's disease.[25] More often, ataxia occurs without a family history and appears to be sporadic. Even in the absence of a family history, a panel of DNA diagnostic tests is sometimes obtained to search for one of the known ataxia gene mutations; the cost of this testing is generally less than that of two or three magnetic resonance imaging (MRI) scans. Friedreich's ataxia and SCA-6 in particular can occur in the absence of an affected family member.[26] Some families lose track of chronically ill relatives, and sometimes paternity is uncertain. Hereditary ataxias can be considered in three groups, autosomal dominant, autosomal recessive and those with another genetic mechanism (including X-linked and mitochondrial).

Autosomal dominant cerebellar ataxia

The dominantly inherited ataxias have provoked a great deal of controversy regarding their classification. A form of hereditary ataxia distinct from Friedreich's was recognized by Marie in the nineteenth century.[2] Most of these disorders were classified as familial forms of olivopontocerebellar atrophy by Konigsmark and Weiner as recently as 1970.[27] In the late 1980s, Anita Harding recognized the fundamental similarities and overlapping manifestation of this group of disorders.[28] She pointed out that these diseases are often indistinguishable based on symptoms and physical examination alone.[28] Over the last decade, genetic markers have been identified to account for more than half of the families with adult onset ataxia and a dominant pattern of inheritance.[29] These mutations are designated SCA-1, SCA-2, etc. (SCA for spinoccrebellar ataxia). Classification of these diseases based on their genetic markers has been more successful than older classifications based on clinical expression and neuropathology. Affected family members that share a gene mutation can truly be said to have the same disease, even if the symptoms are different.

In addition to progressive ataxia, these diseases typically produce dysarthria, ocular motility disorders and sometimes upper motor neuron signs or extrapyramidal features. Cognitive impairment is described with some of the SCAs. The typical age of onset for the CAG trinucleotide repeat mutations is in the mid-thirties. There is a great deal of overlap in these disorders and they cannot reliably be distinguished based on clinical features in a single affected individual. Some differences emerge when groups of patients are compared. Patients with SCA-2 often have a degree of postural tremor and a prominent oculomotor abnormality. Progression to a wheelchair often occurs over a decade.[30] SCA-3 patients have several distinct phenotypes. They often present with stumbling, gait imbalance and falls. Young onset patients are described with a larger number of CAG repeats, prominent dystonia and extrapyramidal signs, and an aggressive natural history.[31] Later onset patients (type III) have ataxia with distal atrophy and sensory loss, and a slow progression. SCA-6 also appears to be a more benign disorder, with progression over 20–30 years.[32] Some patients have onset in their fifties and a relatively pure dysarthria and ataxia. A few patients have discrete episodes of vertigo, ataxia or nausea, which is interesting as the mutation affects the CACNA1A calcium channel. (Episodic ataxia type 2 and familial hemiplegic migraine are also caused by mutations in the same calcium channel.) SCA-3 appears to be the commonest of these mutations worldwide, followed by SCA-2, SCA-6 and SCA-1.[25]

Friedreich's ataxia and related disorders

In 1861, Friedreich described a form of locomotor ataxia distinct from tabes dorsalis.[1] Friedreich's ataxia is the most common form of hereditary ataxia, affecting two individuals per 100 000. The disorder is autosomal recessive, the product of an expanded GAA trinucleotide repeat on chromosome 9. The carrier frequency is estimated to be as high as 1:120 and spontaneous expansions may arise from long, normal alleles.

The typical form of Friedreich's ataxia begins between age 8 years and 15 years, although onset up to age 25 years is accepted in diagnostic guidelines.[33] In addition to progressive ataxia, patients develop absent reflexes in the legs and an extensor plantar response. There is loss of joint position and vibration sense in the legs. Dysarthria may not be evident at time of diagnosis, but is usually present within 5 years. Other features outwith the nervous system help identify typical or classic Friedreich's ataxia: high arched feet (pes cavus deformity), scoliosis and hypertrophic cardiomyopathy. Mild diabetes is identified in 20 per cent of cases. Imaging of the nervous system and neuropathological examination reveal Friedreich's to be primarily a spinal ataxia, with modest changes in the cerebellar output nuclei.

The Friedreich's ataxia mutation on chromosome 9 was identified by Pandolfo and colleagues in 1996.[34] The normal frataxin protein is involved with mitochondrial metabolism. Yeast with frataxin mutations have deficiencies of complex I, II, III and aconitase activity, and are vulnerable to oxidant stress. Iron accumulates in the mitochondria of heart cells in patients with Friedreich's ataxia. Understanding the pathway from gene mutation to cell injury in Friedreich's ataxia brings the promise of therapeutic intervention to retard disease progression. Clinical trials are now being organized, based on the principal of oxidative stress reduction.

Knowledge of the genetic mutation for Friedreich's ataxia has also changed our defining concept of the disorder. Patients with genetically confirmed Friedreich's can present after age 25 years, in some instances, up to age 60 years. These patients with late onset Friedreich's typically have a small GAA repeat and may remain ambulatory 50 years after onset of their symptoms. Many of these patients lack orthopedic features such as scoliosis and pes cavus, most have a normal electrocardiogram, and many have retained spinal reflexes.[35]

Ataxia with vitamin E deficiency is similar to Friedreich's ataxia in its clinical manifestations. The gene abnormality affects the α-tocopherol transfer protein and interferes with the incorporation of vitamin E into lipoprotein packets. Patients have vitamin E deficiency despite a normal diet. Daily oral replacement of vitamin E arrests the progression of the neurological signs.

Sporadic ataxias

A truncal ataxia with cerebellar gait was described in chronic alcoholics by Victor et al.[36] Neuropathological examination in alcoholic cerebellar degeneration reveals a restricted form of cerebellar atrophy with cell loss in the anterior vermis, generally sparing the cerebellar hemispheres. This atrophy can also be appreciated on mid-sagittal MRI. It is not clear whether this is fundamentally a nutritional disorder, as opposed to a direct toxic effect of alcohol on the cerebellum. No clear dose–response relationship has been established.

Olivopontocerebellar atrophy, described in 1900 by Dejerine and Thomas is characterized pathologically by cell loss in the cerebellum and brainstem, including the substantia nigra, inferior olive and pontine base.[37] There is commonly a degree of associated parkinsonism. Both patients described by Dejerine and Thomas developed urinary incontinence. Other symptoms of autonomic failure may appear with progression of the disease. Average survival is 5–7 years from the time of diagnosis. Graham and Oppenheimer[38] have called attention to the overlap with striatonigral degeneration and Shy–Drager syndrome, and these diseases are now considered as part of a broader neurodegenerative disorder, multiple system atrophy. A substantial number of patients with sporadic neurodegenerative ataxia will evolve features of multiple system atrophy over time. In other patients, neurodegeneration remains restricted to the cerebellum and progression is slow over decades. There is no definitive test to identify multiple system atrophy at an early stage, although SPECT imaging with dopamine transporter ligands and sphincter EMG have been used for this purpose.[39]

Measurement of ataxia

A reliable semiquantitative measure of ataxia is needed to follow patients over time and to support clinical trials and intervention studies. Because the fundamental property of ataxia is its irregularity, and because the diseases are so heterogeneous, the production of an ataxia rating scale has been a challenge. Several clinical trials have used some form of ataxia rating.[40,41] The Cooperative Ataxia Group in North America has been working on a rating scale under the sponsorship of the National Ataxia Foundation, but a finalized, validated version is not yet available.

Observational gait analysis provides a useful functional assessment, though it is difficult to standardize. Some ataxia patients adopt a slow, cautious gait, while others career about. In the National Institutes of Health (NIH) ataxia rating scale,[41] gait ataxia was rated mild (1+) if the patient did not use or require a cane, moderate (2+) if the patient used or should use a cane, severe (3+) if the patient used or should use a walker and disabling (4+) if the patient was wheelchair bound. Workers at the NIH have also experimented with a 'gait gauntlet', in which the patient is required to progressively narrow their gait without stepping out of boundaries provided by convergent lines. The course is standardized and the distance successfully navigated is recorded over a series of trials.

Pharmacotherapy of ataxia

Clinical trials using physostigmine, γ-aminobutyric acid (GABA) agonists and thyrotropin-releasing hormone (TRH) for symptomatic treatment of ataxia patients have been inconsistent or disappointing.[40,42,43] Recently, the serotonergic nerve terminal networks in the cerebellar cortex have attracted interest as a point of therapeutic leverage.[44] Trimethoprim and tetrahydrobiopterin have been explored in placebo controlled trials for patients with Machado-Joseph disease.[45,46] While some patients report subjective improvements, it has been difficult to demonstrate benefit. Results have been similar in trials with buspirone, a 5-hydroxytryptamine receptor agonist ($5HT_{1a}$), for Friedreich's ataxia (J.-S. Lou, unpublished data). Anecdotal improvements have been reported with buspirone in some patients with Machado-Joseph disease, provided gait ataxia is mild to begin with.[47] Part of the problem is that the neurodegenerative ataxias differ in how they prune the cerebellar circuit anatomy.

Another approach to the problem is to identify and test a neuroprotective agent, a drug which will retard disease progression. Therapeutic trials are underway, involving an antioxidant for Friedreich's ataxia.

Rehabilitation strategies

Can the disturbances in gait and balance described above be improved with physical training? This is an interesting question, as the cerebellum is known to be involved in motor learning.[48] The cerebellum compares sensory information from muscle spindles and mechanoreceptors to motor output during movement, and is considered important in refining motor performance.[49] It stands to reason that patients might have difficulty relearning postural control when these circuits are damaged.

Programs have been described for rehabilitation of balance and gait in ataxia patients.[50,51] A contemporary approach provides incremental challenge in a structured way, while complexities of postural control are mastered. Case reports suggest that some ataxic patients benefit from this form of gait training.[52] Gill-Body et al.[53] used kinematic studies before and after treatment to document improvements in two patients: one with cerebrotendinous xanthomatosis and one with a cerebellar astrocytoma. A prospective, randomized clinical trial of an ataxia gait and balance training program modeled on vestibular rehabilitation is in progress at Massachusetts General Hospital in Boston, MA, USA.

SENSORY ATAXIA

Physiology

Walking on a flat surface in a well-illuminated room does not require much sensory feedback from the lower limbs. However, sensory information is critical for walking on irregular ground across a poorly lit area. Under these circumstances, control of posture during locomotion depends on high-quality afferent information from the vestibular system, vision, plantar touch and musculo-articular proprioception. There is evidence that cervical mechanoreceptors may also contribute to postural control. Proprioceptive information from joint capsules, tendons and plantar touch travels the dorsal column pathway. Muscle spindle afferents may also play a role in the regulation of dynamic balance; this information is carried in the spinocerebellar pathways.[54] There is usually a healthy redundancy of sensory information about posture. In younger patients, proprioceptive loss must be severe to affect motor performance. In the elderly, the threshold is reduced for imbalance in the face of somatosensory deficits. It is not clear whether this phenomenon is related to normal aging, or the presence of subclinical changes in other sensory systems.

Elegant physiology studies document problems in coordination of interjoint movement in the absence of proprioception. Marsden et al.[55] studied a young man with subacute sensory neuropathy and virtually absent proprioceptive feedback from the limbs. His motor performance demonstrated a reasonable degree of dexterity, but was dependent on visual guidance; he had difficulty with new motor learning. He purchased a new car, but was unable to master the gearshift. Sainburg et al.[56] studied gestural movements of the upper limbs in two patients with large fiber neuropathy and documented a lack of synchrony and finesse related to poor coordination of interactional forces generated during complex multijoint movements.

Lajoie et al.[57] studied the kinematics of walking in a patient with advanced sensory neuropathy who had absent proprioception below the neck. The patient walked with a widened base of support, reduced stride and increased cycle time. A forward tilt of the head was observed, to allow visual monitoring of the performance. Surface EMG demonstrated increased activation of the vastus lateralis, producing knee extension at the point of heel contact. Co-contraction with the medial hamstring was evident, effectively bracing the leg during stance. Consequently the gait appeared more mechanical and less fluid. For this patient, the strategy for walking in the absence of proprioception used three elements: (1) a widened base of support and reduced stride (an adaptation to compensate for perceived imbalance); (2) direct visual monitoring of stepping; and (3) stiffening of the trunk and knee joint during movement (particularly during the stance phase), which reduces the number of degrees of freedom and simplifies the task.

Clinical features

Sensory ataxia is one of the commonest gait and balance disorders in clinical practice. It is not clear how much

Table 10.2 *Discriminating sensory ataxia from cerebellar*

	Cerebellar ataxia	Sensory ataxia
Stance	Wide-based	Narrow
Velocity	Slow	± Slow
Stride	Irregular, lurching	High stepping, regular, visually dependent, may be timid or cautious
Romberg	±	Unsteady
Heel to shin	Abnormal	Normal
Turns	Veers away	Minimally unsteady
Postural instability	Mild	Variable, may be severe
Falls	Uncommon early	Frequent

proprioceptive loss is necessary to cause gait difficulty; older patients tolerate these deficits less well. Patients are typically insecure in their balance and walk with an abbreviated stride. While cadence may be regular, progression deviates from a linear path. A Romberg test is positive and gait proceeds under visual guidance. More severely affected patients look at their feet as they walk and have difficulty getting about in the dark. Falls are common in these patients, as is fear of falling. The features that discriminate sensory ataxia from cerebellar are summarized in Table 10.2.

Differential diagnosis

Tabetic neurosyphilis is a classic cause of sensory ataxia, although the disease is no longer common. Vitamin B_{12} deficiency can present with sensory ataxia, particularly in older patients. A number of peripheral neuropathies preferentially affect the dorsal root ganglia or large Ia afferents. Subacute sensory neuropathy was initially described by Denny-Brown;[58] the disorder can be autoimmune or paraneoplastic. Ataxic neuropathy can occur with paraproteinemias, or sometimes as an idiopathic disorder.[59] Patients with Guillain–Barré syndrome often have striking sensory ataxia at the time of presentation and may have it as a residual deficit.[60] In some variants, such as the Miller–Fisher syndrome, the mechanism for the ataxia may not be purely peripheral.[61] A toxic neuropathy has been described from chronic ingestion of megadose pyridoxine.[62] Cisplatin neuropathy is a particularly common cause of the syndrome in cancer patients. (Small fiber neuropathies affecting primarily pain and autonomic function do not usually produce sensory ataxia.)

Treatment and rehabilitation strategies

Sensory balance training programs designed for patients with vestibular deficits have been applied to older adults at risk for falls.[63] These programs produce measurable improvements in balance stability and reduce risk for falls in frail elderly subjects.[64] Patients with sensory ataxia are also at risk for falls and injury, and often benefit from this approach. Some form of regular practice is generally necessary so that the gains can be maintained. Other issues include the use of appropriate footwear and assistive devices.

ACKNOWLEDGEMENT

The author would like to thank Bradford Dickerson for helpful suggestions in preparing this chapter.

REFERENCES

1. Friedreich N. Uber degenerative Atrophie der spinalen Hinterstrange. *Virchows Arch Pathol Anat Physiol* 1863;**22**:1–26.
2. Marie P. sur l'heredoataxie cerebelleuse, *Sem Med (Paris)* 1893;**13**:444–7.
3. Holmes G, Clinical symptoms of cerebellar disease and their interpretation, the Croonian Lectures, *Lancet* 1922;ii:59–65.
4. Sudarsky L, Ronthal M. Gait disorders among elderly patients: a survey study of 50 patients, *Arch Neurol* 1983;**40**:740–3.
5. Sudarsky L. Clinical approach to gait disorders of aging. In: Masdeu JC, Sudarsky L, Wolfson L, eds. *Gait disorders of aging: falls and therapeutic strategies.* Philadelphia: Lippincott-Raven, 1997;147–57.
6. Rakic P, Sidman RL. Weaver mutant mouse cerebellum: defective neuronal migration secondary to specific abnormality of Bergman glia, *Proc Natl Acad Sci USA* 1973;**70**:240–4.
7. Rakic P. Synaptic specificity in the cerebellar cortex: study of anomalous circuits induced by single gene mutations in mice. *Cold Spring Harb Symp Quant Biol* 1975;**40**:333–46.
8. deLahunta A, Averill DR. Hereditary cerebellar cortical and extrapyramidal nuclear abiotrophy in Kerry blue terriers, *J Am Vet Med Assoc* 1976;**168**:1119–24.
9. Mori S, Neurophysiology of locomotion. In: Masdeu JC, Sudarsky L, Wolfson L, eds. *Gait disorders of aging: falls and therapeutic strategies.* Philadelphia: Lippincott-Raven, 1997;55–78.
10. Mori S, Matsui T, Kuze B, et al. Stimulation of a restricted region in the midline cerebellar white matter evokes coordinated quadrupedal locomotion in the decerebrate cat. *J Neurophysiol* 1999;**82**:290–300.
11. Clark HB, Burright EN, Yunis WS, et al. Purkinje cell expression of a mutant allele of SCA-1 in transgenic mice leads to disparate effects on motor behaviors. *J Neurosci* 1997;**17**:7385–95.
12. Burk K, Dichgans J. Spinocerebellar ataxia type 2. In: Klockgether T, ed. *Handbook of ataxia disorders.* New York: Marcel Dekker, 2000;363–84.
13. Warrick JM, Paulson HL, Gray-Board GL, et al. Expanded polyglutamine protein forms nuclear inclusions and causes neuronal degeneration in *Drosophila. Cell* 1998;**93**:939–49.
14. Ouchi Y, Okada H, Yoshikawa E, et al. Brain activation during maintenance of standing postures in humans. *Brain* 1999;**122**:329–38.
15. Baloh RW, Jacobson KM, Beykirch K, Honrubia V. Static and dynamic posturography in patients with vestibular and cerebellar lesions, *Arch Neurol* 1998;**55**:649–54.
16. Gatev P, Thomas S, Lou JS, et al. Effects of diminished and conflicting sensory information on balance in patients with cerebellar deficits, *Mov Disord* 1996;**11**:654–64.
17. Diener HC, Nutt JG. Vestibular and cerebellar disorders of equilibrium and gait. In Masdeu JC, Sudarsky L, Wolfson L, eds. *Gait disorders of aging: falls and therapeutic strategies.* Philadelphia: Lippincott-Raven, 1997;261–72.
18. Cueman-Hudson C, Krebs DE. Frontal plane dynamic stability and coordination in subjects with cerebellar degeneration. *Exp Brain Res* 2000;**132**:103–13.

19. Diener HC, Dichgans J, Bacher M, Guschlbauer B. Characteristic alterations of long loop reflexes in patients with Friedreich's ataxia and late atrophy of the anterior cerebellar lobe. *J Neurol Neurosurg Psychiatry* 1984;**47**:679–85.

20. Friedemann JJ, Noth J, Diener HC, Bacher M. Long latency EMG responses in hand and leg muscles: cerebellar disorders. *J Neurol Neurosurg Psychiatry* 1987;**50**:71–7.

21. Timmann D, Horak FB. Prediction and set-dependent scaling of early postural responses in cerebellar patients. *Brain* 1997;**120**:327–37.

22. Bronstein AM, Hood JD, Gresty MA, Panagi C. Visual control of balance in cerebellar and Parkinsonian syndromes. *Brain* 1990;**113**:767–79.

23. Palliyath S, Hallett M, Thomas SL, Lebiedowska MK. Gait in patients with cerebellar ataxia. *Mov Disord* 1998;**13**:958–64.

24. Price BH, Richardson EP. The neurologic illness of Eugene O'Neill. *N Engl J Med* 2000;**342**:1126–33.

25. Pulst S, Perlman S. Hereditary ataxia. In: Pulst S, ed. *Neurogenetics*. Philadelphia: FA Davis, 2000;231–63.

26. Zhogbi HY. CAG repeats in SCA6, *Neurology* 1997;**49**:1196–9.

27. Konigsmark BW, Weiner LP. The olivopontocerebellar atrophies: a review. *Medicine* 1970;**49**:227–41.

28. Harding AE. *The hereditary ataxias and related disorders*. Edinburgh: Churchill Livingstone, 1994.

29. Rosenberg RN. Autosomal dominant cerebellar phenotypes: the genotype has settled the issue. *Neurology* 1995;**45**:1–5.

30. Burk K, Stevanin G, Didierjean O, et al. Clinical and genetic analysis of three German kindreds with autosomal dominant cerebellar ataxia type I linked to the SCA-2 locus. *J Neurol* 1997;**244**:256–61.

31. Sudarsky L, Corwin L, Dawson D. Machado–Joseph disease in New England. *Mov Disord* 1992;**7**:204–8.

32. Geschwind DH, Perlman S, Figueroa KP, et al. Spinocerebellar ataxia type 6: frequency of the mutation and genotype–phenotype correlations, *Neurology* 1997;**49**:1247–51.

33. Koenig M, Durr A. Friedreich's ataxia. In: Klockgether T, ed. *Handbook of ataxia disorders*. New York: Marcel Dekker, 2000;151–61.

34. Campuzano V, Montermini L, Molto MD, et al. Friedreich ataxia: autosomal recessive disease caused by an intronic GAA triplet repeat expansion, *Science* 1996;**271**:1423–7.

35. Durr A, Cossee M, Agid Y, et al. Clinical and genetic abnormalities in patients with Friedreich's ataxia, *N Engl J Med* 1996;**335**:1169–75.

36. Victor M, Adams RD, Mancall EL. A restricted form of cerebellar cortical degeneration occurring in alcoholic patients, *Arch Neurol* 1959;**1**:579–688.

37. Dejerine J, Thomas A. L'atrophie olivo-ponto-cerebelleuse. *Nouv Iconogr Salpetriere* 1900;**13**:330–70.

38. Graham JG, Oppenheimer DR. Orthostatic hypotension and nicotine sensitivity in a case of multiple system atrophy, *J Neurol Neurosurg Psychiatry* 1969;**32**:28–34.

39. Wenning GK, Ben Shlomo Y, Magalhaes M, et al. Clinical features and natural history of mulitple system atrophy. *Brain* 1994;**117**:835–45.

40. Kark RAP, Budelli MA, Wachsner R. Double blind, triple crossover trial of low doses of oral physostigmine in inherited ataxias. *Neurology* 1981;**31**:288–292.

41. Lou J, Goldfarb L, McShane L, et al. Use of buspirone for treatment of cerebellar ataxia, *Arch Neurol* 1995;**52**:982–8.

42. Lewitt PA, Ehrenkranz JRL. TRH and spinocerebellar degeneration, *Lancet* 1982;**ii**:981.

43. Oertel WH. Neurotransmitters in the cerebellum: scientific aspects and clinical relevance. In: Harding AE, Deufel T, eds. *Inherited ataxias. Advances in neurology*. New York: Raven Press, 1993;33–75.

44. Trouillas P, Fuxe K. *Serotonin, the cerebellum and ataxia*. New York: Raven Press, 1993.

45. Schols L, Schulte T, Mattern R, et al. Double-blind, placebo-controlled crossover study of trimethoprim-sulfamethoxazole in spinocerebellar ataxia type 3. *Mov Disord* 1998;**13(S2)**:216.

46. Sakai T, Antoku Y, Matsuishi T, Iwashita H. Tetrahydropbiopterin double blind, crossover trial in Machado–Joseph disease. *J Neurol Sci* 1996;**136**:71–2.

47. Friedman JH. Machado-Joseph disease/spinocerebellar ataxia 3 responsive to buspirone. *Mov Disord* 1997;**12**:613–14.

48. Ghilardi M, Ghez C, Dhawan V, et al. Patterns of regional brain activation associated with different forms of motor learning. *Brain Res* 2000;**871**:127–45.

49. Ito M, *The cerebellum and neural control*. New York: Raven Press, 1984.

50. Brandt T, Krafczyks S, Mahbenden I. Postural imbalance with head extension: improvement by training as a model for ataxia therapy. *Ann N Y Acad Sci* 1981;**74**:636–49.

51. Balliet R, Harbst KB, Kim D, Stewart RV. Retraining of functional gait through the reduction of upper extremity weight bearing in chronic cerebellar ataxia. *Int Rehabil Med* 1987;**8**:148–53.

52. Sliwa JA, Thatcher S, Tet J. Paraneoplastic subacute cerebellar degeneration: functional improvement and role of rehabilitation. *Arch Phys Med Rehabil* 1994;**75**:355–7.

53. Gill-Body KM, Popat RA, Parker SW, Krebs DE. Rehabilitation of balance in two patients with cerebellar dysfunction. *Phys Ther* 1997;**77**:534–52.

54. Sabin T. Peripheral neuropathy: disorders of proprioception. In: Masdeu JC, Sudarsky L, Wolfson L, eds. *Gait disorders of aging: falls and therapeutic strategies*. Philadelphia: Lippincott-Raven, 1997.

55. Marsden CD, Rothwell JC, Day BL. The use of peripheral feedback in the control of movement. In: Evarts E, Wise S, Bousfield D, eds. *The motor system in neurobiology*. Amsterdam: Elsevier, 1985.

56. Sainburg RL, Poizner H, Ghez C. Loss of proprioception produces deficits in interjoint coordination, *J Neurophysiol* 1993;**70**:2136–47.

57. Lajoie Y, Teasdale N, Cole JD, et al. Gait of a deafferented subject without large myelinated sensory fibers below the neck. *Neurology* 1996;**47**:109–15.

58. Denny-Brown D. Primary sensory neuropathy with muscular changes associated with carcinoma. *J Neurol Neurosurg Psychiatry* 1948;**11**:73–87.

59. Dalakis MC. Chronic idiopathic ataxic neuropathy. *Ann Neurol* 1986;**19**:545–54.

60. Sobue G, Senda Y, Matsuoka Y, Sobue I. Sensory ataxia: a residual disability of Guillain–Barré syndrome. *Arch Neurol* 1983;**40**:86–9.

61. Ropper AH, Shahani BT. Proposed mechanism of ataxia in Fisher's syndrome. *Arch Neurol* 1983;**40**:537–8.

62. Schaumburg H, Kaplan J. Sensory neuropathy from pyridoxine abuse: a new megavitamin syndrome. *N Engl J Med* 1983;**309**:445–8.

63. Tinetti ME, Baker DI, McAvay G, et al. A multifactorial intervention to reduce the risk of falling among elderly people living in the community, *N Engl J Med* 1994;**331**:821–7.

64. Whipple RH. Improving balance in older adults: identifying the significant training stimuli. In: Masdeu JC, Sudarsky L, Wolfson L, eds. *Gait disorders of aging: falls and therapeutic strategies*. Philadelphia: Lippincott-Raven, 1997;355–79.

11

Gait and balance in basal ganglia disorders

BASTIAAN R. BLOEM AND KAILASH P. BHATIA

INTRODUCTION

Scope and aims

In this chapter, we first establish why disorders of the basal ganglia frequently lead to balance and gait disturbances. Following general guidelines of a clinical approach to basal ganglia disorders, we sketch the presentation and possible treatments of different types of basal ganglia disorders. This part of the chapter is subdivided into sections, each dealing with different categories of balance and gait disorders, namely hypokinetic–rigid syndromes, dystonia, chorea, tremor, myoclonus and paroxysmal dyskinesias. A separate section deals with isolated balance and gait disorders (i.e. without additional signs of basal ganglia disease).

Historical clinical observations

Basal ganglia disorders are traditionally associated with disturbances of gait, posture and balance. However, what

indications are there to suggest that the basal ganglia are so intimately involved in regulating axial motor functions? The oldest line of evidence stems from a traditional neurological approach: normal functions of a given part of the nervous system can be inferred from observations on patients with 'selective' lesions in the same area. Classical historical descriptions typically mention gait and balance disturbances as prominent features of basal ganglia disorders. This is perhaps not surprising because axial motor impairment is easily discernible to the naked clinical eye, unlike, for example, sensory disorders which require more careful physical examination. Indeed, disorders of posture and gait have been described as sequelae to selective lesions involving virtually any of the basal ganglia nuclei (Table 11.1). An exception is perhaps the caudate nucleus where lesions typically cause behavioral problems, rather than balance or gait impairment.[1]

Idiopathic Parkinson's disease (PD) and other forms of parkinsonism, where abnormal posture and gait are clearly noticeable, represent another good example. When James Parkinson wrote his classical description of PD, he

Table 11.1 *Examples of 'selective' lesions within the basal ganglia, leading to disorders of gait or postural stability in humans*

Area	Examples of focal lesion	References
Substantia nigra	Toxic (MPTP)	2, 3
Putamen	Vascular	4
Globus pallidus	Vascular; post-infectious; toxic; iatrogenic (pallidotomy)[a]	4–6
Subthalamic nucleus	Vascular; iatrogenic (subthalamic stimulation or subthalamotomy)	7, 8
Thalamus	Vascular; tumor; iatrogenic (thalamotomy)[a]	9, 10

[a]Particularly when surgery is performed bilaterally.

noted that '... the utmost care is necessary to prevent falls'.[11] Later studies showed that PD is caused by loss of dopamine-producing cells within the substantia nigra, suggesting that central dopaminergic pathways are involved in normal postural control. This impression was corroborated by the more recent description of young drug addicts in California, USA, with intravenous exposure to a self-synthesized heroin analogue called MPTP (1-methyl-4-phenyl-1,2,3,6-tetrahydropyridine).[2,3] MPTP proved to be a potent neurotoxin with a main predilection for nigrostriatal neurons in the substantia nigra, and it caused a subacute hypokinetic–rigid syndrome that strongly resembled severe PD. Significantly, patients with MPTP-induced parkinsonism had severe disturbances of gait and posture.

Postencephalitic parkinsonism was also associated with severe gait and balance problems.[5] The globus pallidus bears the brunt of the damage in this disorder, which suggests that it plays a critical role in the regulation of gait and balance. Supporting evidence for this assumption stems from observations on patients with strategically located vascular or neurodegenerative lesions within the globus pallidus (Table 11.1). Such patients have prominent postural instability and often 'fall like a log'.

Animal models

A second and rather substantial line of evidence comes from experimental studies in animals with lesions in (or stimulation of) selective parts of the basal ganglia. Perhaps best known are the experiments by Denny-Brown,[12] who observed marked disturbances of posture and balance in monkeys with bilateral electrolytic lesions of the globus pallidus, and possibly some surrounding structures. Another well-known animal model is that of parkinsonism induced by MPTP, which causes fairly selective nigral cell death in many different species, including monkeys. Animals exposed to MPTP develop a parkinsonian syndrome with prominent disorders of posture and balance.[3] A recent animal model involves selective lesions of the dorsal mesencephalon, where the pedunculopontine nucleus (PPN) is situated. Destruction of the PPN causes a prominent akinetic syndrome in monkeys.[13] Conversely, chemical or electrical stimulation of the dorsal mesencephalon leads to initiation and maintenance of stepping movements in rats and cats.[14]

Functions and connections of the basal ganglia

A third and final line of evidence is provided by current theories about the normal functions of the basal ganglia. Many of these functions are deemed relevant for control of posture and gait. Many of these theories are based in part upon the above-mentioned 'lesion studies' in human patients and experimental animals. Note, however, that lesion studies alone were generally inconclusive because of the complex parallel organization of multiple basal ganglia circuitries, allowing one part to compensate for a deficit elsewhere.[1]

The traditional model of the basal ganglia mainly emphasizes the 'ascending' thalamocortical projections to the motor cortex and supplementary motor area (Fig. 11.1). Dopamine is the key neurotransmitter within this circuit, but glutamate and gamma-amino butyric acid (GABA) also play an important role. This part of the basal ganglia circuit is responsible for the automatic execution of centrally initiated movements, in particular the running of sequential submovements within a learned motor plan.[16] This could be relevant for the initiation and maintenance of rhythmic stepping movements under routine everyday conditions. A second important basal ganglia function involves the flexible adaptation of motor behavior whenever the environmental context changes.[1] Of particular interest is the 'comparator' or adapter function, whereby the basal ganglia compare the original motor plan (the efferent copy) to the actual ongoing movement (Fig. 11.2). For this purpose, the basal ganglia receive abundant afferent proprioceptive information. It is mainly the globus pallidus that assists in processing this afferent somatosensory information.[17] This comparator function helps subjects to employ predictive motor strategies and to shift their motor or cognitive set, according to the demands of the actual task at hand. Obviously, it is also important for the regulation of posture and gait in our constantly changing environment.

In more recent years, increasing attention has been paid to the 'descending' projections of the basal ganglia to the brainstem. This descending basal ganglia loop is involved in preparing the spinal cord for the moment it receives volitional commands from the motor cortex (gain control function). The brainstem loop contributes to control of automatic motor processes involving mainly axial structures, such as standing, walking and regulation of muscle tone. Brainstem mechanisms also play an important role in moderating startle responses.[18] Figure 11.3 illustrates that the subthalamic nucleus projects directly and indirectly (via the internal globus pallidus and substantia nigra pars reticulata) to the PPN within the dorsal mesencephalon. This nucleus consists of a mainly cholinergic pars compacta and a mixed cholinergic/glutaminergic pars dissipatus.[14] The central connections of the PPN in humans are largely unknown, but have been inferred from observations in rodents and monkeys. This seems to be influenced by both descending projections from the basal ganglia and ascending 'feedback' projections from the spinal cord. In turn, the PPN likely projects to portions of the lower brainstem and spinal cord that are involved in controlling axial and proximal limb musculature.[14] The PPN appears to be the site of a 'mesencephalic locomotor center', for various

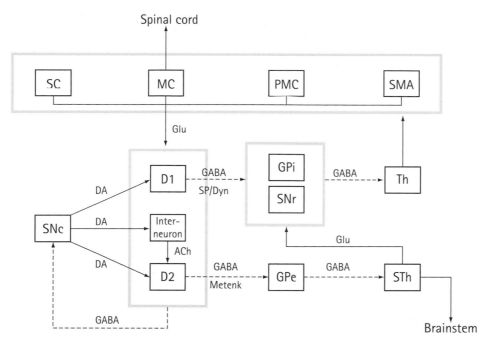

Figure 11.1 *Schematic illustration of the functional relationships among the basal ganglia, and their projections to the spinal cord via loops involving the cortex (modified from ref. 15, with permission of the authors and publisher). Abbreviations: ACh, acetylcholine; DA, dopamine; Dyn, dynorphin; GABA, gamma-amino butyric acid; Glu, glutamate; GPe, globus pallidus, pars externa; GPi, globus pallidus, pars interna; MC, motor cortex; Metenk, metenkephalin; PMC, premotor cortex; SC, sensory cortex; SMA, supplementary motor area; SNc, substantia nigra, pars compacta; SNr, substantia nigra, pars reticulata; SP, substance P; STh, nucleus subthalamicus; Th, thalamus.*

reasons. First, the aforementioned lesion and stimulation studies in animals suggest that the PPN contains a pattern generator for locomotion. Second, the PPN could modulate gait through processing of incoming sensory information from the spinal cord, thus helping

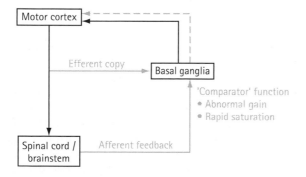

Figure 11.2 *The function of the basal ganglia as a 'comparator'. The basal ganglia permit the motor cortex to launch a particular motor program, which is executed at the level of the spinal cord (chain of events shown in black arrows). The basal ganglia receive proprioceptive feedback from the ongoing movement, and when a discrepancy between the original motor plan and the actual ongoing movement is detected, corrective signals are sent back to motor cortical regions (chain of events shown in gray arrows).*

to adapt gait to external events.[14] Finally, by linking motor behavior to reward systems, the PPN could be evolutionary involved in directing gait towards potentially rewarding targets. A few studies suggest that the PPN might actually be involved in human gait. Thus, blood flow in the dorsal mesencephalon is increased shortly after a period of walking.[19] Furthermore, a patient with a strategically placed vascular lesion in the dorsal mesencephalon (presumably involving the PPN) had severe difficulty in generating stepping movements.[20] Finally, diseases such as PD or progressive supranuclear palsy (PSP), which are characterized by cell loss within the PPN, typically feature gait disorders.

Another potentially important structure in the brainstem is the locus coeruleus (Fig. 11.3). This small pigmented nucleus is situated bilaterally in the pontine tegmentum. In the central nervous system, the locus coeruleus is the main source of the excitatory neurotransmitter norepinephrine. The locus coeruleus innervates widespread areas in the central nervous system, including the spinal cord, the neocortex, the hippocampus and the cerebellum. The locus coeruleus also has a close anatomical relation to the PPN, which can be influenced by noradrenergic projections.[14] Retrograde tracer transport studies in rats have identified a topographic arrangement of these projections within the locus coeruleus. The more caudal and ventral part, which con-

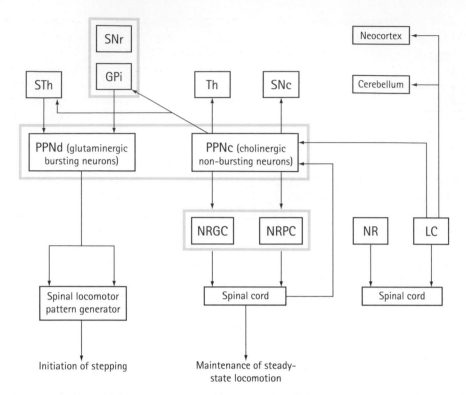

Figure 11.3 *Schematic illustration of brainstem projections to and from the basal ganglia that could be relevant for control of balance and gait.*[14,18] *Note that the existence and importance of rubrospinal projections in humans is debated. Abbreviations: Gpi, globus pallidus, pars interna; LC, locus coeruleus; NR, nucleus ruber; NRGC, nucleus reticularis gigantocellularis; NRPC, nucleus reticularis pontis caudalis; PPNc, pedunculopontine nucleus, pars compacta; PPNd, pedunculopontine nucleus, pars dissipatus; SNc, substantia nigra, pars compacta; SNr, substantia nigra, pars reticulata; STh, nucleus subthalamicus; Th, thalamus.*

sist of densely packed small cells, contain neurons that project to the spinal cord and the cerebellum. The more rostral and dorsal parts, which are formed by large multipolar cells, project mainly to the neocortex.[21] In accord with these widespread projections, the locus coeruleus has rather diverse functions, many of which could be important for balance control. First, studies in acute spinal cats suggest that the locus coeruleus is involved in initiating locomotion. Second, studies in rats, cats and monkeys found evidence that the locus coeruleus is activated in situations demanding immediate attention and coping responses. This function could be relevant when subjects must suddenly handle unexpected balance perturbations. Third, the locus coeruleus has important autonomic functions, and dysfunction might contribute to orthostatic hypotension in neurodegenerative disorders such as multiple system atrophy (MSA). Fourth, the coeruleospinal pathway controls bulbar and spinal motor neurons, and thus assists in regulating motor output from the motor cortex (including gain control of limb reflexes).[22,23] As we shall see later, disturbed gain control of automatic (presumably spinal) responses in leg muscles contributes to balance impairment in various basal ganglia disorders, possibly owing to loss of descending coeruleospinal influence. Finally, given its widespread projections, the locus coeruleus may play a

coordinating role in linking different brain functions. Since balance control requires a linkage between many different brain areas and separate functional systems, the locus coeruleus could be an adequate 'coordinator'. Dysfunction might well lead to imbalance.

CLINICAL IMPACT

These considerations indicate that gait and balance impairment are sensitive features of basal ganglia disorders (i.e. balance and gait are often abnormal when basal ganglia lesions are present). However, the specificity of finding a balance or gait disorder is much lower, and the type of abnormality does not always predict the site of the lesion. For example, hypokinetic-rigid gait disorders often point to a lesion in the substantia nigra, but may also occur following postsynaptic lesions in the striatum. Furthermore, gait and balance impairment are by no means exclusive features of basal ganglia disorders, as is illustrated in, for example, Chapter 10 on the cerebellum.

The extent to which balance and gait problems influence the overall clinical presentation varies widely across different basal ganglia disorders. They can be the primary or even sole manifestation of basal ganglia disease, as in primary orthostatic tremor or acute vascular lesions of the basal ganglia. In other disorders, gait and balance are affected early in the course of the disease, but other signs emerge later. Examples include PSP, MSA, corticobasal degeneration, Lewy body dementia or dopa-responsive dystonia. A gait disorder can also dominate the clinical presentation of vascular parkinsonism for many years. For most basal ganglia disorders, gait and balance problems are a late manifestation of the disease. The most common example of this category is PD. This is reflected by disease progression according to the Hoehn and Yahr stages,[24] which indicates that postural instability is initially absent (stage 1 and 2), emerges in stage 2.5 and becomes the most significant determinant of further progression from stage 3 to stage 5. Parkinson's disease patients share this opinion, because they typically volunteer tremor as their most significant problem in early stages of the disease. However, as the disease progresses further, gait and balance disorders become increasingly important.[25]

GENERAL CLINICAL ASSESSMENT

History taking

History taking is a vital element of the general clinical assessment. Table 11.2 lists several key elements of the interview. Note that many patients fail to volunteer their problems of gait and balance because they feel this is normal for their age. Other patients do not wish to bother their clinician with a problem which they themselves perceive to be untreatable. Others simply forget about their balance problems because of an associated memory impairment. This amnesia is not rare and occurs in, for example, PSP, vascular parkinsonism and Alzheimer's disease. We have the impression that patients with PD also underreport their number of falls.[27,28] Yet, asking for information on prior falls is important because of the association with future falls (see below). Enquiry about falls in the previous 12 months is perhaps least confounded by amnesia. Actively interviewing spouses, carers or other eyewitnesses about falls is often necessary. A critical element of the interview relates to balance confidence and fear of falls, as related to the degree of actually measured postural instability. Patients with an excessive fear may suffer from unnecessary immobilization.[28] Conversely, patients that are overly confident are at increased risk of sustaining falls and injuries, a situation commonly encountered in patients with PSP.

Physical examination

POSTURE AND BALANCE

A battery of clinical tests is needed to capture the complex nature of balance problems in patients with basal

Table 11.2 *History taking in patients with basal ganglia disorders*

Balance and falls	Subjective instability
	Latency since onset of disease
	Frequency of (near-)falls[a]
	Fall circumstances[b]
	Preceding loss of consciousness
	Injuries
	Ability to stand up after fall
	Fear of falls
	Motor recklessness
Gait	Slowing
	(Asymmetrically) reduced armswing
	Stumbling
	Kinesia paradoxica
Freezing	Circumstances (starting, turning, narrow spaces, reaching destination)
	Compensatory tricks (visual, auditory, mental)
	Relation to falls
Use of walking aids	Difficulties in use
	If none: why not? Social embarrassment?
General aspects	Interview of partner or other carer
	Impact on quality of life
	Positive/negative influence of medication
	Relation to clinical condition ('on–off', dyskinesias)
	Use of psychoactive medication?

[a]Near-falls include any loss of balance without the subject hitting the floor or other lower surface (fall arrested by seeking support).
[b]Particularly turning around and 'dual-tasking'.
Table modified from Bloem and Commisaris,[26] with permission of the publisher.

ganglia disorders. Various relevant elements are listed in Table 11.3. It is important to investigate both 'static' and more 'dynamic' components of balance.[29,30] Static components are judged by visual inspection of the patient in rest (seated and standing; frontal and lateral view). The severity of involuntary movements such as dyskinesias (induced by dopaminergic medication) or chorea (as in Huntington's disease) can be estimated in seated patients, but the influence on balance only becomes evident during standing and walking.

Dynamic balance control has several components (Table 11.3). Righting reactions are needed to change posture (e.g. when rising from a chair or bed). Supporting reactions are required to maintain the achieved position. Anticipatory reactions are automatic and predictive adaptations that prevent instability caused by self-initiated movements, such as lifting heavy objects. Reactive postural responses protect against external perturbations, such as a slap on the shoulders. The so-called defensive reactions, which are evoked by

imminent falls, are perhaps the most important element of the normal balance repertoire. Examples include taking corrective steps and making protective arm movements (to grasp for support, or to cushion the impact of an impending fall). Evaluation of these defensive reactions is often difficult in a clinical setting because patients must be brought close to (or even beyond) their limits of stability. Quantified assessment (see later) is more suited for this purpose.

Functional 'everyday' tests should be performed whenever possible. Useful tests include turning in a standing position, rising from a chair and sitting down, getting in and out of a bed and rolling over in bed. Such tests provide insight into daily life performance. Various groups have made attempts to standardize the execution and scoring of such tests.[31,32]

The retropulsion test deserves special comment. This test is commonly used to probe the reactive and defensive postural reactions in clinical practice. The investigator, standing behind the patient, suddenly pulls the

Table 11.3 *Physical examination of gait and balance problems in patients with basal ganglia disorders*

Posture	Seated and standing
	Frontal and lateral view
	Retro-, antero- or laterocollis
	Pisa syndrome
	Camptocormia
	Dyskinesias
Balance	Righting reactions (rising from chair)
	Supporting reactions (quiet stance, eyes open / closed)
	Anticipatory reactions (lifting object from floor; arm raising)
	Reactive/protective postural responses (retropulsion test)[a]
Walking[b]	Gait speed
	Armswing
	Increased or manifest arm tremor while walking
	Step height and length
	Stance width
	Striatal toe upon walking
	Standardized (generic) rating scales (e.g. Tinetti Mobility Index)
Freezing[c]	Gait ignition
	Festination
	Instability while turning[d]
	Compensatory tricks
Other functional tasks	Turning while recumbent
	Climbing stairs
Performing multiple tasks simultaneously	'Stops walking when talking'[e]
	Avoiding obstacles
	Carrying object in hands
	Combinations of the above
Quantifiable tests	'Functional reach' test[40]
	'Get up and go' or 'sit-stand-walk test'[39]

[a]Difficult to standardize and score.
[b]Speed of performance less important than safety.
[c]Often difficult to assess during clinical examination.
[d]Instruct to execute slowly and abruptly.
[e]Usually normal in Parkinson's disease.[35]
Table modified from Bloem and Commissaris.[26]

shoulders and judges the balance reactions. Others prefer to face the patient and push against the sternum, but a disadvantage is that the patient can be supported less easily when balance is lost. The normal balance reaction consists of rapid trunk flexion from the hips, combined with stretching the arms in front. If needed, healthy persons may take corrective backward steps. It is unclear how many steps can still be regarded as 'normal', and different groups have used either one, two or three steps as their cut-off value for normality. Note that corrective steps are important defensive reactions and equating more steps with greater balance impairment may not be correct. Indeed, we have occasionally seen healthy persons taking up to six corrective steps.[33] A problem does arise when the corrective steps are slow or small, leading to retropulsion. Pushing the patient sideways or forward may cause lateropulsion or propulsion, respectively. Severely affected patients entirely fail to step and fall 'like a log' into the arms of the investigator. We recommend taking the speed and quality of balance reactions into account (rather than merely counting the number of corrective steps) and to consider a slow response as abnormal even if only one or two steps are taken. A drawback to the retropulsion test is the variability in execution, introduced by differences in posture of both the patient and the investigator.[34] We usually deliver one shoulder pull without specific prior warning, as this best mimics daily life circumstances where falls are usually unexpected events. We then repeat the test several times and consider failure to 'habituate' to the test as another sign of balance impairment. As such, the retropulsion test indexes the degree of postural instability. However, the test fails to predict falls, at least in PD.[28]

Asking patients to perform several tasks concurrently while walking or standing is particularly informative. The best-known example is the 'stops walking while talking test' (starting a routine conversation during a stroll with the patient). Failure to walk and talk at the same time predicts falls in the elderly, but not in PD.[35] Patients may have more difficulty when two motor tasks are combined (e.g. walking and carrying a cup of tea). Balance problems increase as the combined task becomes more complex.[36,37]

GAIT

Most consulting rooms are too small to properly judge gait disorders. Therefore, the walk from the waiting room can be used to obtain a first impression. We often consult a physiotherapist, since they can investigate patients in much larger and standardized training rooms. Physiotherapists are also able to assess important elements that cannot be investigated in a consulting room, such as climbing stairs. Gait assessment involves evaluation of both initiation, maintenance and cessation of stepping. It is helpful to observe the patient sideways and from behind while walking. Standard rating scales have been developed, but these are not always useful for patients with basal ganglia disorders. For example, the commonly used Tinetti Mobility Index[38] does not score the armswing, a characteristic early gait abnormality in PD.

Ancillary studies

There are many different ways to objectively quantify the nature and severity of gait or balance disorders. Timed tests provide no qualitative information, but can be used to quantify changes in performance following therapeutic intervention. The most commonly used test is the timed up-and-go test. This test is part of the Core Assessment Program for Intracerebral Transplantations (CAPIT), which was specifically developed for use in PD.[39] Assessment of safety is usually more important than speed of performance. Slowed performance is often equated with poor performance, more severe disability and a high risk of falls, but slowing may also reflect prudent behavior due to an adequately perceived imbalance. Such patients may perform everyday tasks much more safely and have a lower risk of falls than patients with a more hasty performance. The same concerns apply to other quantitative tests such as the functional reach test. Intuitively, a reduced ability to flex the trunk and reach forward with feet in place should index functional impairment, yet some patients may simply refuse to stretch out very far because they justly perceive this as being dangerous. A similarly cautious behavior would be advantageous in daily life. This could explain why seemingly poor performance on the functional reach test does not correlate with falls in daily life.[40]

More elaborate quantified assessment techniques include static or dynamic posturography and quantified gait analysis using treadmills or waist-worn accelerometers.[41–44] These techniques have been instrumental in elucidating the underlying pathophysiology of many basal ganglia disorders. However, such studies have yet to prove their benefit for routine clinical management. Some techniques are described in more detail below in the section 'Quantitative gait and balance studies'.

Neuroimaging studies can sometimes reveal abnormalities that were not evident clinically, despite careful history taking and physical examination. For example, patients with a seemingly idiopathic senile gait disorder often have underlying cerebrovascular disease (leukoaraiosis or multiple lacunar infarcts). The same holds for patients with lower-body parkinsonism or gait ignition failure. Computed tomography or magnetic resonance imaging of the brain is also helpful in the diagnostic work-up of patients suspected of having normal pressure hydrocephalus, which may be difficult on clinical grounds alone. Neuroimaging studies can sometimes identify specific abnormalities in patients suspected of having MSA or PSP, but the sensitivity is rather modest. Largely, the same holds true for other ancillary studies such as sphincter electromyography.

SPECIFIC BASAL GANGLIA DISORDERS

The remainder of this chapter focuses on a clinical description of common basal ganglia disorders (Table 11.4). We pay particular attention to idiopathic PD, because this is the most common neurodegenerative disorder involving the basal ganglia. Also, PD has been studied in most detail and many findings may serve as a template for the approach to other basal ganglia disorders.

PARKINSON'S DISEASE

Clinical presentation

GAIT AND FREEZING

Whenever possible, patients with PD should be investigated when their symptomatic treatment is optimally effective, and again when the therapeutic effects have worn off. In early stages (sometimes at onset of the disease), mild gait or postural abnormalities may be present. This includes an asymmetrically reduced or absent arm swing (which can be the sole presenting symptom for several years),[45] a gently stooped posture and difficulties turning around in a standing or recumbent position. As the disease progresses, gait becomes slower and the typical parkinsonian gait emerges with shuffling and short steps, a bilaterally reduced arm swing and slow turns which are executed *en bloc*. The step size becomes asymmetric, particularly in early PD. In early stages of the disease, stance width can be slightly increased, but curiously, gait is typically not wide-based in more advanced stages,[46] in contrast to most other balance disorders. Walking often aggravates or even unveils the typical pill rolling rest tremor of the hands. The so-called 'striatal toe' (extension of the hallux) can be observed in the feet during walking. Simple undisturbed gait is usually performed rather safely (perhaps due to compensatory slowing), unless severe dyskinesias bring the patient beyond the limits of stability. Poorly mobile patients with advanced disease can sometimes respond quickly to environmental events and move unexpectedly well. This phenomenon is termed 'kinesia paradoxica' and is typically triggered by emotional or threatening circumstances.

Even in early stages of PD (and occasionally at first onset), patients may experience brief and sudden moments where the feet subjectively become glued to the

Table 11.4 *Basal ganglia disorders associated with disorders of balance, posture and gait*

Hypokinetic rigid syndromes	Parkinson's disease
	Progressive supranuclear palsy
	Multiple system atrophy (MSA-P phenotype)[a]
	Corticobasal degeneration
	Dementia with Lewy bodies
	Alzheimer's disease with extrapyramidal features
	Vascular 'lower-body half' parkinsonism
	Strategic vascular lesions
	Neuroleptic-induced parkinsonism
	Manganese intoxication
Dystonic features	Generalized dystonia
	Dopa-responsive dystonia
Chorea	Huntington's disease
	Drug-induced dyskinesias
Tremor	Primary orthostatic tremor
Ataxia	Multiple system atrophy (MSA-C phenotype)[b]
Myoclonus	Corticobasal degeneration
	Hyperekplexia (startle disease)
	Myoclonic epilepsy
Paroxysmal dyskinesias	Exercise-induced dystonia
	Kinesigenic choreoathetosis
	Paroxysmal (non-kinesigenic) dystonic choreo-athetosis
'Pure' gait/balance disorders	Senile gait disorder
	Cautious gait disorder
	Primary progressive freezing gait
Other disorders	Amyotrophic lateral sclerosis
	Normal pressure hydrocephalus

[a]Parkinsonian features predominate; previously also termed striatonigral degeneration.
[b]Cerebellar features predominate; previously also termed olivo-ponto-cerebellar atrophy.

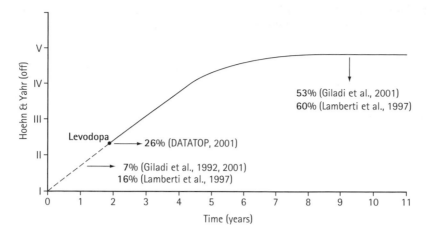

Figure 11.4 *Frequency of gait freezing, as reported in the literature by Giladi et al. in three different surveys[47,49,50] and by Lamberti et al.[52] It is interesting that only a subgroup of patients develops gait freezing. Analysis of the large cohort from the DATATOP study indicates that even those patients who had gait freezing in the first year of their disease had classical PD at long-term follow-up.[50] This figure was kindly provided by Dr Nir Giladi.*

floor ('freezing'). Early freezing episodes most commonly occur among patients presenting with gait or trunk symptoms at onset of the disease.[47] The prevalence of freezing increases with disease duration and progression of disease severity (Fig. 11.4). It is also more common after prolonged dopaminergic treatment, but can occur in drug-naive patients. Note that freezing is not unique for PD and is also common in PSP, vascular parkinsonism and normal pressure hydrocephalus.[48,49] However, freezing is distinctly rare in MSA and drug-induced parkinsonism. Freezing most commonly appears while patients are making turns, but may also occur spontaneously during straight walking, while crossing narrow spaces, when patients try to initiate gait ('hesitation') or when patients reach a target. It may also emerge under stressful circumstances. Shuffling with small steps or trembling of the legs is much more common than complete akinesia.[50] Occasionally, freezing of one leg occurs, particularly in patients with asymmetrical parkinsonism. Freezing episodes are typically brief, usually lasting only several seconds, but may persists for minutes in more advanced stages of the disease. Patients can also have gait festination: i.e. a sudden change in locomotion rhythm owing to an inability to maintain the base of support (the feet) beneath the forward moving trunk during gait, forcing the patient to rapidly take increasingly small steps (hastening) to avoid a fall. Festination leads to propulsion when patients walk forward, or retropulsion when patients lose balance and take corrective steps backward. It may be difficult to distinguish festination from freezing, hence both signs are perhaps best referred to as 'paroxysmal gait disorders'. Patients who have difficulties with gait initiation or maintenance often report the use of simple tricks to promote walking (auditory cues such as listening to rhyth-

mic sounds of a metronome; visual cues such as stepping over small obstacles on the floor; or mental cues such as simple arithmetic).[48,53] Distraction or asking the patient to perform a secondary task (answering questions, carrying an object) interferes with this compensatory strategy and often aggravates the gait disorder, causing patients to slow down or completely stop walking. During history taking, specific enquiry about paroxysmal gait disorders is important because they are notoriously difficult to assess during physical examination. A specific freezing questionnaire has been developed for this purpose.[49]

POSTURE

In early stages of the disease, patients tend to lean a bit backward during quiet stance.[54] In later stages of the disease, body weight shifts into a forward direction owing to development of the characteristically stooped posture, with flexion of the neck, trunk, elbows and knees. However, standing stooped may also reflect an attempt by patients to compensate for their tendency to fall backward. Interestingly, when patients are asked to close their eyes, their body weight shifts backward again,[55] suggesting that patients use visual feedback to actively keep their body weight away from their most feared (backward) fall direction. Patients may thus actively assume (or aggravate) this stooped posture in order to brace themselves against imminent falls, somewhat like Japanese Sumo wrestlers who vigorously attempt to stay upright by stooping forward.[56] An extreme degree of antecollis relative to other body parts, or when the chin touches the chest, is unusual and suggests a diagnosis of MSA.[57,58] In contrast, retroflexion of the neck (retrocollis) suggests a diagnosis of PSP.[59] Some lateral deviation of the trunk may occur, but severe and persistent lateroflex-ion (the so-called 'Pisa syndrome' or pleurothotonus) usually suggests dystonia induced by neuroleptics, the presence of MSA or post-encephalitic parkinsonism.[60–62] Camptocormia (a marked anteflexion of the thoracolumbar spine between 30 and 90 degrees) is rare in idiopathic PD. Some patients with camptocormia also have lateral bending of the spine, but there is no forward flexion of the neck.[63] Camptocormia is apparent on standing, worsens while walking, but decreases while sitting and even disappears when patients are lying down. This last feature separates camptocormia from the fixed kyphoscoliosis seen in patients with degenerative changes of the spine. The Romberg test is typically normal in PD.

BALANCE AND FALLS

Postural stability is preserved early in the course of the disease and falls never occur at onset of the disease in idiopathic (pathologically confirmed) PD. In one series of pathologically confirmed cases, recurrent falls (retrospectively ascertained) never occurred in the first two years of the disease.[64] Over a time period of about three years after onset of the very first symptoms, the patients gradually progress to bilateral disease (Hoehn and Yahr stage 2), but balance is still preserved.[65] Postural instability usually develops after an additional 2–3 years (Hoehn and Yahr stage 3), although an occasional patient may not reach this stage even 17 years into the illness. Falls take even longer to develop and emerge, on average, some 10 years after onset of the disease.[64] Interestingly, for the tremor-dominant type of PD, postural instability and falls appear to be late feature. Eventually, however, most patients will fall. Rarely balance problems and falls

have been reported to be the presenting feature of PD.[66] However, without post-mortem confirmation, it is possible that such patients could have had a different disorder (possibly PSP).

Until recently, falls in PD were ascertained retrospectively through interviews of patients or carers. Because asking for prior falls is unreliable (see General Clinical Assessment), the actual fall rates long remained uncertain. However, four prospective surveys have been completed recently (Table 11.5). The overall incidence of persons with at least one fall ranged from 39 to 68 per cent and from 25 to 50 per cent for recurrent (twice or more) fallers. These fall rates clearly exceed those seen in healthy subjects (Fig. 11.5). The incidence is even higher when near-falls are accommodated.[27,68] Interestingly, falls are common even in rather early stages of the disease when clinical tests show little balance impairment.[28] It appears as if falls are most common in moderately affected patients who are somewhat unstable, yet sufficiently mobile to actually sustain falls. We feel that the falling rates may level off in later stages of the disease due to disease progression and immobility.[69] Indeed, patients in Hoehn and Yahr stage 5 are bound to their bed or wheelchair for most of the time, making falls unlikely. Furthermore, patients probably also compensate for their gradually developing and worsening balance problems. Examples of such compensatory strategies, as well as their effects on postural control, are listed in Table 11.6.

Various studies have examined the fall circumstances.[28,40,67,68] Most falls occur when patients are in their best clinical condition ('on' state), possibly reflecting the increased mobility. This observation also underscores that antiparkinson medication usually

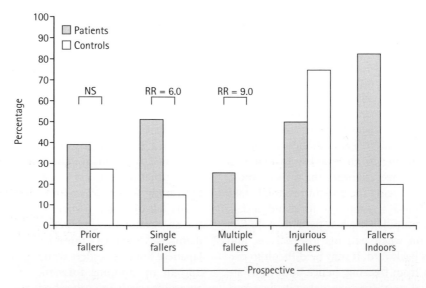

Figure 11.5 *Fall rates in Parkinson's disease, as described by Bloem et al.[28] Note that although patients tended to report more historical falls, there was no significant difference with healthy controls, possibly because many falls were forgotten or simply not reported. In contrast, prospectively measured fall rates are considerably higher among patients compared to controls. NS, no significant difference; RR, relative risk.*

Table 11.5 *Comparison of prospective studies of falls in Parkinson's disease*

	Gray and Hildebrand[27]	Bloem et al.[28]	Ashburn et al.[40]	Wood et al.[67]
Demographics				
Number of patients	118	61	63	109
Mean age (yrs)	70.6 (43–90)[a]	61 (39–80)	71 (46–86)	74.7 ± 7.9
Proportion of men	62.0%	64.4%	52.4%	47.7%
Duration of disease (yrs)	9.1 (1–25)[a]	7.1 ± 4.8	NA	3 (1–31)
Hoehn & Yahr stage	2.6 ± 0.5[a]	2.3 ± 0.7	2.8 ± 0.7	2.0 (1.0–4.0)
MMSE	27.8 ± 2.9[a]	28.1 ± 2.0	NA	NA
Control group studied	No	Yes	No	No
History taking				
Period	3 months	6 months	1 year	1 year
Prior faller	53.4%	39.0%	63.5%	61.4%
Fear of falls	NA	45.8%	36.5%	NA
Prospective follow-up				
Period	12 weeks	6 months	3 months	1 year
Ascertainment	Diary plus regular telephone calls	Postcards plus regular telephone calls	Telephone call at end of follow-up	Postcards plus regular telephone calls
Lost to follow-up	None	$n = 2$	$n = 6$	$n = 8$
Faller (at least once)	59.3%[b]	50.8%	38.6%	68.3%
Recurrent faller	41.5%[b]	25.4%	15.8%	50.5%
Injurious faller	NA	25.4%	NA	NA
Injurious falls	40.0%	62.0%	NA	NA
Indoor falls	Usually on carpet	82.7%	NA	NA
Predictors of falls				
Prior falls	+[c]	+	+[d]	+
Fear of falls	–	–	+	NA
Disease severity	+ (mainly HY 3)[c]	+ (mainly HY 3)	+	+ (HY 3 and 4)
Disease duration	+	+	NA	+
Reduced arm swing	NA	–	–	+

[a]This study analyzed both complete falls and near-falls.
[b]No statistical correction for influence of other variables was performed.
[c]Two or more prior falls had a better combined sensitivity and specificity than at least one prior fall.
[d]But no longer significant after correction for other variables.
HY, Hoehn and Yahr; NA, not available.

provides little or no improvement of postural instability. In fact, dopaminergic medication can cause dyskinesias that may be sufficiently severe to perturb patients. Figures 11.5 and 11.6 illustrate the type of falls in PD, as identified in one study. Most falls occur indoors (particularly in the bedroom). Obvious environmental factors (loose rugs and doorsteps) contribute to only a minority of falls. Most falls result from the underlying balance impairment ('intrinsic' falls) and seem to occur under seemingly harmless circumstances. Falls often involve movements of the trunk, in particular sudden turning movements (Fig. 11.6).

Table 11.6 *Examples of compensatory strategies*

Strategy	Beneficial effect	Adverse effect
Stiffening	Less static sway; reduce degrees of freedom	Poorer dynamic postural control
Adaptations in posture		
Adopting a stooped posture	Reduce backward falls	May cause stiffness and festination
Wide-based stance	Improved lateral stability[a]	Regular gait less efficient
Adaptations in gait		
Reduced walking speed	Falls with lower energy	None
Increased double-limb support	Less instability during swing phase	None
Use of external cues	Reduce freezing and akinesia	Loss of automaticity
Posture-first strategy[b]	Fewer falls	Inflexibility in complex circumstances

[a]Absent in advanced Parkinson's disease.
[b]Avoiding dual tasking may, at first sight, appear to reflect loss of central processing capacity.

Changes in posture ('transfers'), such as rising from a chair, are also commonly responsible. Trips or slips (leading to base-of-support falls) are much less common. Attempts to simultaneously perform two independent tasks (e.g. walking and carrying something) contribute to many falls. Falls caused by preceding loss of consciousness are rare.

Falls can have devastating consequences. Hip fractures appear in about 25 per cent of patients within 10 years after diagnosis of the disease.[70] Fracture development is facilitated by a coexistent osteoporosis (caused by immobilization and perhaps endocrine disorders).[71] Parkinson's disease patients with hip fractures face an unusually high morbidity and mortality risk, and commonly require admission to a nursing home. Fractures of the wrist seem less common, perhaps because the hands are not stretched out quickly enough after a fall. A recent study showed that PD patients may quickly initiate arm muscle responses when they fall, but this is not helpful because the arms are adducted to the trunk.[72] Minor injuries such as bruises or skin lacerations are even more common and represent a major source of discomfort to patients. Injuries are typically caused by propulsion, freezing, dyskinesias and turning movements. A common, yet frequently overlooked consequence is a fear of future falls, which may lead to restriction of daily activities in many patients.[28] This could explain why the large majority of falls occur indoors: patients drastically reduce their outdoor walks. The resultant immobility makes patients highly dependent for performance of everyday activities. Staying indoors perhaps explains why patients mostly suffer relatively 'innocent' falls (no major injury), because soft carpets cushion the impact of indoor falls. Furthermore, patients usually sustain falls with a relatively low energy because they walk slowly. Consequently, the proportion of fallers that sustain injuries is higher among healthy subjects than among patients (Fig. 11.5).

It is difficult to predict who is most at risk of falling (Table 11.5). Various factors are related to 'faller' status, but many of these are interrelated. The presence of prior falls, disease severity (Hoehn and Yahr stage 3 being most prominently associated with falls) and disease duration appear to be the most consistent predictors of falls. In three surveys, falls were independently predicted by asking for earlier falls and by disease severity. In one study, prior falls had a sensitivity and specificity of both 86 per cent in predicting renewed falls.[40] The fourth study did not perform a multiple logistic regression analysis, but again identified prior falls as a considerable risk factor (the relative risk that we calculated from their data was 8.1). Fear of falls was associated with future falls in only one of three studies that addressed this aspect. Daily use of alcohol is another risk factor for falls in PD.[27] Finally, patients taking benzodiazepines have a fivefold increased risk of falls. It thus seems that patients with Hoehn and Yahr stage 3–4 PD[24] who have sustained at least one prior fall are at greatest risk of falls in the near future.

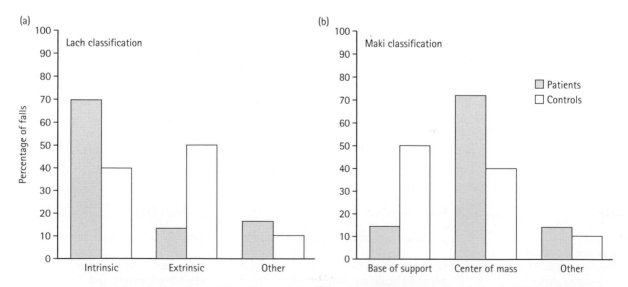

Figure 11.6 *Types of falls in Parkinson's disease, as described by Bloem et al.[28] Falls were scored using two different classification systems. (a) 'Extrinsic' falls were caused by an environmental cause (e.g. collisions), 'intrinsic' falls by mobility or balance disorders, misperception of the environment or loss of consciousness. The remaining falls were labeled as 'other', including falls that occurred while the person was not in a bipedal stance (e.g. fall from a chair). (b) 'Base of support falls' were caused by, for example, trips or slips, 'center of mass falls' including self-induced perturbations (e.g. bending, reaching or turning), externally applied perturbations (e.g. a push or collision) and falls without obvious perturbation (with or without loss of consciousness). The remaining falls were again labeled as 'other'.*

Prognosis

Parkinson's disease patients with gait and balance impairment have a rather poor prognosis (Fig. 11.7). Independence is markedly diminished and the quality of life is strongly reduced. Development of gait and balance problems is often paralleled by the appearance of other debilitating signs, such as dementia and dysphagia. The disease also appears to progress at a faster pace once balance problems are present,[73] and overall survival is reduced. From the moment when recurrent falls occur, median survival of PD patients is reduced to about 6 years and this does not differ from other hypokinetic–rigid syndromes with a much poorer overall survival.[64] This increased mortality is only partly explained by the occurrence of lethal falls. A more important factor is immobilization, which reduces general fitness and thus increases the risk of cardiovascular disease. These physical problems are aggravated by a fear of falls, which can be incapacitating in its own right. Although this fear may in part be understandable in light of the actual balance impairment, for many patients the fear becomes excessive and leads to unnecessary immobilization. This loss of mobility in turn causes loss of independence and deprives the patients of their social contacts. Furthermore, reduced mobility is associated with various other cumbersome complications, including constipation, pressure sores, poorer sleep quality and, significantly, osteoporosis, which further increases the fracture risk in case of falls.

Quantitative gait and balance studies

Quantitative analyses of gait revealed many aspects that were already evident to the naked clinical eye. However, these studies have been instrumental in pinpointing a reduced step length and an increased stride-to-stride variability as the primary gait abnormalities.[74,75] Electromyographic studies showed that muscle activation patterns in the lower legs are more variable and have a reduced left-right symmetry. Furthermore, there is a reduced activation of triceps surae during the stance phase of the step cycle (leading to a weaker push-off), as well as increased activity in the tibialis anterior during the swing phase (leading to a weaker heel strike).[43] Co-contraction of antagonistic muscles, perhaps compounded by secondary joint changes, explains why the range of joint motion (in the ankles, hips, pelvis, trunk and neck) is reduced during walking.[76,77]

Balance control has been studied in detail using static posturography (analysis of quiet unperturbed stance) and dynamic posturography (quantified evaluation of balance reactions following self-inflicted or externally induced postural perturbations). Such studies have identified a host of abnormalities (Table 11.7). Many groups have used dynamic posturography to study whether changes in automatic postural responses contribute to disequilibrium in PD. It appears that this is the case, as will be illustrated for a relatively simple experimental condition where subjects must resist a sudden toe-up rotational movement of a supporting forceplate (Fig. 11.8a). Healthy subjects respond to such sudden postural perturbations

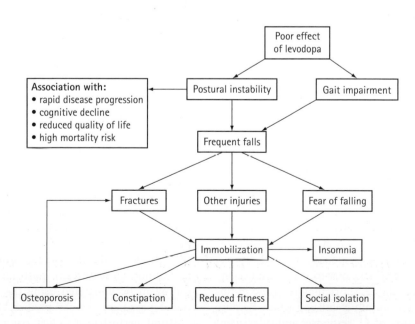

Figure 11.7 *The vicious circle of falls and balance impairment, illustrated for patients with Parkinson's disease. Similar mechanisms apply to patients with other basal ganglia disorders, in particular patients with atypical parkinsonian syndromes such as progressive supranuclear palsy.*

Table 11.7 *Several distinguishing balance control abnormalities in Parkinson's disease*[41–43,78,79]

Passive postural reactions	Enhanced joint stiffness
	Reduced multisegmental flexibility
	Altered viscoelastic muscle properties
	Excessive background muscle activity
Automatic postural responses	Increased size of destabilizing responses
	Decreased size of posturally stabilizing responses
	Co-contraction of antagonist muscles
	Impaired adaptability ('inflexibility')[a]
	Increased use of hip strategy
	Slow, small and multiple-step compensatory stepping movements
	Early but abnormally directed protective arm movements
Voluntary postural responses	Delayed onset
	Inadequate amplitude
Anticipatory postural responses	Inadequate amplitude
	Poor timing
Cognitive postural control	Impaired dual tasking strategies[b]
	Fear of falling
	Excessive balance confidence

[a]Inability to scale the response magnitude according to the demands of the actual postural task at hand (e.g. the stimulus velocity)
[b]Inability to lend priority to postural tasks over other secondary tasks of lesser importance.

by activating a highly coordinated set of muscle contractions, with reciprocal activation of antagonist muscles. For example, early occurring responses can be seen in the stretched triceps surae, followed by an antagonistic response in the shortened tibialis anterior. The earliest activity (short latency or SL response, onset latency around 40 ms) is presumably a monosynaptic spinal stretch reflex, but the later responses are 'automatic' in nature (that is, they are to some extent affected by will, but occur too early to be purely volitional). These automatic postural responses are often termed medium latency (ML, onset latency around 70–80 ms) stretch response in triceps surae and long latency (LL, onset latency around 110 ms) response in the shortened tibialis anterior muscle. The center of foot pressure (CFP) trace shows an early upward deflection because the pressure on the forefeet is initially increased by the toe-up rotation (Fig. 11.8c). This upward deflection also reflects the intrinsic stiffness of the ankle joint and viscoelastic 'spring-like' properties of the stretched triceps surae. Because the toe-up rotations propel the center of gravity (COG) backward (Fig. 11.8d), the CFP subsequently shows a negative deflection because body weight is shifted towards the heels (Fig. 11.8c). The extent of this negative deflection also reflects the combined action of automatic responses: the ML stretch response actually aggravates the posterior sway induced by the platform, whereas the LL shortening response in tibialis anterior exerts a posturally stabilizing action. Because of the stabilizing action of LL responses and subsequent voluntary postural corrections, the backward displacement of the COG is reversed (Fig. 11.8d).

When PD patients are confronted with identical toe-up rotational perturbations, several differences emerge.[80] First, patients have enlarged ML stretch responses and this enlargement of a destabilizing response is thought to induce postural instability (Fig. 11.8a,b). Second, patients have LL responses that are smaller than normal and this reduction of a normally stabilizing response might further lead to postural instability (Fig. 11.8a,b). Indeed, patients are more unstable on the moving platform than controls, as reflected by a larger posterior sway (Fig. 11.8d). Third, the initial forward displacement of the CFP is increased in PD, presumably owing to increased 'intrinsic' ankle stiffness because the CFP traces divert very early (well before automatic postural responses become biomechanically active) (Fig. 11.8c). Finally, the posterior reversal of CFP is delayed and this conceivably reflects insufficiency of later-occurring (possibly voluntary) postural corrections (Fig. 11.8c). Interestingly, comparable abnormalities appear when patients are exposed to sudden horizontal translations of a supporting forceplate.[81] Furthermore, this impaired gain control of postural responses occurs not only in lower leg muscles, but also in muscles spanning the pelvis, trunk and arms.[72]

Reduced flexibility is perhaps one of the most important abnormal features of postural control in PD. This can again be illustrated using the simple toe-up rotational paradigm. Under predictable conditions, small postural perturbations elicit comparably small posturally stabilizing LL responses in healthy subjects (both young and old), while larger perturbations elicit larger

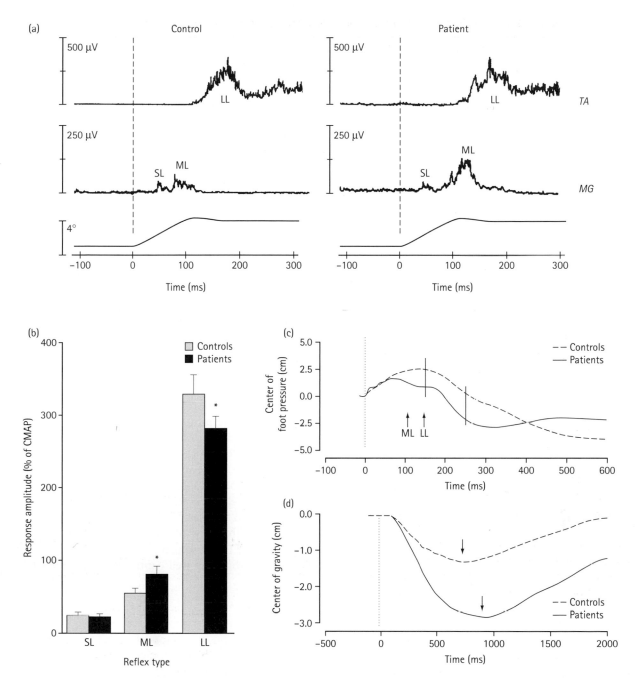

Figure 11.8 *(a) Automatic postural responses to toe-up rotational perturbations (4° amplitude) of a normal subject and a patient with Parkinson's disease (PD) (average of 20 serial perturbations, left leg). The bottom trace indicates the forceplate movement. The first measured platform movement is indicated by a vertical dotted line. SL, short latency; ML, medium latency; LL, long latency. (b) Mean (SEM) normalized amplitudes of automatic postural responses, expressed as a percentage of the compound motor action potential (CMAP), in PD patients and controls; *P < 0.05. (c) Changes in the center of foot pressure (CFP, average of 20 serial perturbations). The first measured platform movement is indicated by a vertical dotted line. Increasing plantarflexion force on the platform is represented by an upward displacement of the CFP trace, whereas increasing dorsiflexion force is represented by a backward displacement. This figure also shows the onset of force recruited by ML and LL responses (calculated as the average onset latency plus 30 ms to account for the electromechanical coupling delay). (d) Displacement of the center of gravity (COG, average of 20 serial perturbations). The first measured platform movement is indicated by a vertical dotted line. Peak backward sway (marked by arrows) and the COG position after 2 s are markedly shifted backward in the patient. (Data in this figure were modified from ref. 80, with permission of the publisher.)*

responses (Fig. 11.9a). When young healthy subjects receive a random mixture of small and large perturbations, they select a 'default' postural response that is sufficiently large to cope with the largest possible perturbation (worst-case scenario). Older subjects also select a default response, albeit one that matches the smaller perturbation size. In other words, healthy subjects can modify the strength of their postural responses according to the demands of the task at hand.[82] This ability is lost in PD.[83] Thus, PD patients have lost the ability to scale their postural responses under predictable conditions (they cannot modify the size of postural responses even though the magnitude of the perturbation is known in advance). Furthermore, they are unable to select a default response during unpredictable conditions, leading to a 'fixed' response size under all conditions (Fig. 11.9b). Similar signs of inflexibility have been observed under many different experimental conditions.[54,84,85] The inability to properly modulate the size of postural responses is another reflection of abnormal gain control.

A salient consequence of postural inflexibility is body stiffening. We have already mentioned the reduced joint motion during walking, as well as the ankle stiffness in patients exposed to toe-up rotational perturbations of an underlying movable platform. A further example is that sway oscillations are reduced in PD during quiet stance or in response to slow platform movements, unless violent tremors or dyskinesias are present.[54,84] More recent studies using multidirectional postural perturbations observed a similar stiffness at the level of the trunk, in particular when patients were tilted laterally.[72] This stiffness interferes with the normal compensatory hinging movements at the hips and trunk that help to stabilize posture by keeping the center of gravity away from the fall direction. These early compensatory movements are reversed in PD, causing patients to fall 'like a log' into the perturbation direction. This stiffness during lateral falls may well explain the high incidence of hip fractures in PD. A commonly accepted explanation for this 'inflexibility' is an increased muscle stiffness, which could be caused by rigidity (reflected by tonically enhanced background muscle activity), secondary changes in intrinsic muscle properties or co-contraction of agonist and antagonist muscles.

More recent observations suggest that stiffening could also represent an active and purposely selected compensatory strategy. Voluntary joint stiffening could have certain advantages (Table 11.6). First, stiffening would reduce the degrees of freedom that need to be controlled and thus facilitate postural control. Second, stiffening would maximize stability under relatively static (unperturbed) conditions, for example when standing on the edge of a cliff. Third, for postural perturbations applied to lower body segments (legs or trunk), stiffening would facilitate the biomechanical transmission of the perturbation characteristics to the head and thus improve the sensory detection of the impending fall through the use of visual and vestibular signals. This would be important for PD patients because they rely more on, for example, visual feedback to improve their motor control.[86,87] It is important to note that 'decisions' to stiffen up are made, in particular, by persons that are afraid to fall. Interestingly, stiffening strategies with elements reminiscent of those observed in PD could be induced in healthy subjects that were placed on an elevated platform and asked to make voluntary rises to the toes.[88] Stiffening in these subjects was associated with a physiological arousal and a subjective fear of falling. Parkinsonian patients often have a fear of falling, and this may well contribute to their postural inflexibility.

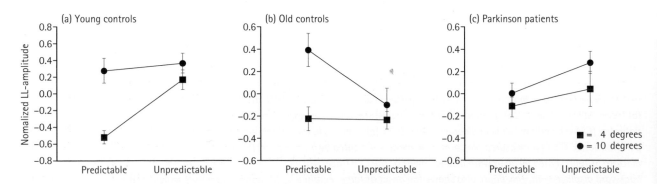

Figure 11.9 *Response amplitude scaling of tibialis anterior long latency (LL) responses for 10 young healthy subjects (a), 13 elderly healthy subjects (b) and 12 patients with Parkinson's disease (c). All subjects were exposed to sudden toe-up rotational movements of supporting forceplate, the size of which could be varied between 4° or 10° amplitude either predictably (serial presentation of identically sized stimuli) or unpredictably (random mix of small and large perturbations). The graphs show the grand mean and SEM for normalized LL response amplitudes for each of the two levels of both independent variables: forceplate amplitude (4° and 10°) and degree of predictability ('predictable' or 'unpredictable'). (Data in this figure were modified from refs 82 and 83, with permission of the publisher.)*

Table 11.8 *Primary disease-related factors (as opposed to the secondary compensatory strategies outlined in Table 11.6) involved in the pathophysiology underlying gait and balance impairment in PD*

Cortical dysfunction	Impaired motor planning
	Difficulty with sequential submovements
	Difficulty set-shifting/'inflexibility'
	Impairment during multiple tasking
	Improper risk assessment
Subcortical deficits	Dopaminergic lesions (substantia nigra)
	Non-dopaminergic lesions:
	adrenergic locus coeruleus
	cholinergic/glutaminergic PPN
	cholinergic basal nucleus of Meynert
	serotonergic raphe nuclei
	nucleus reticularis gigantocellularis
	others
Brainstem involvement	Problems with gait initiation/maintenance
	Abnormal modulation of startle responses
Spinal abnormalities	Reduced reciprocal inhibition
	Increased autogenic inhibition
Sensory processing abnormalities	Impairment of reflex gain control
	Postural 'unawareness'

Pathophysiology

The pathophysiology of gait and balance impairment in PD is complex, for various reasons. Some underlying factors are summarized in Table 11.8.

First, dysfunction occurs at various hierarchical levels of the central nervous system: the cortex, the brainstem and the spinal cord. A reduced excitability of various cortical areas (primary motor cortex, premotor cortex and supplementary motor area) leads to disturbed voluntary motor control (Fig. 11.1). This causes problems in motor planning, such that otherwise preserved motor programs are called up too late, and this is manifested by, for example, gait akinesia.[89] Another problem relates to the impaired ability to run sequential submovements,[16] and this interferes with generating repetitive stepping movements. In addition, various brainstem centers are affected (Fig. 11.3), including alleged locomotor regions in the mesencephalon and various reticular nuclei. Physiological studies suggest that the nucleus reticularis gigantocellularis and nucleus reticularis pontis caudalis are hypoactive in PD, owing to excessive inhibition or abnormal cell loss.[23] The cortical and reticular abnormalities lead, via corticospinal and reticulospinal projections, to secondary changes in spinal interneuronal mechanisms and alpha motor neurons. This includes a reduced reciprocal inhibition and increased autogenic inhibition.[18] This might be the neurophysiological substrate underlying dysfunction of the putative spinal pattern generator and lead to gait akinesia.

Second, there is increasing evidence to suggest that sensory processing abnormalities also contribute to balance and gait problems.[90] It seems as if PD patients incorrectly handle sensory feedback, including proprioceptive, visual and possibly also vestibular cues. This sensory processing deficit presumably relates to dysfunction of the globus pallidus or thalamus, which both receive abundant afferent information. Focal lesions here can induce postural unawareness. Sensory processing abnormalities could explain, for example, the curious observation that patients often appear to be unaware of their stooped posture. Abnormal central processing of somatosensory information might also underlie the disturbed gain control of automatic postural responses and the problems with gait initiation.[91] Finally, it could clarify why difficulty turning around in bed is such a prominent feature of the disease, because rolling over provides massive tactile feedback from the trunk and legs. Some investigators felt that the inability to roll over in bed was a form of apraxia,[92] but we suspect that lack of sensory feedback, combined with an inability to execute the sequential submovements of turning, are more likely explanations.

Third, cognitive deficits and subcortical dementia (bradyphrenia, difficulties in set-shifting and frontal lobe dysfunction) compound the motor problems.[93] This causes problems in planning of adequate motor strategies and partly underlies the difficulty experienced by patients in adapting their postural responses to the actual task at hand.[83] Furthermore, although walking and standing normally require little conscious attention, many patients compensate their balance disorder by using conscious strategies, such as visual cues or mental arithmetic. Such purposeful compensatory strategies fail when concurrent dementia develops (or when psychotropic medication causes cognitive impairment). A particular problem relates to the patients' inability to execute two or more tasks simultaneously (one of them being a balance or gait task). During complex tasks, healthy subjects purposely lend priority to complete certain task components at the expense of others. This strategy, which is chosen particularly if the postural task is perceived as hazardous, has been termed 'posture first'. Parkinson's disease patients have difficulty in employing a 'posture first' strategy, but instead attempt to perform all tasks simultaneously.[37] However, because of their balance impairment and restricted processing resources (conceivably involving frontal lobe dysfunction), neither task is executed very successfully. This 'risky' behavior might well lead to falls in daily life, where dual tasks often play a role.

Fourth, central dopaminergic deficits only partly explain the observed balance and gait problems. Neuropathological and biochemical studies suggest that non-dopaminergic lesions emerge at about the same time as gait and balance problems develop. The most commonly implicated lesions include the adrenergic locus coeruleus and the cholinergic/glutaminergic PPN (Fig. 11.3). Postmortem brain studies identified substantial cell loss within the locus coeruleus, particularly the caudal part that projects mainly to the spinal cord and cerebellum.[23,94] Consistent with this cell loss in the locus coeruleus, various cerebrospinal fluid (CSF) analyses and postmortem brain studies have shown reduced norepinephrine levels in PD. There is a relation between the reduced concentration of norepinephrine and the severity of gait and postural disturbances, and levels of norepinephrine are significantly reduced in PD patients with freezing of gait.[95] Gait abnormalities in PD may also be linked to dysfunction of the PPN due to excessive inhibition from the internal globus pallidus and substantia nigra pars reticulata. Cell loss within the cholinergic portion of the PPN of PD patients further compounds the problem.[96] Finally, considerable loss of pigmented neurons occurs in the nucleus reticularis gigantocellularis and raphe nuclei of patients with PD.[23]

We have mentioned the different compensatory strategies that are used by PD patients to make up for their underlying 'primary' motor deficits (see Table 11.6). This considerably complicates interpretation of the clinical presentation and underlying pathophysiology. The use of external cues to improve gait performance deserves separate mention because this apparently permits patients to bypass their defective basal ganglia circuitry. A possible neuroanatomical explanation is that, for example, the visual cortex can access motor pathways via indirect projections involving the cerebellum, rather than the basal ganglia.[97] Such circuitries could also underlie the phenomenon of kinesia paradoxica.

Table 11.9 *Options to treat gait impairment and postural stability in PD*

Pharmacotherapy	Increase dopaminergic treatment for off-period symptoms
	Consider reducing medication for on-period symptoms
	Eliminate benzodiazepines whenever possible
	Freezing:
	reduce dopaminergic treatment (on-period freezing)
	serotonin reuptake inhibitors
	selegiline
	botulinum toxin into calf muscles
Stereotactic neurosurgery	Young patient with mild and dopa-responsive axial symptoms
	Avoid thalamic surgery and bilateral pallidotomy
Physiotherapy	Practice transfers
	Improve cardiovascular fitness
	Gait training (e.g. use of cues)
	Chaining technique
	Train use of walking aids
	Reduce fear
	Interaction with others
Occupational therapy	Remove domestic hazards?
	Proper footwear
	Walking aids
Other measures	Avoid daily alcohol
	Treat symptomatic orthostatic hypotension
	Electronic warning system
Avoid injuries	Hip or wrist protectors
	Shock-absorbing surface
	Restriction of unsupervised activities
	Treat osteoporosis

Treatment

PHARMACOTHERAPY

Various treatment options are summarized in Table 11.9. The first approach is to carefully evaluate whether the balance and gait problems show any particular relation to the dose cycle. Symptoms that present mainly during off-periods call for an increased dose of antiparkinson medication, and this leads to improvement in some patients.[98] However, the 'axial' features of PD (gait, balance, falls, turning in bed) usually do not ameliorate with antiparkinson medication and are sometimes caused or aggravated by therapy (Table 11.10). Furthermore, dopaminergic therapy can cause dyskinesias or orthostatic hypotension and thus produce falls. Even if antiparkinson medication markedly improves the bradykinesia and rigidity, falls may paradoxically increase because the resultant increase in mobility makes patients more liable to fall. In the appropriate situation it may therefore be necessary to reduce, rather than increase, the dose of antiparkinson medication. Benzodiazepines must be avoided whenever possible.[28]

'Non-dopaminergic' drugs (aimed at correcting adrenergic or cholinergic deficits) have been studied experimentally, but none are available for daily practice. The compound (D)L-threo-dihydroxyphenylserine (DOPS), a synthetic precursor of norepinephrine, has been studied most extensively. It can restore plasma norepinephrine levels in patients with PD,[99] but it is uncertain whether CSF concentrations are also increased. Several investigators reported a beneficial effect of DOPS on various 'non-dopaminergic' manifestations of PD, including freezing, gait impairment, retropulsion and postural instability.[100,101] However, another study found no improvement of gait freezing in a single-dose, placebo-controlled study in six PD patients.[102] Note that most studies were small, poorly controlled and did not objectively quantify the effects.

Paroxysmal gait disorders (freezing and gait festination) require a separate approach. They can develop in patients that have never been treated with levodopa and occur mainly during off-periods in treated patients.[50] These observations suggest that a lack of central

Table 11.10 *Adverse effects of drug therapy on gait and postural stability in Parkinson's disease*

Falls due to drug-induced dyskinesias [a]
Falls due to improved mobility
On-period freezing
Orthostatic hypotension
Leg edema interfering with gait
Blurred vision
Hallucinations/psychosis leading to hazardous behavior
Falls related to benzodiazepines

[a]This includes excessive choreatic movements and, in some patients, dystonic posturing of the feet or trunk (camptocormia).

dopamine is responsible. Indeed, off-period freezing typically improves with dopaminergic drug treatment. Dopamine receptor agonists may aggravate gait freezing, so these are best avoided. Patients with on-period freezing can benefit from a dose reduction of dopaminergic therapy. Occasional patients are helped by selective serotonin reuptake inhibitors such as fluoxetine, possibly via an indirect effect on anxiety. A recent report suggests that selegiline is a good symptomatic treatment, at least early in the course of PD.[50] One uncontrolled study reported improvement of gait freezing following injections of botulinum toxin into calf muscles, perhaps because freezing is a form of dystonia.[103] Finally, poorly controlled studies showed that freezing may improve when central noradrenergic systems are stimulated,[100,101] suggesting a role for underlying non-dopaminergic brain lesions.

STEREOTACTIC NEUROSURGERY

Stereotactic neurosurgery of the basal ganglia is a promising new treatment for PD. Various approaches have been investigated, including different targets (thalamus, internal globus pallidus, or subthalamic nucleus) and different techniques (lesions vs. electrical stimulation; unilateral vs. bilateral interventions). Thalamic surgery may occasionally improve gait in PD, but the risk of postural deficits is considerable, particularly following bilateral approaches.[10] Stereotactic deep brain surgery aimed at the internal globus pallidus or subthalamic nucleus effectively reduces appendicular symptoms (tremor, rigidity and akinesia of the extremities) in advanced PD, but the effects on axial symptoms (gait impairment and postural instability) are less well documented. Gait and postural instability can improve, but clinical experience suggests that these axial symptoms respond less consistently than appendicular symptoms. Bilateral interventions seem more effective than unilateral interventions.[104,105] A problem is that the effects on axial symptoms vary considerably among individual patients, and some patients do not improve at all.[106] Also, the duration of improvement for axial symptoms is shorter than for appendicular symptoms, particularly after pallidotomy or pallidal stimulation. A practical concern is that globus pallidus interventions occasionally aggravate gait and balance impairment, and this risk seems greatest with bilateral approaches. At present, patients with marked gait and balance impairment that respond poorly to antiparkinson medication appear unsuitable candidates for stereotactic neurosurgery. For younger patients with milder axial symptoms that respond well to dopaminergic therapy, deep-brain surgery can be considered.

PHYSIOTHERAPY

There is widespread hope and, indeed, belief that PD patients may benefit from physiotherapy. This is particularly true for the axial signs that respond poorly to pharmacotherapy. Clinical experience and scientific studies (albeit often uncontrolled or inadequately designed) suggest that physiotherapists can teach patients to make safer 'transfers' (e.g. getting in and out of bed), improve cardiovascular fitness and provide gait training.[107] An important role is to facilitate the use of walking aids. Specific designs are available for PD patients, such as the inverted cane. A physiotherapist can also teach patients strategies to improve their gait velocity and to overcome freezing, using visual, rhythmic acoustic or even mental stimuli.[86] Patients can be instructed to avoid dual tasking in daily life and to split complex movements into sequential components that are easier to execute separately ('chaining').[31] However, owing to shortcomings in study design, there is presently little experimental evidence to support (or refute) any beneficial effects of physiotherapy in PD.[108,109] New insights are expected to come from two large clinical trials (the RESCUE study and the PROMISE study).

OCCUPATIONAL THERAPY

Occupational therapists often operate in concert with physiotherapists to achieve similar goals, albeit through different means. Removing domestic hazards is presumably not very effective because most falls in PD are unrelated to environmental circumstances.[28] However, individual patients with obvious extrinsic falls may benefit. Proper footwear with sturdy soles can be recommended. Slightly raised heels may help reduce retropulsion.

OTHER MEASURES

Patients should be asked about the use of walking aids. Some patients refuse to use walking aids because of social embarrassment, whereas others simply put them away because they do not know how to use them. Wheeled rollators occasionally cause or aggravate propulsion because patients with impaired hand function cannot use the handbrakes.

Daily alcohol should be avoided as this increases the risk of falling.[28] Symptomatic orthostatic hypotension is rare in PD, but if present, various therapeutic approaches are possible (see Chapter 16). Patients must be asked about fear of falls and self-confidence in performing everyday activities. Excessive fear leads to unnecessary immobilization, but patients that are overly confident (possibly owing to coexistent cognitive deficits) are at risk of falls resulting from hazardous behavior. In the latter group, the benefit of restricting the patient's activities (which may help to reduce falls) must be weighed against the loss of mobility and independence.

When gait and balance problems become very difficult to treat, the main priority shifts towards prevention of secondary consequences, such as injuries caused by falls. Wearing special hip protectors sewn into undergarments can reduce hip fractures. Note that compliance is often inadequate. Osteoporosis is not uncommon in PD and can be treated in various ways.[71] Patients that are unable to independently stand up after a fall should wear an electronic warning system around the neck or wrist.

OTHER HYPOKINETIC–RIGID SYNDROMES

Progressive supranuclear palsy

Progressive supranuclear palsy (PSP) is a rapidly progressive neurodegenerative disorder of unknown origin characterized, in its complete form, by atypical parkinsonism, supranuclear vertical gaze palsy, pseudobulbar palsy and dementia. The onset is never before the fourth decade. Neuropathological confirmation is required for a definite diagnosis. Development of postural instability and recurrent falls early in the course of the disease are an important feature that help to distinguish PSP from PD.[110,111] In fact, recurrent falls within the first year after disease onset are required for a diagnosis of probable PSP. Postural instability and falls are the most common initial symptom and are particularly frequent when supranuclear vertical gaze palsy also develops (usually several years later). Recurrent falls are more often present at onset of the disease than in any other hypokinetic–rigid syndrome (Table 11.11). Even for patients with an initially preserved balance, falls develop after a shorter latency from onset of first symptoms than in any other hypokinetic–rigid syndrome. However, onset latency to falls overlaps considerably with other conditions, even with PD. Note, for example, that about one-third of patients do not fall within the first year after symptom onset. As a result of this overlap with related conditions, the presence of falls within the first year has an only moderate positive predictive value (68 per cent) for the diagnosis of PSP.[64]

A typical feature is the frequent occurrence of seemingly 'spontaneous' or unprovoked falls and the clear preponderance for backward falls.[115] Falls may also be caused by temporary visual impairment due to blepharospasm. Diplopia can also hamper gait. Patients may fall while climbing or descending stairs because the vertical gaze palsy and retrocollis (neck held stiffly in extension) impairs proper judgment of step height. Injuries appear much more common than in PD, not only because postural instability is more severe, but also owing to 'motor recklessness': many patients with PSP move abruptly and seem unable to properly judge the risk of their actions. The same motor recklessness also underlies the high incidence of car accidents in this disorder. Eventually, the falling frequency tapers off because severely affected patients move only with much assistance or become completely immobilized ('wheelchair sign').

Table 11.11 *Features differentiating gait and balance problems in Parkinson's disease (PD), progressive supranuclear palsy (PSP), multiple system atrophy (MSA), corticobasal degeneration (CBDG) and dementia with Lewy bodies (DLB)*[58,59,64,112–114]

Symptom or sign	PD	PSP	MSA	CBDG	DLB
Presenting symptom[a]					
Postural instability	–	++	MSA-C ++, MSA-P +	+[b]	–
Gait disorder	+	+	+	+	+
Falls within first year	–	++	+	+	–
Symptom at follow-up					
Postural instability	++	+++	+++	+++	
Gait disorder	++	+++	+++	+++	
Falls	++	+++	+++	++	++
Fractures	+	++	+	+	
Wheelchair sign	–	++	+	+	
Falls					
Latency to falls[c]	118 (24–209)	6 (0–156)	24 (0–97)	37 (0–78)	48 (24–287)
Syncopal falls[d]	±	±	+	±	+
Commonest fall direction	Forward	Backward	?	Backward	?
Reckless behavior	±	++	–	-	+
Survival after onset of recurrent falls[c]	73 (8–137)	48 (10 – 114)	27 (12–68)	56 (5–76)	27 (2–97)
Survival predicted by instability or falls	+	+	–	–	
Posture					
Pisa syndrome[e]			++	+	
Retrocollis		++			
Antecollis			++		
Camptocormia	+				
Gait					
Early asymmetry	+	–		++[f]	+
Wide-based stance	–	++	MSA-C ++, MSA-P +	+	–
Reduced arm movements	Asymmetric	–		Asymmetric[f]	Asymmetric
Freezing	+	++[g]	–	+	+
Beneficial effect L-dopa	±	–	±	–	±

Symbols: ?, unknown; –, absent; ±, rare; +, common; ++, very common; +++, nearly always; empty columns indicate that this feature is not described in the literature (possibly because it is rare).
[a]Even more common during the first visit to a clinician.
[b]But rare in one study.[112]
[c]Median (range) in months.[64]
[d]Due to symptomatic orthostatic hypotension.
[e]Including laterocollis.
[f]Often unilateral dystonia, apraxia or myoclonus.
[g]Present earlier and in more severe form compared to Parkinson's disease.
MSA-C, MSA phenotype in which cerebellar features predominate; MSA-P, MSA phenotype in which parkinsonian features predominate.

Standing posture is usually less stooped than in PD. The neck is held stiffly in extension (retrocollis), but this is not an early feature.[59] Axial rigidity of the neck is higher than in the trunk, whereas the opposite pattern occurs in PD.[116] Gait can be relatively normal in an initial stage when falls are already common. When gait does become affected, the pattern resembles severe PD, with some exceptions (there is less asymmetry, the feet are placed more widely apart and the associated arm movements can be preserved). Freezing episodes are very common and, compared with PD, are more severe at early stages of the disease.[49]

Quantified analyses using dynamic posturography revealed a marked reduction of the limits of stability.[117] Patients with PSP were highly dependent on visual feedback, even when this information was incorrect. Whether this is any different from PD remained unclear because there was no control group of Parkinson patients matched for severity of balance impairment. A somewhat unexpected finding was the frequent absence of monosynaptic spinal stretch responses in the lower legs, possibly reflecting involvement of the spinal cord or peripheral nervous system. This does not occur in PD.

Because of the widespread pathology in PSP, it is impossible to pinpoint a particular lesion as being responsible for the postural deficits and falls. The unusually high rate of fractures suggests that 'motor recklessness' (related to frontal dementia) plays a role. In addition, lesions in the cholinergic/glutaminergic PPN have been implicated. In this respect, it is interesting that postural control can improve quite dramatically in occasional patients taking amitriptyline,[118,119] perhaps by correcting the cholinergic deficit caused by cell loss in the PPN or basal nucleus of Meynert. However, these observations must be corroborated by controlled studies involving large numbers of patients. Progressive supranuclear palsy is also characterized by accelerated cell loss in the adrenergic locus coeruleus,[120] and this likely contributes to the treatment-resistant postural disturbances. Involvement of the locus coeruleus may explain the observed therapeutic effects of idazoxan, a selective α_2-adrenoreceptor inhibitor that restores the central norepinephrine deficit. Treatment with idazoxan for 4 weeks in a double-blind crossover study of nine patients with PSP improved clinical ratings of gait and postural instability.[121] Unfortunately, this drug has been withdrawn because of toxicity. Adequate doses of levodopa (up to 1 g/day, if needed) are occasionally effective for a brief period, but most patients have dopa-resistant balance problems. Such patients sometimes benefit from a dopamine receptor agonist. Blepharospasm and neck dystonia (retrocollis) may be alleviated by botulinum toxin injections. Prostheses (crutches) mounted on glasses can also reduce blepharospasm. Some patients benefit from the use of spectacles fitted with prism glasses, which may help to prevent falls related to vertical gaze palsy. Walking aids can be helpful in early stages of the disease. If nothing really helps, the focus should shift to injury prevention, and activities without strict supervision must be avoided. Table 11.12 summarizes the specific problems and therapies in PSP.

Multiple system atrophy

Multiple system atrophy is an adult-onset neurodegenerative disorder of unknown origin, characterized clinically by a variable combination of autonomic failure, parkinsonism, cerebellar ataxia and pyramidal signs. As in PSP, a definite diagnosis can be made only after neuropathological examination. Based upon clinical grounds, MSA can be separated into a phenotype where cerebellar features predominate (MSA-C) and a phenotype where Parkinsonian features predominate (MSA-P). Gait and balance disorders may occur early in the course of both MSA phenotypes (Table 11.11).

They can even be the presenting symptoms, but such patients are more likely to have PSP. During the first visit to a neurologist, postural instability is more often present for patients with the MSA-C phenotype (79 per cent) than for patients with the MSA-P phenotype (30 per cent).[58] This suggests that cerebellar ataxia plays an important role in causing balance and gait problems. Compared with PSP, postural instability and falls are less helpful in distinguishing early stage MSA from PD.[122] In fact, balance impairment and falls are not mandatory to establish a clinical diagnosis of MSA. In many patients, postural instability and falls develop years after onset of the disease. A distinctive feature of MSA is the presence of syncopal falls (due to symptomatic orthostatic hypotension), which occur in about 15 per cent of patients.[58] Such falls are rare in other hypokinetic–rigid syndromes, unless they are caused by coexistent disorders such as cardiac arrhythmia. About half of pathologically proven MSA patients develop a disproportionate antecollis, usually in the middle or late stages of the disease.[57,58] Occasional patients develop antecollis subacutely over a period of 2 weeks. The neck is held in a relatively fixed and severely flexed position, but flexion elsewhere is minimal. This antecollis is not caused by weakness of neck muscles (as in dropping head syndrome), but probably represents a form of dystonia. External correction of head position with braces is therefore unsuccessful.

Patients with the MSA-P phenotype have a shuffling gait with festination and a reduced arm swing, similar to patients with PD. However, in contrast to PD, gait is much more impaired early in the course of the disease.[123,124] Patients with the MSA-C phenotype have an ataxic gait disorder, but gait stance is not necessarily widened. In later stages of the disease, a mixed pattern of hypokinetic–rigid and cerebellar features can be observed. Freezing episodes seem rare in this disorder.[49]

The underlying pathophysiology of postural and gait disorders in MSA has been studied in some detail.[125,126] Histopathological changes are present not only in the basal ganglia (substantia nigra and striatum), but also in the locus coeruleus PPN, cerebellar cortex, pontine nuclei, inferior olives and intermediolateral columns. Of these lesions, putaminal damage correlates best with

Table 11.12 *Specific causes of falls in progressive supranuclear palsy, as well as possible treatment strategies*

Cause	Treatment
Severe postural instability	Levodopa; amitriptyline; walking aids
Blepharospasm	Botulinum toxin; prostheses (crutches) mounted on glasses
Vertical gaze palsy	Spectacles fitted with prism glasses
Diplopia	Eye patch
Retrocollis	Botulinum toxin
Motor recklessness	Restriction of activities

early loss of balance. Pathology involving the olivopontocerebellar pathways may partly explain the gait impairment and falls, particularly in patients with the MSA-C phenotype. However, most patients lack distinctive cerebellar features, suggesting that other lesions are also important. Postural hypotension is associated with degeneration of the intermediolateral cell column.

Antiparkinson medication is generally ineffective, but an adequately dosed levodopa trial (up to 1 g/day, if needed) must always be given because occasional patients respond favorably for several years. A concern is that postural hypotension may increase with levodopa therapy, and MSA patients generally tolerate levodopa less well than patients with PD. As in PSP, some dopa-resistant patients do respond transiently to a dopamine receptor agonist. Symptomatic orthostatic hypotension can be treated using various different approaches (see Chapter 16). Botulinum toxin usually does not alleviate the antecollis and carries the risk of inducing dysphagia.[127]

Corticobasal degeneration

After asymmetrical arm symptoms, mild gait and balance disorders are the second most common presenting symptom of corticobasal degeneration.[113,114] Gait disorders at onset of the disease are rarely severe. The onset of gait symptoms is usually unilaterally. Involvement of one arm is most common and leads to an asymmetrical arm-swing or arm dystonia during walking. Gait may also be affected by asymmetrical leg involvement, such as unilateral leg rigidity or apraxia. Limb myoclonus may occasionally lead to gait or balance problems. Similar to PSP, gait can be broad-based, possibly owing to coexistent ataxia. A frontal gait disorder with freezing and shuffling may develop in later stages of the disease. Other gait features are aspecific and include slowness and small steps. Occasional patients develop laterocollis. Many patients eventually become wheelchair-bound. Some patients have postural instability without specific leg difficulties, suggesting an isolated disturbance of equilibrium. Retrospectively ascertained falls occur in about two-thirds of patients, but this estimate is probably unreliable because some patients also develop dementia. The actual frequency of falls and, in particular, near-falls is therefore likely higher. Patients with symptom onset in the legs develop falls earlier than patients with initial arm symptoms. Falls due to autonomic dysfunction are rare.

Disturbances of balance and gait are less often present during the first visit to a neurologist than in PSP, but eventually develop in almost all patients (Table 11.11). In contrast to PSP, even when patients fall early in the course of the disease, the legs are asymmetrically affected. Similar to MSA, balance impairment and falls are not mandatory to establish a clinical diagnosis of corticobasal degeneration.

Levodopa and other dopaminergic drugs can be helpful initially in about 30 per cent of cases but the effect is not sustained.[113,128] This applies particularly to the gait and balance disorders.

Dementia with Lewy bodies

This disorder classically presents as progressive mental decline with fluctuating cognition and visual hallucinations, as well as a hypokinetic–rigid syndrome. The presence of recurrent falls (at any stage of the disease) is a supportive criterion for the diagnosis.[129] Falls never occur at symptom onset in dementia with Lewy bodies. However, almost 80 per cent of patients eventually fall repeatedly in the course of their disease (Table 11.11). Some falls are related to syncopal attacks. Gait has hypokinetic–rigid features, mainly shuffling with festination.[130] Some patients have a markedly flexed posture.

Little is known about the underlying pathophysiology. Balance and gait impairment are probably caused, in part, by the extrapyramidal signs such as rigidity or bradykinesia. Dopamine depletion in the basal ganglia is equally severe as in PD.[131] In addition, cortical atrophy and cortical Lewy bodies (leading to cognitive deterioration) may contribute to the balance problems.

Levodopa can alleviate the hypokinetic–rigid features, but treatment benefits must be weighed against the risk of exacerbating psychiatric symptoms. Neuroleptics must be avoided because of hypersensitivity. Cholinesterase inhibitors alleviate behavioral disturbances, but motor scores are not improved.

Alzheimer's disease

Patients with Alzheimer's disease are at risk of falls.[132,133] In the study of Buchner and Larson,[133] 17 per cent of patients fell during a 3-year period and an additional 33 per cent lost the ability to walk. Fall rates are even higher among institutionalized patients, where some 78 per cent of patients falls yearly. Furthermore, the fracture rate (involving mainly the hips) is considerably higher than for the general population. Hip fractures in Alzheimer patients invariably lead to nursing home admission.

As in dementia with Lewy bodies, falling is presumably related in part to the behavioral problems. Lack of insight and wandering behavior may explain the unusually high incidence of hip fractures. In addition, concurrent extrapyramidal signs, which are common in otherwise typical Alzheimer's disease,[134] play a role. Patients walk slowly with a shorter step length, a greater step-to-step variability, a reduced armswing and a greater sway path. Simultaneous execution of a secondary task further impairs gait.[135] The gait abnormalities progress as the dementia worsens. A stooped posture is common and static postural sway is increased. Such parkinsonian signs are related to the presence of cell loss, gliosis and Lewy bodies in the substantia nigra, as well as reduction of monoamine metabolites in the cerebrospinal fluid. Cell loss in the nucleus basalis of Meynert and locus coeruleus may also contribute. One study reported that postural and gait abnormalities were associated with decreased frontal cerebral blood flow, as measured with single photon emission computed tomography.[136] Note that the subgroup of Alzheimer patients with concurrent extrapyramidal signs has a poor prognosis, characterized by severe intellectual and functional decline, plus an increased risk of nursing home admission or death.[137] Finally, concurrent illnesses and adverse effects of drugs commonly contribute to falls in Alzheimer's disease.

Treatment of balance and gait disorders in Alzheimer's disease is difficult (Table 11.13). Withdrawing medication (particularly psychoactive and antihypertensive drugs) is nearly always more effective than adding new drugs. A judicious trial of levodopa may be tried in patients with prominent extrapyramidal signs.[138] Neuroleptics often aggravate the extrapyramidal signs and are best avoided. Cholinesterase inhibitors provide modest cognitive improvement. Treatment of any co-morbid illness is important. Restriction of physical activities prevents wandering behavior and thus helps to reduce injurious falls.

Table 11.13 *Treatment options for balance and gait disorders in Alzheimer patients with concurrent extrapyramidal signs*

Withdraw medication whenever possible
Avoid neuroleptics
Consider levodopa
Cholinesterase inhibitors (for cognitive impairment)
Treat co-morbid illnesses
Restrict activities (for wandering behavior)

Vascular 'lower-body half' parkinsonism

'Arteriosclerotic' or vascular parkinsonism is a hypokinetic–rigid syndrome thought to be caused by cerebrovascular disease. Because the symptoms and signs predominate in the legs, this disorder is also referred to as 'lower body' parkinsonism. Vascular parkinsonism can develop acutely or with an insidious onset.[139,140] The acute syndrome mainly involves infarcts in the putamen, globus pallidus or thalamus, whereas the gradual form is associated with diffuse white matter changes.

Lower body parkinsonism classically presents as a shuffling gait with short steps, frequent falls, mild involvement of the upper limbs, absent resting tremor and poor or absent levodopa responsiveness. Typical cases can usually be distinguished from patients with PD (Table 11.14). However, occasional patients with a more atypical clinical presentation can resemble PD (with upper limb involvement) or even PSP.[141,142] A variant involves patients with an exaggerated arm swing and excessive trunk sway, in an apparent attempt to overcome start hesitation. In early stages, diffuse white matter lesions can also cause an isolated 'senile' gait disorder that later progresses to full-blown Binswanger's disease with more incapacitating gait impairment, dementia, spasticity and urinary incontinence.[143–145] Such patients are also at risk of developing other cardiovascular morbidity and mortality.

Most patients fulfil the following inclusion criteria: (1) older than 60 years, because older age at onset favors a vascular cause; (2) parkinsonism (such as rigidity and bradykinesia) predominantly on the lower body, with only mild involvement of the upper limbs; (3) a frontal gait disorder; (4) absent or minimal response to adequate levodopa treatment; (5) neuroradiological evidence of vascular disease (see below); and (6) presence of clear risk factors for cerebrovascular disease. A definite diagnosis of vascular parkinsonism requires postmortem neuropathological examination. Computed tomography and, in particular, magnetic resonance imaging of the brain can reveal cerebrovascular lesions

Table 11.14 *Several differences between 'typical' vascular parkinsonism and idiopathic Parkinson's disease*[144–147]

Feature	Vascular parkinsonism	Parkinson's disease
Base of support	Often wide	Narrow
Posture (knees and trunk)	Upright	Stooped
Festination	Absent	Present
Protective arm movements	Intact	Impaired
Upper motor neuron signs	Present	Absent
Pseudobulbar signs	Common	Uncommon
Involvement of upper body	Absent	Present
Facial involvement	Absent	Present
Vascular co-morbidity and mortality	High	Low
Progression to dementia and urinary incontinence	Yes	No
Response to levodopa	Usually poor	Gratifying

such as white matter changes and lacunar infarcts in the basal ganglia, but such lesions may also coexist in otherwise typical idiopathic PD. Single photon emission computed tomography using the cocaine derivative β-CIT – a ligand with a high-affinity for presynaptic dopamine transporters – reveals preservation of the presynaptic dopaminergic circuitry in the majority of patients, with little overlap with PD.[148]

The pathophysiology underlying vascular parkinsonism is incompletely understood. Mechanisms other than nigrostriatal dopamine loss seem important because pigmented neurons in the substantia nigra are only slightly reduced.[149] Deep periventricular white matter lesions may disrupt the connections between primary motor cortex and supplementary motor cortex with the cerebellum and basal ganglia, thus resulting in 'lower body' parkinsonism.

Timely recognition of vascular parkinsonism during life is important in light of the possibilities for secondary prevention. A trial of adequate levodopa doses should be given because some 25 per cent of patients may improve.[140]

ACUTE VASCULAR LESIONS OF THE BASAL GANGLIA

Acute vascular lesions of the basal ganglia can lead to bilateral lower body parkinsonism.[139,140] In other patients, acute unilateral lesions of the dorsolateral thalamus or globus pallidus may produce gait freezing and severe dysequilibrium, with a falling tendency backwards or contralateral to the lesion ('thalamic or lenticular astasia'). Balance or gait difficulties seem more rare following vascular lesions of the subthalamic nucleus. Upper limb movements are relatively preserved in most patients. Loss of strength is not a major cause of the postural instability, but patients seem to be unaware of their 'drift' to one side, which even occurs when they are seated. This creates an impression as if patients are actively pushing themselves to the side, hence the term 'pusher' syndrome. Some patients have obvious contralateral neglect, but this is not a consistent feature. Patients usually recover over days to months, unless bilateral lesions are present.[4,9] During the recovery period, patients are at risk of sustaining falls.

These observations underscore the prominent somatosensory role played by the basal ganglia (in particular the globus pallidus and thalamus), mainly in relaying afferent feedback back to relevant sensory and motor cortical areas.[90] As stated above, we suspect that a similar 'postural neglect' also plays a role in neurodegenerative disorders such as PD. Interestingly, we have occasionally seen an iatrogenic 'pusher' pattern in PD patients following stereotactic pallidotomy.

Neuroleptic–induced parkinsonism

Patients with neuroleptic-induced parkinsonism have only mild gait impairment. The lower limbs are relatively spared compared with the upper limbs, which usually show tremor. Gait freezing is rare in this disorder. Postural responses are also spared in most patients, not only clinically but also during quantified assessments using dynamic posturography.[150–152] However, axial dystonia such as the Pisa syndrome is not rare, particularly among psychogeriatric patients that are given neuroleptics. This syndrome usually develops within a month after start of neuroleptic treatment and may occur either in isolation or accompanied by drug-induced parkinsonism.[61] Anticholinergics are not helpful, but the dystonia disappears after cessation of neuroleptic treatment.

Akinetic rigid syndrome due to manganese intoxication

Manganese intoxication can result in a syndrome of parkinsonism and dystonia.[153] Classically, these patients tend to walk on their toes (this is called the 'cock-walk'). They often have marked postural instability. Once present, these extrapyramidal findings are likely to be irreversible and even progress after termination of the exposure to manganese. Clinical features are usually sufficient to distinguish these patients from those with PD. Magnetic resonance imaging (MRI) of the brain may reveal signal changes in the globus pallidus, striatum and midbrain. Positron emission tomography (PET) reveals normal presynaptic and postsynaptic nigrostriatal dopaminergic function. The primary site of neurological damage has been shown by pathological studies to be the globus pallidus. The neurological syndrome does not respond to levodopa.

DYSTONIA

Patients with dystonia require specific attention because their gait or balance impairment can be task-specific. For example, patients may have severe gait impairment due to leg dystonia, but can easily walk backwards or even run. This is easily misinterpreted as a psychogenic sign. To complicate matters further, some forms of dystonia concur with psychiatric manifestations (e.g. in Wilson's disease). Dystonia is classified by etiology (primary, where no particular cause can be identified and which is often familial; or secondary due to environmental insult or heredo-degenerative disease), by affected body parts and by age of onset. The dystonic features can be generalized (as in Oppenheim's primary generalized dystonia), segmental (involving one or adjacent contiguous body parts) or focal. Young-onset dystonia tends to spread and generalize, while adult-onset dystonia tends to remain focal or segmental. It is important to distinguish between primary and secondary types of dystonia. Examples of secondary dystonia that were mentioned above include the Pisa syndrome (in patients treated with neuroleptics) and the severe anterocollis of patients with MSA. Patients presenting with primary leg dystonia have a poor overall prognosis because symptoms tend to generalize. In these patients, stiffening due to excessive co-contraction hampers gait and postural stability. In more advanced stages, debilitating contractures secondary to immobilization develop often. Rarely, adult-onset primary dystonia can mainly affect the trunk and sometimes the neck (axial dystonia), but the prognosis in these cases is not bad and the dystonia does not spread to involve the legs.[154] However, axial forms of dystonia, including dystonic scoliosis, hyperlordosis or torticollis, can interfere with walking and standing. This is particularly true if extensor or flexor spasms are present.

It is particularly important to recognize dopa-responsive dystonia, a clinical syndrome of childhood-onset dystonia associated with hypokinetic–rigid features. This autosomal dominant disease typically presents with foot dystonia (equinovarus) or a stiff gait disorder.[155] The leg disability gradually increases over time and postural instability also develops. Progression to generalized dystonia occurs in about 75 per cent of patients, but gait and balance problems remain the primary source of disability. Almost 40 per cent of untreated patients eventually become partly or completely wheelchair-bound. The stiff gait pattern accompanied by postural instability can be difficult to differentiate from juvenile parkinsonism.[156] The symptoms of dopa-responsive dystonia (including gait and balance impairment) usually respond very well to low doses of levodopa. Other drugs (such as anticholinergics or carbamazepine) are less effective.

CHOREA

Choreatic movements can be sufficiently severe to cause postural imbalance and lead to falls. As mentioned earlier, this can be seen in PD due to levodopa-induced dyskinesias which are typically choreic. The classic example of chorea is Huntington's disease. This is an autosomal dominant disorder in which behavioral changes and frontostriatal cognitive impairment (culminating in dementia) occur apart from florid chorea. In his original description of the disease, George Huntington noted that patients may suffer from '… chorea to such an extent that they can hardly walk'.[157] The stepping height and length are irregular because of the unpredictable involuntary movements, leading to frequent stumbling and falls. Stance width is increased. Huntington patients have difficulty adapting their gait to

specific circumstances.[158] Other patients have bizarre stereotypical gait patterns that are sometimes interpreted as psychogenic, particularly in advanced stages of the disease. Dystonia, rigidity and hypokinesia may contribute to balance and gait problems in patients with juvenile onset (less than 20 years of age) or older patients with longstanding disease. Indeed, careful gait analysis reveals PD-like features in most patients, including a reduced gait velocity and a shortened stride length.[158]

Not surprisingly, quantitative analyses indicate that gait variability and postural sway are increased in Huntington's disease.[75,159,160] A disturbed control of automatic postural responses in leg muscles (delayed onset and abnormal size) partially explains the postural abnormalities in Huntington's disease. Patients with Huntington's disease can scale their automatic responses to the postural task at hand, unlike PD patients. Habituation of postural responses is preserved.

Antidopaminergic agents such as neuroleptics can reduce chorea, but often at the expense of worsening voluntary motor performance. The effects of drug therapy on gait and balance have not been studied specifically. It is unknown whether gait rehabilitation is helpful, although expectations are high.

TREMOR

Primary orthostatic tremor

Patients with primary orthostatic tremor can only stand upright for brief periods of time. Posture and balance do not change much objectively, but patients typically report a subjective feeling of increasing instability that develops seconds after assuming quiet stance. Equally characteristic is the disappearance of this feeling when the patient sits down or walks away. Another feature is that patients rarely fall, despite severe subjective instability. Surface electromyograph (EMG) can detect the 16 Hz (range 12–18 Hz) tremor with alternating bursts in antagonistic leg muscles that is pathognomonic of this disease.[161] This particular tremor is often barely visible to the naked eye, although patients may manifest a discernable leg or trunk tremor with a lower frequency. Muscle palpation can readily disclose a fine rapid tremor. Upon prolonged standing, more violent shaking of the legs or trunk can develop.

Electrophysiological examination is essential to detect the 16 Hz tremor and differentiate primary orthostatic tremor from other conditions associated with leg shaking while standing, such as myoclonus, cerebellar ataxia or spastic clonus. Essential tremor has a lower frequency of 6–8 Hz. Electromyograph studies showed that orthostatic tremor can also arise in the upper extremities when patients support their weight with the arms.[161] Power spectrum analysis of body sway during quiet stance on a force platform also reveals a characteristic 16 Hz oscillation.[162] Overall body sway is increased compared with controls but, interestingly, this correlates poorly with subjective ratings of instability.[162,163] During walking, the 16 Hz tremor persists in the trunk and weight-bearing leg, even though subjective instability is absent. Tremor bursts are highly synchronized between homologous muscle groups of both legs (and between the arms and legs when standing on all fours).

The dissociation between objective sway measurements and subjective ratings of unsteadiness formed the basis for an interesting hypothesis about the underlying pathophysiology. Thus, Fung and colleagues[163] speculated that the high-frequency tremor from coherently firing muscles might disrupt proprioceptive feedback from the legs, much like muscle vibration (Fig. 11.10). Patients could compensate for the perceived instability by co-contracting leg muscles, thus hoping to increase stability by stiffening their joints. Indeed, such stiffening strategies are commonly used to compensate for postural instability (Table 11.6). However, because patients can only activate muscles through a frequency of 12–18 Hz, this in turn increases the tremulous feedback and aggravates the subjective unsteadiness. Sitting down or walking away is the only way to disrupt this vicious circle. An attractive element of this hypothesis is that it explains the peculiar discrepancy between severe subjective instability and low frequency of true falls.

Clonazepam or primidone are usually effective in reducing orthostatic tremor.[161] Some patients may respond to levodopa. Unlike essential tremor, propranolol is rarely helpful.

MYOCLONUS

Various disorders of the basal ganglia are characterized by myoclonus, but myoclonus can also occur with lesions in other parts of the central and even peripheral nervous system. Some forms of myoclonus can lead to falls. Two examples in this category include hyperekplexia (startle disease) and myoclonic epilepsy. Both disorders are described in more detail in Chapter 16, which deals with falls owing to (or mimicking) loss of consciousness.

PAROXYSMAL DYSKINESIAS

A separate category involves patients with episodic balance or gait problems due to paroxysmal dyskinesias. There are three main types: paroxysmal exercise-induced dystonia, paroxysmal kinesigenic choreoathetosis and paroxysmal (non-kinesigenic) dystonic choreoathetosis.[164]

Paroxysmal exercise–induced dystonia

Paroxysmal exercise-induced dystonia is characterized by attacks of dystonia that are induced by prolonged exercise, such as walking or running. The attacks typically last up to 2 h, provided that subjects stop exercising. Patients have dystonia, which can be painful, and because the legs or feet are invariably involved, walking becomes difficult. Both legs can be affected simultaneously, whereas involvement of one arm leads to hemidystonia. Occasional patients also have involvement of the lower trunk. Anticholinergics sometimes prevent the attacks, but antiepileptic drugs and levodopa are usually not helpful.

Paroxysmal kinesigenic choreoathetosis

Patients with paroxysmal kinesigenic choreoathetosis have attacks with more complex symptoms, including dystonia, chorea or hemiballismus. Symptoms are usually unilateral. A hallmark is the induction of attacks following sudden (often stereotypical) movements, most commonly rising from a chair. Startle, hyperventilation or exercise may also provoke the attacks. Falls may occur as a result of the unexpected occurrence during self-initiated movements. The disorder is usually familial and starts in childhood or adolescence. Attacks occur frequently, but each individual episode is brief (typically less than two minutes). Antiepileptics (particularly carbamazepine) are usually very effective in preventing paroxysmal kinesigenic choreoathetosis.

Paroxysmal (non–kinesigenic) dystonic choreoathetosis

Paroxysmal (non-kinesigenic) dystonic choreoathetosis also starts in childhood or adolescence, but here the attacks often occur spontaneously. Alcohol, coffee or

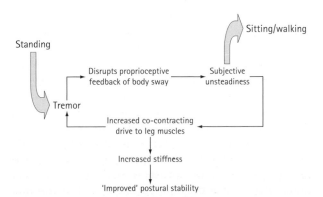

Figure 11.10 *The vicious circle of balance impairment in patients with primary orthostatic tremor, according to Fung et al.[162] This figure was kindly provided by Dr Brian Day.*

emotions may also act as triggers. Symptoms include dystonia, chorea or hemiballismus. Involvement of the legs disturbs gait and may lead to falls. The episodes last much longer than in kinesigenic dystonia (minutes to days), but are less frequent. Familial cases have been linked to a locus on chromosome 2q. In sporadic cases, it is important not to miss underlying disorders such as (vascular) lesions of the basal ganglia.[165] Benzodiazepines can prevent the attacks, but carbamazepine is not usually effective.

'ISOLATED' GAIT AND BALANCE DISORDERS

Senile and cautious gait disorders

The 'senile gait disorder' is an age-related condition characterized clinically by a variable mixture of extrapyramidal features (small and slow steps, *en bloc* turns) and ataxic features (staggering with a wide base).[166,167] Balance reactions can be mildly impaired. Because no apparent cause can be found upon clinical examination, this gait disorder is often regarded as an unavoidable (and untreatable!) feature of the 'normal' aging process.

However, there is increasing evidence to refute this concept. First, many elderly persons continue to enjoy a completely normal gait beyond the eighth decade.[167] Being old and walking poorly are therefore not synonymous. Second, survival analyses suggest that persons with senile gait disorders have an increased mortality compared with age-matched persons whose gait was fully preserved.[145] Cardiovascular disease was the leading cause of death in subjects with senile gait disorders, suggesting that cerebrovascular disease (leukoaraiosis, multiple cerebral infarcts) caused the gait problems. Indeed, seemingly 'idiopathic' senile gait disorders can be the initial manifestation of overt multi-infarct dementia and Binswanger's disease. Furthermore, neuroimaging studies have identified white matter vascular lesions in patients with 'idiopathic' balance or gait disorders.[168] As such, the senile gait disorder can be regarded as a variant of lower body vascular parkinsonism. Third, the senile gait disorder shares many features of what Nutt and colleagues called the 'cautious gait disorder': reduced walking velocity, normal base of support, short steps and turns *en bloc*, without start hesitation, shuffling or freezing.[29] Most persons with a cautious gait have a fear of falls because they perceive some form of postural threat, either internal (an underlying balance disorder) or external (e.g. a slippery floor). It is actually not uncommon for this fear of falls to be disproportional ('fall phobia'), leading to unnecessary immobilization and loss of independence.

Therefore, 'idiopathic' senile gait disorders should not be accepted as an inevitable, benign concomitant of the normal aging process, but rather as a possible marker for underlying disorders. A search for potentially treatable diseases seems warranted, in particular cerebrovascular disorders. Many patients also have concurrent cardiac or other vascular diseases that contribute to the overall mortality.[145] Identification of underlying cardiovascular disorders may have practical implications and strategies of secondary prevention should be considered. There is sufficient time for secondary prevention, as mortality is not increased in the first 5 years after the initial diagnosis of multi-infarct dementia.[143] Although there is no accepted treatment for leukoaraiosis and early multi-infarct dementia, aggressive treatment of hypertension and management of other cardiovascular risk factors may delay or even arrest further physical and mental decline. Perhaps prophylactic treatment with antiplatelet agents should be initiated, but no controlled studies support this. Note that the effects of secondary prevention are difficult to predict in very old subjects, given the complex relation between common risk factors (such as hypertension or cholesterol) and cardiovascular disease in this age group. However, even very old subjects benefit from antihypertensive treatment because this prevents disability from stroke. Finally, subjects should be stimulated to exercise (e.g. by taking daily walks), as this improves overall fitness and decreases cardiovascular morbidity and mortality.

Primary progressive freezing gait ('gait ignition failure')

This disorder mainly occurs in subjects over 60 years of age. Patients present with gradually progressive gait freezing of variable severity, ranging from motor blocks only when confronted with obstacles to being wheelchair-bound.[169] Start hesitation varies from a slightly delayed initiation to a completely frozen state. Mobility of the trunk is reduced while walking, but balance is preserved and patients rarely report falls. Gait is slow and often has a shuffling character because lateral weight shifts are inadequate, but becomes more normal after patients have taken a few steps ('slipped clutch phenomenon'). Patients compensate by using visual cues or by concentrating on walking, so any distraction (e.g. dual tasking) reinstates the underlying gait difficulties. Significantly, the neurological examination is otherwise normal and patients can imitate normal walking movements as long as they are seated or recumbent. Climbing stairs also causes less problems than simple walking on an even surface. Imaging studies of the brain can be entirely normal, but most patients have (often vascular) lesions in the basal ganglia. It is not a pure basal ganglia disorder, because patients can also have cortical atrophy, periventricular white matter abnormalities, or both.[169] The disorder somewhat resembles vascular parkinsonism, but patients do not have excessive vascular risk factors and rarely develop parkinsonism or dementia. Levodopa is generally ineffective, even when prescribed in adequate doses. One patient with isolated akinesia and gait freezing that responded well to levodopa later proved to have Lewy body PD at postmortem examination.[170]

OTHER DISORDERS

Patients with amyotrophic lateral sclerosis may occasionally develop backward falls and retropulsion, even rather early in the course of the disease (within 6 months).[171] Interestingly, lateropulsion or propulsion appears absent. These patients also have mild other extrapyramidal signs in the face or hands. These postural abnormalities seem related to the presence of basal ganglia lesions, including the substantia nigra, locus coeruleus and globus pallidus.

The signs of normal pressure hydrocephalus may relate in part to basal ganglia dysfunction.[172] Patients presenting with a classical triad of a gait disorder with largely preserved arm movements, urinary incontinence and frontal dementia can usually be distinguished without difficulty from PD. However, this distinction can be difficult in more atypical cases. Several helpful distinguishing features are listed in Table 11.15. The increased stance width possibly reflects the severity of the underlying balance deficit, while the reduced foot clearance might be caused by primitive grasp reflexes of the feet. Freezing is not uncommon. Tapping of cerebrospinal fluid helps to improve the gait velocity, but step width remains broad.[48] External visual or auditory cues have only limited benefit in patients with normal pressure hydrocephalus.

Finally, it is useful to realize that hysterical (psychogenic) gait or balance disorders can mimic diseases of the basal ganglia. Examples include dystonia and chorea, or even complete astasia–abasia.[173,174] Camptocormia can occasionally be the sole presentation of a psychogenic balance or gait disorder.

CONCLUSIONS

Disorders of the basal ganglia are closely intertwined with gait and balance impairment. All different categories of basal ganglia disorders can, to a varying extent, affect the ability to walk and stand. A proper diagnosis is often possible, using careful history taking and proper physical examination. Abnormalities of posture, balance and gait can be helpful features in the differential diagnosis of basal ganglia disorders (Table 11.9). Key elements that aid in this differential diagnosis are:

- the nature of the gait or balance disorder;
- the timing of their first appearance in the course of the disease;

Table 11.15 *Comparison of the gait disorder characteristics in Parkinson's disease and normal pressure hydrocephalus (NPH)*[48]

Feature	Parkinson's disease	NPH
Reduced gait velocity	+	++
Reduced stride length	++	++
Reduced cadence	+	+
Increased variability	+	+
Freezing	+	+
Reduced arm movements	+	–
Increased step width	–	+
Outward rotation feet	–	+
Reduced foot clearance	+	++
Reduced range of joint motion in legs	+	++
Stooped posture	+	±
Beneficial effect of external cues	++	±

Symbols: –, absent; ±, rare; +, moderately present; ++, markedly present.

- the associated symptoms and signs; and
- the response to (pharmacological) treatment.

We hope that this chapter provides some useful background information to help clinicians in making this differential diagnosis. Irrespective of the nature of the underlying disease process, the presence of gait and balance impairment has a significant impact on the overall clinical presentation. The quality of life is markedly affected and survival is often significantly reduced. The response to treatment varies considerably among different basal ganglia disorders, some often being nearly resistant to intervention (as in, e.g. PSP), others showing a gratifying therapeutic response (as in, e.g. dopa-responsive dystonia and paroxysmal kinesigenic choreoathetosis). Even when treatment of the underlying condition proves difficult, prevention of fall-associated injuries must be considered.

ACKNOWLEDGEMENTS

We thank Dr D. J. Beckley for his critical comments. Dr J. E. Visser is gratefully acknowledged for this assistance in preparing some of the figures. B. R. Bloem was supported by a research grant of the Prinses Beatrix Fonds.

REFERENCES

1. Bhatia KP, Marsden CD. The behavioural and motor consequences of focal lesions of the basal ganglia in man. *Brain* 1994;**117**:859–76.
2. Langston JW, Ballard JW, Tetrud JW, Irwin I. Chronic parkinsonism in humans due to a product of meperidine-analog synthesis. *Science* 1983;**219**:979–80.

3. Bloem BR, Roos RA. Neurotoxicity of designer drugs and related compounds. In: Vinken PJ, Bruyn GW, Klawans HL, de Wolff FA, eds. *Handbook of clinical neurology, vol. 21 (65): intoxications of the nervous system, part II*. Amsterdam: Elsevier, 1995;363–414.

4. Labadie EL, Awerbuch GI, Hamilton RH, Rapcsak SZ. Falling and postural deficits due to acute unilateral basal ganglia lesions. *Arch Neurol* 1989;46:492–3.

5. Martin JP. *The basal ganglia and posture*. London: Pitman Medical Publishing, 1967.

6. Aizawa H, Kwak S, Shimizu T, et al. A case of adult onset pure pallidal degeneration. Clinical manifestations and neuropathological observations. *J Neurosci* 1991;102:76–82.

7. Volkmann J, Allert N, Voges J, et al. Safety and efficacy of pallidal or subthalamic nucleus stimulation in advanced PD. *Neurology* 2001;56:548–51.

8. Su PC, Tseng HM, Liou, HH. Postural asymmetries following unilateral subthalomotomy for advanced Parkinson's disease. *Mov Disord* 2002;17:191–4.

9. Masdeu JC, Gorelick PB. Thalamic astasia: inability to stand after unilateral thalamic lesions. *Ann Neurol* 1988;23:596–603.

10. Speelman JD. *Parkinson's disease and stereotaxic neurosurgery*. Thesis. Amsterdam: Academic Medical Center, 1991.

11. Parkinson J. *An essay on the shaking palsy*. London: Sherwood, Neely and Jones, 1817.

12. Denny-Brown D. *The basal ganglia, and their relation to disorders of movement*. Oxford: Oxford University Press, 1962.

13. Munro-Davies LE, Winter J, Aziz TZ, Stein JF. The role of the pedunculopontine region in basal-ganglia mechanisms of akinesia. *Exp Brain Res* 1999;129:511–17.

14. Pahapill PA, Lozano AM. The pedunculopontine nucleus and Parkinson's disease. *Brain* 2000;123:1767–83.

15. van Vugt JP, Roos RA. Huntington's disease – options for controlling symptoms. *CNS Drugs* 1999;11:105–23.

16. Marsden CD. The mysterious motor function of the basal ganglia: the Robert Wartenberg Lecture. *Neurology* 1982;32:514–39.

17. Filion M, Tremblay L, Bedard PJ. Abnormal influences of passive limb movement on the activity of globus pallidus neurons in parkinsonian monkeys. *Brain Res* 1988;444:165–76.

18. Delwaide PJ, Pepin JL, de Pasqua V, Maertens de Noordhout A. Projections from basal ganglia to tegmentum: a subcortical route for explaining the pathophysiology of Parkinson's disease signs? *J Neurol* 2000;247(Suppl 2):II/75–81.

19. Hanakawa T, Katsumi Y, Fukuyama H, et al. Mechanisms underlying gait disturbance in Parkinson's disease. A single photon emission computed tomography study. *Brain* 1999;122:1271–82.

20. Masdeu JC, Alampur U, Cavaliere R, Tavoulareas G. Astasia and gait failure with damage of the pontomesencephalic locomotor region. *Ann Neurol* 1994;35:619–21.

21. German DC, Manaye KF, White CL III, et al. Disease-specific patterns of locus coeruleus cell loss. *Ann Neurol* 1992;32:667–76.

22. Pompeiano O. The role of noradrenergic locus coeruleus neurons in the dynamic control of posture during the vestibulospinal reflexes. In: Shimazu H, Shinoda Y, eds. *Vestibular and brain stem control of eye, head and body movements*. Basel: Karger, 1992;91–110

23. Braak H, Rub U, Sandmann-Keil D, et al. Parkinson's disease: affection of brain stem nuclei controlling premotor and motor neurons of the somatomotor system. *Acta Neuropathol (Berl)* 2000;99:489–95.

24. Hoehn MM, Yahr MD. Parkinsonism: onset, progression, and mortality. *Neurology* 1967;17:427–42.

25. Wendell CM, Hauser RA, Nagaria MH, et al. Chief complaints of patients with Parkinson's disease. *Neurology* 1999;52(Suppl 2):A90–1.

26. Bloem BR, Commissaris, DACM. Balance and gait problems in Parkinson's disease. In: Overstall PW, ed. *Falls and bone disease – CD ROM*. Hereford: Kiss of Life Multimedia Ltd, 2002.

27. Gray P, Hildebrand, K. Fall risk factors in Parkinson's disease. *J Neurosci Nurs* 2000;32:222–228.

28. Bloem BR, Grimbergen YAM, Cramer M, et al. Prospective assessment of falls in Parkinson's disease. *J Neurol* 2001;248:950–8.

29. Nutt JG, Marsden CD, Thompson PD. Human walking and higher-level gait disorders, particularly in the elderly. *Neurology* 1993;43:268–79.

30. Smithson F, Morris ME, Iansek R. Performance on clinical tests of balance in Parkinson's disease. *Phys Ther* 1998;78:577–92.

31. Kamsma YPT, Brouwer WH, Lakke JPWF. Training of compensation strategies for impaired gross motor skills in Parkinson's disease. *Physiother Theory Pract* 1995;11:209–229.

32. Nieuwboer A, de Weerdt W, Dom R, et al. Development of an activity scale for individuals with advanced Parkinson disease: reliability and 'on-off' variability. *Phys Ther* 2000;80:1087–96.

33. Bloem BR, Lammers GJ, Overeem S, et al. Outcome assessment of retropulsion tests in Parkinson's disease. *Mov Disord* 2000;15(Suppl. 3):179.

34. Bloem BR, Beckley DJ, van Hilten JJ, Roos RA. Clinimetrics of postural instability in Parkinson's disease. *J Neurol* 1998;245:669–673.

35. Bloem BR, Grimbergen YAM, Cramer M, Valkenburg VV. 'Stops walking when talking' does not predict falls in Parkinson's disease. *Ann Neurol* 2000;48:268.

36. Bond JM, Morris, ME. Goal-directed secondary motor tasks: their effects on gait in subjects with Parkinson disease. *Arch Phys Med Rehabil* 2000;81:110–16.

37. Bloem BR, Valkenburg VV, Slabbekoorn M, van Dijk JG. The Multiple Tasks Test. Strategies in Parkinson's disease. *Exp Brain Res* 2001;137:478–86.

38. Tinetti ME. Performance-oriented assessment of mobility problems in elderly patients. *J Am Geriatr Soc* 1986;34:119–26.

39. Langston JW, Widner H, Goetz CG, et al. Core assessment program for intracerebral transplantations (CAPIT). *Mov Disord* 1992;7:2–13.

40. Ashburn A, Stack E, Pickering R, Ward C. Predicting fallers in a community-based sample of people with Parkinson's disease. *Gerontology* 2001;47:277–81.

41. Bloem BR. *Postural reflexes in Parkinson's disease*. Delft: Eburon, 1994.

42. Horak FB, Frank JS, Nutt JG. Effects of dopamine on postural control in parkinsonian subjects: scaling set, and tone. *J Neurophysiol* 1996;75:2380–96.

43. Dietz V. Neurophysiology of gait disorders: present and future applications. *Electroencephalogr Clin Neurophysiol* 1997;**103**:333–55.

44. Adkin AL, Allum JHJ, Carpenter MG, Bloem BR. Clinical evaluation of postural instability in Parkinson's disease using quantifiable trunk sway measures in freely moving subjects. *Mov Disord* 2000;**15**(Suppl 3):81.

45. Lees AJ. When did Ray Kennedy's Parkinson's disease begin? *Mov Disord* 1992;**7**:110–16.

46. Charlett A, Weller C, Purkiss AG, et al. Breadth of base while walking: effect of ageing and Parkinsonism. *Age Ageing* 1998;**27**:49–54.

47. Giladi N, McMahoon D, Przedborski S, et al. Motor blocks in Parkinson's disease. *Neurology* 1992;**42**:333–9.

48. Stolze H, Kuhtz-Buschbeck JP, Drucke H, et al. Comparative analysis of the gait disorder of normal pressure hydrocephalus and Parkinson's disease. *J Neurol Neurosurg Psychiatry* 2001;**70**:289–97.

49. Giladi, N. Freezing of gait. Clinical overview. *Adv Neurol* 2001;**87**:191–7.

50. Giladi N, Mcdermott MP, Fahn S, et al. Freezing of gait in PD: prospective assessment in the DATATOP cohort. *Neurology* 2001;**56**:1712–21.

51. Giladi N, Treves TA, Simon ES, et al. Freezing of gait in patients with advanced Parkinson's disease. *J Neural Transm* 2001;**108**:53–61.

52. Lamberti P, Armenise S, Castaldo V, et al. Freezing gait in Parkinson's disease. *Eur Neurol* 1997;**38**:297–301.

53. Lewis GN, Byblow WD, Walt, SE. Stride length regulation in Parkinson's disease: the use of extrinsic, visual cues. *Brain* 2000;**123**:2077–90.

54. Schieppati M, Nardone A. Free and supported stance in Parkinson's disease. *Brain* 1991;**114**:1227–44.

55. Kitamura J, Nakagawa H, Iinuma K, et al. Visual influence on center of contact pressure in advanced Parkinson's disease. *Arch Phys Med Rehabil* 1993;**74**:1107–12.

56. Bloem BR, van Dijk JG, Beckley DJ. Are automatic postural responses in patients with Parkinson's disease abnormal due to their stooped posture? *Exp Brain Res* 1999;**124**:481–8.

57. Quinn NP. Disproportionate antecollis in multiple system atrophy. *Lancet* 1989;**i**:844.

58. Wenning GK, Ben-Shlomo Y, Magalhaes M, et al. Clinical features and natural history of multiple system atrophy. An analysis of 100 cases. *Brain* 1994;**117**:835–45.

59. Litvan I, Mangone CA, Mckee A, et al. Natural history of progressive supranuclear palsy (Steele–Richardson–Olszewski syndrome) and clinical predictors of survival: a clinicopathological study. *J Neurol Neurosurg Psychiatry* 1996;**61**:615–20.

60. Martin JP. Curvature of the spine in post-encephalitic parkinsonism. *J Neurol Neurosurg Psychiatry* 1965;**28**:395–400.

61. Yassa R, Nastase C, Cvejic J, Laberge G. The Pisa syndrome (or pleurothotonus): prevalence in a psychogeriatric population. *Biol Psychiatry* 1991;**29**:942–5.

62. Colosimo C. Pisa syndrome in a patient with multiple system atrophy. *Mov Disord* 1998;**13**:607–9.

63. Djaldetti R, Mosberg-Galili R, Sroka H, et al. Camptocormia (bent spine) in patients with Parkinson's disease – characterization and possible pathogenesis of an unusual phenomenon. *Mov Disord* 1999;**14**:443–7.

64. Wenning GK, Ebersbach G, Verny M, et al. Progression of

falls in postmortem-confined parkinsonian disorders. *Mov Disord* 1999;**14**:947–50.

65. Muller J, Wenning GK, Jellinger K, et al. Progression of Hoehn and Yahr stages in Parkinsonian disorders: a clinicopathologic study. *Neurology* 2000;**55**:888–91.

66. Klawans HL, Topel JL. Parkinsonism as a falling sickness. *JAMA* 1974;**230**:1555–7.

67. Wood BH, Bilclough JA, Bowron A, Walker R. 2002. Incidence and prediction of falls in Parkinson's disease – a prospective multidisciplinary study. *J Neurol Neurosurg Psychiatry* 2002;**72**:721–5.

68. Stack E, Ashburn A. Fall events described by people with Parkinson's disease: implications for clinical interviewing and the research agenda. *Physiother Res Int* 1999;**4**:190–200.

69. Bloem BR, van Vugt JP, Beckley DJ. Postural instability and falls in Parkinson's disease. *Adv Neurol* 2001;**87**:209–23.

70. Johnell O, Melton ILJ, Atkinson EJ, et al. Fracture risk in patients with parkinsonism: a population based study in Olmsted County, Minnesota. *Age Ageing* 1992;**21**:32–38.

71. Sato Y, Manabe S, Kuno H, Oizumi K. Amelioration of osteopenia and hypovitaminosis D by 1 alpha-hydroxyvitamin D3 in elderly patients with Parkinson's disease. *J Neurol Neurosurg Psychiatry* 1999;**66**:64–68.

72. Bloem BR, Carpenter MG, Allum JHJ, Honegger F. Trunk control and protective arm responses to multidirectional postural perturbations in Parkinson's disease. In: Duysens J, Smits-Engelsman BCM, Kingma H, eds. *Control of posture and gait*. Maastricht: International Society for Postural and Gait Research, 2001;916–19.

73. Goetz CG, Stebbins GT, Blasucci LM. Differential progression of motor impairment in levodopa-treated Parkinson's disease. *Mov Disord* 2000;**15**:479–84.

74. Morris ME, Iansek R, Matyas TA, Summers JJ. The pathogenesis of gait hypokinesia in Parkinson's disease. *Brain* 1994;**117**:1169–81.

75. Hausdorff JM, Cudkowicz ME, Firtion R, et al. Gait variability and basal ganglia disorders: stride-to-stride variations of gait cycle timing in Parkinson's disease and Huntington's disease. *Mov Disord* 1998;**13**:428–37.

76. van Emmerik RE, Wagenaar RC, Winogrodzka A, Wolters ECh. Identification of axial rigidity during locomotion in Parkinson's disease. *Arch Phys Med Rehabil* 1999;**80**:186–91.

77. Mesure S, Azulay JP, Pouget J, Amblard B. Strategies of segmental stabilization during gait in Parkinson's disease. *Exp Brain Res* 1999;**129**:573–81.

78. Morris ME. Movement disorders in people with Parkinson disease: a model for physical therapy. *Phys Ther* 2000;**80**:578–97.

79. Rogers MW. Disorders of posture, balance, and gait in Parkinson's disease. *Clin Geriatr Med* 1996;**12**:825–45.

80. Bloem BR, Beckley DJ, van Dijk JG, et al. Influence of dopaminergic medication on automatic postural responses and balance impairment in Parkinson's disease. *Mov Disord* 1996;**11**:509–21.

81. Dietz V, Berger W, Horstmann GA. Posture in Parkinson's disease: impairment of reflexes and programming. *Ann Neurol* 1988;**24**:660–9.

82. Beckley DJ, Bloem BR, Remler MP, et al. Long latency postural responses are modified by cognitive set. *Electroencephalogr Clin Neurophysiol* 1991;**81**:353–8.

83. Beckley DJ, Bloem BR, Remler MP. Impaired scaling of long latency postural reflexes in patients with Parkinson's disease. *Electroencephalogr Clin Neurophysiol* 1993;**89**:22–28.

84. Horak FB, Nutt JG, Nashner LM. Postural inflexibility in parkinsonian subjects. *J Neurol Sci* 1992;**111**:46–58.

85. Bloem BR, Beckley DJ, Remler MP, et al. Postural reflexes in Parkinson's disease during 'resist' and 'yield' tasks. *J Neurol Sci* 1995;**129**:109–19.

86. Morris ME, Iansek R, Matyas TA, Summers JJ. Stride length regulation in Parkinson's disease. Normalization strategies and underlying mechanisms. *Brain* 1996;**119**:551–68.

87. Azulay JP, Mesure S, Amblard B, et al. Visual control of locomotion in Parkinson's disease. *Brain* 1999;**122**:111–20.

88. Adkin AL, Frank JS, Peysar GW, Carpenter MG. Fear of falling modifies anticipatory postural control. In: Duysens J, Smits-Engelsman BCM, Kingma H, eds. *Control of posture and gait.* Maastrich: International Society for Postural and Gait Research, 2001;250–3.

89. Rosin R, Topka H, Dichgans J. Gait initiation in Parkinson's disease. *Mov Disord* 1997;**12**:682–90.

90. Wijnberg N, Quinn NP, Bloem BR. Posture in Parkinson patients: a proprioceptive problem? In: Duysens J, Smits-Engelsman BCM, Kingma H, eds. *Control of posture and gait.* Maastricht: International Society for Postural and Gait Research, 2001;758–62.

91. Rogers MW, Chan CW. Motor planning is impaired in Parkinson's disease. *Brain Res* 1988;**438**:271–6.

92. Lakke JPWF. Axial apraxia in Parkinson's disease. *J Neurol Sci* 1985;**69**:37–46.

93. Brown RG, Marsden CD. Dual-task performance and processing resources in normal subjects and patients with Parkinson's disease. *Brain* 1991;**114**:215–31.

94. Hoogendijk WJ, Pool CW, Troost D, et al. Image analyser-assisted morphometry of the locus coeruleus in Alzheimer's disease, Parkinson's disease and amyotrophic lateral sclerosis. *Brain* 1995;**118**:131–43.

95. Tohgi H, Abe T, Saheki M, et al. Concentration of catecholamines and indoleamines in the cerebrospinal fluid of patients with vascular parkinsonism compared with Parkinson's disease patients. *J Neural Transm* 1997;**104**:441–9.

96. Zweig RM, Jankel WR, Hedreen JC, et al. The pedunculopontine nucleus in Parkinson's disease. *Ann Neurol* 1989;**26**:41–6.

97. Manganotti P, Bortolomasi M, Zanette G, et al. Intravenous clomipramine decreases excitability of human motor cortex. A study with paired magnetic stimulation. *J Neurol Sci* 2001;**184**:27–32.

98. Koller WC, Glatt S, Vetere-Overfield B, Hassanein R. Falls and Parkinson's disease. *Clin Neuropharmacol* 1989;**2**:98–105.

99. Azuma T, Suzuki T, Sakoda S, et al. Effect of long-term L-threo-3,4-dihydroxyphenylserine administration on alpha 2-adrenergic receptors in platelet membranes in neurologic disorders. *Acta Neurol Scand* 1991;**84**:46–50.

100. Narabayashi N, Kondo T. Results of a double-blind study of L-threo-DOPS in parkinsonism. In: Fahn S, Marsden CD, Goldstein M, eds. *Recent developments in Parkinson's disease.* New York: Macmillan, 1987;279–91.

101. Tohgi H, Abe T, Takahashi S. The effects of L-threo-3,4-dihydroxyphenylserine on the total norepinephrine and dopamine concentrations in the cerebrospinal fluid and freezing gait in parkinsonian patients. *J Neural Transm Park Dis Dement Sect* 1993;**5**:27–34.

102. Quinn NP, Perlmutter JS, Marsden CD. Acute administration of DL-threoDOPS does not affect the freezing phenomenon in parkinsonian patients. *Neurology* 1984;**34**(Suppl 1):149.

103. Giladi N, Gurevich T, Shabtai H, et al. The effect of botulinum toxin injections to the calf muscles on freezing of gait in parkinsonism: a pilot study. *J Neurol* 2001;**248**:572–6.

104. Kumar R, Lozano AM, Sime E, et al. Comparative effects of unilateral and bilateral subthalamic nucleus deep brain stimulation. *Neurology* 1999;**53**:561–6.

105. Yokoyama T, Sugiyama K, Nishizawa S, et al. Subthalamic nucleus stimulation for gait disturbance in Parkinson's disease. *Neurosurgery* 1999;**45**:41–7.

106. Siegel KL, Metman LV. Effects of bilateral posteroventral pallidotomy on gait of subjects with Parkinson disease. *Arch Neurol* 2000;**57**:198–204.

107. Morris ME, Bruce M, Smithson F, et al. Physiotherapy strategies for people with Parkinson's disease. In: Morris M, Iansek R, eds. *Parkinson's disease: a team approach.* Blackburn: Buscombe Vicprint Ltd, 1997;27–64.

108. de Goede CJT, Keus SHJ, Kwakkel G, Wagenaar RC. The effects of physical therapy in Parkinson's disease: a research synthesis. *Arch Phys Med Rehabil* 2001;**82**:509–15.

109. Deane KHO, Jones D, Playford ED, et al. Physiotherapy versus placebo or no intervention in Parkinson's disease (Cochrane review). In: *The Cochrane Library, issue 2.* Oxford: Update Software, 2001.

110. Daniel SE, de Bruin VMS, Lees AJ. The clinical and pathological spectrum of Steele–Richardson–Olszewski syndrome (progressive supranuclear palsy): a reappraisal. *Brain* 1995;**118**:759–70.

111. Litvan I, Agid Y, Calne D, et al. Clinical research criteria for the diagnosis of progressive supranuclear palsy (Steele–Richardson–Olszewski syndrome): report of the NINDS-SPSP international workshop. *Neurology* 1999;**47**:1–9.

112. Litvan I, Grimes JD, Lang AE, et al. Clinical features differentiating patients with postmortem confirmed progressive supranuclear palsy and corticobasal degeneration. *J Neurol* 1999;**246**(Suppl 2):II/1–5.

113. Wenning GK, Litvan I, Jankovic J, et al. Natural history and survival of 14 patients with corticobasal degeneration confirmed at postmortem examination. *J Neurol Neurosurg Psychiatry* 1998;**64**:184–9.

114. Rinne JO, Lee MS, Thompson PD, Marsden CD. Corticobasal degeneration. A clinical study of 36 cases. *Brain* 1994;**117**:1183–96.

115. Maher ER, Lees AJ. The clinical features and natural history of the Steele–Richardson–Olszewski syndrome (progressive supranuclear palsy). *Neurology* 1986;**36**:1005–8.

116. Tanigawa A, Komiyama A, Hasegawa O. Truncal muscle tonus in progressive supranuclear palsy. *J Neurol Neurosurg Psychiatry* 1998;**64**:190–6.

117. Ondo WG, Warrior D, Overby A, et al. Computerized posturography analysis of progressive supranuclear palsy: a case–control comparison with Parkinson's disease and healthy controls. *Arch Neurol* 2000;**57**:1464–1469.

118. Kvale JN. Amitriptyline in the management of progressive supranuclear palsy. *Arch Neurol* 1982;**39**:387–8.

119. Newman GC. Treatment of progressive supranuclear palsy with tricyclic antidepressants. *Neurology* 1985;**35**:1189–93.

120. Jellinger KA. Pathology of Parkinson's disease. Changes other than the nigrostriatal pathway. *Mol Chem Neuropathol* 1991;**14**:153–197.

121. Ghika J, Tennis M, Hoffman E, et al. Idazoxan treatment in progressive supranuclear palsy. *Neurology* 1991;**41**:986–91.

122. Wenning GK, Ben-Shlomo Y, Hughes A, et al. What clinical features are most useful to distinguish definite multiple system atrophy from Parkinson's disease? *J Neurol Neurosurg Psychiatry* 2000;**68**:434–40.

123. Fearnley JM, Lees AJ. Striatonigral degeneration. A clinicopathological study. *Brain* 1990;**113**:1823–42.

124. Litvan I, Goetz CG, Jankovic J, et al. What is the accuracy of the clinical diagnosis of multiple system atrophy? A clinicopathologic study. *Arch Neurol* 1997;**54**:937–944.

125. Wenning GK, Ben Shlomo Y, Magalhaes M, et al. Clinicopathological study of 35 cases of multiple system atrophy. *J Neurol Neurosurg Psychiatry* 1995;**58**:160–6.

126. Wenning GK, Tison F, Ben Shlomo Y, et al. 1997. Multiple system atrophy: a review of 203 pathologically proven cases. *Mov Disord* 1997;**12**:133–47.

127. Rivest J, Quinn NP, Marsden CD. Dystonia in Parkinson's disease, multiple system atrophy, and progressive supranuclear palsy. *Neurology* 1990;**40**:1571–8.

128. Kompoliti K, Goetz CG, Boeve BF, et al. Clinical presentation and pharmacological therapy in corticobasal degeneration. *Arch Neurol* 1998;**55**:957–61.

129. McKeith IG, Galasko D, Kosaka K, et al. Consensus guidelines for the clinical and pathologic diagnosis of dementia with Lewy bodies (DLB): report of the consortium on DLB international workshop. *Neurology* 1996;**47**:1113–24.

130. Hohl U, Tiraboschi P, Hansen LA, et al. Diagnostic accuracy of dementia with Lewy bodies. *Arch Neurol* 2000;**57**:347–51.

131. Langlais PJ, Thal L, Hansen L, et al. Neurotransmitters in basal ganglia and cortex of Alzheimer's disease with and without Lewy bodies. *Neurology* 1993;**43**:1927–34.

132. Brody EM, Kleban MH, Moss MS, Kleban F. Predictors of falls among institutionalized women with Alzheimer's disease. *J Am Geriatr Soc* 1984;**32**:877–82.

133. Buchner DM, Larson EB. Falls and fractures in patients with Alzheimer-type dementia. *JAMA* 1987;**257**:1492–5.

134. Funkenstein HH, Albert MS, Cook NR, et al. Extrapyramidal signs and other neurologic findings in clinically diagnosed Alzheimer's disease. A community-based study. *Arch Neurol* 1993;**50**:51–6.

135. Camicioli RM, Howieson DB, Lehman S, Kaye JA. Talking while walking. The effect of a dual task in aging and Alzheimer's disease. *Neurology* 1997;**48**:955–8.

136. Nakamura T, Meguro K, Yamazaki H, et al. Postural and gait disturbance correlated with decreased frontal cerebral blood flow in Alzheimer disease. *Alzheimer Dis Assoc Disord* 1997;**11**:132–9.

137. Stern Y, Albert M, Brandt J, et al. Utility of extrapyramidal signs and psychosis as predictors of cognitive and functional decline, nursing home admission, and death in Alzheimer's disease: prospective analyses from the Predictors Study. *Neurology* 1994;**44**:2300–7.

138. Rajput AH, Rozdilsky B, Rajput A, Ang L. Levodopa efficacy and pathological basis of Parkinson syndrome. *Clin Neuropharmacol* 1990;**13**:553–8.

139. Zijlmans JC, Thijssen HO, Vogels OJ, et al. MRI in patients with suspected vascular parkinsonism. *Neurology* 1995;**45**:2183–8.

140. Winnikates J, Jankovic J. Clinical correlates of vascular parkinsonism. *Arch Neurol* 1999;**56**:98–102.

141. Dubinsky RM, Jankovic J. Progressive supranuclear palsy and a multi-infarct state. *Neurology* 1987;**37**:570–6.

142. Hughes AJ, Daniel SE, Kilford L, Lees AJ. Accuracy of clinical diagnosis of idiopathic Parkinson's disease: a clinico-pathological study of 100 cases. *J Neurol Neurosurg Psychiatry* 1992;**55**:181–4.

143. Kotsoris H, Barclay LL, Kheyfets S, et al. Urinary and gait disturbances as markers for early multi-infarct dementia. *Stroke* 1987;**18**:138–41.

144. Thompson PD, Marsden CD. Gait disorder of subcortical arteriosclerotic encephalopathy: Binswanger's disease. *Mov Disord* 1987;**2**:1–8.

145. Bloem BR, Gussekloo J, Lagaay AM, et al. Idiopathic senile gait disorders are signs of subclinical disease. *J Am Geriatr Soc* 2000;**48**:1098–101.

146. Trenkwalder C, Paulus W, Krafczyk S, et al. Postural stability differentiates 'lower body' from idiopathic parkinsonism. *Acta Neurol Scand* 1995;**91**:444–52.

147. Zijlmans JC, Poels PJ, Duysens J, et al. Quantitative gait analysis in patients with vascular parkinsonism. *Mov Disord* 1996;**11**:501–8.

148. Gerschlager W, Bencsits G, Pirker W, et al. [^{123}I]\beta;-SPECT distinguishes vascular parkinsonism from Parkinson's disease. *Mov Disord* 2002;**17**:518–23.

149. Yamanouchi H, Nagura H. Neurological signs and frontal white matter lesions in vascular parkinsonism: a clinicopathologic study. *Stroke* 1997;**28**:965–9.

150. Beckley DJ, Bloem BR, Singh J, et al. Postural reflexes in psychotic patients on long-term neuroleptic medication. *Clin Neurol Neurosurg* 1991;**93**:119–22.

151. Bloem BR, Beckley DJ, van Vugt JP, et al. Long latency postural reflexes are under supraspinal dopaminergic control. *Mov Disord* 1995;**10**:580–8.

152. Hassin-Baer S, Sirota P, Korczyn AD, et al. Clinical characteristics of neuroleptic-induced parkinsonism. *J Neur Transm* 2001;**108**:1299–308.

153. Pal PK, Samii A, Calne DB. Manganese neurotoxicity: a review of clinical features, imaging and pathology. *Neurotoxicology* 1999;**20**:227–38.

154. Bhatia KP, Quinn NP, Marsden CD. Clinical features and natural history of axial predominant adult onset primary dystonia. *J Neurol Neurosurg Psychiatry* 1997;**63**:788–91.

155. Nygaard TG, Marsden CD, Fahn S. Dopa-responsive dystonia: long-term treatment response and prognosis. *Neurology* 1991;**41**:174–81.

156. Jankovic J, Fahn S. Dystonic disorders. In: Jankovic J, Tolosa E, eds. *Parkinson's disease and movement disorders.* Baltimore: Williams and Wilkins, 1998;513–51.

157. Huntington, G. On chorea. *Med Surg Rep* 1872;**26**:320–1.

158. Churchyard AJ, Morris ME, Georgiou N, et al. Gait dysfunction in Huntington's disease: parkinsonism and a disorder of timing. Implications for movement rehabilitation. *Adv Neurol* 2001;**87**:375–85.

159. Huttunen J, Hömberg V. EMG responses in leg muscles to postural perturbations in Huntington's disease. *J Neurol Neurosurg Psychiatry* 1990;**53**:55–62.

160. Tian J-R, Herdman SJ, Zee DS, Folstein SE. Postural stability in patients with Huntington's disease. *Neurology* 1992;**42**:1232–8.

161. Britton TC, Thompson PD, van der Kamp W, et al. Primary orthostatic tremor: further observations in six cases. *J Neurol* 1992;**239**:209–17.

162. Yarrow K, Brown P, Gresty MA, Bronstein AM. Force platform recordings in the diagnosis of primary orthostatic tremor. *Gait Posture* 2001;**13**:27–34.

163. Fung VSC, Sauner D, Day BL. A dissociation between subjective and objective unsteadiness in orthostatic tremor. *Brain* 2001;**124**:322–30.

164. Bhatia KP. The paroxysmal dyskinesias. *J Neurol* 1999;**246**:149–155.

165. Lee MS, Marsden CD. Movement disorders following lesions of the thalamus or subthalamic region. *Mov Disord* 1994;**9**:493–507.

166. Elble RJ, Hughes L, Higgins C. The syndrome of senile gait. *J Neurol* 1992;**239**:71–75.

167. Bloem BR, Haan J, Lagaay AM, et al. Investigation of gait in elderly subjects over 88 years of age. *J Geriatr Psychiatry Neurol* 1992;**5**:78–84.

168. Kerber KA, Enrietto JA, Jacobson KM, Baloh RW. Disequilibrium in older people: a prospective study. *Neurology* 1998;**51**:574–80.

169. Achiron A, Ziv I, Goren M, et al. Primary progressive freezing gait. *Mov Disord* 1993;**8**:293–7.

170. Quinn NP, Luthert P, Honavar M, Marsden CD. Pure akinesia due to Lewy body Parkinson's disease: a case with pathology. *Mov Disord* 1989;**4**:85–89.

171. Desai J, Swash M. Extrapyramidal involvement in amyotrophic lateral sclerosis: backward falls and retropulsion. *J Neurol Neurosurg Psychiatry* 1999;**67**:214–16.

172. Curran T, Lang AE. Parkinsonian syndromes associated with hydrocephalus: case reports, a review of the literature, and pathophysiological hypotheses. *Mov Disord* 1994;**9**:508–20.

173. Keane JR. Hysterical gait disorders: 60 cases. *Neurology* 1989;**39**:586–9.

174. Sinel M, Eisenberg MS. Two unusual gait disturbances: astasia abasia and camptocormia. *Arch Phys Med Rehabil* 1990;**71**:1078–80.

12

Spastic movement disorders

VOLKER DIETZ

INTRODUCTION

Spasticity produces numerous physical signs. These have little relationship to the patient's disability, which is caused by impairment by a movement disorder. On the basis of the clinical signs, a widely accepted conclusion was drawn for the pathophysiology and treatment of spasticity: exaggerated reflexes are responsible for muscle hypertonia and, consequently, the movement disorder. Drug therapy is therefore usually directed at reducing the activity of stretch reflexes. The function of these reflexes during natural movements and the connection between exaggerated reflexes and movement disorder is frequently not considered. This chapter focuses on the pathophysiological basis of spastic movement disorder in children and adults with the therapeutic consequences and current drug therapy. The physiological changes during the transition from spinal shock to spasticity after an acute spinal cord injury will be discussed first.

FROM SPINAL SHOCK TO SPASTICITY

More than 100 years ago the term 'spinal shock' was introduced to describe the clinical state in patients with acute spinal cord injury (SCI) presenting muscle paralysis with flaccid muscle tone and loss of tendon reflexes below the level of lesion.[1] Although complete loss of sensorimotor function persists, spinal shock ends after some weeks and during the following months a 'spastic syndrome' develops with exaggerated tendon reflexes, increased muscle tone and involuntary muscle spasms. The development of a spastic syndrome is a common finding in surgically or pathologically confirmed complete spinal cord transection (i.e. changes in the excitability of spinal cord neuronal circuits occur independently of supraspinal influences).[2] In a recent study clinical and electrophysiological parameters were systematically assessed in patients after an acute SCI.[3]

The period of spinal shock is electrophysiologically associated with a reduced excitability of alpha-motoneurons (MN) reflected by a low persistence of F-waves (the F-wave results from the antidromic excitation of MN following supramaximal electrical stimulation of a peripheral nerve), which is in line with previous studies.[4,5] This observation may be related to the clinical signs found at this stage: the loss of tendon reflexes and muscle hypotonia. The neurophysiological basis of the reduced alpha-MN excitability may result from the sudden loss of tonic input and/or trophic support from supraspinal to spinal neuronal centers.

In contrast to the neuronal depression reported above, H-reflexes can be elicited at an early stage after SCI,[3] which is in accord with earlier reports.[6-8] The discrepancy between preserved H-reflex and the loss of tendon reflexes as a typical clinical sign might at least partly be due to a reduced activity of gamma-MN.

While H-reflex was present early and F-wave persistence was low (but usually F-waves could be recorded), there was a loss of flexor reflex activity in the tibialis anterior (TA) early after SCI.[3] The latter observation indicates a suppression of interneuronal (IN) activity mediating this polysynaptic reflex (for review see ref. 9).

The recovery from spinal shock is clinically reflected by an increase in the excitability of tendon tap reflexes and in muscle tone (assessed by the Ashworth scale) as well as more frequently occurring muscle spasms (assessed by the Penn spasm frequency scale).[3] These clinical changes were associated in electrophysiological recordings with an increase in F-wave persistence and flexor reflex activity.[3] There was only a minor change in H-reflex excitability during this period. It may be suggested that the increase in tendon tap reflex excitability is at least partly due to a recovery of alpha-MN and probably also of gamma-MN function mediating this reflex. There was also an increase in flexor reflex activity which should not only be due to recovery of alpha-MN excitability, but also to the resolving depression of spinal interneuronal function. The pathway underlying the flexor reflex is a polysynaptic spinal one and allows the integration of inputs from muscles, joints and cutaneous afferents on common interneurons.[9]

The changes in flexor reflex excitability may be at least partly reflected in the appearance of muscle spasms. The increase in muscle tone may be caused by a more general recovery of spinal neuronal (alpha-MN and IN) activity. Nevertheless, for both clinical parameters reflecting recovery from spinal shock (Penn spasm frequency and Ashworth scale)[3] it cannot be ruled out that factors other than the neuronal activity described here, as well as changes of muscle biomechanics, contribute to the development of spasticity.

Clinically, the development of the spastic syndrome is characterized by exaggerated muscle tendon tap reflexes, increased muscle tone and involuntary muscle contractions. The onset of spastic signs is difficult to determine because there is a smooth transition to a clearly established spasticity.

During this stage, both M-wave and flexor reflex amplitudes remained about stable in tetraplegic or decreased in amplitude in paraplegic patients (i.e. developed even opposite to the clinical signs).[3] A slight increase of H/M ratio, which was in line with an earlier study,[10] might contribute to exaggerated tendon tap reflexes. However, a correlation of this increase with the spastic state must be considered cautiously: (1) the high H/M ratio can express a decrease of M-wave rather than an increase in reflex excitability; (2) short latency reflex hyperexcitability was shown to be little related to spastic muscle tone.[11]

The fact that the decrease of M-wave and flexor reflex amplitude was more pronounced in paraplegic than in tetraplegic patients indicates that several weeks after an SCI, secondary degenerations of spinal tracts occur including pre-motoneuronal circuits and alpha-MN. Direct damage of alpha-MN as an underlying cause is rather unlikely because M-wave amplitude increases up to the fourth week after SCI. Therefore, secondary degenerations are likely to depend on the level of lesion (i.e. are less pronounced with higher level of lesion). The phenomenon of transynaptic degeneration of alpha-MN due to degeneration of terminal synapses on a cell after SCI was claimed earlier.[12]

On the basis of the observations made in the study of Hiersemenzel and co-workers[3] clinical signs of increasing spasticity, such as muscle tone and spasms, can hardly be related to the electrophysiological recordings. Secondary changes of motor units might contribute to

the syndrome of spasticity, especially in respect to muscle tone and spasms (see below).

CENTRAL PROGRAMS AND REFLEXES DURING SPASTIC MOVEMENT

The neuronal regulation of functional movements, such as gait, is achieved by a complex interaction of spinal and supraspinal mechanisms: the rhythmic activation of leg muscles by spinal interneuronal circuits is modulated and adapted to the actual needs by a multisensory afferent input. The spinal programming as well as the reflex activity are under supraspinal control. Disturbances of this supraspinal control lead to characteristic gait impairments seen in cerebellar and extrapyramidal disorders as well as in spastic paresis (for review see ref. 13).

The electrical leg muscle activity which results from a close interaction between these different mechanisms, is transferred to a functionally modulated muscle tension by the mechanical muscle fiber properties.[14]

Several findings suggest that the central programming in spastic patients is basically preserved. Gait analysis[12] shows that neither the timing nor the reciprocal mode of activation of the antagonistic leg muscles differs between healthy subjects and patients with severe spasticity. A similar observation was made for the compensatory leg muscle activation following feet displacement during stance:[15] the timing of the triphasic pattern, which is assumed to be centrally programmed,[16] is preserved in patients with spastic paresis.

Exaggerated reflexes are frequently thought to be responsible for the spastic movement disorder, without considering the functional significance of the different reflex mechanisms involved in the regulation of complex movements. The analysis of the compensatory responses following feet displacement during stance in patients with spastic hemiparesis shows that in the unaffected leg, small monosynaptic reflex potentials are followed by a strong polysynaptic electromyographic response; in the spastic leg, the monosynaptic reflex potential is larger but the functionally essential polysynaptic reflex response, however, is absent.[15,17] The overall activity of the spastic muscle is reduced compared with the healthy muscle, despite exaggerated monosynaptic reflexes

REFLEX EFFECTS AND SPASTIC MUSCLE TONE

In patients with spastic hemiparesis a different tension development of triceps surae takes place during the stance phase of gait;[17] in the unaffected leg the tension development correlates with the modulation of electromyographic activity (the same is true in healthy subjects), while in the spastic leg, tension development is connected to the stretching period of the tonically activated (with small electromyographic amplitude) muscle (see Fig. 12.1). There is no visible influence of mono-synaptic reflex potential on muscle tension.

Investigations of functional movements in spastic patients have led to the conclusion that spastic muscle tone can hardly be explained by an increased activity of motoneurons. Instead, a transformation of motor units occurs, with the consequence that regulation of muscle tension takes place on a lower level of neuronal organization.[11,18] Such a transformation of motor units is functionally meaningful, since it enables the patient to support the body weight during gait; fast active movements, however, become impossible. A time interval of several weeks between the occurrence of an acute stroke and the development of spastic muscle tone is needed for such a muscle transformation.[19]

There are additional findings that support the suggestion that changes in the mechanical muscle fiber properties occur in spasticity: (1) contraction times in hand muscles[20] as well as in the triceps surae[21] are prolonged; (2) torque motor experiments applied to the triceps surae indicate a peripheral contribution to spastic muscle tone;[22] (3) histochemistry and morphometry of spastic muscle reveal specific changes of muscle fibers.[19,23]

SPECIFIC ASPECTS OF GAIT DISORDER IN CHILDREN WITH CEREBRAL PALSY

As in spastic adults, studies on children with cerebral palsy were frequently restricted to physical signs of spas-

ticity.[24-26] This may also be due to the fact that about half of the children with cerebral palsy could not yet walk at an age of 6 years.[27]

The leg-muscle activity during functional movements, such as locomotion, of children with congenital cerebral palsy has characteristic signs of impaired maturation of the normal gait pattern.[28] The pattern recorded in children with cerebral palsy of around 10 years of age mainly consists of a coactivation of antagonistic leg muscles during the stance phase of a gait cycle and a general reduction in electromyograph (EMG) amplitude. In contrast, when the cerebral lesion is acquired at a later stage and the reciprocal mode of leg muscle activity is already established (i.e. at around 4 years), reciprocal activation of antagonistic leg muscles is preserved during spastic gait.

Although neurophysiological studies indicate that muscle tone in children with cerebral palsy represents an inhomogeneous condition,[24] there are typical features, such as the coactivation of all antagonistic leg muscles during the stance phase of gait, associated with a reduced and tonic mode of leg extensor muscle activation (starting before ground contact), and the appearance of isolated electromyographic potentials after ground contact.[29] These potentials are probably monosynaptic stretch reflex potentials mediated by group I afferents, since they appear with a short latency after the onset of gastrocnemius stretch. This pattern closely resembles the pattern of stepping in newborn infants.[29-31] Also, a myotatic reflex irradiation, usually observed in children with cerebral palsy, is present in non-disabled infants under 2 years of age.[32-34] Both an abnormal corticospinal

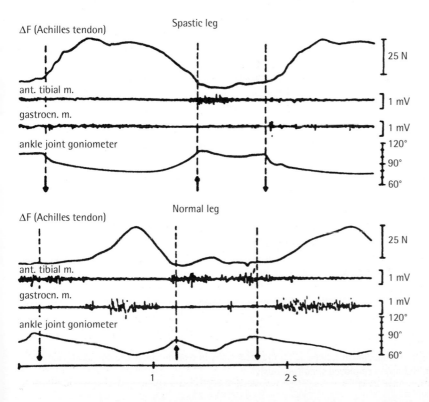

Figure 12.1 *Gait recordings of a step cycle during slow gait of a patient with spastic hemiparesis; the spastic leg is shown above and normal one below. From top to bottom in each recording: changes in tension recorded from the Achilles tendon, tibialis anterior and gastrocnemius electromyographs, potentiometer signal of the ankle joint. Vertical lines with arrows indicate touch down and lift up of the foot. Reproduced from* J Neurol Neurosurg Psychiatry, *1984,* **47,** *1029–33, with permission from the BMJ publishing group.*

input and a deficient modulation of spinal interneuronal circuits with impairment of reciprocal inhibition may contribute to the coactivation pattern.[35,36]

From 4 years of age onwards, the monosynaptic reflex potentials disappear, the polysynaptic reflex response becomes more phasic and stronger, and a reciprocal mode of leg muscle activation becomes established. These changes represent a shift from the predominance of the rigid and functionally ineffective monosynaptic stretch reflexes to that of the polysynaptic spinal reflexes. According to kinematographic analysis, this shift is reflected in a stick-like usage of the legs in the early stage of stepping, while in older children the body is rolled off over the standing leg.

Little is known about the natural evolution of cerebral palsy. There are only a few controlled studies documenting the positive effect of a treatment or training program.[37,38] It appears that children with cerebral palsy have a delayed development of infant stepping and supported locomotion, and fail to develop the plantigrade gait.

DRUG THERAPY OF SPASTICITY

Drug therapy should usually be restricted to immobilized patients, as the reduction of spastic muscle tone is associated with paresis (i.e. is achieved on the cost of muscle power).

As a rule, the use of only one substance at a time is recommended, at least to begin with. There are patients that do best with modest doses of two medications which have different modes of action (baclofen and tizanidine, for example) so combination therapy may eventually be necessary. Because relief of spasms and muscle hypertonia may only be achieved at the cost of reduced muscle power, doses (see Table 12.1) should be kept to minimum effective levels, especially in mobile patients. Almost all antispastic drugs may induce side-effects, often consisting of drowsiness and nausea (for synopsis, see Table 12.2).

Drugs of first choice

The best antispastic effects are reported for baclofen, tizanidine and benzodiazepines (e.g. clonazepam). Therefore, these are the drugs of first choice for spastic patients. They are most effective in spasticity of spinal origin such as with multiple sclerosis and traumatic or neoplastic spinal cord lesions.[39]

Baclofen acts as a γ-amino butyric acid (GABA)-B agonist on a spinal level pre- and post-synaptically (less so on the former compared with the latter).

Table 12.1 *Dosage in drug therapy for spasticity*

Substance	Tablets	Beginning	Increase	Maximal
Primary choice				
Baclofen	5, 10, 25 mg	2 × 5 mg/day	2 × 5 mg/week	4 × 20 mg up to 150 mg
Clonazepam	0.5, 2 mg	2 × 0.5 mg/day	3 × 0.5 mg/week	3 × 2 mg
Secondary choice				
Tizanidine	2, 4, 6 mg	3 × 2 mg/day	4–8 mg/week	24 mg/day
Clonidine	0.075, 0.15, 0.3 mg	2 × 0.075 mg/day	0.075 mg/week	3 × 0.15 mg/day
Diazepam	2, 5, 10 mg	2 × 2 mg/day	2 × 4 mg/week	c. 3 × 20 mg
Tetrazepam	50 mg	1 × 25 mg/day	25 mg/day	4 × 50 to 8 × 50 mg
Memantine	10 mg	1 × 10 mg/day	2 × 10 mg/week	3 × 20 mg
Dantrolene	25, 50 mg	2 × 25 mg/day	2 × 25 mg/week	4 × 5 to 4 × 100 mg

Table 12.2 *Side-effects in drug therapy for spasticity*

Drug	Side-effects
Common effects	Sedation, drowsiness, nausea, muscle weakness
Baclofen	Nausea, vomiting, diarrhea, psychosis and confusion (also after sudden withdrawal), ataxia, depression of respiratory and cardiovascular systems, headache (especially when kidneys are malfunctioning)
Tizanidine or clonidine	Arterial hypotension (especially when hypotensive therapy is simultaneously performed), mouth dryness, indigestion
Clonazepam or diazepam	Increased appetite, loss of libido, impaired menstruation, ataxia potentiated with alcohol; long-term effects: dependency, development of tolerance, sleeplessness, timidity, hallucinations
Memantine	Agitation, pressure in the head, mouth dryness; contraindication: patients with liver dysfunction, confusion, pregnancy
Dantrolene	Nausea, vomiting, anorexia, diarrhea, hepatic failure (especially in women above the age of 35 years or when estrogen therapy is employed simultaneously)

Monosynaptic stretch reflexes are depressed more effectively than polysynaptic reflexes but flexor spasms are particularly reduced. Baclofen can also alleviate pain, particularly painful spasms, in patients with spasticity.[40] Baclofen should be introduced slowly because of possible induction of drowsiness and hallucinations. It should be withdrawn slowly so as not to produce a rebound increase in spasms (see Tables 12.1 and 12.2).

Tizanidine is an imidazoline derivative closely related to clonidine. Both are thought to act on α_2-adrenergic receptors in spasticity of supraspinal origin. It is suggested that these substances reduce the activity of polysynaptic reflexes, in many ways similar to the action of baclofen.[41,42] Clonidine and tizanidine also have effects upon the cord which are generally inhibitory; in part at least, they reduce the release of glutamate (and perhaps other excitatory amino acids). Clonidine and presumably tizanidine produce marked inhibition of short latency responses in alpha-MN to group II activity in the spinal cat.[43] Tizanidine also results in non-opiate analgesia by actions on α_2-receptors in the spinal dorsal horn which inhibit release of substance P. This would diminish flexor reflex afferent (FRA)-mediated actions. Thus, it comes as no surprise that clonidine alleviates spastic dystonia and reduces the frequency and severity of spasms in patients with spinal cord injury.[44]

Benzodiazepines (e.g. clonazepam) amplify the inhibitory action of GABA-A at a pre- and post-synaptic level. Thereby, excitatory actions become dampened with a negative rebound. It is believed that increasing presynaptic inhibition in the spinal cord of patients with spasticity should reduce the release of excitatory transmitters from afferent fibers and thereby reduce the gain of monosynaptic and polysynaptic stretch reflexes and flexor reflexes. One can assume that these compounds work directly on the spinal cord.[45] For diazepam, serious side-effects such as development of tolerance, dependency and drowsiness are reported.[39] These side-effects are somewhat less pronounced with clonazepam. Again, withdrawal must occur slowly (see Tables 12.1 and 12.2). Cumulative effects were observed with diazepam and other benzodiazepines that have longer half-lives.

Drugs of second choice

Memantine represents an amantadine derivative which seems to act primarily as an N-methyl-D-aspartate (NMDA)-receptor antagonist.[46] A few studies report efficacy on spasticity following brain lesions.

Glycine reduces experimentally induced hypertonia in animals because of its inhibitory action on neurons in the central nervous system. Oral administration of the simple amino acid glycine can alleviate the symptoms of spasticity. Similarly, an antispastic effect was described for L-threonine,[47] which is thought to modify spinal glycinergic transmission.

Cannabinoids may have significant beneficial effects on spasticity in a dosage (5 mg) which is well below the amount that induces altered states of consciousness.[48,49] On the basis of animal experiments they are thought to attenuate mono- and polysynaptic reflexes.

Dantrolene acts primarily in the muscle itself, producing peripheral paresis because it reduces release of calcium ions from the sarcoplasmic reticulum, thereby preventing activation of the contractile apparatus. It is effective in all forms of spasticity because of its peripheral target. The use of dantrolene is restricted because its generalized paretic effects are frequently not well tolerated by patients.[50] In addition, severe side-effects such as toxic liver necrosis are reported, especially in women above the age of 35 years and when used in combination with estrogen.

Recently, gabapentin was shown to have a beneficial effect on spastic symptoms in patients with multiple sclerosis.[51]

EFFECT OF LOCOMOTOR TRAINING IN PARAPLEGIC PATIENTS

The aim of several recent studies was to show that the degree to which locomotor electromyographic activity and movements can be both elicited and trained in leg muscles of complete and incomplete paraplegic patients.[52,53] The induction of complex bilateral leg muscle activation combined with coordinated stepping movements in incomplete and complete paraplegics was achieved by partly unloading (up to 60 per cent) patients that were on a moving treadmill. The leg movements had to be assisted from externally during the first phases of the training in the incomplete paraplegic patients (Fig. 12.2) and during the whole training period (3–5 months) in all complete paraplegic patients. Compared with healthy subjects, paraplegic patients displayed a less dynamic mode of muscle activation. This may be due to the impaired function of polysynaptic and monosynaptic spinal reflexes in patients with a spinal lesion.[12] In other respects, such as the timing, the pattern of leg muscle electromyographic activity was similar to that seen in healthy subjects. Different amplitude levels of leg extensor (the main antigravity muscle during gait) electromyographic activity occurred in the different subject groups which largely exceeded the inter-individual variability. The amplitude level of electromyographic activity was considerably smaller in complete compared with the incomplete paraplegics and in the latter group compared with the healthy subjects. Despite the reduced level of electromyographic activity spastic symptoms (e.g. increased muscle tone, exaggerated reflexes) were present in both patient groups. This underlines earlier notions claiming that alterations of mechanical muscle fiber properties of the tonically active muscle are mainly

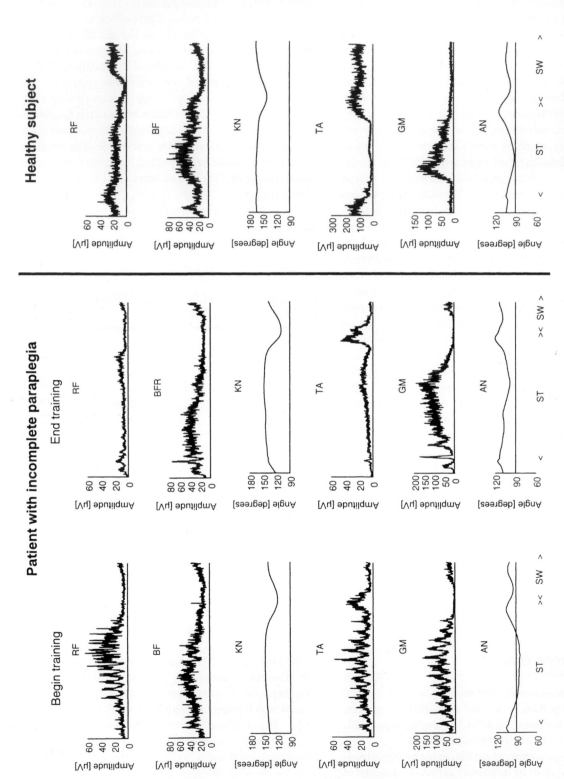

Figure 12.2 Rectified and averaged (n = 20) electromyographic activity of lower and upper leg muscles during slow locomotion (around 1.3 km/h) of a healthy subject (right) and an incompletely paraplegic patients (left). For the patient the recordings at the beginning and after a daily performed locomotor training over 5 months are displayed. The amount of unloading for the healthy subject was 40 of 80 kg. RF, rectus femoris; BF, biceps femoris; KN, knee joint; TA, tibialis anterior; GM, gastrocnemius medialis; AN, ankle joint; ST, stance; SW, swing phase. (Reproduced from Dietz V, Colombo G, Jensen L, Baumgartner L. Locomotor capacity of spinal cord in paraplegic patients. Ann Neurol 1995;**37**:574–82, Copyright © 1995 John Wiley & Sons, Inc. Reprinted by permission of John Wiley & Sons, Inc.)

responsible for the clinical signs of spasticity. Restoration of gait in non-ambulatory patients with hemiparesis has been achieved by such training with partial body-weight support.[54,55]

During the course of a daily locomotor training program, the amplitude of gastrocnemius electromyographic activity increased significantly during the stance phase, while an inappropriate tibialis anterior activation decreased. These training effects were seen in both groups, incomplete and complete paraplegic patients. This was related to a greater weight-bearing function of the extensors. The slope of increase was similar in incomplete and complete paraplegics. This indicates that the isolated human spinal cord contains the capacity not only to generate a locomotor pattern, but also 'to learn'. Nevertheless, apart from positive effects upon, for example the cardiovascular and musculoskeletal systems, only incomplete paraplegic patients benefited from the training program with respect to the performance of unsupported stepping movements on solid ground.[52,53] In comparison with leg extensor EMG, only a small effect of training on leg flexor EMG amplitude was seen, which may be due to a differential neuronal control of leg flexor and extensor muscles during locomotion. The successive reloading of the body during the training may serve as a stimulus for extensor load receptors, which have been shown to be essential for leg extensor activation during locomotion in cat[56] and humans.[57,58] The lower gain of the extensor EMG in complete paraplegic patients may be due to a loss of input from descending noradrenergic pathways to spinal locomotor centers.[59]

CONCLUSIONS

The spastic movement disorder is usually thought to result from exaggerated stretch reflexes. As a consequence, therapeutic measures aim largely to reduce reflex activity. However, physiological investigations of functional movements (e.g. gait) have revealed that the disinhibition of the monosynaptic reflexes is accompanied by a loss of the functionally essential polysynaptic spinal reflexes. Overall electromyographic activity in leg muscles during gait is reduced. The centrally programmed reciprocal activation of antagonistic leg muscles is preserved. Development of tension by the calf muscles is normally determined by modulated gastrocnemius activity. In the spastic leg, calf muscle tension is associated with the stretching of the tonically activated muscle. It is concluded that a central (cerebral or spinal) lesion, associated with paresis, is followed by a transformation of motor units such that tension development in the muscles is basically changed. This regulation of muscle tension is efficient in so far as it enables the patient to support body weight during stance and gait. Recent studies indicate that spinal locomotor centers can also be activated and trained in paraplegic patients. Patients with incomplete paraplegia profit from the training program in that their walking ability on a stationary surface is improved.

REFERENCES

1. Bastian HC. On the symptomatology of total transverse lesions of the spinal cord, with special reference to the condition of the various reflexes. *Med Chir Trans (Lond)* 1890;**73**:151–217.
2. Kuhn R. Functional capacity of isolated human spinal cord. *Brain* 1950;**73**:1–51.
3. Hiersemenzel LP, Curt A, Dietz V. From spinal shock to spasticity: neuronal adaptation to a spinal cord injury. *Neurology* 2000;**54**:1574–82.
4. Leis AA, Stetkarova I, Beric A, Stokic DS. The relative sensitivity of F wave and H reflex to changes in motoneuronal excitability. *Muscle Nerve* 1996;**19**:1342–4.
5. Curt A, Keck ME, Dietz V. Clinical value of F-wave recordings in traumatic cervical spinal cord injury. *Electroencephalogr Clin Neurophysiol* 1997;**105**:189–93.
6. Diamantopoulos E. Excitability of motor neurones in spinal shock in man. *J Neurol Neurosurg Psychiatry* 1967;**30**:427–31.
7. Weaver R, Landau W, Higgins J. Fusimotor function. Part 2: evidence of fusimotor depression in human spinal shock. *Arch Neurol* 1963;**9**:127–32.
8. Ashby P, Verrier M, Lightfoot E. Segmental reflex pathways in spinal shock and spinal spasticity in man. *J Neurol Neurosurg Psychiatry* 1974;**37**:1352–60.
9. Lundberg A. Multisensory control of spinal reflex pathways in reflex control of posture and movement. In: Granit R, Pompeiano O, eds. *Progress in brain research*, Vol 50. Amsterdam: Elsevier, 1979;12–28.
10. Faist M, Mazevet D, Dietz V, Pierrot-Deseilligny E. A quantitative assessment of presynaptic inhibition of Ia afferents in spastics. Differences in hemiplegics and paraplegics. *Brain* 1997;**117**:1449–55.
11. O'Dwyer NJ, Ada L. Reflex hyperexcitability and muscle contracture in relation to spastic hypertonia. *Curr Opin Neurol* 1996;**9**:451–5.
12. Dietz V, Quintern J, Berger W. Electrophysiological studies of gait in spasticity and rigidity. Evidence that altered mechanical properties of muscle contribute to hypertonia. *Brain* 1981;**104**:431–49.
13. Dietz V. Human neuronal control of functional movements. Interaction between central programs and afferent input. *Physiol Rev* 1992;**72**:33–69.
14. Gollhofer A, Schmidtbleicher D, Dietz V. Regulation of muscle stiffness in human locomotion. *Int J Sports Med* 1984;**5**:19–22.
15. Berger W, Horstmann GA, Dietz V. Spastic paresis: impaired spinal reflexes and intact motor programs. *J Neurol Neurosurg Psychiatry* 1988;**51**:568–71.
16. Dietz V, Quintern J, Sillem M. Stumbling reactions in man: significance of proprioceptive and pre-programmed mechanisms. *J Physiol (Lond)* 1987;**386**:149–63.
17. Berger W, Horstmann GA, Dietz V. Tension development and muscle activation in the leg during gait in spastic

hemiparesis: the independence of muscle hypertonia and exaggerated stretch reflexes. *J Neurol Neurosurg Psychiatry* 1984;**47**:1029–33.

18. O'Dwyer NJ, Ada, L, Neilson PD. Spasticity and muscle contracture following stroke. *Brain* 1996;**119**:1737–49.

19. Dietz V, Ketelsen UP, Berger W, Quintern J. Motor unit involvement in spastic paresis: relationship between leg muscle activation and histochemistry. *J Neurol Sci* 1986;**75**:89–103.

20. Young JL, Mayer RF. Physiological alterations of motor units in hemiplegia. *J Neurol Sci* 1982;**54**:401–12.

21. Dietz V, Berger W. Inter-limb coordination of posture in patients with spastic paresis: impaired function of spinal reflexes. *Brain* 1984;**107**:965–78.

22. Sinkjaer T, Toft E, Larsen K, et al. Non-reflex and reflex mediated ankle joint stiffness in multiple sclerosis patients with spasticity. *Muscle Nerve* 1993;**16**:69–76.

23. Edström L. Selective changes in the size of red and white muscle fibres in upper motor lesions and Parkinsonism. *J Neurol Sci* 1970;**11**:537–50.

24. Brown JK, Rodda J, Walsh EG, Wright GW. Neurophysiology of lower-limb function in hemiplegic children. *Dev Med Child Neurol* 1991;**33**:1037–47.

25. Brouwer B, Wheeldon RK, Stradiotto-Parker N, Allum J. Reflex excitability and isometric force production in cerebral palsy: the effect of serial casting. *Dev Med Child Neurol* 1998;**40**:168–75.

26. Lin JP, Brown JK, Brotherstone R. Assessment of spasticity in hemiplegic cerebral palsy. II: Distal lower-limb reflex excitability and function. *Dev Med Child Neurol* 1994;**36**:290–303.

27. Trahan J, Marcoux S. Factors associated with the inability of children with cerebral palsy to walk at six years: a retrospective study. *Dev Med Child Neurol* 1995;**36**:787–95.

28. Berger W, Quintern J, Dietz V. Pathophysiological aspects of gait in children with cerebral palsy. *Electroencephalogr Clin Neurophysiol* 1982;**53**:538–48.

29. Dietz V, Berger W. Cerebral palsy and muscle transformation. *Dev Med Child Neurol* 1995;**37**:180–4.

30. Forssberg H, Wallberg H. Infant locomotion: a preliminary movement and electromyographic study. In: Berg K, Eriksson BD, eds. *Children and exercise. IX International series on sport sciences.* Baltimore: University Park Press, 1980;32–49.

31. Leonard CT, Hirschfeld H, Forssberg H. The development of independent walking in children with cerebral palsy. *Dev Med Child Neurol* 1991;**33**:567–77.

32. Leonard CT, Hirschfeld H. Myotatic reflex responses of non-disabled children and children with spastic cerebral palsy. *Dev Med Child Neurol* 1995;**37**:783–99.

33. Mykleburst BM, Gottlieb GL, Agarwal GC. Stretch reflexes of the normal infant. *Dev Med Child Neurol* 1986;**28**:440–9.

34. O'Dwyer NJ, Neilson P, Nash J. Reduction of spasticity in cerebral palsy using feedback of the tonic stretch reflex: a controlled study. *Dev Med Child Neurol* 1994;**36**:770–86.

35. Brouwer B, Smits E. Corticospinal input onto motor neurons projecting to ankle muscles in individuals with cerebral palsy. *Dev Med Child Neurol* 1996;**38**:787–96.

36. Leonard CT, Moritani T, Hirschfeld H, Forssberg H. Deficits in reciprocal inhibition of children with cerebral palsy as revealed by H-reflex testing. *Dev Med Child Neurol* 1990;**32**:974–84.

37. Tardieu C, Lespargot A, Tabary C, Bret MD. For how long must

the soleus muscle be stretched each day to prevent contracture? *Dev Med Child Neurol* 1988;**30**:3–10.

38. McLaughlin JF, Astley SJ, Bjornson KF, et al. Selective dorsal rhizotomy: Efficacy and safety in an investigator masked randomized clinical trial. *Dev Med Child Neurol* 1998;**40**:220–32.

39. Glenn MB, Whyte J. *The practical management of spasticity in children and adults.* Philadelphia and London: Lea & Febiger, 1990.

40. Hattab JR. Review of European clinical trials with baclofen. In Feldman RG, Young RR, Koella WP, eds. *Spasticity: disordered motor control.* Chicago: Year Book Publishers, 1980;71–85.

41. Bes A, Eyssette M, Pierrot-Deseilligny E, et al. A multi-centre, double-blind trial of tizanidine, a new antispastic agent, in spasticity associated with hemiplegia. *Curr Med Res Opin* 1988;**10**:709–18.

42. Stien R, Nordal HJ, Oftedal SI, Slettebo M. The treatment of spasticity in multiple sclerosis: a double-blind clinical trial of a new antispastic drug tizanidine compared with baclofen. *Acta Neurol Scand* 1987;**75**:190–4.

43. Schomburg ED, Steffens H. The effect of DOPA and clonidine on reflex pathways from group II afferents to alpha-motoneurons in the cat. *Exp Brain Res* 1988;**71**:442–6.

44. Shefner JM, Berman SA, Sarkarati M, Young RR. Recurrent inhibition is increased in patients with spinal cord injury. *Neurology* 1992;**42**:2162–8.

45. Davidoff RA. Antispasticity drugs: Mechanisms of action. *Ann Neurol* 1985;**17**:107–16.

46. Seif el Nasr M, Peruche B, Rossberg C, et al. Neuroprotective effect of memantine demonstrated *in vivo* and *in vitro. Eur J Pharmacol* 1990;**185**:19–24.

47. Lee A, Patterson V. Double-blind study of L-threonine in patients with spinal spasticity. *Acta Neurol Scand* 1993;**88**:334–8.

48. Meinck H-M, Schönle PW, Conrad B. Cannabinoids on spasticity and ataxia in multiple sclerosis. *J Neurol* 1989;**236**:120–2.

49. Maurer M, Henn V, Dittrich A, Hofmann A. Delta-9-tetrahydrocannabinol shows antispastic and analgesic effects in a single case double-blind trial. *Eur Psychiatr Clin Neurosci* 1990;**240**:1–4.

50. Anderson TP. Rehabilitation of patients with completed stroke. In: Kottke FJ, Stillwell GK, Lehmann JF, eds. *Krusen's handbook of physical medicine and rehabilitation*, 3rd edn. Philadelphia: WB Saunders, 1982;583–603.

51. Cutter NC, Scott DD, Johnson JC, Whiteneck G. Gabapentin effect on spasticity in multiple sclerosis: a placebo-controlled, randomized trial. *Arch Phys Med Rehabil* 2000;**81**:164–9.

52. Dietz V, Colombo G, Jensen L. Locomotor activity in spinal man. *Lancet* 1994;**344**:1260–3.

53. Dietz V, Colombo G, Jensen L, Baumgartner L. Locomotor capacity of spinal cord in paraplegic patients. *Ann Neurol* 1995;**37**:574–82.

54. Hesse S, Bertelt Ch, Schaffrin A, et al. Restoration of gait in nonambulatory hemiparetic patients by treadmill training with partial body-weight support. *Arch Phys Med Rehabil* 1994;**75**:1087–93.

55. Hesse S, Helm B, Krajnik J, et al. Treadmill training with partial body weight support: Influence of body weight release on the gait of hemiparetic patients. *J Neurol Rehabil* 1997;**11**:15–20.

56. Pearson KG, Collins DF. Reversal of the influence of group Ib-

afferents from plantaris on activity in medial gastrocnemius muscle locomotor activity. *J Neurophysiol* 1993;**7**:1009–17.

57. Dietz V, Gollhofer A, Kleiber M, Trippel M. Regulation of bipedal stance: dependency on 'load' receptors. *Exp Brain Res* 1992;**89**;229–31.

58. Harkema, SJ. Requejo PS, Hurley SL, et al. Human lumbosacral

spinal cord interprets loading during stepping. *J Neurophysiol* 1997;**77**:797–811.

59. Barbeau H, Rossignol S. Enhancement of locomotor recovery following spinal cord injury. *Curr Opinion Neurol* 1994;**7**:517–24.

13

Frontal and higher level gait disorders

PHILIP D. THOMPSON AND JOHN G. NUTT

THE CONCEPT OF FRONTAL AND HIGHER LEVEL GAIT DISORDERS

Experimental studies of locomotion in quadrupeds indicate a prominent role of brainstem structures and spinal cord networks. The role of the cerebral cortex appears relatively small compared with that of subcortical structures, although the cortex and corticospinal tract are important for adept placement of the feet during locomotion. The applicability and scope for any generalization of these studies to human bipedal locomotion has frequently been questioned. This conundrum is well illustrated by the concept of frontal and higher level gait disorders. Experimental models of locomotion do not predict the complex range of gait disturbances encountered in diseases of the frontal lobes and the subcortical circuits connecting the frontal lobes, basal ganglia, cerebellum and brainstem. The mechanisms of these gait disturbances are poorly understood, and in many cases it is simply the association with frontal pathology that leads to the designation 'frontal gait disorder'. As a result, the nomenclature and classification of frontal gait disorders remains the subject of debate.[1] The term 'higher level' gait disorder has also been used to describe gait disorders associated with disease of the frontal lobes and their connections, distinguishing these gait patterns from middle-level disorders caused by lesions of the corticospinal tracts (paraparesis or hemiparesis), the cerebellum (ataxia), or basal ganglia (parkinsonian and dyskinetic gaits) and lower level disorders affecting the peripheral neuromuscular apparatus.[1]

Frontal gait disorders are estimated to account for 20–30 per cent of cases of significant walking difficulties in the elderly,[1,2] although they may occur at any age.

CLINICAL SIGNS OF FRONTAL GAIT DISORDERS

The clinical features of frontal gait disorders are characterized by variable combinations of disequilibrium, locomotor (stepping) abnormalities and difficulties with gait ignition (Table 13.1).

Initial complaints are often non-specific, with a slowing of walking speed and general loss of walking efficiency, and the diagnosis may not be suspected in the early stages. The patient may report that extra effort is required to initiate stepping or maintain normal stride length and stepping while walking. There may be a subtle loss of the normal fluidity of body motion; leg movements appear stiff and turning may be accomplished *en*

Table 13.1 *Summary of clinical features of a frontal gait disorder*

Upright trunk posture
Wide stance base
Start hesitation
Short shuffling steps
Slow walking speed
Stiff leg movement
Exaggerated arm swing
Freezing
Impaired or aberrant postural reflexes
Falls

bloc. These early symptoms can be interpreted as a loss of the normal automatic control of leg and trunk movement during walking and a requirement for additional voluntary effort to maintain locomotion. In other cases, the initial symptoms may be unsteadiness and imbalance, with the need for greater care to avert the threat of falls. There may be little to find on examination in these early stages except for a subtle loss of the normal fluency of walking, but no other definite abnormal neurological signs.

As the gait disorder evolves, imbalance and unsteadiness become more pronounced and the stance base becomes slightly wider than normal. The initiation of walking is hesitant, with a series of short shuffling steps (start hesitation). Once underway, the stride lengthens but is shorter than normal. A burst of small shuffling steps may interrupt the normal stepping rhythm. Freezing (sudden cessation of stepping) and shuffling may occur spontaneously but typically appear when turning a corner, encountering an obstacle, or with distraction and diversion of attention away from the task of walking. During walking, the normal rhythmic flow of trunk and limb motion is lost. Unlike parkinsonism, arm swing is normal or even exaggerated, reminiscent of a 'military two-step' gait. There may be exaggerated lateral sway of the trunk with each step.

With progression of the underlying condition, start hesitation, shuffling and unsteadiness become more pronounced. Gait ignition becomes increasingly difficult with repetitive small foot movements that fail to initiate a step (the slipping clutch phenomenon) progressing to the 'magnetic foot' in which the feet are stuck to the floor and cannot be moved while standing. Exaggerated upper truncal movement and arm swing may be employed to shift the body weight to one side and free the opposite foot, allowing the leg to swing forward and step. Postural and righting reactions are impaired, either slowed or inappropriate, causing unsteadiness while standing and walking. On attempting to rise from sitting, the legs may extend before being positioned under the body. When standing, the trunk may hyperextend. The loss of normal postural responses is a common cause of falls, particularly backwards, when arising from a seated position, attempting the first step, encountering an unexpected obstacle while walking or experiencing the slightest postural perturbation. With support, the patient may be able to take a step, but once underway shuffling becomes even more pronounced, with hesitant and disorganized steps. Festination, as seen in Parkinson's disease, is unusual. A few steps of propulsion or retropulsion prompt the patient to seek support of nearby objects or to sit down because they may fall. Fear of falling may lead to additional slowness and caution when walking and avoidance of crowded areas or open spaces. Patients occasionally adopt a crouched flexed posture of the trunk in an effort to compensate for the disequilibrium.

In contrast to the difficulty using the legs to step and walk while standing, patients may be able to move their legs with greater facility when seated or lying supine.[3,4] The patient may be able to mimic stepping movements of the legs when lying or seated and some can propel themselves in a wheelchair with bilateral alternating movements of the legs. Other leg movements such as bicycling may also appear relatively preserved compared with the difficulty walking. However, close examination usually reveals slowness in the initiation of complex and repetitive movement and movement execution is clumsy.[4] This is most evident when performing repetitive sequences of movement such as bilateral alternating movements of the legs and feet, but simple leg movements such as drawing a number on the floor with the foot or kicking an imaginary ball may also be performed poorly. There may also be a degree of heel–shin ataxia although this is generally not as marked as that associated with cerebellar ataxia.

With further progression, postural responses, truncal control and balance are increasingly disrupted and falls are common. Clinical observations on the evolution of dysequilibrium in patients with frontal gait disorder suggest this is partly related to a progressive loss of control of truncal posture and declining truncal mobility. Consequently, the capacity for independent lower limb movement, as in stepping, is compromised when the trunk cannot be stabilized. This situation resembles the 9- to 15-month-old infant who is capable of stepping movements but cannot do so to walk because of poor truncal control. Conversely, the inability to make steps of normal size interferes with attempts to recover from postural perturbations by stepping, leading to more falls.

The disorder of truncal balance progresses with increasing loss of truncal mobility, making standing and walking impossible. Poor control of truncal movements may interfere with the ability to sit in a chair or turn over while lying in bed.

Facial expression and upper limb movement may be relatively normal. Upper motor neuron signs are variably present. Frontal release signs, such as grasp reflexes, may be accompanied by other signs of frontal lobe disease, including slowing of cognitive and motor responses, rigidity or gegenhalten, perseveration, slowness in initiating and difficulty maintaining repetitive upper limb or hand movements and urinary incontinence.

DIFFERENTIAL DIAGNOSIS

The major difficulties in diagnosis arise in the early stages of a frontal gait disorder. The clinical presentation may be mistaken for Parkinson's disease when the disorder of stepping predominates or a cerebellar syndrome when unsteadiness is the major complaint. Eventually, with disease progression, both features are evident in frontal gait disorder. Several clinical clues are useful in differentiating between these conditions and are supported by the results from kinematic analyses of gait discussed below. Prominent start hesitation, shuffling and freezing, wide stance base, falls, lower half predominance with sparing of the upper limb movement and facial expression are valuable clues to the diagnosis of a frontal gait disorder. The preservation of arm swing and excessive lateral movements of the trunk during walking are further signs of a frontal gait disorder. In addition, the presence of upper motor neuron signs including a pseudobulbar palsy and the failure to respond to levodopa distinguish this syndrome from Parkinson's disease. A resting tremor is uncommon in frontal gait disorder.

When unsteadiness and imbalance are prominent, the presence of shuffling steps, start hesitation and impaired postural reactions suggest a frontal gait disorder rather than a cerebellar ataxia. Falls are more common in frontal gait disorder. A combination of ataxia, parkinsonism and falls also may occur in multiple system atrophy. Parkinsonism in multiple system atrophy is generalized without the lower body predominance seen in frontal gait disorder. Magnetic resonance imaging can be helpful in distinguishing between these conditions by demonstrating atrophy of the cerebellum in cerebellar degenerations, putaminal atrophy in multiple system atrophy, frontal lobe disease or hydrocephalus in frontal gait disorders.

When falls and disequilibrium are the presenting feature the differential diagnosis includes Steele–Richardson–Olszewski syndrome with characteristic vertical supranuclear gaze palsy, a feature not seen in frontal gait disorder.

QUANTITATIVE ANALYSIS OF FRONTAL GAIT DISORDERS

Detailed kinematic analysis of frontal gait disorders caused by subcortical arteriosclerotic encephalopathy reaffirm these clinical observations. During gait initiation, the early postural shifts transferring weight towards the supporting leg, that are necessary to allow the stepping or stride limb to swing into motion, were more variable in amplitude and direction than in normal, elderly age-matched, subjects.[5] Instead of phasic patterns of muscle activation in gastrocnemius, vastus lateralis and hamstrings at the initiation of gait, tonic muscle activity was observed, perhaps contributing to the flexed 'stiff' leg posture and restricted leg movement. Activation of tibialis anterior, heralding the shift of body weight as gait begins was also more variable. These effects lead to a delay in the transition from standing to walking. The abnormal postural adjustments contributed to a delay in the transition from standing to walking and were accompanied by several unsuccessful attempts to start walking. Voluntary attempts to

compensate for faulty postural mechanisms and prevent a possible fall lead to further interruption of the normal sequence at gait initiation. Overall, it was concluded that impaired postural control was a significant factor in the delayed gait initiation.[5] In a study of Parkinson's disease, subcortical arteriosclerotic encephalopathy and cerebellar ataxia, slow walking speeds and short steps were observed in all groups, but an increased variability in the amplitude and timing of steps emphasized the ataxic elements in the last two.[6]

Patients with hydrocephalus walk slowly with short steps, widened base and increased body sway.[7–9] All measures, particularly increased body sway are improved by ventricular drainage.

Functional imaging (using $^{15}O_2$ positron emission tomography) revealed focal hypometabolism of the medial frontal lobes in two cases in whom a frontal gait disturbance was the initial feature of Alzheimer's disease and corticobasal degeneration.[10]

CAUSES OF FRONTAL GAIT DISORDERS

The commonest conditions causing a frontal gait disorder are subcortical arteriosclerotic encephalopathy (Binswanger's disease) and hydrocephalus (Table 13.2). The gait disturbance in these conditions can be very similar[11] and clinical recognition of the underlying cause is greatly simplified by magnetic resonance imaging of the brain.

Table 13.2 *Causes of a frontal gait disturbance*

Multiple lacunar infarcts (Binswanger's disease)
Anterior cerebral artery infarction
Hydrocephalus
Frontal lobe tumors (glioma, meningioma)
Demyelination (multiple sclerosis)
Corticobasal degeneration
Subdural hematoma
Fronto-temporal dementia
Infections (encephalitis, abscess)

Subcortical arteriosclerotic encephalopathy

The typical features of Binswanger's disease include a history of stroke or repeated stroke-like episodes, a stepwise evolution and the accumulation of neurological deficits. Upper motor neuron signs and pseudobulbar palsy often accompany the gait disturbance. It is increasingly recognized that many patients do not have an obvious history of strokes or a stepwise course. Nevertheless, imaging, particularly magnetic resonance imaging discloses numerous, often confluent, areas of altered signal in the periventricular and subcortical white matter of the

Table 13.3 *Terms used to describe the clinical features of frontal and higher gait disorders*

Magnetic apraxia
Slipping clutch phenomenon
Marché à petits pas
Arteriosclerotic parkinsonism
Lower-half parkinsonism
Lower-body parkinsonism
Parkinsonian ataxia
Frontal ataxia
Gait apraxia
Trepidant abasia
Astasia–abasia

cerebral hemispheres consistent with small-vessel ischemia. Descriptions of this clinical picture include 'marché à petits pas',[12] 'arteriosclerotic parkinsonism',[13] 'lower half parkinsonism',[11] 'parkinsonian ataxia',[11] and 'lower body parkinsonism'[14] (Table 13.3).

Hydrocephalus

A gait disturbance is a well-recognized presenting feature of hydrocephalus and may occur before cognitive changes or incontinence develop. The evolution of the gait disturbance with progression of hydrocephalus may be striking.[15] Initially, the gait appears ataxic and hypokinetic. Later, increasing difficulty initiating stepping and 'magnetic feet' appear to be accompanied by loss of truncal balance. The latter may become so severe the patient is unable to sit. Early intervention with ventricular drainage and shunting may reverse these features.

With advancing hydrocephalus, the clinical deficits may extend beyond a gait disorder to include soft speech and a marked reduction in spontaneous movement, with a loss of normal facial expression. Mutism ('akinetic mutism') and other frontal lobe release signs are often associated features.[16]

In several descriptions of the parkinsonism that may accompany hydrocephalus, upper body parkinsonism with typical resting tremor have been described in addition to ataxia and lower-half parkinsonism.[17] In some cases, the parkinsonism has been levodopa responsive, suggesting additional structural or functional disruption of the nigrostriatal system.[17,18]

Other causes of frontal gait disorders

A frontal gait disorder may be the presenting feature of corticobasal degeneration and other cortical degenerations.[10,19] Frontal lobe tumors, or other mass lesions such as an abscess, encephalitis and demyelination may also present with a frontal gait disturbance. In some cases there is no clinical or imaging evidence of any underlying abnormality and a degenerative frontal lobe disorder is postulated.

NATURE OF THE DISTURBANCE IN FRONTAL GAIT DISORDERS

Many descriptions of the gait accompanying frontal lobe disease focus on specific but different elements of the complex gait disturbance (Table 13.3). These reports, highlighting fragments of the clinical picture of a frontal gait disorder, serve to emphasize the variation in clinical presentation of a frontal gait disturbance.

Early descriptions of frontal gait syndromes emphasized the ataxic elements (referred to as frontal ataxia or frontal dysequilibrium). Involvement of frontoponto-cerebellar pathways was considered the most likely mechanism.[20] Subsequently, the relative preservation of leg movements when lying or sitting, in contrast to the difficulties walking, prompted the designations gait apraxia and truncal apraxia.[21] Denny Brown[3] postulated that mesial frontal lobe disease released grasp reflexes in the feet and 'tonic innervation', resulting in the feet being 'glued' to the floor (magnetic apraxia). Meyer and Barron[4] defined gait apraxia as 'the loss of ability to properly use the lower limbs in the act of walking which cannot be accounted for by demonstrable sensory impairment or motor weakness'. They emphasized the combination of ataxia, slow shuffling steps, rigidity (gegenhalten) and brisk reflexes as the essential features of gait apraxia. The finding of slow, small leg movements and rigidity distinguished gait apraxia from cerebellar ataxia. These authors viewed apraxia of gait as a failure of the normal mechanisms of initiation of movement.[4] This difficulty was compounded by the basic requirement of coordinated action of both legs in bilateral simultaneous movement during walking and provided an explanation for the improvement in the performance of leg movements when seated or lying down, or using only one limb at a time. In this cogent review, Meyer and Barron[4] concluded that frontal lobe disease produced a striking disorder of gait but were careful to not to draw any anatomical correlations because their cases like many of those already in the literature had diffuse cerebral disease.

There are several reservations about the use of the term apraxia in the context of gait disorders. First, the term does not take into account the many different requirements that are critical for the performance of normal gait. These requirements include the need to stand, the ability to maintain an upright posture, negotiate the postural adjustments necessary to initiate stepping and the capacity to sustain a rhythmic stepping action of both legs. The term apraxia neglects the role of the frontal lobes in initiating and adapting voluntary movement by modulating the brainstem and spinal cord networks that generate postural responses and locomotor limb movements. Second, leg movements are not necessarily normal when performing other tasks when seated or lying.

In other descriptions of the disorder of gait accompanying frontal lobe disease, the breakdown of stepping mechanisms has been emphasized. The term 'marché à petits pas' is attributed to Dejerine[12] who described the syndrome of small shuffling steps and pseudobulbar palsy with sparing of upper limb function associated with multiple lacunar strokes. Critchley[13] later used the term 'atherosclerotic parkinsonism' to describe a similar phenomenon. A disorder of step initiation has also been described. Isolated gait ignition failure[22] or primary progressive freezing gait[23] refer to syndromes in which start hesitation and freezing are the major features. Once walking is underway, step size and rhythm are normal. Postural reflexes and balance are preserved. In one case of isolated gait ignition failure, functional imaging with positron emission tomography revealed hypometabolism in the inferomedial frontal lobes.[22] Occasionally, gait ignition failure is the first sign of a frontal gait disorder and can be the presenting feature of hydrocephalus or Binswanger's disease.

MECHANISMS OF FRONTAL GAIT DISORDERS

One proposed mechanism for the predominant lower body (trunk and leg) involvement in the periventricular pathologies of hydrocephalus[24] and Binswanger's disease[25] is vulnerability of the long corticospinal fibers controlling leg and trunk movement as they descend close to the lateral ventricles. However, upper motor neuron signs are not always seen and it is possible that a number of other projections to and from cortical motor areas and basal ganglia, cerebellum, brainstem and spinal cord may be affected. Particularly important connections include the basal ganglia ouflow from the pallidum via thalamus, which may contribute to the hypokinetic elements of gait, the frontal projections to brainstem locomotor centers, which may cause failure of gait ignition[1,22] and the frontal projections to brainstem reticular nuclei and the cerebellum, which may account for disequilibrium.

A further question is whether there are any differences between the disequilibrium seen in frontal gait disorders and the disturbance of truncal balance in syndromes of the flocculonodular lobe and anterior lobe of the cerebellum. Superficially, the disequilibrium in frontal gait disorders resembles a cerebellar truncal ataxia without appendicular ataxia, although freezing and shuffling are not features of the latter. However, as pointed out by Fulton,[26] the flocculonodular and anterior lobe syndromes should be regarded as disturbances of balance and equilibrium rather than ataxia. In both flocculonodular and anterior lobe syndromes, there may also be impairment of postural reflexes consistent with disequilibrium. Falls, particularly backwards, are a feature of the flocculonodular syndrome, while abnormal

postural reflexes with increased extensor tone, exaggerated supporting reactions and truncal oscillations are seen in anterior lobe lesions. Both the flocculonodular and anterior lobes of the cerebellum project to the fastigial nucleus which, in turn, projects to the reticulospinal and vestibulospinal systems, thereby influencing postural muscle tone and locomotion.[27] The fastigial nucleus also projects to the motor and premotor cortical areas via the thalamus.[27] The pontomedullary reticular formation receives projections from area 6, providing the capacity for frontal motor areas to influence postural tone and locomotion through reticulospinal projections.

The interaction of higher motor centers, the fastigial nucleus and brainstem nuclei in the voluntary and automatic control of posture and locomotion was highlighted recently by Mori et al.[27] The extent of this network of structures controlling posture and locomotion, encompassing the frontal lobes, basal ganglia, cerebellum and brainstem reticular nuclei, suggests a degree of redundancy. Accordingly, it is unlikely that isolated or discrete lesions of the central nervous system will produce the elements of a frontal gait disorder. Rather, the lesions would need to be dispersed to interrupt a critical number of the connections between these structures and possibly progressive to reduce the scope for compensation and become symptomatic. Many of these connections lie in the frontal periventricular white matter, which may account for the association of pathologies in this area with the 'frontal gait disorder'.

A final question is whether frontal gait disorder includes basal ganglia dysfunction. Although we have emphasized the major clinical differences between frontal gait disorder and parkinsonism, there are several reported examples of generalized parkinsonism and resting tremor associated with hydrocephalus or frontal tumors. In some, levodopa responsiveness and pretectal signs have suggested a functional or structural disruption of the nigrostriatal system, as a consequence of rostral midbrain compression.[17,18,28] Finally, normal pressure hydrocephalus in the elderly may be accompanied by idiopathic Parkinson's disease in some cases.[17,29,30] Nevertheless, these cases are rare.

CONCLUSION

Frontal gait disorders are characterized by varying combinations of disequilibrium, gait ignition failure and locomotor hypokinesia. Many of the terms used to describe the patterns of gait associated with frontal lobe disease have focused on one aspect of this complex disorder. This spectrum of gait abnormalities associated with frontal lobe disease may be interpreted as a consequence of the breakdown in higher-order control of truncal and limb posture while standing and walking, and the initiation and maintenance of locomotion. This higher-order control is related to the interaction of the frontal motor areas with subcortical structures including the basal ganglia, cerebellum and brainstem.

REFERENCES

1. Nutt JG, Marsden CD, Thompson PD. Human walking and higher level gait disorders, particularly in the elderly. *Neurology* 1993;**43**:268-79.

2. Sudarsky L, Ronthal M. Gait disorders among elderly patients: a survey of 50 patients. *Arch Neurol* 1983;**40**:740-3.

3. Denny Brown D. The nature of apraxia. *J Nerv Ment Dis* 1958;**126**:9-31.

4. Meyer JS, Barron D. Apraxia of gait: a clinico-pathological study. *Brain* 1960;**83**:61-84.

5. Elble R, Cousins R, Leffler K, Hughes L. Gait initiation by patients with lower-half parkinsonism. *Brain* 1996;**119**:1705-16.

6. Ebersbach G, Sojer M, Valldeoriola F, et al. Comparative analysis of gait in Parkinson's disease, cerebellar ataxia and subcortical arteriosclerotic encephalopathy. *Brain* 1999;**122**:1349-55.

7. Knutsson E, Lying-Tunell U. Gait apraxia in normal pressure hydrocephalus: Patterns of muscle activation. *Neurology* 1985;**35**:155-60.

8. Sorensen, PS, Jansen EC, Gjerris F. Motor disturbances in normal pressure hydrocephalus. Special reference to stance and gait. *Arch Neurol* 1986;**43**:34-8.

9. Sudarsky L, Simon S. Gait disorder in late-life hydrocephalus. *Arch Neurol* 1987;**44**:267-7.

10. Rossor MN, Tyrell PJ, Warrington EK, et al. Progressive frontal gait disturbance with atypical Alzheimer's disease and corticobasal degeneration. *J Neurol Neurosurg Psychiatry* 1999;**26**:345-52.

11. Thompson PD, Marsden CD. Gait disorder of subcortical arteriosclerotic encephalopathy: Binswanger's disease. *Mov Disord* 1987;**2**:1-8.

12. Dejerine J. *Semeiologie du systeme nerveux*. Paris: Masson, 1926;301.

13. Critchley M. Arteriosclerotic parkinsonism. *Brain* 1929;**52**:23-83.

14. Fitzgerald PM, Jankovic J. Lower body parkinsonism: evidence for a vascular aetiology. *Mov Disord* 1989;**4**:249-60.

15. Messert B, Baker NH. Syndrome of progressive spastic ataxia and apraxia associated with occult hydrocephalus. *Neurology* 1966;**16**:440-52.

16. Messert B, Henke TK, Langheim W. Syndrome of akinetic mutism associated with obstructive hydrocephalus. *Neurology* 1966;**16**:635-49.

17. Curran T, Lang AE. Parkinsonian syndromes associated with hydrocephalus: case reports, a review of the literature and pathophysiological hypotheses. *Mov Disord* 1994;**9**:508-20.

18. Zeidler M, Dorman PJ, Ferguson IT, Bateman DE. . Parkinsonism associated with obstructive hydrocephalus due to idiopathic aqueductal stenosis. *J Neurol Neurosurg Psychiatry* 1998;**64**:657-9.

19. Petrovici I. Apraxia of gait and trunk movements. *J Neurol Sci* 1968;**7**:229-43.

20. Bruns L. . Uber Störugen des Gleichgewichtes bei Stirnhirntumoren. *Dtsch Med Wochenschr* 1892;**18**:138-40.

21. van Bogaert L, Martin P. Sur deux signes du syndrome de desequilibration frontale: l'apraxie de la marche et l'atonie statique. *Encephale* 1929;**24**:11-18.

22. Atchison PR, Thompson PD, Frackowiak RSJ, Marsden CD. The syndrome of isolated gait ignition failure: a report of six cases. *Mov Disord* 1993;**8**:285-92.

23. Achiron A, Ziv I, Goren M, et al. Primary progressive freezing gait. *Mov Disord* 1993;**8**:293-7.

24. Yakovlev PI. Paraplegias of hydrocephalus. *Am J Ment Defic* 1947;**51**:561-76.

25. Ishii N, Nishihara Y, Imamura T. Why do frontal lobe symptoms predominate in vascular dementia with lacunes? *Neurology* 1986;**36**:340-345.

26. Fulton JF. *The physiology of the nervous system*, 3rd edn. New York: Oxford University Press, 1949;528-9.

27. Mori S, Matsuyama K, Mori F, Nakajima K. Supraspinal sites that induce locomotion in the vertebrate central nervous system. In: Ruzick E, Hallett M, Jankovic J, eds. *Gait disorders. Advances in neurology*, vol 87. Philadelphia: Lippincott, Williams and Wilkins, 2001;25-40.

28. Jankovic J, Newmark M, Peter P. Parkinsonism and acquired hydrocephalus. *Mov Disord* 1986;**1**:59-64.

29. Lobo Antunes J, Fahn S, Cote L. Normal pressure hydrocephalus and Parkinson's disease. *J Neural Trans Suppl* 1983;**19**:225-31.

30. Krauss JK, Regel JP, Droste DW, et al. Movement disorders in adult hydrocephalus. *Mov Disord* 1997;**12**:53-60.

14

Cerebrovascular disease and hydrocephalus

JOSÉ MASDEU

CEREBROVASCULAR DISEASE

Vascular disease of the brain ranks among the top three causes of gait impairment in the older adult.[1,2] In addition to the obviously spastic gait of someone that has had a stroke, cerebrovascular disease is an important cause of progressive gait impairment in older patients, many of whom have never had a typical stroke syndrome. Because the etiology and rehabilitation aspects of the spastic gait, with isometric weakness of the leg, are reviewed in Chapter 12, this chapter will rather focus on cerebrovascular disease as the cause of progressive gait and postural impairment, but with preserved isometric strength. Vascular disease causing this syndrome most often affects the supratentorial compartment in the form of lacunar disease or ischemic disease of the white matter. Less often, it involves the posterior circulation, affecting vestibular or cerebellar structures and, very rarely, other brainstem structures important for gait, such as the mesencephalic locomotor center or substantia nigra.

Gait impairment in the elderly as the result of lacunar disease was described by Lhermitte in a monograph on 'senile paraplegia' published in 1907.[3] In 1948, Critchley described a common gait abnormality of aging and ascribed it to vascular disease of the brain, reflecting the views of the time.[4] He stated:

> There exists a large group of cases where the gait in old people becomes considerably disordered, although the motor power of the legs is comparatively well preserved. A paradoxical state of affairs is the result: testing of the individual movements of the legs while the patient reclines upon the couch shows little, if any, reduction in the strength. The tonus may not be grossly altered and the reflexes may betray only minor deviations. Sensory tests show no unusual features. But when the patient is instructed to get out of bed and to walk, remarkable defects may be witnessed. The patient, first of all, appears most reluctant to make the attempt. His stance is bowed and uncertain. He props himself against the end of the bed and seeks the aid of the bystanders. Encouraged to take a few steps, he advances warily and hesitatingly. Clutching the arms of two supporters, he takes short, shuffling steps. The legs tend to crumble by giving way suddenly at the knee joints. Progression, as far as it is possible, is slow and tottery. The patient veers to one side or the other. Frequently the legs cross, so that one foot gets in the way of the other.

In the 1960s and 1970s, the characterization of Parkinson's disease turned the attention of neurologists to dopaminergic dysfunction in order to explain syndromes of the elderly resembling Dr Critchley's masterly description quoted above. Even recently, the term 'lower-body parkinsonism' has been coined to designate a similar gait pattern in patients that probably do not have a parkinsonian disorder, but have instead vascular disease of the brain.[5-7] Despite its decline in diagnostic popularity, stroke can still be listed among the most frequent and yet often forgotten causes of impaired gait and balance. What is overlooked is not sizeable infarction resulting in sudden leg weakness, but the accumulation over time of the effect of chronic ischemia or minor episodes of vascular disease of the brain, which give rise to the more subtle and progressive changes in ambulation described by Critchley.[4] Gait impairment may be the consequence of the ischemic white matter disorder that has been termed Binswanger's disease or subcortical arteriosclerotic encephalopathy.[8] In addition, in recent years lacunar strokes or acute hemorrhage have been recognized to cause acute impairment of the ability to stand and walk but with little or no change in volitional isometric strength of the muscles of the lower extremities.

Ischemic brain disease tends to follow one of three patterns, discernible by clinical evaluation and with the help of neuroimaging procedures: (1) cortical infarcts, most often related to embolic disease; (2) subcortical disease, often in the form of widespread lacunes and white matter changes, most often related to arteriolar disease; and (3) a mixture of the two patterns, often related to atheromatous disease of the major vessels.[9,10] The second and third types of cerebrovascular disease are more prone than the first one to cause gait and balance impairment, once a critical amount of cumulative damage has affected gait-critical structures. Subcortical infarcts, strategically located, may impair equilibrium and gait with little or no limb weakness on isometric testing. These lesions tend to affect structures such as the paracentral white matter, or the basal ganglia, with an important role in gait and balance mechanisms. The disturbances of mobility caused by cerebellar or vestibular cerebrovascular lesions are well known. Striking abnormalities of gait and balance have been described with lesions in the thalamus, in the basal ganglia, in the infratentorial compartment, and in the pedunculopontine region.

This chapter reviews the evidence for vascular disease causing ambulation impairment, indicates the most frequent types of pathology and localization and summarizes their current management. Detailed descriptions of the management of cerebrovascular disease can be found elsewhere.[9,10] Clinical manifestations of vascular disease depend on the localization of the ischemic or hemorrhagic insult. Logically, gait impairment will result from damage of brain structures critical for ambulation. Localization of vascular disease is emphasized because diagnostic and therapeutic decisions often depend on localization. Vascular diseases of the supratentorial structures are discussed first, and afterwards those in the posterior fossa, ending the vascular section with a discussion of the role of cerebrovascular disease in the genesis of drop attacks.

Supratentorial vascular lesions

Since the advent of computed tomography (CT) and, particularly, magnetic resonance imaging (MRI), the ubiquitous changes observed in the white matter of older individuals have mesmerized both clinicians and radiologists. The clinical significance of these changes is still to be fully elucidated, but the best data point to gait and balance impairment rather than cognitive deterioration as the main clinical correlate of white matter disease of the elderly. Lacunar events, easily imaged with CT or MRI in the chronic stage, albeit elusive acutely, are often responsible for the sudden onset of impaired balance and gait in an older individual, particularly when the

lesion affects structures that play a key role in ambulation, such as the thalami, basal ganglia or projection fibers from the paracentral lobule. White matter disease and lacunar strokes will be reviewed in sequence.

WHITE MATTER DISEASE OF THE ELDERLY

Neuroimaging findings

Neuroimaging findings are considered before the clinical findings because they alert clinicians to the presence of this disorder and are paramount for the diagnosis. White matter changes on CT or MRI are very frequent in older people. On MRI, some degree of white matter changes is present in about 45 per cent of asymptomatic subjects with a mean age of 55 years.[11] Since these changes are unusual below age 50 and their severity and prevalence increase with age, it is clear that they are somehow related to the aging process.[12-16] On CT, the density of the centrum semiovale decreases with age.[17]

White matter hypodensity of the elderly, subtle on CT, has striking visual characteristics when imaged by MRI.[12,18-20] Areas of the periventricular white matter hypodense on CT appear markedly hyperintense on T2-weighted images, and hypointense on T1-weighted images (Fig. 14.1). However, high-intensity areas on T2 MRI are often undetected on CT. On T2 MRI images, it may be difficult to differentiate functionally normal areas of increased water content because of dilation of perivascular spaces with normal aging or transependymal cerebrospinal fluid (CSF) absorption, from areas of tissue damage because both have increased intensity values.[20-22] On proton-density images, areas of increased water content appear isointense or slightly hypointense, whereas areas of gliosis are hyperintense. For this reason it seems preferable to make the diagnosis of white matter disease only when the abnormalities are visible not only on T2-weighted images but also on proton-density or T1-weighted images.[23] Diffusion-tensor imaging has shown an age-related loss of regional white matter coherence, which correlates with gait, balance, and interhemispheric transfer test scores.[24]

Clinical correlates

There is ample evidence that white matter disease of aging causes gait impairment. Disorders of gait were pronounced among 41 well-documented cases of progressive arteriopathic white matter disease described with histology since 1978 (23 males, 18 females; mean age of onset 60 ± 9.7 years; mean length of illness 5.8 ± 4.2 years).[8,13,25-30] Impairment of ambulation preceded cognitive impairment in 43 per cent of the cases, whereas dementia developed before gait impairment in only 17 per cent; in 20 per cent the impairments evolved simultaneously, and in 20 per cent insufficient data precluded timing of gait abnormality versus dementia. Two of the cases where dementia occurred first had amyloid angiopathy and senile changes in the cortex.[25] Neuroimaging studies, both with CT[31-33] and MRI[34] have

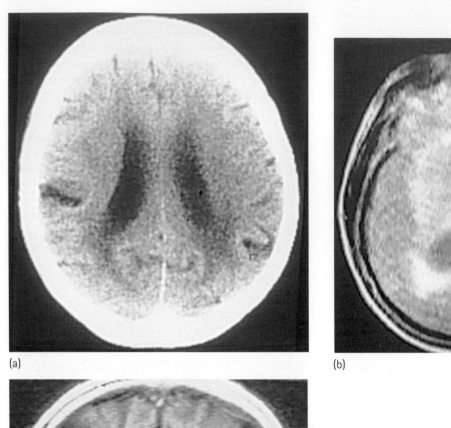

(a)

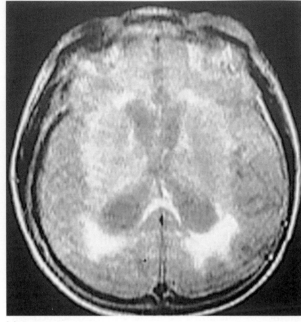

(b)

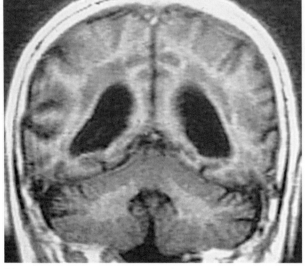

(c)

Figure 14.1 *White matter changes of the elderly. Computed tomography (CT) and magnetic resonance imaging (MRI) of a normotensive 79-year-old woman with normal mentation but slow, hesitating gait and a propensity to falling. Areas of low density on CT (a), particularly in the periatrial white matter, appear of high intensity on proton-density MRI (b), and of low intensity on T1-weighted MRI (c).*

also confirmed the relationship between impaired gait or balance and the presence of white matter disease or 'leuko-araiosis.' Periventricular white matter changes were present in the cases of 'lower body parkinsonism' described in elderly subjects by Thompson and Marsden[35] and by FitzGerald and Jankovic.[5] In controlled studies of elderly prone to falling, impaired gait and balance has been shown to correlate with the presence of white matter disease on CT or MRI.[31,36–46]

Characteristically, patients with severe white matter changes have an unsteady gait with features of parkinsonism and ataxia.[5,35] However, unlike patients with cerebellar ataxia, they seldom broaden their base of support on standing or walking. Their performance resembles Critchley's[4] description of the gait of some elderly people quoted at the beginning of this chapter. Disequilibrium dominates the clinical picture and predisposes these patients to falls.[31,37] Whereas they have difficulty walking, they are often able to use their feet on finer volitional tasks, such as drawing a cross or a circle. Long-tract findings, including Babinski signs and hyperreflexia, are not necessarily present. Paratonia is generally pronounced in the legs, but less so in the upper extremities. As in Parkinson's disease, by attending to their gait, the patient can make the steps longer and improve their balance.

Pathology, pathogenesis and risk factors

Because the histology underlying the white matter neuroimaging changes remains elusive, Hachinski proposed the descriptive term 'leuko-araiosis' for the CT findings.[47] Several authors have reported normal histology, but vascular or ischemic disease has been present in cases with pronounced white matter changes on T1-weighted MRI or CT.[30,48–55]

The mechanisms by which periventricular white matter disease may interfere with normal gait and balance need further clarification. Long-loop reflexes, essential for adequate gait and balance, are mediated by ascending fibers from the ventrolateral nucleus of the thalamus to the paracentral lobule and by descending corticospinal fibers. These fibers may be affected as they traverse the periventricular region. With arteriolosclerotic or amyloid arteriopathic disease of the white matter the periventricular fibers are predominantly affected.[25] The periventricular region represents the arterial end and border zone for the perforating medullary vessels.[56] Thus, it can sustain acute or chronic ischemic damage as a result of arteriolar disease, hemorheologic factors, anoxia or hypotension. The subcortical U-fibers are generally spared because their angioarchitecture is part of the cortical rather than the deep medullary supply.[57]

Cerebrovascular disease and hypertension are frequent correlates of subcortical arteriosclerotic encephalopathy, including white matter disease, studied in people in their 60s.[18,58–61] Blood pressure control seems to reduce the likelihood of developing white matter lesions.[61–63] In the elderly population, isolated systolic hypertension, caused by a reduction in connective tissue elasticity of large blood vessels, is common.[64] It is defined by systolic readings of greater than or equal to 160 mmHg and diastolic readings less than 90 mmHg. The prevalence of isolated systolic hypertension is about 7 per cent in those over age 60 years and increases with age to nearly 20 per cent in those over age 80 years.[65] Prevalence is greater in women and non-whites.

Although in both cases the white matter is affected, subcortical arteriosclerotic encephalopathy or Binswanger's disease may differ pathogenetically from white matter disease of the elderly.[47] Hypertension or left-ventricular hypertrophy, commonly reported in association with subcortical arteriosclerotic encephalopathy in patients in their 60s,[60] may not be present in subjects in their 80s with white matter changes.[31,45] At least in part, the absence of association might be explained because severely hypertensive patients may suffer a greater degree of cardiac and cerebrovascular disease earlier in life and not survive into the age groups included in gait studies, typically the late 70s or 80s. Factors other than hypertension may be important in the genesis of white matter disease in the more advanced decades. Cerebral hypoperfusion from episodic hypotension or cardiac dysrhythmias has been implicated.[66,67] Plasma viscosity was increased in a group of eight patients with CT diagnosis of subcortical arteriosclerotic encephalopathy (mean age 62 years).[68] Possibly owing to increased distal arteriolar resistance, cerebral blood flow velocity, measured with transcranial Doppler, is reduced in elderly with white matter abnormalities.[69] Some of the neuronal and white matter damage may be mediated by matrix metalloproteinases.[54] Particularly when asymmetrical, white matter disease can be related to chronic hypoperfusion from carotid artery stenosis. These patients typically have a history of several episodes of mild unilateral weakness and may have frank infarcts in the distal territory of the middle cerebral artery, particularly in the white matter lateral to the head of the caudate nucleus or in the white matter underlying the middle frontal and superior temporal gyri. Carotid artery stenosis can be easily detected with MR angiography or carotid duplex studies. Cardiovascular and hematologic risk factors should be explored in an effort to identify potentially treatable causes of white matter disease of the elderly.

Amyloid angiopathy has been described in the genesis of white matter disease in some elderly individuals.[25,27] In addition to white matter changes, amyloid angiopathy results in subcortical or thalamic hemorrhages (Fig. 14.2). Most of these individuals were normotensive. In

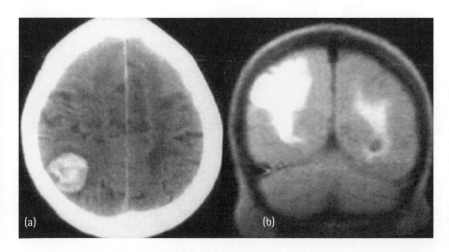

(a)　　　　　　　　　　　　　(b)

Figure 14.2 *Amyloid angiopathy. (a) Computed tomography scan of a 79-year-old woman showing a recent hemorrhage in the right supramarginal gyrus. (b) On T2-weighted magnetic resonance imaging, the lesion appears bright because of the high methemoglobin content and the abnormal white matter is hyperintense on both hemispheres.*

some individuals there is a strong genetic component. The α_1-antichymotrypsin T allele has been associated with cerebral amyloid angiopathy.[70]

A genetically better characterized ischemic leuko-encephalopathy is cerebral autosomal dominant arterio-pathy with subcortical infarcts and leukoencephalopathy (CADASIL).[71,72] Both CT and MRI show an abnormal white matter: hypodense on CT, hyperintense on T2-weighted MR images and hypointense on T1-weighted MR images (Fig. 14.3). The temporal and anterior

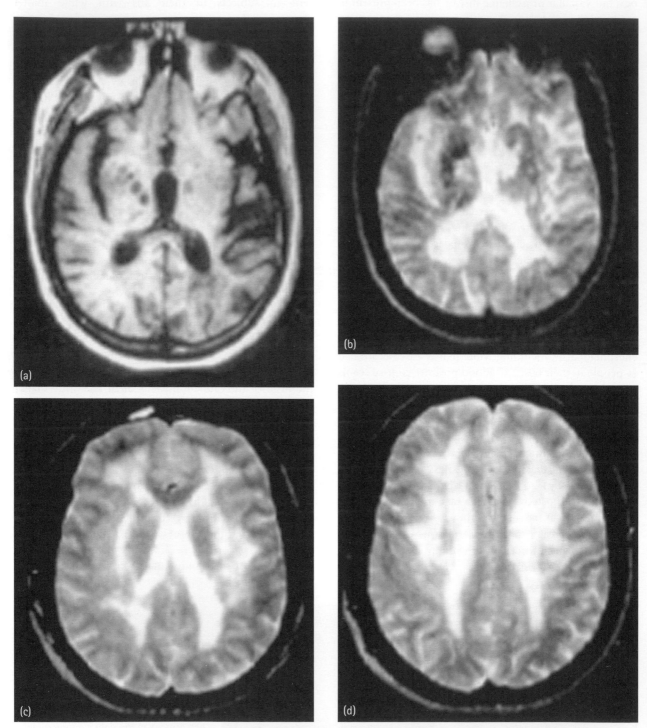

Figure 14.3 *Cerebral autosomal dominant arteriopathy with subcortical infarcts and leukoencephalopathy (CADASIL). (a,b) T1-weighted and T2-weighted magnetic resonance images of a 40-year-old who had sustained several strokes, leaving him with a quadriparesis. CADASIL was confirmed by brain biopsy and genetic typing. (c,d). T2-weighted magnetic resonance images of an asymptomatic, 40-year-old relative of the previous patient at 50 per cent genetic risk of having CADASIL, showing abnormally hyperintense periventricular white matter. (Reprinted from Sabbadini G, Francia A, Calandriello L, et al. Cerebral autosomal dominant arteriopathy with subcortical infarcts and leucoencephalopathy (CADASIL). Clinical, neuroimaging, pathological and genetic study of a large Italian family.* Brain *1995;* **118***:207–15, by permission of Oxford University Press.)*

frontal white matter and the subcortical arcuate fibers tend to be more affected by CADASIL than by sporadic subcortical arteriosclerotic encephalopathy.[73] Imaging changes are often present in presymptomatic individuals.[72] CADASIL has been mapped to a mutation of the Notch 3 gene, on chromosome 19.[74-76] A periodic acid–Schiff (PAS)-positive, granular material is deposited in the media of the arterioles of the brain and other organs, including skin.[77] When positive, a skin biopsy is helpful, but there are genetically proven cases with negative skin biopsy.[78] CADASIL is associated with another vascular risk factor, namely hyperhomocysteinemia.[79]

Hyperhomocysteinemia may be associated with lacunar disease and white matter lesions in the elderly.[80] Because white matter disease can be caused by impaired cobalamin metabolism, which also causes hyperhomocysteinemia, in some cases the white matter damage might be metabolic, with a variable vascular component.[81]

Treatment

As discussed above, chronic hypertension may be a risk factor for ischemic white matter disease.[60,61] There is no direct evidence that blood pressure control lessens the progression of white matter changes in the elderly but treated hypertensives may have less white matter changes than untreated hypertensives.[62] Clearly, treatment of hypertension prevents ischemic brain disease, even in the elderly.[87] Hypertension control in patients aged 40–69 years at the start of follow-up effected stroke reduction in a large longitudinal study.[83] In the Systolic Hypertension in the Elderly Program, treated subjects over the age of 60 years with isolated systolic hypertension had a 36 per cent reduction in stroke risk compared with those in the placebo group.[84]

In the treatment of hypertension, the mean perfusion pressure must be carefully monitored in older patients. Daily fluctuations in blood pressure, such as postprandial hypotension, may result in unwanted hypotensive episodes with overtreatment.[85] Chronic hypotension may cause selective necrosis of oligodendrocytes because these cells are particularly prone to ischemic injury.[86] The existence of an optimal window for patients with target-organ damage, such as white matter lesions, is highlighted by studies showing that midrange blood pressure contributes to optimal function. In a prospective observational study of 29 hypertensive patients with arteriosclerotic encephalopathy, maintenance of systolic blood pressure between 135 mmHg and 150 mmHg was associated with stabilization of cognition, while lowering of systolic blood pressure below 135 mmHg was associated with decline.[87] The Joint National Committee on high blood pressure[82] has stratified patients with hypertension based on target organ damage. Data and guidelines are needed regarding the management of hypertension for patients falling into this group.

Precautions for detection and evaluation of hypertension in the elderly include multiple blood pressure measurements in the fasting state, and sitting and supine blood pressure measurements before and during therapy. Pseudohypertension due to stress may be recorded in a doctor's office in older patients with denervation supersensitivity of sympathetic receptors. For this reason, 24-h ambulatory blood pressure monitoring can be used to obtain a more accurate picture of the response to medication.[88]

In the treatment of hypertension, the decision to treat must be on an individual patient basis.[82] For mild to moderate systolic hypertension, the most common form of hypertension in the older adult,[64] hygienic measures may be sufficient. These include weight reduction if overweight, limiting daily alcohol intake, moderate intensity physical activity (e.g. 30–45 minutes of brisk walking daily or a similar activity compatible with the patient's gait disorder, such as using a stationary bicycle), reduction of sodium intake (no more than 6 g of sodium chloride daily), maintaining adequate potassium, calcium and magnesium intake, avoiding smoking, and reducing the dietary saturated fat and cholesterol intake.

When medication is needed, the 'low and slow' approach to therapy is helpful in minimizing adverse effects. In ordinary hypertension, the goal is to maintain a diastolic blood pressure below 90 mmHg. For isolated systolic hypertension, a reasonable goal is a 20 mmHg reduction in systolic pressure, provided that hypotension is avoided.[65]

Low-dose diuretics, for example chlorthalidone, 12.5 or 25 mg/day, have been documented to be effective in blood pressure control. Other agents, such as beta-blockers, angiotensin-converting enzyme (ACE) inhibitors, and calcium channel blockers, are best used as 'Step 2' agents.[65,82,88,89]

A greater than 70 per cent carotid stenosis should be considered an indication for carotid endarterectomy in symptomatic patients.[90] This study proved the benefit of therapy in patients with definite transient ischemic attacks or stroke, but patients with only slowly progressive gait impairment were not included. More doubtful is the role of carotid endarterectomy in asymptomatic patients. It may help one out of 19 patients with carotid stenosis greater than 60 per cent provided that the combined morbidity from angiography and surgery at a given institution does not exceed 3 per cent.[91,92]

Hyperhomocysteinemia might be a greater risk factor for arteriolopathic white matter disease than for other types of stroke.[80] Although there are no prospective studies proving the use of homocysteine-lowering agents in the prevention of white matter disease, given their safety and low cost, use of folic acid and B vitamins might be considered for patients with known elevated homocysteine levels.[92]

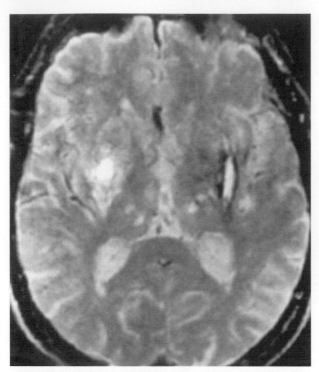

Figure 14.4 *Subcortical disequilibrium with lacunar disease. Magnetic resonance image of a 73-year-old man, a chronic hypertensive, with a transient episode of mild left-sided weakness but progressive gait impairment, with unsteadiness and a tendency to sustaining falls. In addition to multiple thalamic lacunes and a larger infarct in the right lenticular nucleus, there is an organizing hematoma in the left external capsular region.*

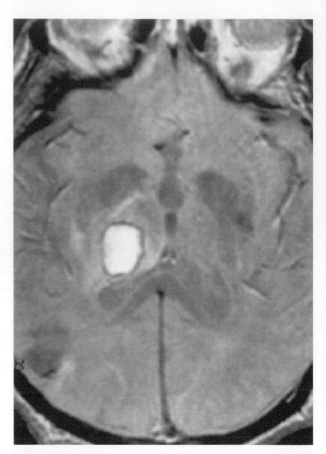

Figure 14.5 *Thalamic hematoma. Magnetic resonance image of an 86-year-old man with a transient mild left hemiparesis but inability to walk for 8 weeks, despite recovery of isometric strength. A right thalamic hematoma involves the ventrolateral and ventral posterior nuclei, as well as the pulvinar.*

Acute vascular disease

Several vascular syndromes have been described in which the patients had pronounced abnormalities of their ability to stand and walk, despite having strong leg muscles. The patients' gait differed somewhat from cerebellar gait in that it was not, or only minimally, broad-based. The outstanding feature was unsteadiness or disequilibrium. Patients tended to topple over after their knees suddenly buckled under them or fell 'like a log', without activating ankle or hip strategies to break the fall. Because most of the lesions involved subcortical structures, this disorder has been called 'subcortical disequilibrium'.[93] Lesions of the thalamus, suprathalamic white matter and basal ganglia may cause this syndrome (Fig. 14.4).

THALAMIC ASTASIA

Inability to stand or walk despite minimal weakness has been recorded acutely with thalamic infarction[94–96] and hemorrhage (Fig. 14.5), particularly when the superior portion of the ventrolateral nucleus or the suprathalamic white matter was involved (Fig. 14.6).[96–98] Alert, with normal or near normal strength on isometric muscle testing

and a variable degree of sensory loss, these patients could not stand and some with larger lesions could not even sit up unassisted. They fell backwards or toward the side contralateral to the lesion. Paying attention to the movement of the feet, or timing it with maneuvers such as chanting 'one, two; one, two' improved both stability and gait (Fig. 14.7). These patients appeared to have a deficit of overlearned motor activity of an axial and postural nature. In the vascular cases, the deficit improved in a few days or weeks. However, these patients had a tendency to sustain falls during the rehabilitation period. It is important to note that this syndrome is transient, perhaps because it is generally unilateral. Chronic stroke patients with bilateral thalamic lesions severe enough to cause permanent astasia would be too hypokinetic to carry on volitional motor activity.

It is reasonable to ask whether the term I originally used for this syndrome, 'thalamic astasia', is still appropriate. It may be countered that this term has often been used to indicate psychogenic imbalance. However, as Dr P. Gorelick and I wrote in the original article, we refrained from using more classical neurological terms,

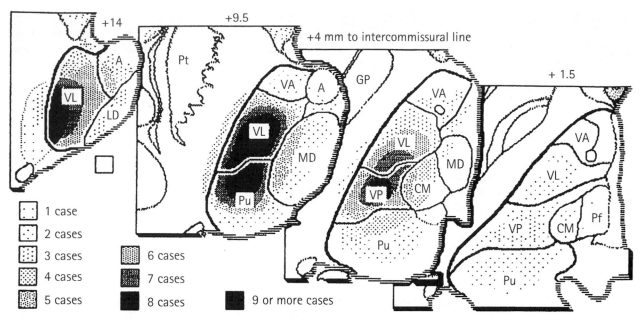

Figure 14.6 *Thalamic astasia. Horizontal sections of the thalamus showing the regional frequency distribution of lesions in the patients with thalamic astasia reported by Masdeu and Gorelick.[96] Note that anterior is on top, posterior at the bottom, medial to the right and lateral to the left. The most rostral section is at the left and the most caudal at the right.*

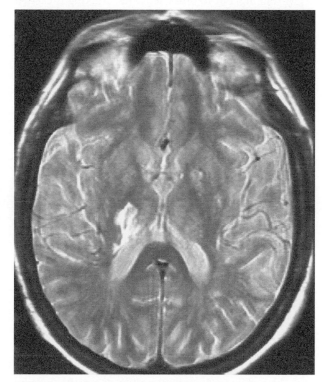

Figure 14.7 *Brain magnetic resonance imaging of a 67-year-old man. Note infarction in the ventrolateral, ventral posterior and pulvinar nuclei of the right thalamus.*

word *stasis*, meaning station. Dorland's Medical Dictionary[99] defines astasia as 'motor incoordination with inability to stand.' It seems appropriate to apply this term to the syndrome displayed by our patients. Regarding psychogenic imbalance, DeJong[100] remarked, "the term astasia-asbasia has been given to the type of gait disturbance which is sometimes observed in hysterical individuals. These words, however, actually mean 'inability to stand and walk,' and it is better to use the term hysterical dysbasia ..." when referring to psychogenic disturbances of gait.

It could be asked whether thalamic astasia is caused by motor neglect affecting the lower limbs, or leg akinesia. Thalamic akinesia has been reported in patients with right thalamic[94,95,101] or left thalamic[102,103] lesions. This deficit of motor control differs from non-dominant parietal neglect, resulting in hemispatial neglect, anosognosia, tactile alloesthesia, topographic disorientation and hemiasomatognosia, which is often present to a mild degree in patients with right thalamic lesions. Similarly, a language disturbance is present in those with left thalamic lesions. Lateralizing manifestations of thalamic disease reflect the diverse specialization of the cortex and subcortical structures targeted by fibers originating in the thalami or coursing through them. These lateralizing findings confound the analysis and interpretation of the akinesia associated with thalamic astasia, a finding that is probably common to lesions of either thalamic nuclear complex and which therefore probably represents a more basic motor disorder.

Thalamic akinesia may be partly related to damage of pallido-thalamic and thalamo-striatal connections. Bilateral pallidal damage causes akinesia.[104,105] Some of

such as ataxia, because the disturbance differs from cerebellar ataxia in that the gait is not broad-based or lurching.[96] It resembles the marked balance impairment of patients with vestibulo-cerebellar disease. The term astasia is derived from the Greek negative particle *a*, and the

the clinical findings in patients with thalamic astasia mimic the deficits resulting from basal ganglia disease, namely proximal hypokinesia, poor performance of automatic associated movements and impairment in postural reflexes. They also share with parkinsonian patients a tendency to keep their hips and knees flexed. However, patients with thalamic astasia, like some of the patients with the so-called lower-body parkinsonism, have greater instability than patients with Parkinson's disease.[7]

Involvement of vestibular pathways has been postulated by Brandt and Dieterich to explain the syndrome of thalamic astasia.[106] They documented an ocular tilt reaction, ocular torsion and tilts of the perceived visual vertical in a study of 35 patients with thalamic infarction.[107] Interestingly, only five patients had 'ataxia' and these belonged to the group of 17 patients with posterolateral infarcts. The lesions were smaller and more caudally located than in the patients described with thalamic astasia. Vestibular eye findings were most prominent in patients with paramedian thalamic infarction, likely from involvement of important vestibulo-ocular structures at the thalamo-mesencephalic junction, such as the rostral nucleus of the medial longitudinal fasciculus and the nucleus of Cajal. In contrast, patients with thalamic astasia tended to have lesions in the laterodorsal thalamus, involving the ventrolateral nucleus and suprathalamic white matter.[96] The unsteadiness of thalamic astasia resembles vestibular unsteadiness. In this regard, Karnath and co-workers[108] have described a tendency for some patients with hemispheric strokes to push forcibly toward the hemiparetic side, therefore falling to that side (the 'pusher syndrome'). These patients also had tilts of the perceived visual vertical. A lesion in the superolateral thalamus and suprathalamic white matter distinguished these patients from controls with hemispheric strokes who did not have the 'pusher syndrome.' From this work, they concluded that there is a supratentorial graviceptive center in the laterosuperior portion of the thalamus.[108] Whether through the interruption of vestibulocortical pathways or by damage to a different graviceptive center, superolateral thalamic lesions cause a syndrome that resembles vestibular disequilibrium.

The lesions in patients with thalamic astasia tended to cluster in the ventrolateral nucleus (Fig. 14.6).[96] The ventrolateral nucleus of the thalamus consists of two portions.[109,110] The smaller anterior portion (VLa) receives projections from the medial globus pallidus via the thalamic fasciculus and projects to area 6 of the frontal cortex. The larger posterior portion (VLp) receives cerebellar, spinothalamic and vestibular afferents and projects in a somatotopic fashion to area 4 of the precentral gyrus. Medial neurons project to the lateral part of the precentral gyrus, whereas laterosuperior ones project to the medial portion of the precentral gyrus, where the trunk and leg are represented. Fibers destined for the leg region course in the posterior limb of the internal capsule and then ascend in the more medial portion of the corona radiata, near the wall of the lateral ventricle. These fibers were probably involved in cases of ataxic hemiparesis with capsular lesions.[111–114] Impairment of gait in the elderly with periventricular white matter disease might be related to involvement of this pathway.[31] Through the fastigial projection, VLp receives information from the vestibulo-cerebellum.[115] Bilateral representation of this projection, affected in our patients at the level of the thalamus, may be one of the factors explaining the transient nature of thalamic astasia.

Studies of cerebral perfusion in patients with thalamic astasia have shown decreased perfusion of the lesioned thalamus, but also of the ipsilateral frontal lobe and contralateral cerebellum (J. Masdeu, unpublished observations). In some cases, cerebellar perfusion was specifically decreased in the vermian and paravermian cerebellar cortex. These studies suggest that the thalamus plays a major role in the activation of frontal cortex, particularly as regards activities that are carried out in the background, without the need for the individual to directly attend to them. This is the case with gait. When normal individuals walk, they do not pay attention to the act of walking, but to other activities. Walking is carried out by 'automatic pilot' that is impaired in patients with thalamic astasia. For this reason, as these patients recover, they can appear quite normal in the constrained framework of a doctor's examination, because they compensate for their deficit by paying attention to their gait. It is in the familiar context of their daily life, when they switch back to using the 'automatic pilot,' that they tend to sustain falls.

CAPSULAR AND BASAL GANGLIA LESIONS

A syndrome of instability with vascular disease has been reported in patients with lesions in the internal capsule or corona radiata who had the syndrome of unilateral ataxia and crural paresis (ataxic hemiparesis).[111–114] A tendency to fall despite good strength was recorded by Groothuis et al.[116] in a patient with a small medial capsular hemorrhage involving the most lateral portion of the ventrolateral nucleus of the thalamus and by Labadie and co-workers in patients with acute lesions in the basal ganglia.[117] Multiple bilateral lacunas involving the basal ganglia can be attended by gait impairment (Fig. 14.4). The impairment of balance resembles the syndrome after lesions of the ventrolateral nucleus of the thalamus. Acutely, the patients fall with a slow, tilting motion, like a falling log, in a lateral or diagonal trajectory. The patients are not aware that they are about to fall and make no protective movements. Within a few days after the acute event, the patients realize that they are falling, but are unable to perform full corrective movements, such as tilting their body, moving their feet or arms, or reaching for nearby objects. As in the thalamic cases, these patients recover their ability to ambulate independently in 3–6 weeks. Recovery was slower when the patient had bilateral basal ganglionic lesions. Bilateral lesions of the globus pallidus can also result in disequilibrium.[104,105] Gait impairment is a prominent component of many degenerative disorders of the basal ganglia, including Cockayne's disease.[118] However, unilateral chronic lesions of the putamen in young individuals seldom lead to disequilibrium, at least to any clinically relevant degree.[119] Studies of bilateral basal ganglia lesions in older individuals are confounded by lesions in other areas of the brain. It is possible that multiple lesions to somewhat redundant circuits supporting gait and posture may need to be lesioned to result in a clinical syndrome from lenticular nucleus lesions. The lesions of subcortical arteriosclerotic encephalopathy are often bilateral, but are accompanied by white matter lesions, which can cause gait unsteadiness by themselves.[120,121] Unlike in the case of the globus pallidus,[122] massive bilateral lesions of the striatum are rare with vascular disease. Smaller lesions are likely to cause a transient disorder, easily overlooked.[117] Better clinico-radiological correlation studies are needed to understand the role of the striatum in the genesis of central disequilibrium. The availability of functional studies with positron-emission tomography (PET) and single photon emission computed tomography (SPECT) may help this process.

MANAGEMENT OF LACUNAR STROKE

Blood pressure should not be lowered aggressively in a patient with acute ischemic stroke. Often, there is a mild to moderate transient rise in blood pressure after stroke that may have a protective effect on perfusion of the ischemic area.[84] The motor deficit is managed with early physical therapy.[123] The physical therapist should be mindful of the particular kind of deficit these patients have. Strategies that rely of the volitional control of motor activity such as standing and walking, not normally under the control of the will, are likely to be successful. With small unilateral lesions, even automatic strategies will eventually recover.

Progression of the gait impairment in these patients is predicated on the basis of accumulation of lacunas. Whereas they recover easily from one single lesion, they become more and more unsteady as lesions accumulate, particularly when they affect parallel critical areas of both hemispheres. For this reason, the medical interventions for these patients involve mainly prevention of risk factors for lacunar stroke. Control of hypertension was discussed above under the management of white matter lesions. Cigarette smoking should be discontinued and excessive alcohol consumption eliminated. Patients with known coronary heart disease and elevated low-density lipoprotein (LDL) cholesterol levels should be considered for treatment with a statin.[92] An active lifestyle with physical exercise protects from both coronary artery disease and stroke. Postmenopausal women need not discontinue estrogen intake.[84]

Although we know that antithrombotic therapy is effective for the prevention of stroke, no prospective trials have addressed specifically lacunar stroke. A subgroup analysis in the French AICLA trial suggested a benefit of aspirin in these patients.[84] The recommended dose of aspirin is a tablet (325 mg) per day. In a small study, triflusal compared favorably with this dose of aspirin.[124] In addition, evidence-based guidelines support the use of clopidogrel (75 mg daily) and extended-release dipyridamole plus aspirin as acceptable options for the prevention of stroke after non-cardioembolic transient ischemic attack (TIA) or stroke.[92]

OTHER SUPRATENTORIAL VASCULAR LESIONS

Gait impairment, in the form of difficulty taking the first steps (freezing) and unsteadiness, can occur with bilateral lesions of the medial frontal region. Damage of this region may result from infarction in the territory of the anterior cerebral artery or from bilateral, high convexity subdural hematomas that compress the medial frontal cortex (Fig. 14.8).

Infratentorial lesions

Infratentorial lesions often cause impairment of balance and gait. Two major classical syndromes are cerebellar ataxia and vestibular disequilibrium. Since gait and balance impairment related to lesions of these structures is reviewed in Chapters 9 and 10, only vascular lesions will be summarily described here. Less often reported are disequilibrium syndromes arising from midbrain or high pontine lesions in the mesencephalic locomotor region, and these will be described here in greater detail.

Ponto–mesencephalic gait failure

The laterodorsal region of the midbrain contains the mesencephalic locomotor region, which plays an important role in locomotion in animals.[125] Stimulation of this region in the cat induces rapid walking, followed by running. This area contains the nucleus cuneiformis and the cholinergic pedunculopontine nucleus. In humans, loss of neurons in the pedunculopontine nucleus has been found in progressive supranuclear palsy and Parkinson's disease, but not in patients with Alzheimer's disease, implying perhaps a role of this nucleus in ambulatory mechanisms[126] (Fig. 14.9). The patient with a hemorrhage in the area of the pedunculopontine nucleus whose MRI is shown in Fig. 14.9 had the acute onset of inability to walk, without hemiparesis or sensory loss.[127] She was waiting for a bus after her weekly 6 h of casino

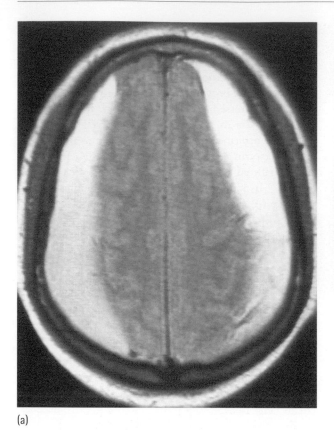

(a)

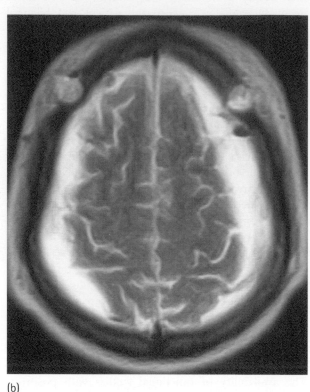

(b)

Figure 14.8 *Subdural hematomas compressing the medial frontal region before surgery (a) in a 68-year-old man with a 3-month history of slowly progressive gait impairment. The gait problem had prompted a referral to an orthopedic surgeon, on the suspicion that it was related to arthrosis of the knee. (b) After surgery, the sulci of the paracentral lobule are no longer compressed.*

playing when she became nauseated and fell to the floor; she was alert but unable to stand or walk. She could draw a circle with either leg when sitting down, but did not generate regular stepping movements with her feet and was unable to stand without support. Holding on to a walker and stooped forward, she walked with short, shuffling, irregular steps. Her base of ambulation was only minimally wide. Regular stepping was not initiated either in attempted walking or in response to loss of her balance. The steps were of irregular amplitude and direction, sometimes directed laterally. The left foot seemed to step less readily than the right. Often, there would be two steps with one foot while the other remained motionless. There was no cadence or rhythmicity to this patient's gait. Her performance bore striking resemblance to the gait failure experienced by many elderly individuals, which in most cases does not have a clear anatomic correlate.[93] They lack the ability to generate spontaneous, rhythmic stepping movements.

The connectivity of the pedunculopontine region suggests an important role in motor behavior for this area. It receives projections from the deep cerebellar nuclei, substantia nigra and globus pallidus, as well as from the nucleus locus coeruleus and the raphe nuclei, and projects to the substantia nigra, globus pallidus, subthalamic nucleus, ventrolateral nucleus of the thalamus

and motor cortex, as well as to pontomedullary reticular nuclei known to influence the pattern generators in the spinal cord.[125,128,129] In addition to the effects of electrical stimulation mentioned above, the results of injection in this area of putative neurotransmitters suggest a role for the pedunculopontine area in locomotion. Spontaneous locomotion, which occurs in the precollicular–premammillary transected cat, can be blocked by the injection of γ-aminobutyric acid (GABA). In contrast, by giving increasing amounts of GABA antagonists or substance P, the step cycle frequency can be increased from a walk to a trot to a gallop.[130] Lesions of the pedunculopontine nucleus lead to a reduction of locomotor activity in experimental animals.[131]

Imaging studies in patients with sudden dysfunction of the mesencephalic locomotor center have shown hemorrhagic or ischemic lesions.[132–134] Like the woman described at the beginning of this section, these patients are generally hypertensive, with small vessel disease causing white matter changes and lacunes in the basal ganglia and thalami. Therefore, their impairment could be caused by damage of several overlapping brain mechanisms subserving gait and balance in the human brain. Management of small-vessel disease of the brain was discussed in the sections on white matter disease and lacunar stroke.

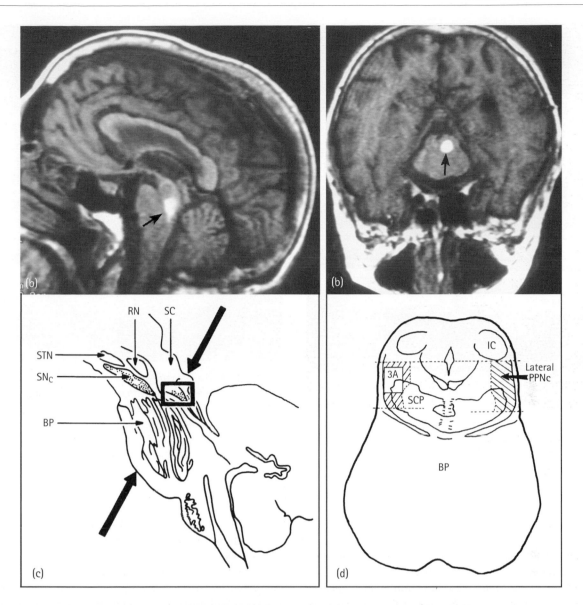

Figure 14.9 *Mesencephalic gait failure. Magnetic resonance imaging of an 83-year-old woman with gait failure after a hemorrhage in the locomotor mesencephalic region. Lesion is shown in the sagittal (a) and coronal (b) planes, arrow. Below each magnetic resonance image, note the location of the pedunculopontine nucleus in the human brainstem, at the junction of the pons and midbrain (c,d) (reprinted with permission from Zweig, 1987). Some of the labels are: RN, red nucleus; SC, superior culliculus; STN, subthalamic nucleus; SNc, substantia nigra, pars compacta; BP, basis pontis; PPNc, pedunculo-pontine nucleus. (Reproduced from Masdeu J, Alampus G, Cavaliere R, Tavoulareas G, Astasia and gait failure with damage of the pontomesencephalic locomotor region. Ann Neurol 1994; 35: 619–21, copyright © 1994. Reprinted by permission of John Wiley & Sons, Inc.)*

BASIS PONTIS

Kwa and co-workers[135] studied 17 atherosclerotic patients that had pontine hyperintense lesions on MRI but no supratentorial white matter lesions. These patients were identified in an ongoing prospective cohort study of 229 atherosclerotic patients who presented initially with non-disabling ischemic stroke, myocardial infarction or peripheral arterial disease. Controls were patients from the same cohort with neither pontine nor supratentorial white matter lesions. Disequilibrium was ascertained by a questionnaire, asking the patients 'Did you suffer from dizziness or unsteadiness (on walking or standing) during the past year?' Twelve of the 17 patients (71 per cent) with pontine lesions complained of disequilibrium versus five of the 17 controls (29 per cent) – a significant difference. There was a trend for abnormal tandem-walking tests to be more frequent in patients than they were in controls. Babinski signs were equally distributed between the two groups. In the disorder recorded by these authors, the disequilibrium was less severe than with large, strategically placed, cerebellar or vestibular lesions.

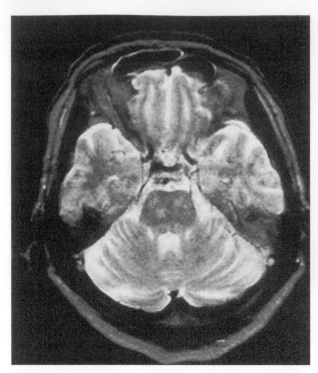

Figure 14.10 *Ischemic rarefaction of the basis pontis. Note the high-intensity lesions that correlated with impaired balance in the series of Kwa et al.,[135] from whose report this figure is reproduced.*

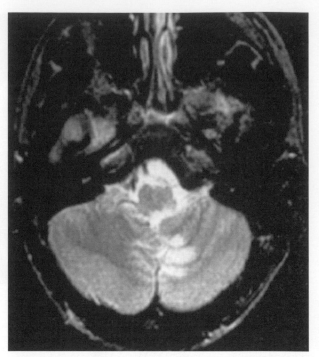

Figure 14.11 *Wallenberg syndrome. Magnetic resonance image of a 31-year-old man with a left lateral medullary infarction after spontaneous dissection of the left vertebral artery. The cerebellar tonsil is also affected.*

As described by Kwa and co-workers,[135] the lesions were foci of hyperintensity on T2-weighted images of the basis pontis (Fig. 14.10). The lesions did not appear in the mesencephalon or in the medulla and tended to spare the tegmentum of the pons containing vestibular pathways. The disequilibrium could be explained by involvement of structures known to participate in balance mechanisms. Alternatively, the finding may uncover new balance-mediating structures. Abnormal areas in the basis pontis overlapped the pontine nuclei, part of the fronto-ponto-cerebellar pathway. Infarcts in the basis pontis, particularly its anterolateral portion, can cause bilateral leg ataxia in addition to contralateral leg paresis.[135,136] Because the lesions were likely to be ischemic, it is possible that, even in the absence of abnormal signal intensity, some of the vestibular structures were also involved.

Vestibular lesions

Vestibular lesions are extensively discussed in Chapter 9. The discussion in the present chapter is restricted to vascular lesions of the central vestibular system. Vestibular involvement occurs in the lateral medullary or Wallenberg syndrome, caused by infarction in the territory of the vertebral or the postero-inferior cerebellar arteries (Fig. 14.11). These patients tend to fall to the side of the infarct. Their gait is broad-based and lurching.

Removal of vision by environmental darkness or impaired eyesight impacts negatively on their ability to ambulate and predisposes them to falls. Initially, most of these patients have a prominent headache and are nauseated. In addition to the impairment of balance and ataxia ipsilateral to the lesion, they have a crossed sensory loss (on the ipsilateral face and contralateral body), an ipsilateral Horner's syndrome and ipsilateral palatal weakness with hoarseness and dysphagia. These findings reflect involvement of the vestibular nuclei and inferior cerebellar peduncle, trigeminal pathways, spinothalamic tract, sympathetic pathways projecting from the hypothalamus to the low cervical segments, and nucleus ambiguus of the glossopharyngeal and vagus nerves. They also have central vestibular nystagmus or oculoparetic nystagmus if the lesion extends upwards into the lower pons.

Atherosclerotic vascular disease of the vertebral or posterior-inferior cerebellar arteries may occlude these vessels and is responsible for this syndrome in about half of the cases.[137] Vascular reconstruction may help some of these patients.[138] Most of the rest are due to cardiogenic emboli. Spontaneous dissection of the arterial wall is a frequent cause in younger,[139] but not in older patients, where temporal arteritis should be suspected, particularly in the very old with a high erythrocyte sedimentation rate.[140] In a small autopsy series of patients with temporal or giant cell arteritis, the vertebral arteries were found to be affected in all cases.[141] Polymyalgia rheumatica may be present but is not a universal finding. The superficial temporal arteries are often tender and swollen, with a faint pulse. Temporal arteritis responds to treatment with steroids or other immunomodulators. Oral prednisone often works well. The dose will depend on the response, but patients on starting doses of 40 mg/day or less have fewer complications.[142] Long-term therapy is often needed.

More controversial in the genesis of brainstem ischemia is the role played by compression by overgrown bone of the vertebral arteries as they transverse the vertebral foramina of the cervical vertebrae. Sheehan and co-workers[143] popularized this mechanism by publishing a study of 26 patients with angiographic demonstration of kinking or stenosis of the vertebral artery at the vertebral foramina. Many of their patients had dizziness evoked by head turning or extension in addition to frank strokes at different levels of the neuraxis. Localization was based on the clinical findings because this study antedated CT. For this reason, and given the frequency of spondylotic narrowing of the vertebral foramina and of peripheral vestibular disease causing dizziness in older individuals with or without strokes, the cause–effect of the angiographic changes to the production of ischemic damage is far from proven. Recent studies on this topic are scant. Sakai and co-workers[144] reported on a 58-year-old man who, on SPECT, had reduced perfusion in the left cerebellum and the right occipital region during an attack of vertebrobasilar insufficiency. Angiography demonstrated compression of the left vertebral artery by osteophytes when the patient turned his head to the left.[144] Unless this mechanism of ischemia is clearly proven for an individual patient, surgical decompression of the vertebral artery at the vertebral foramina is not recommended.[10]

Cerebellar lesions

Cerebellar infarction or hemorrhage, particularly when affecting the flocculonodular lobe, or vestibulocerebellum, can present with acute or progressive impairment of balance and gait. Although most often patients with cerebellar lesions tend to fall to the side of the lesion, some patients with lesions in the tonsillar area develop increased tone (and increased reflexes) in the ipsilateral side and fall to the contralateral side. This was the case with the 64-year-old whose CT is shown in Fig. 14.12. Because gait mechanisms are heavily represented in the anterior cerebellar lobule, gait impairment is the most frequent presentation of infarcts in the area of the superior cerebellar artery.[137] In the older age group, infarction in the area of the posterior inferior cerebellar artery is caused by atheromatous vascular disease as often as by embolic disease. Presumed cerebral embolism was the predominant stroke mechanism in patients with superior cerebellar artery distribution infarcts.[137]

Daily medication with aspirin, 325 mg, may reduce

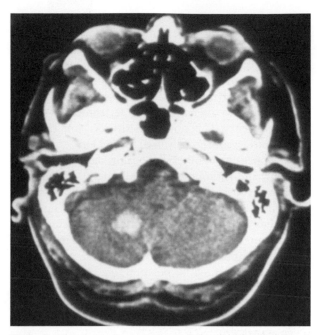

Figure 14.12 *Cerebellar hematoma. Computed tomography of a 64-year-old man with sudden onset of inability to walk and a tendency to fall to the left side. A hemorrhage involves the right supratonsilar region.*

the risk of additional strokes in patients with atherothrombotic disease.[84] Chronic anticoagulation is indicated for patients at risk of repeated embolic events from a cardiac source, such as those with lone atrial fibrillation.[84]

The clinical presentation of cerebellar hemorrhage may be acute, subacute, or chronic.[145,146] Variations in location, size, and development of the hematoma, brainstem compression, fourth ventricular penetration and development of hydrocephalus result in variations in the mode of presentation of cerebellar hemorrhage. These hemorrhages most frequently occur in the region of the dentate nucleus. Patients present with occipital or frontal headache, dizziness, vertigo, nausea, repeated vomiting, and inability to stand or walk. They often have truncal or limb ataxia, ipsilateral gaze palsy and small reactive pupils. Horizontal gaze paresis, paretic nystagmus and facial weakness are also frequent. Frank hemiparesis is absent. Ocular bobbing and skew deviation may be present. Not all patients present such a dramatic picture. Those with small (usually less than 3 cm diameter) cerebellar hematomas may present only with vomiting and with no headaches, gait instability, or limb ataxia.

Hypertension is the predominant risk factor for cerebellar hemorrhage, particularly in the elderly. The management of hypertension was discussed above, under white matter disease. Cavernous angioma, a more common lesion in younger patients, is seldom responsible for intracerebellar hemorrhages in the elderly. Its surgical management is described by Ojemann et al.[147]

DROP ATTACKS

Drop attacks are discussed more extensively in Chapter 16 and are mentioned in the geriatric literature as a major cause of falls and as a common event affecting older people.[148] Drop attacks are discussed in this chapter because they are often ascribed to vertebrobasilar vascular insufficiency. This notion merits revision. The term 'drop attack' was originally used by Sheldon[149] to describe what happens to an otherwise healthy older person, who suddenly and without warning falls to the ground without loss of consciousness. Although fully alert, the victim frequently experiences difficulty in standing up again and needs help to do so. In addition to the demands on postural mechanisms required to arise from the floor to the standing position, some of these patients may have more than a brief loss of postural tone. As described by Sheldon, 'the sudden loss of strength and muscle tone in the legs and trunk may last several hours.'[149] Injuries are common.

Vertebrobasilar ischemia as a major cause of drop attacks received particular support from the work of Sheehan and co-workers, published before CT became available.[143] They reported brainstem ischemia caused by osteophyte encroachment on the vertebral arteries at the vertebral foramina.[143] Of 26 patients with angiographic demonstration of kinking or stenosis of the vertebral artery at the vertebral foramina, six had drop attacks. These patients had other neurological findings and most of them could have suffered the lacunar or hemorrhagic syndromes described earlier in this chapter. For example, a severely hypertensive 63-year-old man fell without losing consciousness. He got to his feet, but for some time he was noted to 'stagger around' and had to hold on to the furniture while walking. Eventually, he improved, but 10 years later he collapsed while walking on the street, remaining alert but unable to walk. The eventual clinical outcome was not described. Another patient, a 68-year-old diabetic woman, fell without losing consciousness and was unable to get up. Shortly after admission to the hospital she became able to walk but was ataxic for several days. In reporting these cases, Sheehan and co-workers emphasized the presence of dizziness with head turning and vertebral changes on angiography.[143] Dizziness with head turning is more likely related to peripheral vestibular dysfunction, which is common in the elderly, than to brain stem ischemia, in which dizziness is generally accompanied by diplopia or other brainstem findings. Cervical spondylosis occurs regularly with aging. Therefore, the link between vertebrobasilar ischemia and drop attacks, as reported by Sheehan and co-workers,[143] remains unproven.

In rare cases, drop attacks are caused by ischemia of the pyramids and may herald infarction in the vertebrobasilar territory. One such case was described by Brust and co-workers.[150] Two episodes of sudden unexpected falls without associated neurological findings preceded infarction of the corticospinal tracts at the pons and medulla and eventual death. At autopsy there was bilateral vertebral artery occlusion. This was an unusual case because ischemia in the vertebrobasilar territory often presents with other neurological manifestations, such as numbness, diplopia or vertigo, in addition to sudden loss of postural tone in the legs. In terms of cerebrovascular disease, lacunar strokes of the basal ganglia, thalamus or suprathalamic white matter are much more likely to cause sudden inability to stand or walk, as described above, because these lesions are much more common than ischemia of the pyramids in the medulla.

Many events meeting the clinical definition of drop attacks are not caused by vascular disease of the brain. Meissner and co-workers[151] reviewed 108 patients diagnosed with drop attacks at the Mayo Clinic (Rochester, MN, USA) between 1976 and 1983; mean age was 70 years. In the majority (64 per cent) of the patients the mechanism was unknown. Some of them may have had falls on the basis of one of the vascular syndromes described in this chapter; these were poorly recognized until more recently. Cardiac causes were present in 12 per cent, clear-cut cerebrovascular insufficiency in 8 per cent, combined cardiac and cerebrovascular disease in 7 per cent, seizures in 5 per cent vestibular disease in 3 per cent, and in one case the falls were felt to be psychogenic. Among the patients with cerebrovascular disease, the two with persistent drop attacks had carotid artery disease. About 80 per cent of the patients were symptom-free at a mean follow-up of 6.5 years. Neurological findings on examination, cardiac arrhythmias and congestive heart failure increased the risk of death on follow-up. The stroke rate in the overall group, approximately 0.5 per cent per year, was not significantly different from that in a normal age- and sex-matched population. However, small vessel disease and disease of the white matter evolve over a longer period of time than covered in this study. In addition, progressive vascular disease of these structures may not have been classified as stroke because it would have presented with gait or balance impairment but without hemiparesis or some other of the classic features of cerebrovascular disease. Other causes of drop attacks include hydrocephalus and intraventricular tumors.[152]

Vertebrobasilar ischemia is not currently accepted as a frequent cause of drop attacks. Two recent editions of standard stroke textbooks do not even list drop attack in their index[9,153] and another lists the term only to argue against its purported vertebrobasilar basis.[10] However, the vascular syndromes described in this chapter, including white matter ischemic disease and lacunar or hemorrhagic stroke of the basal ganglia, thalamus or suprathalamic white matter, result in disequilibrium with a propensity towards falling. Falls are often precipitated by sudden buckling of the knees, mimicking a drop attack. In many instances there is no history of stroke, despite the evidence on neuroimaging studies. It is likely that at least some of the patients described previously with drop attacks probably had a propensity to falling on the basis of subcortical disequilibrium, caused by one of the vascular syndromes described above.

LATE–LIFE HYDROCEPHALUS

Although not a frequent cause of gait disorders in older people, symptomatic hydrocephalus presents initially with a gait disorder and it should be recognized because it is potentially treatable.[154] Particularly after CT became available, several authors found enlarged ventricles frequently to be present in patients with gait disorders.[155] From this finding they concluded that symptomatic hydrocephalus was common and shunting procedures multiplied. However, even in series with carefully selected patients, some failed to improve after shunting, suggesting that hydrocephalus was not the cause of their gait disorder.[156] For this reason, it is important to apply more sensitive diagnostic criteria in the work-up of these patients.[157]

Clinical syndrome

The classical syndrome consists of slowly progressive gait impairment, with instability.[158] At the bedside, or even with a force platform, it is difficult to distinguish between the gait disorder caused by subcortical arteriosclerotic encephalopathy and that caused by hydrocephalus.[159] Urinary incontinence may be present, but is not necessary for the diagnosis. Only very late in the course of the disorder might the patient have cognitive slowness or impaired attention. Onset of cognitive impairment before gait disturbance suggests a different process.[157]

Neuroimaging findings

The diagnosis is made with CT or MRI, which show enlarged ventricles (Fig 14.13). Often, the cortical sulci are compressed. However, in many patients they may be enlarged, sometimes greatly so.[160,161] Sulcal enlargement involves in particular the basal cisterns, Sylvian fissures and other major sulci on the convexity of the hemispheres. Typically, the sulci in the high parietal convexity and medial aspect of the parietal lobe are compressed (Fig. 14.14).

Cerebrovascular disease, in the form of lacunar strokes or abnormal white matter on CT or MRI, is more frequent in patients with hydrocephalus than in controls.[162] It predicts a poorer outcome after shunting in some large studies,[163] but not in smaller ones.[164] When the clinical or CT–MR diagnosis is dubious, a pattern of decreased perfusion or metabolism in the association cortex of the parietal lobes on SPECT or PET predicts a poor outcome.[157] This pattern is usually seen in Alzheimer's disease and Parkinson's with dementia.

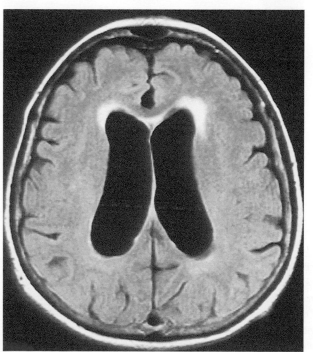

(a)

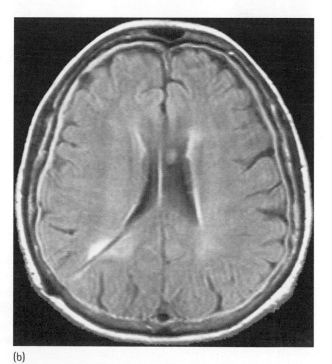

(b)

Figure 14.13 *Magnetic resonance imaging of a 76-year-old woman. Note the ventricular dilation in the presurgical scan (a), corrected by a ventriculo-peritoneal shunt (b).*

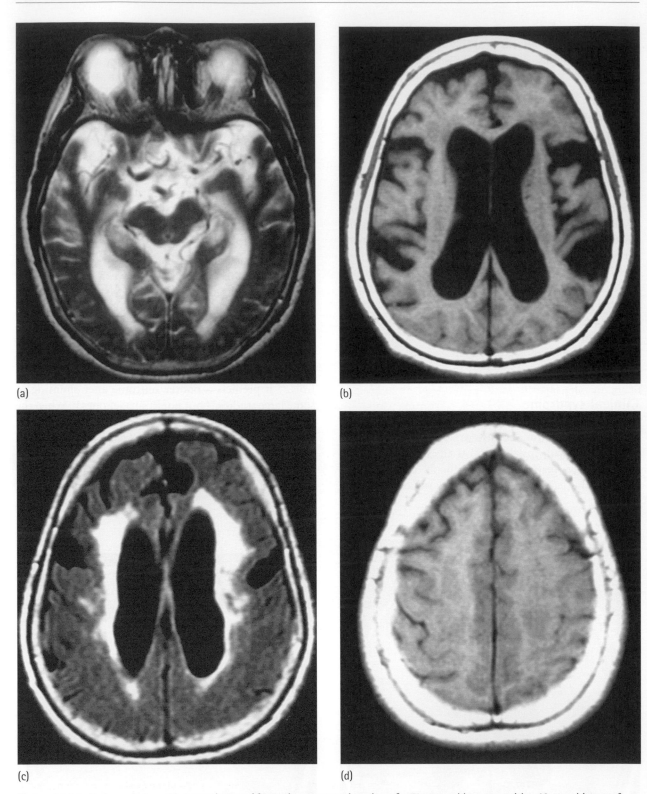

Figure 14.14 *Hydrocephalus with megacisterns. Magnetic resonance imaging of a 71-year-old woman with a 10-year history of progressive difficulty walking. Unable to walk for about 1 year before this scan was obtained. Doubly incontinent. Very friendly, witty; mild memory impairment. (a) Axial T2 section though the suprasellar cistern. (b) Axial T1 section through the lateral ventricles; note the large size of the Sylvian fissures. (c) Axial FLAIR section through the lateral ventricles; note high signal in the peri-ependymal region, corresponding probably to transependymal CSF resorption and gliosis. (d) Supraventricular axial T1 section. Note that the sulci in the high parietal convexity are compressed. The patient became able to walk after ventriculoperitoneal shunting.*

Cerebrospinal fluid dynamics

Cerebrospinal fluid flow may be abnormal in symptomatic hydrocephalus, and therefore help with the diagnosis. It can be evaluated by MRI or by manometric methods through lumbar puncture. Magnetic resonance imaging allows for quantitative phase-contrast CSF velocity imaging. Patients with CSF stroke volumes greater than 42 µl responded favorably to CSF shunting.[165] Some groups have found cerebrospinal-fluid manometrics to be not predictive of which patients will improve after shunting.[166] However, other groups have found values greater than 18 mmHg/ml/min of resistance to outflow of cerebrospinal fluid, obtained by lumbar constant flow infusion, to be highly predictive of a positive outcome after shunting.[167]

Pathogenesis

Hydrocephalus causes stretching of the periventricular thalamocortical fibers that run in the subependymal region of the lateral ventricles. It may also affect these fibers by altering the local extracellular milieu. The extracellular space is enlarged, with edema, and there is demyelination and subependymal gliosis.[168] The involvement of these fibers, also preferentially affected in subcortical arteriosclerotic encephalopathy, explains the clinical similarity of these disorders.

Treatment

Ventriculo-peritoneal shunting is the procedure of choice to treat symptomatic hydrocephalus. A feared complication is infection of the shunt. In addition, because this is a disorder with higher prevalence in the older population, who are prone to having brain atrophy as well, shunting may favor the development of subdural collections, which may become symptomatic. However, in the Dutch Normal-Pressure Hydrocephalus Study, subdural effusions occurred in 71 per cent of patients treated with a low-pressure shunt and in 34 per cent with a medium-pressure shunt; but their influence on patient outcome was limited.[169] Indeed, the functional outcome was better in those treated with a low-pressure shunt. Newer shunts are being developed to try to avoid excessive shunting when the patient is in the upright position, with the consequent risk of subdural effusions and the low intracranial pressure syndrome.[170]

CONCLUSION

Vascular lesions are a frequent cause of disorders of stance and gait, particularly in the elderly. Both ischemic and hemorrhagic disease can cause gait impairment and both can present with a sudden onset of symptoms or in a slowly progressive, or, more typically, in an incremen-

Table 14.1 *Vascular gait syndromes*

	Structure(s) involved	Type of stance and gait impairment	Typical associated signs and symptoms
Slowly progressive, or incremental, step-wise progression	High convexity subdural hematoma	Gait apraxia Hand grasp	Bradyphrenia
	Hemispheric white matter disease	Unsteady, prone to falls	Lower body parkinsonism
	Small, multiple basal ganglia or lateral thalamic lacunes	Narrow base	
	Basis pontis	Unsteady	
Sudden onset	Medial frontal	Gait apraxia, freezing	Bradyphrenia; hand and foot grasp
	Hemispheric, suprathalamic white matter; putamen	Marked unsteadiness, narrow base	Lower body parkinsonism
	Lateral thalamus	Marked unsteadiness, narrow base	Contralateral axial muscle dysfunction Contralateral sensory loss (often)
	Mesencephalic locomotor center	Marked unsteadiness	Pseudo-six
	Vestibular nucleus	Disrupted stepping pattern Unsteadiness, 'pulling' to one side Worse with eyes closed	Gaze palsy, nystagmus, Horner syndrome Cerebellar ataxia Ipsilateral face and contralateral body numbness
	Cerebellum	Broad-based, unsteady, lurching	Heel-to-shin dysmetria

tal, step-wise fashion. The sudden onset is characteristic of larger lesions. However, the accumulation over time of small ischemic or hemorrhagic lesions, indicated by MRI or CT, may give the impression of a slowly progressive process. Ischemic disease of the white matter may be slowly progressive, because the oligodendrocytes may suffer chronic, sublethal ischemic damage that interferes with the normal production of myelin. Subdural hematomas may cause acute compression of the frontal lobe, owing to a fresh hemorrhage into the hematoma, or slowly compress this structure, as the hematoma grows slowly. Thus, the tempo of the clinical manifestations of vascular disease varies depending on the size and nature of the damage. Another important factor that defines the manifestations of vascular brain lesions is the localization of the lesion, namely, the structure or structures damaged by the vascular lesion. The most common vascular syndromes are summarized in Table 14.1.

The latter portion of this chapter is dedicated to the gait and equilibrium disorder caused by hydrocephalus. The clinical disorder shares many of the features of the slowly progressive vascular disorder of the white matter, but its treatment is much more effective. Although severe hydrocephalus may cause bradyphrenia and other attentional and executive function disorders, postural and gait impairment are the most characteristic and earliest manifestations of symptomatic hydrocephalus in the adult. The disorder is verified with CT or MRI. The perfusion pattern on SPECT and the tests of CSF infusion may help diagnose cases with less clear-cut clinical and imaging findings.

REFERENCES

1. Fuh JL, Lin KN, Wang SJ, et al. Neurologic diseases presenting with gait impairment in the elderly. *J Geriatr Psychiatry Neurol* 1994;**7**:89–92.
2. Sudarsky L. Clinical approach to gait disorders of aging: an overview. In: Masdeu J, Sudarsky L, Wolfson L, eds. *Gait disorders of aging. Falls and therapeutic strategies*. Philadelphia: Lippincott and Raven, 1997;147–57.
3. Lhermitte J. *Étude sur la paraplégies des vieillards*. Paris: Maretheux, 1907.
4. Critchley M. On senile disorders of gait, including the so-called 'senile paraplegia'. *Geriatrics* 1948;**3**:364–70.
5. FitzGerald P, Jankovic J. Lower body parkinsonism: evidence for vascular etiology. *Mov Disord* 1987;**4**:249–60.
6. Masdeu J, Wolfson L. Lower body (vascular) parkinsonism. *Arch Neurol* 1990;**47**:748.
7. Trenkwalder C, Paulus W, Krafczyk S, Hawken M, Oertel WH, Brandt T. Postural stability differentiates 'lower body' from idiopathic parkinsonism. *Acta Neurol Scand* 1995;**91**:444–52.
8. Caplan L, Schoene W. Clinical features of subcortical arteriosclerotic encephalopathy (Binswanger disease). *Neurology* 1978;**28**:1206–15.
9. Caplan L. *Caplan's Stroke. A clinical approach*, 3rd edn. Boston: Butterworth-Heinemann, 2000.
10. Barnett H, Mohr J, Stein B, Yatsu F. *Stroke. Pathophysiology, diagnosis and management*, 3rd edn. New York: Churchill Livingstone, 1998.
11. Fazekas F, Schmidt R, Offenbacher H, et al. Prevalence of white matter and periventricular magnetic resonance hyperintensities in asymptomatic volunteers. *J Neuroimag* 1991;**1**:27–30.
12. Gerard G, Weisberg L. MRI periventricular lesions in adults. *Neurology* 1986;**36**:998–1001.
13. Goto K, Ishii N, Fukasawa H. Diffuse white-matter disease in the geriatric population: a clinical, neuropathological, and CT study. *Radiology* 1981;**141**:687–95.
14. McQuinn B, O'Leary D. CT periventricular lucencies: association with systemic disease states and with sub-acute arteriosclerotic encephalopathy (SAE, 'Binswanger's disease'). *Stroke* 1986;**17**:135.
15. Pullicino P, Eskin T, Ketonen L. Prevalence of Binswanger's disease. *Lancet* 1983;**l**:939.
16. Meyer JS, Kawamura J, Terayama Y. White matter lesions in the elderly. *J Neurol Sci* 1992;**110**:1–7.
17. Zatz L, Jernigan T, Ahumada AJ. White matter changes in cerebral computed tomography related to aging. *J Comput Assist Tomogr* 1982;**6**:l9–23.
18. Awad I, Spetzler R, Hodak J, Awad C, Carey R. Incidental subcortical lesions identified on magnetic resonance imaging in the elderly. I. Correlation with age and cerebrovascular risk factors. *Stroke* 1986;**17**:1084–9.
19. Brant-Zawadzki M, Fein G, van Dyke C, et al. MR imaging of the aging brain: patchy white-matter lesions and dementia. *Am J Neuroradiol* 1985;**6**:675–82.
20. Zimmerman R, Fleming C, Lee B, et al. Periventricular hyperintensity as seen by magnetic resonance: prevalence and significance. *Am J Rad* 1986;**146**:443–50.
21. Awad I, Johnson P, Spetzler R, Hodak J. Incidental subcortical lesions identified on magnetic resonance imaging in the elderly. II. Postmortem pathological correlations. *Stroke* 1986;**17**:1090–7.
22. Kirkpatrick J, Hayman L. White-matter lesions on MR imaging of clinically healthy brains of elderly subjects: possible pathologic basis. *Radiology* 1987;**162**:509–11.
23. Gass A, Oster M, Cohen S, et al. Assessment of T2- and T1-weighted MRI brain lesion load in patients with subcortical vascular encephalopathy. *Neuroradiology* 1998;**40**:503–6.
24. Sullivan EV, Adalsteinsson E, Hedehus M, et al. Equivalent disruption of regional white matter microstructure in ageing healthy men and women. *Neuroreport* 2001;**12**:99–104.
25. Dubas F, Gray F, Roullet E, Escourolle R. Leucoencéphalopathies artériopathiques (17 cas anatomo-cliniques). *Rev Neurol (Paris)* 1985;**141**:93–l08.
26. Dupuis M, Brucher J, Gonsette R. Obsevation anatomo-clinique d'une encéphalopathie sous-corticale artérioscléreuse ('maladie de Binswanger') avec hypodensité de la substance blanche au scanner cérébral. *Acta Neurol Belg* 1984;**84**:131–40.
27. Gray F, Dubas F, Roullet E, Escourolle R. Leukoencephalopathy in diffuse hemorrhagic cerebral amyloid angiopathy. *Ann Neurol* 1985;**18**:54–9.
28. Huang K, Wu L, Luo Y. Binswanger's disease: progressive subcortical encephalopathy or multi-infarct dementia? *Can J Neurol Sci* 1985;**12**:88–94.

29. Janota I. Dementia, deep white matter damage and hypertension: 'Binswanger's disease'. *Psychol Med* 1981;**11**:39–48.

30. Rosenberg G, Kornfeld M, Stovring J, Bicknell J. Subcortical arteriosclerotic encephalopathy (Binswanger): computerized tomography. *Neurology* 1979;**29**:1102–6.

31. Masdeu JC, Wolfson L, Lantos G, et al. Brain white-matter changes in the elderly prone to falling. *Arch Neurol* 1989;**46**:1292–6.

32. Steingart A, Hachinski V, Lau C. Cognitive and neurologic findings in subjects with diffuse white matter lucencies on computed tomographic scan (leuko-araiosis). *Arch Neurol* 1987;**44**:32–35.

33. George A, de Leon M, Gentes C, et al. Leukoencephalopathy in normal and pathologic aging: CT of brain lucencies. *Am J Neuradiol* 1986;**7**:561–6.

34. Hendrie H, Farlow M, Austrom M, et al. Foci of increased T2 signal intensity on brain MR scans of healthy elderly subjects. *Am J Neuroradiol* 1989;**10**:703–7.

35. Thompson P, Marsden C. Gait disorder of subcortical arteriosclerotic encephalopathy: Binswanger's disease. *Mov Disord* 1987;**2**:1–8.

36. Baloh RW, Yue Q, Socotch TM, Jacobson KM. White matter lesions and disequilibrium in older people. I. Case-control comparison. *Arch Neurol* 1995;**52**:970–974.

37. Hennerici MG, Oster M, Cohen S, et al. Are gait disturbances and white matter degeneration early indicators of vascular dementia? *Dementia* 1994;**5**:197–202.

38. Tell GS, Lefkowitz DS, Diehr P, Elster AD. Relationship between balance and abnormalities in cerebral magnetic resonance imaging in older adults. *Arch Neurol* 1998;**55**:73–9.

39. Camicioli R, Moore MM, Sexton G, et al. Age-related brain changes associated with motor function in healthy older people. *J Am Geriatr Soc* 1999;**47**:330–4.

40. van Zagten M, Lodder J, Kessels F. Gait disorder and parkinsonian signs in patients with stroke related to small deep infarcts and white matter lesions. *Mov Disord* 1998;**13**:89–95.

41. Kerber KA, Enrietto JA, Jacobson KM, Baloh RW. Disequilibrium in older people: a prospective study. *Neurology* 1998;**51**:574–80.

42. Brooks WM, Wesley MH, Kodituwakku PW, et al. 1H-MRS differentiates white matter hyperintensities in subcortical arteriosclerotic encephalopathy from those in normal elderly. *Stroke* 1997;**28**:1940–3.

43. Briley DP, Wasay M, Sergent S, Thomas S. Cerebral white matter changes (leukoaraiosis), stroke, and gait disturbance. *J Am Geriatr Soc* 1997;**45**:1434–1438.

44. Sohn YH, Kim JS. The influence of white matter hyperintensities on the clinical features of Parkinson's disease. *Yonsei Med J* 1998;**39**:50–5.

45. Whitman GT, Tang Y, Lin A, et al. A prospective study of cerebral white matter abnormalities in older people with gait dysfunction. *Neurology* 2001;**57**:990–4.

46. Guttmann CR, Benson R, Warfield SK, et al. White matter abnormalities in mobility-impaired older persons. *Neurology* 2000;**54**:1277–83.

47. Hachinski V, Potter P, Merskey H. Leuko-araiosis. *Arch Neurol* 1987;**44**:21–3.

48. Braffman B, Zimmerman R, Trojanowski J, et al. Pathologic correlation with gross and histopathology. 2. Hyperintense white-matter foci in the elderly. *Am J Neuroradiol* 1988;**9**:629–36.

49. Kinkel W, Jacobs L, Polachini I, et al. Subcortical arteriosclerotic encephalopathy (Binswanger's disease). Computed tomographic, nuclear magnetic resonance, and clinical correlations. *Arch Neurol* 1985;**42**:951–9.

50. Johnson K, Davis K, Buonanno F, et al. Comparison of magnetic resonance and roentgen ray computed tomography in dementia. *Arch Neurol* 1987;**44**:1075–80.

51. Lotz P, Ballinger W, Quisling R. Subcortical arteriosclerotic encephalopathy: CT spectrum and pathologic correlation. *Am J Radiol* 1986;**147**:1209–14.

52. Marshall V, Bradley W, Marshall C, et al. Deep white matter infarction: correlation of MR imaging and histopathologic findings. *Radiology* 1988;**167**:517–22.

53. Rezek D, Morris J, Fulling K, Gado M. Periventricular white matter lucencies in senile dementia of the Alzheimer type and in normal aging. *Neurology* 1987;**37**:1365–8.

54. Rosenberg GA, Sullivan N, Esiri MM. White matter damage is associated with matrix metalloproteinases in vascular dementia. *Stroke* 2001;**32**:1162–8.

55. Yamanouchi H. Loss of white matter oligodendrocytes and astrocytes in progressive subcortical vascular encephalopathy of Binswanger type. *Acta Neurol Scand* 1991;**83**:301–5.

56. De Reuck J, Crevits L, De-Coster W, et al. Pathogenesis of Binswanger chronic progressive subcortical encephalopathy. *Neurology* 1980;**30**:920–8.

57. De Reuck J. The cortico-subcortical arterial angioarchitecture in the human brain. *Acta Neurol Belg* 1972;**72**:323–9.

58. Skoog I. Risk factors for vascular dementia: a review. *Dementia* 1994;**5**:137–44.

59. van Swieten JC, Geyskes GG, et al. Hypertension in the elderly is associated with white matter lesions and cognitive decline. *Ann Neurol* 1991;**30**:825–30.

60. Longstreth WT Jr, Manolio TA, Arnold A, et al. Clinical correlates of white matter findings on cranial magnetic resonance imaging of 3301 elderly people. The Cardiovascular Health Study. *Stroke* 1996;**27**:1274–82.

61. Schmidt R, Fazekas F, Kapeller P, Schmidt H, Hartung HP. MRI white matter hyperintensities: three-year follow-up of the Austrian Stroke Prevention Study. *Neurology* 1999;**53**:132–9.

62. Dufouil C, de Kersaint-Gilly A, Besancon V, et al. Longitudinal study of blood pressure and white matter hyperintensities: the EVA MRI Cohort. *Neurology* 2001;**56**:921–6.

63. de Leeuw FE, de Groot JC, Oudkerk M, et al. Hypertension and cerebral white matter lesions in a prospective cohort study. *Brain* 2002;**125**:765–72.

64. Hyman DJ, Pavlik VN. Characteristics of patients with uncontrolled hypertension in the United States. *N Engl J Med* 2001;**345**:479–86.

65. Probstfield JL, Furberg CD. Systolic hypertension in the elderly: controlled or uncontrolled. *Cardiovasc Clin* 1990;**20**:65–84.

66. Brun A, Englund E. A white matter disorder in dementia of the Alzheimer type: a pathoanatomical study. *Ann Neurol* 1986;**19**:253–62.

67. Harrison M, Marshall J. Hypoperfusion in the aetiology of subcortical arteriosclerotic encephalopathy (Binswanger type). *J Neurol Neurosurg Psychiatry* 1984;**47**:754.

68. Schneider R, Wöbker G, Willmes K, et al. Do different ischemic brain lesions have different hemorheological profiles? *Klin Wochenschr* 1986;**64**:357–6l.

69. Tzourio C, Levy C, Dufouil C, et al. Low cerebral blood flow velocity and risk of white matter hyperintensities. *Ann Neurol* 2001;**49**:411–14.

70. Durany N, Ravid R, Riederer P, Cruz-Sanchez FF. Increased frequency of the alpha-1-antichymotrypsin T allele in cerebral amyloid angiopathy. *Neuropathology* 2000;**20**:184–9.

71. Sabbadini G, Francia A, Calandriello L, et al. Cerebral autosomal dominant arteriopathy with subcortical infarcts and leucoencephalopathy (CADASIL). Clinical, neuroimaging, pathological and genetic study of a large Italian family. *Brain* 1995;**118**:207–15.

72. Chabriat H, Vahedi K, Iba-Zizen MT, et al. Clinical spectrum of CADASIL: a study of 7 families. Cerebral autosomal dominant arteriopathy with subcortical infarcts and leukoencephalopathy. *Lancet* 1995;**346**:934–9.

73. Auer DP, Putz B, Gossl C, et al. Differential lesion patterns in CADASIL and sporadic subcortical arteriosclerotic encephalopathy: MR imaging study with statistical parametric group comparison. *Radiology* 2001;**218**:443–51.

74. Kalaria RN. Advances in molecular genetics and pathology of cerebrovascular disorders. *Trends Neurosci* 2001;**24**:392–400.

75. Ducros A, Nagy T, Alamowitch S, et al. Cerebral autosomal dominant arteriopathy with subcortical infarcts and leukoencephalopathy, genetic homogeneity, and mapping of the locus within a 2-cM interval. *Am J Hum Genet* 1996;**58**:171–181.

76. Joutel A, Vahedi K, Corpechot C, et al. Strong clustering and stereotyped nature of Notch3 mutations in CADASIL patients. *Lancet* 1997;**350**:1511–15.

77. Ruchoux MM, Maurage CA. CADASIL: Cerebral autosomal dominant arteriopathy with subcortical infarcts and leukoencephalopathy. *J Neuropathol Exp Neurol* 1997;**56**:947–64.

78. Rubio A, Rifkin D, Powers JM, et al. Phenotypic variability of CADASIL and novel morphologic findings. *Acta Neuropathol* 1997;**94**:247–54.

79. Flemming KD, Nguyen TT, Abu-Lebdeh HS, et al. Hyperhomocysteinemia in patients with cerebral autosomal dominant arteriopathy with subcortical infarcts and leukoencephalopathy (CADASIL). *Mayo Clin Proc* 2001;**76**:1213–18.

80. Vermeer SE, van Dijk EJ, Koudstaal PJ, et al. Homocysteine, silent brain infarcts, and white matter lesions: The Rotterdam Scan Study. *Ann Neurol* 2002;**51**:285–9.

81. Rossi A, Cerone R, Biancheri R, et al. Early-onset combined methylmalonic aciduria and homocystinuria: neuroradiologic findings. *Am J Neuroradiol* 2001;**22**:554–63.

82. National Institutes of Health. *The 6th Report of the Joint National Committee on Prevention, Detection, Evaluation, and Treatment of High Blood Pressure, November 1997. NIH Publication No. 98-40801997.* Washington, DC: NIH, 1997.

83. Lindblad U, Rastam L, Ranstam J. Stroke morbidity in patients treated for hypertension – The Skaraborg Hypertension Project. *J Intern Med* 1993;**233**:155–63.

84. Feinberg WM, Albers GW, Barnett HJ, et al. Guidelines for the management of transient ischemic attacks. From the *Ad Hoc* Committee on Guidelines for the Management of Transient Ischemic Attacks of the Stroke Council of the American Heart Association. *Circulation* 1994;**89**:2950–65.

85. Jansen RW, Lipsitz LA. Postprandial hypotension: epidemiology, pathophysiology, and clinical management. *Ann Intern Med* 1995;**122**:286–95.

86. Utzschneider DA, Kocsis JD, Waxman SG. Differential sensitivity to hypoxia of the peripheral versus central trajectory of primary afferent axons. *Brain Res* 1991;**551**:136–141.

87. Meyer JS, Judd BW, Tawaklna T, Rogers RL, Mortel KF. Improved cognition after control of risk factors for multi-infarct dementia. *JAMA* 1986;**256**:2203–9.

88. Furberg CD, Berglund G, Manolio TA, Psaty BM. Overtreatment and undertreatment of hypertension. *J Intern Med* 1994;**235**:387–97.

89. Kendall MJ, Tse WY, Head A. The treatment of elderly hypertensive patients. *J Clin Pharm Ther* 1993;**18**:9–14.

90. North American Symptomatic Carotid Endarterectomy Trial Collaborators. Beneficial effect of carotid endarterectomy in symptomatic patients with high-grade carotid stenosis. *N Engl J Med* 1991;**325**:445–53.

91. Executive Committee for the Asymptomatic Carotid Atherosclerosis Study. Endarterectomy for asymptomatic carotid artery stenosis. *JAMA* 1995;**273**:1421–8.

92. Goldstein LB, Adams R, Becker K, et al. Primary prevention of ischemic stroke: a statement for healthcare professionals from the Stroke Council of the American Heart Association. *Stroke* 2001;**32**:280–99.

93. Nutt J, Marsden C, Thompson P. Human walking and higher-level gait disorders, particularly in the elderly. *Neurology* 1993;**43**:268–79.

94. Cambier J, Elghozi D. Strube E. Lésions du thalamus droit avec syndrome de l'hémisphère mineur. Discussion du concept de négligence thalamique. *Rev Neurol* 1980;**136**:105–16.

95. Laplane D, Escourolle R, Degos J, et al. La négligence motrice d'origine thalamique. A propos de deux cas. *Rev Neurol (Paris)* 1982;**138**:201–11.

96. Masdeu J, Gorelick P. Thalamic astasia: Inability to stand after unilateral thalamic lesions. *Ann Neurol* 1988;**23**:596–603.

97. Jenkyn L, Alberti A, Peters J. Language dysfunction, somasthetic hemi-inattention, and thalamic hemorrhage in the dominant hemisphere. *Neurology* 1981;**31**:1202.

98. Verma A, Maheshwari M. Hypesthetic-ataxic-hemiparesis in thalamic hemorrhage. *Stroke* 1986;**17**:49–51.

99. Friel J. *Dorland's illustrated medical dictionary*, 25th edn. Philadelphia: Saunders, 1974.

100. DeJong R. Case taking and the neurologic examination. In: Baker A, Joynt R, eds. *Clinical neurology.* Hagerstown: Harper and Row, 1985;48.

101. Watson R, Valenstein E, Heilman K. Thalamic neglect. Possible role of the medial thalamus and nucleus reticularis in behavior. *Arch Neurol* 1981;**38**:501–6.

102. Velasco F, Velasco M. A reticulothalamic system mediating proprioceptive attention and tremor in man. *Neurosurgery* 1979;**4**:30–6.

103. Bogousslavsky J, Miklossy J, Deruaz J, et al. Unilateral left paramedian infarction of thalamus and midbrain: a clinico-pathological study. *J Neurol Neurosurg Psychiatry* 1986;**49**:686–94.

104. Rabitsch W, Brugger SA, Pirker W, et al. Symmetrical necrosis of globus pallidus with severe gait disturbance in a patient with myelodysplastic syndrome given allogeneic marrow transplantation. *Ann Hematol* 1997;**75**:235–7.

105. Haaxma R, van Boxtel A, Brouwer WH, et al. Motor function in a patient with bilateral lesions of the globus pallidus. *Mov Disord* 1995;**10**:761–77.

106. Brandt T, Dieterich M. Vestibular syndromes in the roll plane: topographic diagnosis from brainstem to cortex. *Ann Neurol* 1994;**36**:337–47.

107. Dieterich M, Brandt T. Thalamic infarctions: differential effects on vestibular function in the roll plane (35 patients). *Neurology* 1993;**43**:1732–40.

108. Karnath HO, Ferber S, Dichgans J. The neural representation of postural control in humans. *Proc Natl Acad Sci USA* 2000;**97**:13931–6.

109. Jones EG, Steriade M, McCormick DA. *The thalamus.* New York: Elsevier Science, 1997.

110. van Buren J, Borke R. *Variations and connections of the human thalamus.* Berlin, New York: Springer Verlag, 1972.

111. Fisher C, Cole M. Homolateral ataxia and crural paresis; a vascular syndrome. *J Neurol Neurosurg Psychiatry* 1965;**28**:48–55.

112. Huang C, Lui F. Ataxic-hemiparesis, localization and clinical features. *Stroke* 1984;**15**:363–6.

113. Iragui V, McCutchen C. Capsular ataxic hemiparesis. *Arch Neurol* 1982;**39**:528–9.

114. Sage J, Lepore F. Ataxic hemiparesis from lesions of the corona radiata. *Arch Neurol* 1983;**40**:449–50.

115. Asanuma C, Thach W, Jones E. Distribution of cerebellar terminations and their relation to other afferent terminations in the thalamic ventral lateral region of the monkey. *Brain Res Rev* 1983;**5**:237–65.

116. Groothuis D, Duncan G, Fisher C. The human thalamocortical sensory path in the internal capsule: evidence from a small capsular hemorrhage causing a pure sensory stroke. *Ann Neurol* 1977;**2**:328–33.

117. Labadie E, Awerbuch G, Hamilton R, Rapcsak S. Falling and postural deficits due to acute unilateral basal ganglia lesions. *Arch Neurol* 1989;**261**:492–6.

118. Ozdirim E, Topcu M, Ozon A, Cila A. Cockayne syndrome: review of 25 cases. *Pediatr Neurol* 1996;**15**:312–16.

119. Inagaki M, Koeda T, Takeshita K. Prognosis and MRI after ischemic stroke of the basal ganglia. *Pediatr Neurol* 1992;**8**:104–8.

120. Yamanouchi H, Nagura H. Neurological signs and frontal white matter lesions in vascular parkinsonism. A clinicopathologic study. *Stroke* 1997;**28**:965–969.

121. Chang CM, Yu YL, Ng HK, et al. Vascular pseudoparkinsonism. *Acta Neurol Scand* 1992;**86**:588–92.

122. Feve AP, Fenelon G, Wallays C, et al. Axial motor disturbances after hypoxic lesions of the globus pallidus. *Mov Disord* 1993;**8**:321–326.

123. Schenkman M, Riegger-Krugh C. Physical intervention for elderly patients with gait disorders. In: Masdeu JC, Sudarsky L, Wolfson L, eds. *Gait disorders of aging.* Philadelphia: Lippincott and Raven, 1997;327.

124. Matias-Guiu J, Alvarez-Sabin J, Codina A. Comparative study of the effect of low-dosage acetylsalicylic acid and triflusal in the prevention of cardiovascular events among young adults with ischemic cerebrovascular disease. *Rev Neurol* 1997;**25**:1669–72.

125. Garcia-Rill E. The pedunculopontine nucleus. *Prog Neurobiol* 1991;**36**:363–89.

126. Zweig R, Jankel W, Hedreen J, Mayeux R, Price D. The pedunculopontine nucleus in Parkinson's disease. *Ann Neurol* 1989;**25**:41–6.

127. Masdeu J, Alampur U, Cavaliere R, Tavoulareas G. Astasia and gait failure with damage of the pontomesencephalic locomotor region. *Ann Neurol* 1994;**35**:619–21.

128. Hazrati LN, Parent A. Projection from the deep cerebellar nuclei to the pedunculopontine nucleus in the squirrel monkey. *Brain Res* 1992;**585**:267–71.

129. Moriizumi T, Hattori T. Separate neuronal populations of the rat globus pallidus projecting to the subthalamic nucleus, auditory cortex and pedunculopontine tegmental area. *Neuroscience* 1992;**46**:701–10.

130. Skinner R, Garcia-Rill E. Brainstem modulation of rhythmic functions and behaviors. In: Klemm W, Vertes R, eds. *Brainstem mechanisms and behavior.* New York: John Wiley and Sons, 1990;465–96.

131. Mogenson G, Wu M, Brudzynski S. The role of pedunculopontine nucleus in locomotor activity. *Neurosci Abstr* 1990;**16**:753.

132. Caplan L, Goodwin J. Lateral tegmental brainstem hemorrhages. *Neurology* 1982;**32**:252–60.

133. Felice K, Keilson G, Schwartz W. 'Rubral' gait ataxia. *Neurology* 1990;**40**:1004–5.

134. Sand J, Biller J, Corbett J, et al. Partial dorsal mesencephalic hemorrhages: report of three cases. *Neurology* 1986;**36**:529–533.

135. Kwa VI, Zaal LH, Verbeeten B Jr, Stam J. Disequilibrium in patients with atherosclerosis: relevance of pontine ischemic rarefaction. Amsterdam Vascular Medicine Group. *Neurology* 1998;**51**:570–3.

136. Fisher C. Ataxic hemiparesis. *Arch Neurol* 1978;**35**:126–8.

137. Kase CS, Norrving B, Levine SR, et al. Cerebellar infarction. Clinical and anatomic observations in 66 cases. *Stroke* 1993;**24**:76–83.

138. Van-Schil PE, Ackerstaff RG, Vermeulen FE, et al. Long-term clinical and duplex follow-up after proximal vertebral artery reconstruction. *Angiology* 1992;**43**:961–8.

139. Mokri B, Houser OW, Sandok BA, Piepgras DG. Spontaneous dissections of the vertebral arteries. *Neurology* 1988;**38**:880.

140. Reich KA, Giansiracusa DF, Strongwater SL. Neurologic manifestations of giant cell arteritis. *Am J Med* 1990;**89**:67–72.

141. Wilkinson I, Russell R. Arteries of the head and neck in giant cell arteritis. *Arch Neurol* 1972;**27**:378–91.

142. Nesher G, Sonnenblick M, Friedlander Y. Analysis of steroid related complications and mortality in temporal arteritis: a 15-year survey of 43 patients. *J Rheumatol* 1994;**21**:1283–6.

143. Sheehan S, Bauer R, Meyer J. Vertebral artery compression in cervical spondylosis. Arteriographic demonstration during life of vertebral artery insufficiency due to rotation and extension of the neck. *Neurology* 1960;**10**:968–86.

144. Sakai F, Ishii K, Igarashi H, et al. Regional cerebral blood flow during an attack of vertebrobasilar insufficiency. *Stroke* 1988;**19**:1426–30.

145. Brennan RW, Bergland RM. Acute cerebellar hemorrhage. Analysis of clinical findings and outcome in 12 cases. *Neurology* 1977;**27**:527.

146. Marshall J. Cerebellar vascular syndromes. In: Toole J, ed. *Vascular diseases. Part III.* New York: Elsevier, 1989;89–94.

147. Ojemann RG, Crowell RM, Ogilvy CS. Management of cranial and spinal cavernous angiomas (honored guest lecture). *Clin Neurosurg* 1993;**40**:98–123.

148. Lipsitz LA. The drop attack: a common geriatric symptom. *J Am Geriatr Soc* 1983;**31**:617–20.

149. Sheldon J. On the natural history of falls in old age. *BMJ (Clin Res)* 1960;ii:1685–90.

150. Brust JC, Plank CR, Healton EB, Sanchez GF. The pathology of drop attacks: a case report. *Neurology* 1979;**29**:786–90.

151. Meissner I, Wiebers DO, Swanson JW, O'Fallon WM. The natural history of drop attacks. *Neurology* 1986;**36**:1029–34.

152. Criscuolo GR, Symon L. Intraventricular meningioma. A review of 10 cases of the National Hospital, Queen Square (1974–1985) with reference to the literature. *Acta Neurochir Wien* 1986;**83**:83–91.

153. Bogousslavsky J, Caplan L. *Stroke syndromes*, 2nd edn. Cambridge: Cambridge University Press, 2001.

154. Weiner HL, Constantini S, Cohen H, Wisoff JH. Current treatment of normal-pressure hydrocephalus: comparison of flow-regulated and differential-pressure shunt valves. *Neurosurgery* 1995;**37**:877–84.

155. Fisher C. Hydrocephalus as a cause of disturbances of gait in the elderly. *Neurology* 1982;**32**:1358–63.

156. Graff-Radford N, Godersky J, Jones M. Variables predicting outcome in symptomatic hydrocephalus in the elderly. *Neurology* 1989;**39**:1601–4.

157. Graff-Radford N, Godersky J. A clinical approach to symptomatic hydrocephalus in the elderly. In: Masdeu J, Sudarsky L, Wolfson L, eds. *Gait disorders of aging. Falls and therapeutic strategies.* Philadelphia: Lippincott and Raven; 1997;245–59.

158. Adams R, Fisher C, Hakim S, et al. Symptomatic occult hydrocephalus with 'normal' cerebrospinal fluid pressure. *N Engl J Med* 1965;**273**:117–26.

159. Blomsterwall E, Svantesson U, Carlsson U, et al. Postural disturbance in patients with normal pressure hydrocephalus. *Acta Neurol Scand* 2000;**102**:284–91.

160. Holodny AI, George AE, de Leon MJ, et al. Focal dilation and paradoxical collapse of cortical fissures and sulci in patients with normal-pressure hydrocephalus. *J Neurosurg* 1998;**89**:742–7.

161. Kitagaki H, Mori E, Ishii K, et al. CSF spaces in idiopathic normal pressure hydrocephalus: morphology and volumetry. *Am J Neuroradiol* 1998;**19**:1277–84.

162. Krauss JK, Regel JP, Vach W, et al. White matter lesions in patients with idiopathic normal pressure hydrocephalus and in an age-matched control group: a comparative study. Neurosurgery 1997;**40**:491–6.

163. Boon AJ, Tans JT, Delwel EJ, et al. Dutch Normal-Pressure Hydrocephalus Study: the role of cerebrovascular disease. *J Neurosurg* 1999;**90**:221–6.

164. Tullberg M, Jensen C, Ekholm S, Wikkelso C. Normal pressure hydrocephalus: vascular white matter changes on MR images must not exclude patients from shunt surgery. *Am J Neuroradiol* 2001;**22**:1665–73.

165. Bradley W Jr, Scalzo D, Queralt J, et al. Normal-pressure hydrocephalus: evaluation with cerebrospinal fluid flow measurements at MR imaging. *Radiology* 1996;**198**:523–9.

166. Malm J, Kristensen B, Karlsson T, et al. The predictive value of cerebrospinal fluid dynamic tests in patients with the idiopathic adult hydrocephalus syndrome. *Arch Neurol* 1995;**52**:783–9.

167. Boon AJ, Tans JT, Delwel EJ, et al. Dutch normal-pressure hydrocephalus study: prediction of outcome after shunting by resistance to outflow of cerebrospinal fluid. *J Neurosurg* 1997;**87**:687–93.

168. Bruni JE, Del Bigio MR, Clattenburg RE. Ependyma: normal and pathological. A review of the literature. *Brain Res* 1985;**356**:1–19.

169. Boon AJ, Tans JT, Delwel EJ, et al. Dutch Normal-Pressure Hydrocephalus Study: randomized comparison of low- and medium-pressure shunts. *J Neurosurg* 1998;**88**:490–5.

170. de Jong DA, Delwel EJ, Avezaat CJ. Hydrostatic and hydrodynamic considerations in shunted normal pressure hydrocephalus. *Acta Neurochir (Wien)* 2000;**142**:241–7.

15

Psychiatric aspects of dizziness and imbalance

ROLF G. JACOB, THOMAS BRANDT AND JOSEPH M. FURMAN

A culture's category structures highlight certain connections between concepts and mask possible alternative connections

(M. Turner, *Reading minds. The study of English in the age of cognitive science,* Princeton University Press, Princeton, NJ, USA, 1991)

... we human beings seem strangely unconscious – sometimes almost totally unaware – of many of the common categories that figure in our cognitive activities, rather like the fish slow to discover water.

(AG Amsterdam and Bruner J, *Minding the law,* Harvard University Press, Cambridge MA, USA, 2002)

INTRODUCTION

The interface between psychiatry and neuro-otology previously was dominated by one major concept: 'psychogenic dizziness'. Anchored in the category system of the mind–body dichotomy, this concept explained dizziness that was not judged to be caused by a medical disorder. Because the mind-versus-body category system is binary, by implication, when no cause for the dizziness can be found in the 'body,' its cause must reside in the 'mind.'

As the two quotations introducing this chapter indicate, once a category system is formed it provides a hidden structure for future observations, one that facilitates those consistent with it but blocks those inconsistent with it. Therefore, it is not surprising that phenomena that contradict the 'either mind or body but not both' categorical system have tended to remain unnoticed or been resisted. However, not even Descartes subscribed to

a purely dichotomous mind–body system; his main distinction was not between mental and physical properties of a person, but between mind and physical objects, the latter characterized as having 'length, breadth and depth, admitting of various shapes and various motions.'[1]

In addition, more recent empirical findings and conceptual developments – especially within the field of psychiatry – require us to recognize a number of additional relationships within the interface. There is evidence that patients with dizziness have an increased prevalence of anxiety symptoms, and that, conversely, patients with certain anxiety symptoms have an increased prevalence of vestibular dysfunction. Furthermore, biological models have replaced psychodynamic models for many mental disorders. Thus, in biological psychiatry, most psychiatric disorders are not conceptualized as 'psychogenic.' The move to biology has been reinforced by genetic findings of the heritability of psychiatric disorders and by the successes of drug treatments that target specific neuropharmacological mechanisms.[2]

An outgrowth of the psychiatric move toward a medical model has been a greater emphasis on research. The resulting empirical orientation required the development of a taxonomy that would increase the replicability of psychiatric diagnosis (reliability). For each psychiatric disorder, specific inclusion criteria were formulated. Within this new taxonomy, the lack of a medical explanation for dizziness is no longer a sufficient condition for assigning a psychiatric diagnosis.

When studying the interface between psychiatry and neuro-otology, we also need to acknowledge that there are uncertainties in the otoneurological diagnostic system. A vestibular disorder is diagnosed if the symptoms, signs and other findings fit certain syndromal descriptions. However, many patients have laboratory evidence for vestibular dysfunction without their symptoms and signs conforming to a syndromal pattern. The label 'non-syndromal vestibular disorder' has been proposed for these cases.[3] Conversely, some patients have no laboratory indicators of vestibular dysfunction on routine clinical testing, but their symptoms seem highly suggestive of a balance disorder, such as otolith dysfunction. This category of individuals has been assigned to a category of 'subclinical vestibular disorder'.[3] Finally, there is 'non-vestibular dizziness' (i.e. dizziness attributable to conditions other than vestibular disorders, including certain psychiatric disorders such as panic disorder, and certain medical disorders such as orthostatic hypotension or diabetic neuropathy).

Table 15.1 shows an overview of the interface between balance disorders and psychiatric disorders. There are several partly overlapping relationships, categorized into two classes. The first class concerns dizziness as a symptom of a psychiatric disorder: psychiatric dizziness. Although monosymptomatic dizziness is not a sufficient condition for a psychiatric diagnosis, dizziness can be part of larger symptom clusters that are diagnostic of specific psychiatric disorders. In particular, certain anxi-ety states can present with dizziness in combination with other psychiatric symptoms such as heart palpitations, tremors, and specific cognitions.

The second class comprises six types of interactions between vestibular disorders and psychiatric symptoms. The first type concerns somatopsychic consequences of vestibular dysfunction. Particularly interesting in this regard is a symptom complex that we call 'space and motion discomfort,' which overlaps with agoraphobia and other situational phobic states. The second type concerns psychosomatic relationships; for example, anxiety and associated hyperventilation could affect vestibular compensation, leading to re-emergence of vestibular symptoms in individuals with pre-existing vestibular lesions.

The third type is one in which anxiety and vestibular dysfunction are associated as a result of a neurological linkage (i.e. overlapping neurobiological mechanisms that give rise to both psychiatric and neurological symptoms). For example, dizziness can be migraine-related, and migraines and panic disorder are moderately comorbid conditions.[4]

A fourth type of interaction concerns the general psy-

Table 15.1 *Overview of the interface between psychiatry and neuro-otology*

I. Psychiatric dizziness: dizziness due to a mental disorder
    a. Panic attacks or anxiety
       Panic disorder
       Agoraphobia
       Specific phobia
       ICD-10 generalized anxiety disorder (GAD)
       ICD-10 acute stress disorder
       ICD-10 neurasthenia
    b. Dizziness label used for poor concentration, fatigue or depersonalization.
       Depressive disorders
       DSM-IV GAD
       Post-traumatic stress disorder
       Depersonalization disorder
II. Complex interactions between psychiatric and vestibular disorders
    a. Somatopsychic relationships: psychiatric symptoms possibly explained by vestibular mechanisms
       Dizziness between panic attacks
       Space and motion discomfort
    b. Psychosomatic relationships: psychiatric conditions affecting vestibular disorders
       Hyperventilation and somatosensory function
       Hyperventilation and nystagmus in patients with balance disorders
    c. Neurological linkage: psychiatric and vestibular symptoms as neurologically linked phenomena
       Migraine-related dizziness
    d. Psychiatric consequences of disability caused by vestibular dysfunction
       Depression
       States characterized by chronic anger
    e. Psychiatric potentiation: magnified impact of vestibular symptoms
       Personality disorders
       Anxiety proneness
       Symptom amplification and somatization
    f. Chance concurrence of both a psychiatric and vestibular disorder
III. Self-contained syndromes within otoneurology with suspected psychiatric components
    a. Conversion disorder of stance and gait
    b. Phobic postural vertigo

chological effects of disability. Disability increases the risk of psychiatric disorders; particularly depression and social avoidance. Depression is important to recognize, both because of the increased risk of suicide and because effective treatments are available.

The fifth type of relationship is that of 'psychiatric potentiation' or 'psychiatric overlay'. Some psychiatrically compromised individuals may respond to vestibular symptoms in a way that leads to increased illness impact and chronicity. This relationship may be superimposed on the ones already discussed. For example, behavioral avoidance because of anxiety retards recovery from a vestibular disorder. Certain personality traits seem to be associated with psychiatric overlay; for example, individuals with compulsive personality traits seem to respond more strongly to vestibular symptoms. Similarly, some individuals may be sensitized to symptoms in general such that any somatic symptom is amplified. Amplification may even occur for normal body sensations. The tendency toward symptom amplification constitutes the core problem in patients with somatoform disorders.

The sixth type of interaction is that of a 'non-relationship'. A vestibular disorder and psychiatric disorder may coexist in the same person merely as a statistical chance concurrence. This possibility needs to be mentioned here because of the common practice of diagnosing 'psychogenic dizziness' whenever the symptom of dizziness occurs in the presence of psychiatric symptoms. There is no reason to believe that the presence of a psychiatric disorder would 'immunize' a patient against developing a vestibular disorder. Therefore, by statistical necessity, some psychiatric patients will also have a vestibular disorder, and some patients with a vestibular disorder will also have a psychiatric disorder.

Even in the context of these varying relationships, the status of some syndromes with both psychiatric and vestibular symptoms remains unclear or even controversial. Phobic postural vertigo may involve more than one type of interaction. A disorder referred to as 'psychogenic disorder of stance and gait' may be a variant of a psychiatric condition called conversion disorder. Conversion disorder, one of a few disorders whose etiology is still conceptualized as psychogenic, remains one of the most poorly understood conditions in psychiatry.

PSYCHIATRIC DIAGNOSIS AND PSYCHIATRIC DIZZINESS

The DSM-IV diagnostic system

In 1980, new psychiatric diagnostic rules were codified in the third edition of the *Diagnostic and Statistical Manual of the American Psychiatric Association* (DSM-III).[5]

Compared with the two earlier editions, the DSM-I and DSM-II,[6,7] the changes in the DSM-III were so extensive that it is difficult to compare research finding pre- and post-DSM-III. In addition to the formulation of explicit diagnostic criteria, the other major change was the introduction of a 'multi-axial' diagnostic system. For a complete psychiatric diagnosis, information relevant for each of five 'axes' had to be specified:

Axis I, defined as 'Clinical Disorders' and 'Other conditions that may be the focus of clinical attention' concerns traditional psychiatric disorders such as 'panic disorder,' 'major depressive disorder,' etc.
Axis II specifies conditions that imply enduring dysfunctional predispositions that are not considered to be psychiatric disorders (i.e. characteristics of a person similar to 'temperament' and other traits). This axis includes personality disorders and mental retardation.
Axis III represents 'General Medical Conditions.' Here, medical diagnoses such as 'labyrinthine dysfunction,' would be specified.
Axis IV specifies the 'psychosocial and environmental problems' that are applicable to the patient at the time of the diagnosis. An example would be 'problems with primary support group: marital separation.'
Axis V represents a 'global assessment of function' of a patient; this is done on a 0–100 point scale reflecting (1) the degree of distress from or dangerousness of the symptoms, (2) the severity and number of areas of psychosocial functioning affected (e.g. professional, personal), and (3) degree of impairment in reality testing (e.g. delusions).

An example of a 'complete' DSM-IV diagnosis is shown in Table 15.2.

In addition to introducing diagnostic criteria and multi-axial case formulations, the DSM-III recognized many new diagnoses. For example, within the category of anxiety disorders, there are now 10 distinct disorders, plus a 'not otherwise specified' (NOS) category. In part, this increase in number was accomplished by dividing DSM-II categories into distinct disorders. For example, 'anxiety reaction' (DSM-I) survived as 'anxiety neurosis' (DSM-II) but was divided into two disorders, 'panic disorder' and 'generalized anxiety disorder' in the DSM-III.

The DSM-III stimulated much research that influenced its subsequent revisions, the DSM-III-R[8] and the current version, the DSM-IV.[9] The descriptive parts of the DSM-IV, but not the criteria for diagnosis, were updated in a year 2000 revision, the DSM-IV-TR.[10] The DSM-III and its successors also have had major influences outside of the USA, including the 10th revision of the International Classification of Diseases (ICD-10).[11] The working groups developing the DSM-IV also had extensive contacts with developers of the ICD-10.

Table 15.2 *Example of a complete multi-axial DSM-IV diagnosis*

DSM–IV multi-axial diagnostic formulation	
I. Clinical psychiatric syndromes and V codes	
Panic disorder with agoraphobia	
Generalized anxiety disorder	
Rule out Depression, NOS	
II. Developmental and personality disorders	
None	
III. Physical disorders and conditions	
Rule out labyrinthine dysfunction	
IV. Social stressors	
[x] 1. Problems with primary support group	Specify: husband's illness
[ ] 2. Problems related to the social environment	Specify:
[ ] 3. Educational problems	Specify:
[x] 4. Occupational problems	Specify: new boss
[ ] 5. Housing problems	Specify:
[x] 6. Economic problems	Specify: reduced income
[ ] 7. Problems with access to health care services	Specify:
[ ] 8. Other psychosocial and environmental problems	Specify:
V. Functioning levels	
Past GAF/GAS Score: 75 Current GAF/GAS Score: 45	
(Highest within the last year)	

Specific descriptions and diagnostic rules for psychiatric research for ICD-10 psychiatric disorders have been published.[11,12]

Defining symptoms and associated symptoms

Heuristically, the symptoms of a psychiatric disorder can be classified as 'defining' symptoms and 'associated' symptoms. Defining symptoms are symptoms included among the formal DSM or ICD-10 inclusion criteria of the disorder. Associated symptoms are symptoms that occur commonly in patients with the disorder but are not 'defining.' For example, patients with panic disorder tend to be particularly sensitive to substances such as caffeine, but caffeine sensitivity does not have 'defining' status.

Dizziness is a defining symptom for several psychiatric disorders. However, for a psychiatric origin of dizziness to be considered, it would have to be:[13,14] (a) a member of the set of defining or associated symptoms of the psychiatric disorder; (b) occur simultaneously with a sufficient number of other defining symptoms to fulfill the diagnostic rules for the disorder, and (c) not in itself be related to vestibular dysfunction. We will use the term 'psychiatric dizziness' for dizziness that fulfills these criteria.

Criterion (a), the 'defining symptom' criterion, defines the set of psychiatric disorders that can be considered in the differential diagnosis of dizziness. This list, which will be reviewed in the next section, is dominated by the anxiety disorders. Criterion (b), the requirement of a symptom cluster, indicates that monosymptomatic

dizziness and dizziness that is part of a symptom constellation that is different from the one that defines the disorder would be insufficient grounds for a diagnosis of psychiatric dizziness. Criterion (c), that the symptom is not related to vestibular dysfunction, makes room for the possibility that some symptoms traditionally considered psychiatric might in fact be related to vestibular dysfunction. For example, some patients with panic disorder also report monosymptomatic dizziness even when they are not feeling panicky, and this 'dizziness between panic attacks' has been found to predict abnormalities on vestibular laboratory tests.[15] The latter type of dizziness would not be considered 'psychiatric'. Often patients can learn to distinguish between the two, especially after they have undergone treatment.[16]

A survey of psychiatric disorders for which dizziness is a defining symptom

The top of Table 15.1 lists conditions for which dizziness is listed among their inclusion criteria. These disorders include many of the anxiety disorders, as well as a condition called neurasthenia, which is codified only within the ICD-10 system. The diagnosis of the most important of these anxiety disorders will be discussed below.

Some patients may apply the label of 'dizziness' or its synonyms to subjective states that most individuals would label differently. This can happen because, unlike verbal descriptions of physical objects, the verbal labels that an individual gives to a phenomenological experience are not shaped by a learning history of consensual validation. For example, a patient may describe a state that most would label 'poor concentration' as 'swimming sensations' or 'dizziness.' Difficulty concentrating is a defining symptom of depressive disorders. If, in the patient's lexicon, 'poor concentration' is described as 'dizziness', the symptom referred to would be 'psychiatric,' provided that a sufficient number of other defining symptoms of depressive disorders occur simultaneously. Another example of idiosyncratic labeling may be the symptoms of depersonalization, derealization or 'numbing' often observed in post-traumatic stress disorder.

ANXIETY DISORDERS

The anxiety disorders for which dizziness is a defining symptom in either the DSM-IV or the ICD-10 'research criteria' include panic disorder, phobic disorders, and (for ICD-10 only) generalized anxiety disorder. Figure 15.1 depicts the decision trees for the diagnosis of anxiety disorders that might be the source of psychiatric dizziness.

Panic and phobias

Comparing Fig. 15.1a and b, the classification of anxiety disorders according to the DSM-IV and ICD-10 are similar but not identical. In the diagnostic decision tree, the major difference concerns the status of panic disorder, a condition characterized by panic attacks (i.e. attacks of intense anxiety that lead to an urge to flee the situation). Although both systems provide criteria for identifying panic attacks, the DSM-IV classification system is based on a conviction that panic anxiety is fundamentally different from other forms of anxiety. In the DSM-IV, the presence or absence of spontaneous panic attacks therefore is a primary consideration in the classification of anxiety disorders. When combined with phobic avoidance, the panic–anxiety distinction gives rise to a scheme for reaching an anxiety disorder diagnosis (Table 15.3).

The motivation for making a distinction between psychiatric dizziness and other types of anxiety originally came from findings, later refuted, of differential treatment responsiveness to antidepressants vs. benzodiazepines. Another reason was that many panic attacks did not seem to be triggered by any external event (i.e. they occurred without provocation). The distinction between panic and general anxiety has subsequently been validated by family studies and twin studies in which the prevalence of panic disorder is found to be increased in relatives of probands with panic disorder.[17,18]

The identification of panic attacks in both the DSM-IV and ICD-10 is based upon the nature of the anxiety symptoms (primarily autonomic, along with 'catastrophizing' cognitions), their eliciting stimuli (cued, uncued; see below), and the time course of an individual anxiety episode (i.e. abrupt onset). The actual criteria are detailed in Table 15.4. Thus, panic attacks are symptoms of anxiety that begin suddenly and peak within minutes. They are characterized by a predominance of somatic symptoms that can be attributed to autonomic arousal or hyperventilation, including heart palpitations, tremors, chest pain, dizziness and gastrointestinal distress. These sensations are accompanied by fear of a bodily catastrophic event such as a heart attack and a strong urge to escape the situation, which in turn results in a fear of doing something uncontrolled or embarrassing.

One type of panic attack occurs seemingly without a trigger. This type is called 'uncued,' 'unexpected,' 'spontaneous' or 'out of the blue' panic. The diagnosis of DSM-IV panic disorder (with or without agoraphobia) requires that the patient report a history of spontaneous panic attacks. Similarly in the ICD-10 diagnostic criteria for research, Criterion 'A' requires that 'The individual experiences recurrent panic attacks that are not consistently associated with a specific situation or object and that often occur spontaneously. The panic attacks are not associated with marked exertion or with exposure to dangerous or life-threatening situations.' However, spontaneous panic attacks occur quite commonly in the population.[19] Therefore, a DSM-IV diagnosis of panic disorder requires that the spontaneous attacks have further adverse consequences: either worry about the possibility of future attacks, worry about the implications of an attack (e.g. 'hypochondriasis') or other changes in behavior.

In the DSM-IV, spontaneous panic attacks are contrasted with 'situationally bound' and 'situationally predisposed' panic attacks. Situationally bound or 'cued' attacks occur if, and only if, the individual is exposed to a phobic situation or object. That is, such patients consistently experience panic each time they are facing the phobic situation but not otherwise. Situationally predisposed attacks occur only if the individual is exposed to the phobic situation but not every time. The last two types of panic are not specific for panic disorder but commonly occur in phobias, especially situational phobias of enclosed places (claustrophobia).[20]

Table 15.3 *The DSM-IV panic disorder, generalized anxiety disorder, and phobias*

	No phobic avoidance	Phobic avoidance
Spontaneous panic attacks	Panic disorder without agoraphobia	Panic disorder with agoraphobia
Anxiety or cued or situationally predisposed panic attacks; no history of spontaneous panic attacks	Generalized anxiety disorder	Social phobia Specific phobias

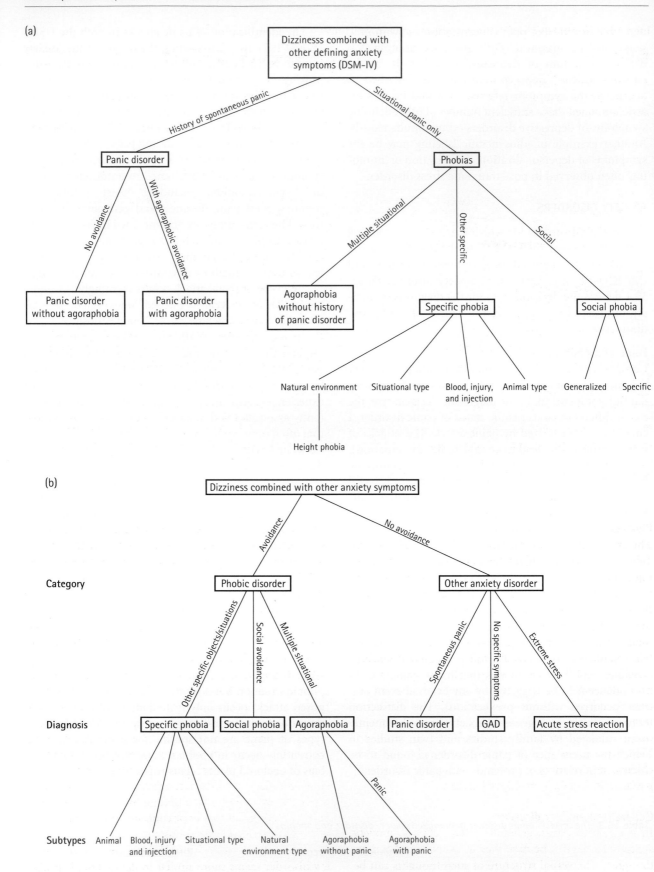

Figure 15.1 *Differential diagnosis of psychiatric dizziness: (a) according to the DSM-IV; (b) according to the ICD-10.*

Table 15.4 *The DSM-IV and ICD-10 defining symptoms of panic attacks*[a]

DSM-IV	ICD-10 (research criteria), criterion B[b]
A discrete period of intense fear or discomfort, in which *four (or more)* of the following symptoms developed abruptly and reached a peak within 10 min	All of the following: (1) It is a discrete episode of intense fear or discomfort (2) It starts abruptly (3) It reaches a maximum within a few minutes and lasts at least some minutes (4) *At least four* of the symptoms listed below must be present, one of which must be from items (a) to (d) (i.e., autonomic arousal symptoms)
(1) Palpitations, pounding heart, or accelerated heart rate	(a) Palpitations, pounding heart, or accelerated heart rate
(2) Sweating	(b) Sweating
(3) Trembling or shaking	(c) Trembling or shaking
(4) Sensations of shortness of breath or smothering sensations	(d) Dry mouth
(5) Feeling of choking	(e) Difficulty breathing
(6) Chest pain or discomfort	(f) Feeling of choking
(7) Nausea, abdominal distress	(g) Chest pain or discomfort
(8) Feeling dizzy, unsteady, lightheaded or faint	(h) Nausea, abdominal distress
(9) Derealization (feelings of unreality), or depersonalization (being detached from oneself)	(i) Feeling dizzy, unsteady, faint, or lightheaded
(10) Fear of losing control or going crazy	(j) Feelings that objects are unreal (derealization), or that the self is distant or 'not really here' (depersonalization)
(11) Fear of dying	(k) Fear of losing control, 'going crazy', or passing out
(12) Chills or hot flushes	(l) Fear of dying
(13) Paresthesias (numbness or tingling sensations)	(m) Hot flushes or cold chills
	(n) Numbness or tingling sensations

[a]The wording of the criteria is from the DSM-IV[9] (reprinted with permission from the *Diagnostic and Statistical Manual of Mental Disorders*, 4th edn, text revision, Copyright 2000 American Psychiatric Association) and the ICD-10 Diagnostic Criteria for Research[12] with permission from the World Health Organization.
[b]Order of symptoms as they appear in the ICD-10 research criteria.[12]

Phobias

The entire set of DSM-IV anxiety disorders appears in Table 15.5. Those disorders that have dizziness as a defining symptom are in italics and include all disorders characterized by panic attacks regardless of variety (i.e. all phobic conditions). Dizziness is particularly noteworthy in two of the phobias. Specific phobia, particularly blood injury and injection type, may lead to the sensations of fainting (as well as to actually fainting). Height phobia, classified as a 'natural environment' subtype, may be associated with 'height vertigo.' In a later section we will argue that height phobia may be part of a symptom pattern called 'Space and Motion Discomfort' that also occurs in patients with vestibular dysfunction. Therefore, dizziness in height phobia may be 'non-psychiatric' according to criterion (c) of our definition of psychiatric dizziness introduced earlier.

Generalized anxiety disorder

In contrast to panic, general anxiety refers to anxiety symptoms that can be described as 'worries' or 'anxious thoughts.' The verbal structure of such thoughts can be characterized by the fact that their content can be brought out crisply by placing the words 'what if' at the beginning of the thought (e.g. 'what if we miss the deadline for this chapter'). A person with generalized anxiety disorder (GAD) thus is the prototypical 'worry wart.' Specifically, generalized anxiety disorder is characterized by excessive worry that the patients find difficult to control. These worries are about several minor issues rather than just one. They occur 'more days than not,' and the duration of the symptoms has to be at least 6 months.

The DSM definition of generalized anxiety disorder underwent a major revision between DSM-III-R and DSM-IV that led to the elimination of the overlap between the defining symptoms of panic disorder and generalized anxiety disorder. Table 15.6 shows DSM-IV criteria for generalized anxiety disorder compared with those of DSM-III-R and ICD-10. DSM-IV generalized anxiety disorder requires at least three of the following six symptoms to accompany the worries: restlessness, fatigue, difficulty concentrating, irritability, muscle tension and sleep disturbance. Dizziness is not included among these symptoms, although 'poor concentration' is. We noted earlier that poor concentration could sometimes be described as dizziness.

As a result of the revision, DSM-IV generalized anxiety disorder seems more similar to depression. It is also quite different from generalized anxiety disorder as diagnosed according to the ICD-10. Comparing the criteria for the DSM-III-R with those of ICD-10 (Table 15.6), it is obvious that the ICD-10 is influenced by the DSM-III-R.

Table 15.5 *The DSM-IV diagnosis of anxiety disorders*[a]

	No phobic avoidance	Phobic avoidance	Subtype	Examples or further subtypes
Spontaneous panic attacks	*300.01 Panic disorder without agoraphobia*	*300.21 Panic disorder with agoraphobia*		
Anxiety or cued or situationally predisposed panic attacks; no history of spontaneous panic attacks	Generalized anxiety disorder	*300.23 Social phobia*	Specific / Generalized	Stage fright
	300.29 Specific phobias	Animal type	Natural environment / Blood injection injury / Situational	Heights, storms, water (generally childhood onset) / Airplanes, elevators, enclosed places
Obsessions or compulsions	300.3 Obsessive compulsive disorder (OCD)			
Severe stress	309.81 Post traumatic stress disorder		Acute	Chronic / With delayed onset
	308.3 Acute stress disorder			
Drug induced	293.84 *Substance induced anxiety disorder*		With generalized anxiety	Onset during intoxication or withdrawal / *With panic* / With OCD symptoms / *With phobia*
Secondary to medical disorders	Anxiety due to a general medical condition[b]		With generalized anxiety	Thyroid, respiratory, or vestibular dysfunction / With panic attacks[b] / With OCD symptoms
(309.xx) Adjustment disorders	309.0 With depressed mood / 309.24 With anxiety / 309.28 With mixed anxiety and depressed mood / 309.3 With disturbance of conduct / 309.4 With mixed dist. of emotions and conduct			

[a]Disorders that include dizziness as a defining symptom are *in italics*. DSM-IV numeric codes are based on those in the ICD-9-CM.

[b]Anxiety caused by to a general medical condition may be related to vestibular dysfunction. Dizziness in this patients would not be considered 'Psychiatric' due to criterion 'c' (see text).

(Reprinted with permission from the *Diagnostic and Statistical Manual of Mental Disorders*, 4th edn, text revision, Copyright 2000 American Psychiatric Association.)

Table 15.6 *Generalized anxiety symptoms in DSM-IV, DSM-III-R and ICD-10*[a]

DSM-IV (1994)	DSM-III-R (1987)	ICD-10 (1993)
The anxiety and worry are associated with three or more of the following six symptoms	At least six of the following 18 symptoms are often present when anxious	At least four of the symptoms below must be present, at least one of which must be from items (1)–(4)
		Autonomic arousal symptoms
	(6) Palpitations or accelerated heart rate (tachycardia)	(1) Palpitations or pounding heart, or accelerated heart rate
	(7) Sweating, or cold clammy hands	(2) Sweating
	(1) Trembling, twitching, or feeling shaky	(3) Trembling or shaking
	(8) Dry mouth	(4) Dry mouth (not due to medication or dehydration)
		Symptoms involving chest or abdomen
	(5) Shortness of breath or smothering sensations	(5) Difficulty breathing
		(6) Feeling of choking
		(7) Chest pain or discomfort
	(10) Nausea, diarrhea, or abdominal distress	(8) Nausea or abdominal distress (e.g., churning in stomach)
	(12) Frequent urination	
		Symptoms involving mental state
	(9) Dizziness or lightheadedness	(9) Feeling dizzy, unsteady, faint, or lightheaded
		(10) Feeling that objects are unreal (derealization), or that the self is distant or 'not really here' (depersonalization)
	(11) Fear of losing control	(12) Fear of dying
		General symptoms
	(11) Flushes (hot flashes) or chills	(13) Hot flushes or cold chills
		(14) Numbness or tingling sensations
		Symptoms of tension
(5) Muscle tension	(2) Muscle tension, aches, or soreness	(15) Muscle tension, aches or pains
(1) Restlessness or feeling keyed up or on edge	(3) Restlessness	(16) Restlessness, inability to relax
	(14) Feeling keyed up or on edge	
	(13) Trouble swallowing or lump in throat	(18) A sensation of lump in the throat, or difficulty swallowing
		Other nonspecific symptoms
	(15) Exaggerated startle response	(19) Exaggerated response to minor surprise or being startled
(3) Difficulty concentrating or mind going blank	(16) Difficulty concentrating or 'mind going blank' because of anxiety	(20) Difficulty in concentrating, or mind 'going blank' because of worrying or anxiety
(4) Irritability	(18) Irritability	(21) Persistent irritability
(6) Sleep disturbance (difficulty falling asleep or restless unsatisfying sleep)	(17) Trouble falling or staying asleep	(22) Difficulty going to sleep because of worrying.
(2) Being easily fatigued	(4) Easy fatiguability	

[a] From the DSM IV[9] (reprinted with permission from the *Diagnostic and Statistical Manual of Mental Disorders*, 4th edn, text revision, Copyright 2000 American Psychiatric Association) and ICD-10 Diagnostic Criteria for Research with permission from the World Health Organization.[12]

The ICD-10 generalized anxiety disorder symptoms are grouped into one of the following categories: (1) autonomic arousal symptoms, (2) symptoms involving chest or abdomen, (3) symptoms involving mental state, (4) general symptoms, (5) symptoms of tension, and (6) other non-specific symptoms. The symptom of dizziness is listed within group 3 (symptoms involving mental state), along with feelings of unsteadiness, faintness or light-headedness.

Psychiatric dizziness and ICD-10 anxiety disorders

Table 15.7 depicts the overall system of anxiety disorders within the ICD-10. The corresponding decision tree is shown in Fig. 15.1b. Reflecting European skepticism of the uniqueness of panic, the primary consideration in the ICD-10 categorical system is the presence or absence of phobia. Conceptualizing panic as 'episodic paroxysmal anxiety,' the ICD-10 view is that panic represents a particularly intense form of anxiety, a form characterized by a predominance of somatic symptoms and abrupt onset.

The overlap between ICD-10 panic and ICD-10 general anxiety can be appreciated when comparing Tables 15.6 and 15.4: the symptoms (a–n) of ICD-10 panic are identical to the first 14 symptoms of ICD-10 generalized anxiety disorder.

The ICD-10 research criteria refer to the list of generalized anxiety disorder symptoms when describing anxiety disorders other than generalized anxiety disorder. Because dizziness is included on this list, these other anxiety disorders can be a source for psychiatric dizziness, including specific phobia, social phobia, acute stress reaction, and possibly some of the adjustment disorders (Table 15.7).

INTERACTIONS BETWEEN PSYCHIATRIC ANXIETY DISORDERS AND VESTIBULAR DISORDERS

The preceding section discussed the conceptually straightforward circumstances in which dizziness could entirely be due to a psychiatric disorder. We will now consider more complex cases where dizziness and anxiety are functionally interrelated. For example, the DSM-IV-TR, in its discussion of anxiety disorder caused by a medical condition, explicitly recognizes that vestibular dysfunction can be a cause of anxiety. This diagnosis would be given if the anxiety symptoms are a direct physiological consequence of the vestibular disorder. The diagnosis is not given if the anxiety symptoms are 'not better accounted for' by a psychiatric disorder (i.e. if the symptoms conform to the typical pattern of one of the main anxiety disorders). The phrase 'direct physiologic consequence' implies a specific relationship rather than just the general 'stress' from being ill. In this case, a diagnosis of adjustment disorder with anxiety (Table 15.5)

would be made. Other medical disorders that can have anxiety as a direct physiological consequence include hyper- and hypothyroidism, congestive heart failure, cardiac arrhythmia, respiratory failure, porphyria and pheochromocytoma.

Anxiety symptoms in patients with vestibular disorders

Several studies have demonstrated the increased prevalence of panic disorder in patients with vestibular dysfunction. For example, Clark and co-workers[21] found that panic attacks and agoraphobic avoidance were more common in patients with vestibular dysfunction than in patients evaluated for mild hearing loss (see Table 15.8). Specifically, 21 of 47 patients (45 per cent) with either peripheral or non-localizing findings on vestibular function tests reported panic attacks; in 10 of these (20 per cent of the sample), the panic attacks occurred at a frequency sufficient for a DSM-III-R diagnosis of panic disorder. The prevalence of anxiety symptoms was significantly higher than in a comparison group of patients evaluated for mild hearing loss. In an earlier study on members of a non-psychiatric self-help group for patients with balance disorders, Clark et al.[22] found that 47 per cent reported panic attacks, and 43 per cent of these (20 per cent of the entire sample) had panic disorder. Furthermore, about two-thirds (69 per cent) of these patients reported that they avoided at least one agoraphobic situation 'most of the time' or 'all the time' while 29 per cent had agoraphobia, defined (in this study) as avoidance of seven or more agoraphobic situations. The most common fears reported were fear of heights and boats.

Although these studies indicate that anxiety symptoms and anxiety disorders are common in patients with vestibular dysfunction, direction of causality cannot be inferred from them because of their cross-sectional designs. A longitudinal study was conducted by Eagger and co-workers,[23] who monitored the emergence of psychiatric symptoms in a follow-up study of 54 otoneurological patients with verified vestibular lesions. Again, the psychiatric condition observed most frequently was panic disorder with or without agoraphobia (41 per cent). Particularly common were fear of falls, heights, darkness or social situations. About two-thirds of the patients had developed their psychiatric symptoms after the onset of their vestibular symptoms. In patients that recovered from their vestibular disorder, the anxiety symptoms tended to be transient, whereas in 60 per cent of those whose symptoms became chronic, the anxiety symptoms persisted.

The Eagger et al.[23] study was limited to patients with laboratory evidence of vestibular dysfunction. However, anxiety disorders including panic disorder also appear to be common in patients with dizziness without syndro-

Table 15.7 *Overview of ICD-10 anxiety disorders*

Characteristics	Class	Specific disorder	Subtype	Examples
Phobic avoidance:	F 40 Phobic disorders	F 40.0 Agoraphobia	F 40.00 Without panic disorder F 40.01 With panic disorder	
		F 40.1 Social phobia		
		F 40.2 Specific phobias	Animal type Nature-forces type Blood, injection and injury Situational type Other	Insects, dogs Storm, water Elevators, tunnels
No phobic avoidance	F 41 Other anxiety disorders	F 41.0 Panic disorder	F 41.00 Moderate F 41.01 Severe	At least four panics in 4 weeks At least four panics per week for a 4-week period
		F 41.1 Generalized anxiety disorder		
		F 41.2 Mixed anxiety and depressive disorder		
Obsessions or compulsions	F 42 Obsessive compulsive disorder	F 42.0 Predominantly obsessional thoughts		
		F 42.1 Predominantly compulsive acts		
		F 42.2 Mixed thoughts and acts		
Stress-related	F 43 Reactions to severe stress and adjustment disorders	F 43.0 Acute stress reaction F43.01 Moderate F 43.02 Severe	F 43.00 Mild	
		F 43.1 Post-traumatic stress disorder		
		F 43.2 Adjustment disorders	F 43.2 Brief depressive reaction F43.21 Prolonged depressive reaction F 43.22 Mixed anxiety and depressive reaction F 43.23 With ... disturbance of other emotions (including anxiety)	

Table 15.8 *Anxiety symptoms in otoneurological patients with vestibular dysfunction*[a]

	Peripheral vestibulopathy (*n* = 37)	Central or non-specific vestibulopathy (*n* = 10)	Hearing loss (*n* = 44)
Panic disorder	22%	20%	0%
Panic attacks but not panic disorder	19%	40%	7%
Agoraphobic avoidance (Mobility inventory score)	1.5	1.4	1.2

[a]Excerpted from Clark et al. [21]

mal vestibular disorders.[24] Stein et al.[25] found no association between symptoms of anxiety and diagnoses of vestibular disorders in a dizziness clinic population, but not all patients received vestibular function tests. Specifically, 32 of 87 patients with a chief complaint of dizziness (37 per cent), who had returned a questionnaire, had elevated fear, anxiety or depression scores. Thirteen subjects (15%) had panic disorder and 10 of these had agoraphobia. Psychiatric morbidity was similar in patients with or without vestibular diagnoses; of the 13 panic patients, six were given a vestibular diagnosis and seven were not.

In a questionnaire-based study with patients with Ménière's syndrome, Hägnebo et al.[26] conducted a factor analysis that revealed that autonomic or respiratory anxiety symptoms (tingling or prickling, sweating, nausea, intense breathing) covaried with vestibular symptoms (lightheadedness, whirling sensations) such that they did not constitute an independent symptom constellation. The results of these studies and others reviewed by Asmundson et al.[27] suggest that anxiety disorders are comorbid with dizziness. Thus, the presence of anxiety symptoms does not reduce the likelihood of a vestibular disorder, as has previously been claimed.[28] Furthermore, the relationship between dizziness and anxiety does not represent a non-specific reaction that would occur to any kind of intrusive symptoms. For example, tinnitus tends have a higher comorbidity with depression than with anxiety.[24]

The excess in comorbidity between dizziness and anxiety has also been established in a primary care population. Questionnaire responses from about 2000 respondents in a population survey of primary care patients indicated that one-third endorsed dizziness, anxiety, or both; 11 per cent reported comorbid anxiety and dizziness, whereas 13 per cent reported dizziness alone, and 10 per cent, anxiety alone. If dizziness and anxiety were not associated with each other, the comorbidity rate would have been close to 5 per cent rather than 11 per cent. The presence of anxiety increased the overall level of concurrent handicap.[29] The presence of vertigo, agoraphobic avoidance, and fainting, which may be a component of panic, were independent predictors of chronic, handicapping dizziness one year later. A subsample of respondents reporting that the dizziness had impacted their lifestyle (handicapping dizziness) was subjected to closer vestibular and psychiatric examinations. The prevalence of psychiatric dysfunction was three times higher than that of normal control subjects; the largest difference between the groups was in the prevalence of phobias. The prevalence of vestibular dysfunction in those with and without abnormal psychiatric test scores (70 per cent vs. 50 per cent) was not statistically significant. These results are again inconsistent with the maxim that the presence of anxiety 'rules out' vestibular dysfunction.

Vestibular dysfunction in patients with anxiety disorders

The preceding section showed that dizziness is comorbid with anxiety both in dizziness clinic and primary care populations. In this section we address the comorbidity between anxiety and vestibular dysfunction in psychiatric patients with anxiety disorders. Vestibular abnormalities have been found to be common in this population.[30,31] A few studies have included comparison groups other than normal controls. In one study, vestibular abnormalities were found to be more common in patients with panic disorder than in those with generalized anxiety disorder.[32,33] In three studies, patients with agoraphobia had a particularly high prevalence of abnormalities on balance tests.[34,15,35]

Among different vestibular tests, the test on which performance of patients with agoraphobia was most consistently impaired was dynamic posturography. Furthermore, the sensory conditions in which their performance was decreased were those that specifically reflect somatosensory dependence in the control of balance. This pattern of posturography findings was described in detail by Jacob et al.[36] and is reproduced in Fig. 15.2.

Two variables predicted vestibular dysfunction independently from psychiatric diagnosis.[15] One of these was a measure of space and motion discomfort to which we will return in a later section. The other was a questionnaire measure of vestibular symptoms such as lightheadedness, veering and feeling like falling. The questionnaire, called the Symptom Questionnaire, included two subscales, one that inquired about the frequency of symptoms occurring during states of panic,

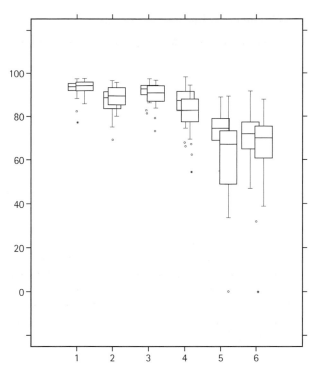

Figure 15.2 *Performance of agoraphobics (foreground) and normal comparison subjects on dynamic posturography. (Reproduced from Jacob RG, Furman JM, Durrant JD, Turner SM. Surface dependence: a balance control strategy in panic disorder with agoraphobia.* Psychosom Med *1997;59:323–30, Lippincott Williams & Wilkins, © 1997.)*

anxiety or stress, and one that specifically inquired about the frequency between such episodes (i.e. when the respondent was a relatively calm state). Interestingly, the dizziness symptoms that predicted vestibular laboratory abnormalities were those occurring between panic attacks (i.e. during anxiety-free intervals). Dizziness occurring when the patient was anxious or panicky was unrelated to vestibular dysfunction. Because panic attacks are frequently accompanied by hyperventilation, it is likely that the dizziness occurring during panic attacks is a consequence of this behavior rather than vestibular dysfunction. This finding matches clinical observations that patients with panic disorder can learn to discriminate between dizziness related to panic and dizziness occurring separately from panic.[16]

Agoraphobics also have impaired balance function on various clinical balance tests such as the Romberg test, heel walking, walking on sides of feet, toe walking, heel-to-toe walking, hopping and standing on tiptoe.[37] They also have impaired spatial orientation (i.e. getting lost more easily in a maze).[38] Recently, Jacob et al.[39] performed clinical examinations of balance function in a small sample of agoraphobic patients that were about to undergo vestibular rehabilitation therapy. The patients had been selected because they had abnormalities on laboratory tests of vestibular function.[39] All of the patients experienced dizziness in response to one or

more of various head movements, body movements, or coordinated head–eye movements. In addition, compared with historical controls, the patients had poor balance on single leg stance with eyes closed (but not with eyes open), with a median stance duration of 10 s.

The comorbidity between vestibular disorders and anxiety disorders raises questions about possible mediating mechanisms. As we stated in the introduction, these possibilities include psychological mediation in the psychosomatic and somatopsychic directions and direct linkage via overlapping neural circuitry underlying both vestibular and anxiety disorders.

Behavioral effects on vestibular or balance function

It is generally accepted that anxiety or 'stress' increases the sensitivity of the vestibular–ocular reflex.[40] However, this has not been true of normal subjects selected for their high trait anxiety.[41,42] Further, in experiments in which stress is induced by some mental task, the observed effects may result from the motor behaviors required to complete the task, rather than the stress itself. Such mental tasks often require the subject to speak out loud. Yardley and co-workers[43] found that an increase in body sway during such a task could be attributed to the behavior of speaking rather than the stress from the task itself.

Two studies on patients with Ménière's disease examined the relationship between stressors occurring during daily activities and dizziness symptoms. In the first study, Anderson and co-workers[44] had patients self-monitor symptoms of 'stress' and discomfort from dizziness, tinnitus and hearing problems. There was a correlation between stress and symptoms for the same day, but no association was found between stress and symptoms recorded on the following day. In the second study, the investigators examined individuals attending a self-help group for anxiety disorders.[45] Although measures were taken more frequently during each day and a greater number of stress attributes were recorded, results indicated that the association between stress and dizziness was primarily concurrent. Thus, these studies do not provide conclusive evidence that stress has a causative role for exacerbation of vestibular symptoms.

Many patients with panic disorder hyperventilate. Sakellari et al.[46] found that hyperventilation increased action potentials in the sural nerve and reduced somatosensory evoked potentials, suggesting that hyperventilation changes somatosensory balance input. In addition, hyperventilation can induce nystagmus in patients with vestibular disorders, and can elicit the original symptoms of dizziness,[47] suggesting that hyperventilation can unmask or reactivate a vestibular lesion. Possible mechanisms for this effect include normalizing conduction defects in the affected nerve and reversing central compensation. This should caution against the use of the hyperventilation test as a diagnostic instrument to rule out vestibular disorders. Overall, the studies discussed in this section indicate that normal stresses of everyday life are unlikely to induce vestibular symptoms. However, hyperventilation, a behavior that often occurs during panic attacks, might induce a vestibular imbalance, especially in individuals with pre-existing vestibular dysfunction.

Anxiety affects higher cortical, cognitive processes and some of these may be relevant for vestibular processes involving higher levels of processing, such as spatial orientation or self-report of motion. This area of research, pioneered by Berthoz and co-workers, is likely to grow.[48,49] These investigators studied the shift in the beating field of nystagmus during rotation. The beating field reflects the average direction of gaze in head coordinates. In normal subjects, the beating field shifts into the direction of rotation. This 'anticipatory' movement enables the subject to fixate their gaze (during the slow phase) on objects that are approaching the subject or that they are approaching. Subjects high in trait anxiety showed a negative gaze shift rather than an anticipatory one.[42] This difference may be an expression of an egocentric orientation strategy or an expression of a generally 'avoidant' perceptual style but the results do not provide evidence of the direction of causality. It would be interesting to examine whether experimentally induced anxiety would have similar effects.

Vestibular effects on autonomic function, respiration and attention

In the preceding section we discussed how behavioral factors such as anxiety affect vestibular function. Is there also evidence of influences in the opposite direction? Anxiety is characterized by increased cardiovascular activity (heart rate and blood pressure), increased respiration rate and by a narrowing of attention to fear relevant stimuli. Vestibular stimulation affects each of these domains. Vestibular influences on autonomic function or respiration have been demonstrated in basic animal research.[50] Teleologically, these influences are thought to enable cardiovascular and respiratory responses to rapid postural changes. The vestibular autonomic interactions are also clinically relevant in humans.[51]

Caloric stimulation leads to an increase in respiration rate.[52] Furthermore, rapid head movements along the pitch axis lead to changes in respiration; this effect was not observed in patients with bilateral vestibular dysfunction.[53] Specifically, the head movements resulted in a shortening of the exhalation phase in the respiratory cycle, a pattern akin to the type of breathing seen in acute anxiety states. The vestibular effects on respiration, in combination with the effects of hyperventilation on vestibular function described in the previous section, could theoretically lead to the build-up of a vicious cycle.

The cardiovascular system in humans tends to be affected in subtle ways by vestibular stimulation. Caloric stimulation decreased heart rate variability, suggesting vagal withdrawal,[52] although this effect may have been secondary to changes in respiration rate. Linear acceleration in a sled leads to transient increases in heart rate,[54] as does sudden head drops.[55] These responses are of brief duration (i.e. extended over a few heartbeats) and do not habituate. The latency of the response is 600 ms (i.e. within the duration of a heartbeat). The cardiac response is diminished or delayed in patients with bilateral vestibular hypofunction. These results point toward the existence of a 'vestibulo-cardiac reflex' in humans.

The activity of maintaining one's balance appears to make demands on a person's attentional resources, particularly if the balancing task is made difficult. Consequently, less attention can be devoted to other mental tasks. Performance on various mental tasks was reduced in normals as well as vestibular patients when they stood on a destabilized support surface compared with sitting.[56] Furthermore, patients with vestibular dysfunction overall had reduced mental task performance. The relationship between impaired balance and decreased attentional resources for other tasks may explain the finding that elderly individuals who 'stop walking when talking' have less safe gait and would move about more slowly than individuals that were able to maintain a conversation while walking.[57] The incidence of falls during a follow-up period was significantly higher in those that stopped walking when talking.

It is unclear whether the effects of vestibular stimulation enumerated in this section could induce an anxiety reaction. Nevertheless, as reviewed in the previous section, anxiety states are frequently observed in vestibular disorders. Even in individuals that already have an anxiety disorder, the onset of a vestibular disorder can exacerbate it. There are likely to be two sources for such anxiety.[58] One source is the meaning that the individual attributes to a new symptom in general (i.e. the relevant belief system). Another component of anxiety is more immediate in nature and stems from our normal reaction to loss of balance. As observed already by John B. Watson (the father of Behaviorism), sudden loss of support, along with blocking of respiration, is a primary anxiogenic stimulus even for preverbal babies.[59] Thus, this second anxiety component is not a response to just symptoms in general but, rather, linked specifically to the vestibular system.

Neurological linkage

Specific neural circuitry subserves the expression of both anxiety and vestibular symptoms. A possible linkage is suggested by basic science work in which it was found that strains of mice bred to be anxiety prone have relatively poor balance function;[60] however, both anxiety and balance improve with drug treatments.[61] A recent study of fear potentiation of the conditioned acoustic startle reflex demonstrates that a neurological disorder can affect parameters of anxiety in humans.[62] Potentiated startle is a commonly used psychophysiological indicator of anxiety. Maschke et al.[62] found that patients with medial cerebellar lesions showed diminished fear potentiation. Anxiety responses are frequently learned via classical conditioning.[63] In patients with cerebellar lesions, classical conditioning was diminished. Recently, a linkage between dizziness and migraines has received recognition.[64] This linkage may also include panic disorder, since patients with migraines have an increased prevalence of both dizziness and panic disorder.[4]

Balaban and Thayer[65] recently reviewed the neurological linkages that exist between the vestibular system and neural circuitry involved in anxiety. These include: (1) monoaminergic inputs to the vestibular system that mediate the effects of anxiety on vestibular function; (2) the parabrachial nucleus network that mediates emotional responses related to disordered vestibular function; and (3) the widely distributed noradrenergic outflow from the locus coeruleus that mediates the overall responsiveness of these systems to novel stimuli.

The parabrachial nucleus is a point of convergence for vestibular information, visceral information (including visceral graviception), and somatic nociception. It has reciprocal connections with the central nucleus of the amygdala and the infralimbic cortex (i.e. structures involved in fear and avoidance conditioning). These structures are, in turn, under the control of higher cortical regions that support cognitive appraisals of incoming stimulation. If the appraisal is one of 'danger', an anxiety state may ensue. Through its connections to brainstem regions controlling respiration and sympathetic and parasympathetic outflow, the parabrachial nucleus may be instrumental in mediating the autonomic concomitants to such anxiety appraisals.

Space and motion discomfort: a unifying theme relating vestibular dysfunction and phobia

Situations in which information from non-vestibular sources relevant for postural control is reduced or misleading often elicit dizziness even in healthy individuals. This form of dizziness is often referred to as 'physiological' vertigo. For example, exposure to heights triggers height vertigo even in normal individuals. Some patients with vestibular disorders have an increased sensitivity to situations that are the same or similar to those that would elicit physiological vertigo in normal controls. This increased sensitivity manifests as discomfort, anxiety, or avoidance behaviors. We will refer to this situational symptom pattern as 'Space and Motion

Discomfort' (SMD).[66] In some cases, SMD may lead to incapacitating avoidance behaviors, and we designate such individuals as suffering from 'Space and Motion Phobia' (SMP).[3]

The types of situations that trigger SMD, like those triggering physiological vertigo, tend to have one or more of the following attributes: (1) unusual motion in the visual surround not matched by vestibular information (e.g. wide-screen movies); (2) situations in which visual feedback for body sway is diminished, including long visual distances (e.g. heights); (3) rich and repetitive visual patterns (e.g. certain wallpaper patterns or shiny surfaces);[23,67] (4) neck extension (e.g. looking up at tall buildings, rinsing hair in shower); (5) unfamiliar bodily accelerations (e.g. boats or roller coasters); (6) unstable or soft support surfaces (e.g. soft carpets, vibrations in the floors of parking garages, bridges or higher levels of shopping malls); and (7) intense vestibular stimulation (e.g. abrupt head movements). A phenomenon related to SMD is visual vertigo.[67] Visual vertigo represents a subset of SMD that involves visual SMD triggers in particular (attributes 1–4 above). The SMD pattern also seems to be similar to the one observed in patients with symptoms of phobic postural vertigo described later in this chapter. Some SMD-inducing situations also can elicit motion sickness. However, SMD tends to occur immediately, whereas motion sickness requires longer exposure.

To measure SMD, Jacob et al.[68] constructed a measure of SMD called the Situational Characteristics Questionnaire (SitQ). This questionnaire includes two subscales measuring SMD, using different item formats, called SMD-I and SMD-II. Another subscale, the Ag-I, is a 'control' scale that measures agoraphobic discomfort not thought to be related to vestibular dysfunction (e.g. being far from an exit in a supermarket). Table 15.9 shows the items on these subscales. The difference between the two SMD scales is that the SMD-I compares different aspects of a situation whereas the SMD-II is in the traditional Likert scale format. The SitQ was administered to a group of unselected patients with vestibular dysfunction and a group of patients being evaluated for mild hearing loss.[66] The results indicated that the vestibular patients had significantly higher levels of SMD than the hearing loss patients.

The overall pattern of results is shown in Fig. 15.3. Both the SMD-I and SMD-II, but not the Ag-I, differentiated between the two groups. Among medical conditions, intolerance of certain situations is not unique for vestibular dysfunction. For example, patients with allergies avoid provocative situations and patients with hyperthyroidism prefer cold environments. In essence, SMD is a 'vestibular' situational symptom constellation. In fact, because most psychiatric anxiety disorders have a typical age of onset before 30 years, onset of SMD, such as fear of heights, in someone above the age of 40 years should raise the suspicion of a medical disorder.

Table 15.9 *Items of the subscales of the Situational Characteristics Questionnaire*[a]

Source (subcale)	Situation	Aspects compared (SMD-I, Ag-I only)	Effect size[b]
SMD-II	Looking up at tall buildings		1.14
	Closing eyes in shower		0.99
	Rolling over in bed		0.87
	Leaning far back in chair		0.78
	Dancing		0.69
	Aerobic exercise		0.66
	Discomfort increases as the day progresses		0.64
	Reading newspaper close to face		0.44
	Riding on roller coasters		0.33
SMD-I	Riding in a car	Reading vs. looking out of the window	0.73
		Back seat vs. front seat	0.55
		Winding vs. straight roads	0.43
		Changing speed vs. steady speed	0.12
		Narrow vs. wide road	0.11
		Bumpy vs. smooth road	0.02
	Tunnels	Looking at lights on side flashing by vs. looking at the light at the end of the tunnel	0.55
		Curved vs. straight	−0.32
	Elevators	Glass vs. standard	0.53
		Stopping vs. moving at steady speed	0.32
	Buses	Moving vs. standing still	0.41
	Supermarkets	Looking at shelves while walking down an aisle vs. looking at the end of the aisle	0.17
Ag-I	Riding in a car	Limited access vs. unlimited access roads	0.17
	Buses	Window seat vs. aisle seat	0.30
		Crowded vs. empty	0.11
	Elevators	Crowded vs. empty	0.37
	Movies	Sitting in middle of row vs. on aisle	0.49
	Supermarkets	Crowded vs. empty	0.37
		Far from exit vs. close to exit	−0.49

[a]Data from Jacob et al.[66]

[b]Effect size: difference between groups divided by the standard deviation of the difference. SMD-I; SMD-II; Ag-I: for subscale designations, see text.

The increased levels of SMD in patients with vestibular disorders may be related to visual or somatosensory dependence that develops to compensate for the vestibular deficit (i.e. 'sensory reweighting').[69] A study examining postural sway in individuals exposed to full-field motion in the visual environment (optic flow stimuli) showed that individuals with SMD may be visually dependent. The patients included in this study had an anxiety disorder as well as SMD. The results indicated that compared with normal healthy comparison sub-

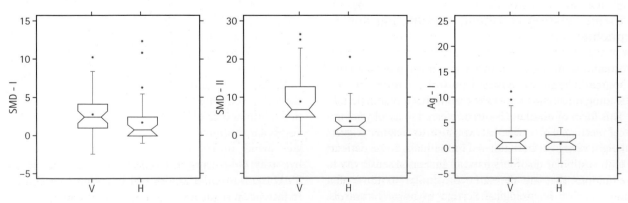

Figure 15.3 *Differences between vestibular disordered and hearing-impaired patients with respect to two measures of space and motion discomfort (SMD-I and SMD-II) and a control scale of non-space related agoraphobic avoidance (Ag-I). (Reproduced from ref. 66.)*

jects, anxiety patients with SMD had increased postural sway responses to movement of the visual surround.[70] Fourier analysis of the frequency of sway suggested that subject's body sway 'entrained' to the motion in the visual surround. The design of this study, however, does not rule out that visual dependence might have been related to anxiety alone rather than to SMD. Findings reported by Viaud-Delmon et al.[41] suggest that normal subjects with high trait anxiety may be visually dependent with respect to spatial orientation. The investigators manipulated the subjects' visual environment via a head-mounted virtual reality display and manipulated their vestibular input by physically rotating them while they sat on a spinning 'robot' device. The subjects were asked to estimate the amount of rotation that had occurred in each trial. A vestibular visual mismatch was introduced such that the virtual environment would move only half as fast as the chair rotation. After this experience, high-trait anxious individuals, more than low-trait anxious subjects adjusted their response to be consistent with the visual input.

Recently, Guerraz et al.[71] examined anxiety levels, spatial orientation and optic flow-induced body sway in patients with visual vertigo not specifically selected for symptoms of anxiety. These patients had been referred for vestibular evaluation and mostly had mild peripheral vestibular disorders. The experiment also included a normal control group and a group of 'labyrinthine defective' subjects whose vestibular disorder was more severe but well compensated. The subjects stood in front of a rod and frame display with a tilted frame, or in front of a rotating disk, while their subjective vertical and amount of lateral body tilt was measured. The results indicated that compared with normal comparison subjects, the visual vertigo patients showed greater deviations on the subjective vertical measure than did the normal subjects in response to the tilted frame or rotating disk. Furthermore, their bodies tilted in the lateral direction by a greater amount. The labyrinthine defective patients' performance was essentially similar to that of the visual vertigo patients. Similarly, their visual vertigo questionnaire scores were comparable to those of the visual vertigo subjects. Questionnaire measures of anxiety indicated that the visual vertigo patients were not any more anxious than the labyrinthine defective patients or the normal subjects. The combination of these findings again suggests that SMD, in its visual vertigo variant, is not an anxiety equivalent, but rather a correlate of vestibular dysfunction.

Among patients with anxiety disorders, patients with agoraphobia have particularly high levels of SMD. This is shown in Fig. 15.4.[66] Similar findings were obtained in a sample of Brazilian agoraphobics.[72] High SMD levels may explain why agoraphobic patients report increased anxiety in certain spatial environments such as elevators, stairs, floors above the ground level, queues or barriers.[73] The subjects represented in Fig. 15.4 also participated in

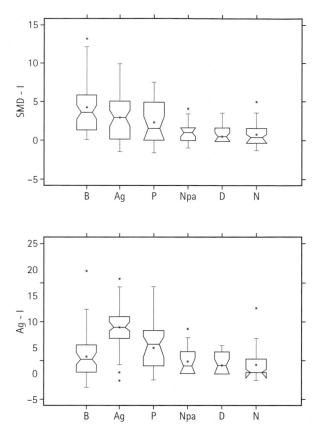

Figure 15.4 *Space and motion discomfort (SMD) levels within the following patient samples: participants within a self-help group of balance disorders (Group B), patients with agoraphobia (Ag), patients with panic disorder with no or mild agoraphobia (P), patients with non-panic anxiety disorders (Npa), patients with depression without anxiety (D) and normal control subjects (N). Note high levels of SMD in agoraphobics and self-help group members as well as the different pattern for the control scale Ag-I for these two groups. (Reproduced from ref. 66.)*

the study, discussed earlier, in which the agoraphobic group had the highest prevalence of abnormal vestibular test findings, and in which levels of SMD proved to be a predictor of vestibular dysfunction even after accounting for the effect of diagnostic group.[15] Figure 15.4 also shows a group of individuals presumed to have vestibular dysfunction (Group B). The members of this group were recruited from a self-help group for balance disorders.[22] This group had high levels of SMD, but unlike the agoraphobics, low levels on the control scale, the Ag-I.

HISTORICAL NOTE

Vestibular syndromes that reflect the situational specificity of SMD have been described in the earlier clinical literature. These include the supermarket syndrome (i.e. intolerance to looking at the shelves while walking down a supermarket aisle),[74] the motorist's disorientation syndrome (i.e. intolerance to driving on open, featureless roads or over the crest of a hill)[75] and space phobia (i.e. anxiety in situations characterized by lack of support or by a paucity of visual cues for orientation in space).[76,77]

A recent historical review[78] (which is the source of the ensuing quotations) indicates that the phenomena subsumed under SMD have been described since antiquity. For example, in the first century AD, Soranus of Ephesis observed that

> dizziness ... is aggravated if the patient watches the flow of a river from a high point or gazes at a potter's wheel.

In the sixteenth century, Andrew Borde noted:

> Such men having this passion [vertigo] let them beware of climbing or going up upon high hills or round stairs.

Willis, in 1692, wrote that vertigo

> is wont to be raised by non-natural things, for by a long turning round of the Body, by looking from an high place, passing over a Bridge, by sailing in a Ship or going in a Coach.

The notion of visual dependence was anticipated in the nineteenth century, when Herbert Mayo, in 1837, noted that vision and the 'muscular sense' (proprioception) were the two main sensory modalities for maintaining balance:

> When in the light, we use vision likewise. We then rest or support ourselves upon visible objects. Of which we know from experience the distance. We lean upon our eyesight as upon crutches.

Mayo also observed the phenomenon of height vertigo:

> This is proved to his conviction, when one unaccustomed to look down heights stands on the top of a tower, resting against the parapet; he knows that he is safe, but he feels insecure; his eyes no longer support him, and he feels as if he would topple over.

The importance of vision was so well known that a special form of vertigo, called visual or ocular vertigo, was recognized. Attributed to eye muscle paralysis, this concept persisted until the early twentieth century. Importantly, a condition called 'Platzschwindel,' ('vertigo in open places') described by Benedikt (1870) was considered to be a consequence of ocular vertigo:

> This rare condition consists thereof, that persons feel well or reasonably well in their rooms or on narrow streets; however, as soon as they arrive at a wider street or especially an open square, they become overcome by vertigo, such that they either fear that they might tumble or develop such a fear, that they do not dare to pass by such a place. If they are in a position to fixate on a specific line or an object that is moving away in from of them, they can overcome the impediment.

The following year, in 1871, Westphal relabeled this condition as 'agoraphobia.' For the next decade, acrimonious discussions took place as to whether agoraphobia was a component of vertigo or a psychiatric disorder. Although the controversy was resolved in favor of psychiatry, the findings reviewed earlier in this section documenting increased prevalence of vestibular and balance dysfunction in agoraphobia raise this same issue once again.

PSYCHIATRIC CONSEQUENCES OF DISABILITY: DEPRESSION

In the preceding section we saw that vestibular symptoms have inherent anxiety components. In addition, vestibular symptoms that are chronic and disabling, like other chronic, distressing or disabling symptoms, may result in depression. Any medical disorder leading to disability or chronic distress, including tinnitus and chronic pain, is likely to lead to depressive states.[24,79–81] Weight loss, sleep disturbances, and poor concentration are signs that should prompt follow-up questions for the other criteria (see Table 15.10). It is important to recognize depressive syndromes, because appropriate treatment with pharmacotherapy can improve the patient's condition and prevent other negative consequences. Although we could not find any documented cases of suicide related to vertigo, such cases have been reported for tinnitus sufferers;[82] in fact, in the elderly, tinnitus was a predictor of suicide.[83]

Table 15.10 *Symptoms and signs of depression*[a]

Symptoms/signs
1. Depressed mood (affect appears sad, weepy)
2. Loss of interest or loss of enjoyment
3. Weight loss or weight gain
4. Insomnia or hypersomnia
5. Psychomotor retardation or agitation
6. Loss of energy
7. Feeling worthless or guilty
8. Trouble concentrating
9. Recurrent thought of death, or suicidal ideation

[a]From DSM-IV[8] (reprinted with permission from the *Diagnostic and Statistical Manual of Mental Disorders*, 4th edn, text revision, Copyright 2000 American Psychiatric Association). To count as a criterion the symptoms must be pervasive and occur on a daily basis.

PSYCHIATRIC POTENTIATION (OVERLAY)

Not all patients develop anxiety or depression in response to vestibular dysfunction. Individuals appear to differ with respect to their ability to cope with dizziness. Certain modes of coping may be more dysfunctional for the task at hand. Some of these dysfunctional coping styles seem to be associated with certain psychiatric clinical or subclinical conditions. Such conditions include personality disorders or traits, particularly obsessive–compulsive personality disorder (OCPD), a condition that is listed on Axis II in DSM-IV. A high prevalence of OCPD has been observed in patients with phobic postural vertigo (PPV) to be discussed later. Table 15.11 describes the main features of OCPD. Many patients do not have fully fledged OCPD but have obsessive–compulsive personality traits, essentially involving a high degree of 'perfectionism.' Dimensional measures of perfectionism reveal several relatively independent subdimensions.[84–86] The most important of these are one that primarily involves 'obsessiveness' (i.e. indecisiveness and high personal standards) and those who are primarily 'compulsive' (i.e. highly organized, as the proverbial 'house-proud housewife').

Table 15.11 *DSM-IV-based characteristics of obsessive–compulsive personality disorder (OCPD)[p]*

1. Getting lost in details
2. Perfectionism that interferes with task completion
3. Excessive devotion to work
4. Overly conscientious or scrupulous
5. Trouble discarding unneeded objects
6. Unwilling to delegate
7. Miserly spending style
8. Rigid and stubborn

[a]For a diagnosis of OCPD, four or more of these characteristics should be manifest in a variety of contexts (e.g. not just in the work setting), with onset in early adulthood.

There may be several reasons why patients with OCPD, or traits thereof, cope poorly with vestibular symptoms. Inherent in the condition is a decreased tolerance of imperfections of any kind. This may cause them to try hard not to be 'dizzy'. However, as a result of their continuous attempts not to be dizzy they might paradoxically increase their awareness of the dizziness. This paradoxical response would be analogous to the one occurring in a person instructed 'not to think about something'. We will further discuss coping in individuals with OCPD traits in the section on PPV.

Another source for dysfunctional modes of coping with dizziness is anxiety proneness, a personality trait of high vulnerability for anxiety disorders. Indicators of anxiety proneness include the presence of an anxiety disorder prior to the onset of a vestibular condition, a family history of anxiety disorders, or the traits of certain personality disorders (again, particularly OCPD). Individuals who are anxiety prone will react with anxiety when faced with new situations or tasks.

Somatization refers to a pervasive tendency toward increased illness behaviors. Individuals with somatizing tendencies will have multiple medical symptoms, either simultaneously or sequentially, often in excess of what would be expected from medical examinations. A group

of psychiatric disorders, the somatoform disorders, include psychiatric conditions that are primarily characterized by somatization.

The mechanisms for somatization are poorly understood. Multiple pathways may be involved. For example, somatization has been related to a trait called alexithymia, or the inability to conceptualize sources of distress in psychological terms. According to this theory, alexithymic individuals use the language of physical symptoms to seek help for problems that other individuals might perceive as interpersonal or environmental. This tendency to convert psychosocial stress into a physical manifestation in order to seek help may also be culturally determined.[87,88] A related explanation for somatization is that it is a form of 'masked depression,' where the symptoms of depression are described in the language of physical symptoms. This concept is supported by observations that, particularly in the primary care setting, the onset of depression is sometimes preceded by an increase in physical complaints.[33]

A model for somatization that is also useful as an explanatory device for patients is that of 'symptom amplification.'[89–91] This concept is illustrated in Fig. 15.5; the theory distinguishes between 'stimuli,' 'sensations,' and 'impact.' Stimuli are physically measurable external

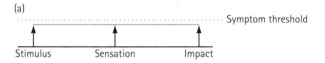

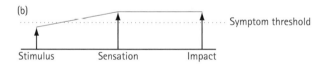

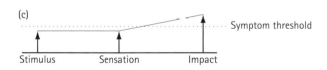

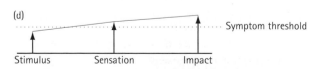

Figure 15.5 *Determinants of illness impact for a given stimulus: (a) normal perception; (b) increased sensations due to vestibular dysfunction; (c) symptom formation as a result of secondary 'amplifying' appraisals; (d) a mixed scenario.*

inputs. Sensations refer to the initial subjective correlate of the stimulus. The impact of the sensation, e.g. whether or not a symptom is reported depends on appraisals of the sensations. Symptom report or illness behavior occurs when the impact exceeds a threshold (horizontal dotted line).

We will discuss symptom amplification employing the development of height phobia from height vertigo as a prototypical scenario. We know from Chapter 9 that normal individuals develop height vertigo, but this does not necessarily raise any concerns (Fig. 15.5a). Second, according to our earlier discussion of SMD, patients with vestibular dysfunction who develop visual dependence become physiologically more responsive to heights. This means that their 'sensations' have become more prominent and may have caused an increase in impact above the threshold level (Fig. 15.5b). Height phobia could therefore be the direct result of the increase in SMD that develops as a result of a vestibular disorder. Third, symptom formation can also occur as a result of psychological elaboration of a normal sensation (Fig. 15.5c). For example, individuals that are anxiety prone may not tolerate even 'normal' levels of height vertigo. Scenarios (b) and (c) in Fig. 15.5 represent the two extremes of a continuum. Scenario (d) in Fig. 15.5 shows one of many possible intermediary cases in which the increase in sensation due to visual dependence remains at a subclinical level but is augmented to exceed the symptom threshold by secondary elaborative processes. This may be the case for some patients with symptoms of PPV, or SMP to be discussed in the next section. Not covered in Fig. 15.5 is yet another scenario, that of 'stoic' individuals who do not complain much even in the presence of severe sensations.

Symptom amplification can be expected in any patient with somatizing tendencies. The psychiatric category of somatoform disorders subsumes several disorders characterized by extreme degrees of somatization. Such patients have a multitude of symptoms either simultaneously or sequentially. Patients who fulfill all of the diagnostic criteria for these disorders are rare, at least in psychiatric settings. We will therefore not cover these disorders further, except for conversion disorder (see next section). Measures of somatization are based on a count of the number of different somatic symptoms during a period of time. For example, in a study of the physiological effects of head movements (pitch, yaw or circular), increases in respiration rate were found to be correlated with the number of different somatic symptoms reported during the preceding two-month period.[92]

CONVERSION DISORDER

Conversion disorder remains an enigmatic disorder for both psychiatrists and neurologists. Neurologists, rather than psychiatrists, see most of the patients. We include a discussion of it here to provide a background for the description of Psychogenic Disorder of Stance and Gait (next section). Historically, conversion was seen as coupled with dissociative phenomena and grouped together under the general label of 'hysteria'.[93] In current terminology, the label 'hysteria' has been abandoned. However, the two psychiatric diagnostic systems, the DSM-III and ICD-10, classify conversion disorder differently. In the DSM-III, conversion disorder is grouped with other disorders involving medically unexplained symptoms under the rubric of somatoform disorders. The ICD-10 retains the classification of conversion disorder as a form of dissociative disorder.

Dissociation is a poorly understood phenomenon that seems to have etiological significance for conversion disorder. In the ICD-10, dissociation is described as involving a 'loss of normal integration between memories of the past, awareness of identity, and immediate sensation, and control of bodily movements'.[11] In the DSM-IV-TR, it is described as 'a disruption in the usually integrated functions of consciousness, memory, identity or perception.' Dissociation includes normal and mild states as well as pathological, severely disturbed states. Normal dissociative states occur during hypnosis or even when watching a highly engaging movie. Pathological dissociative states include those where a patient suddenly becomes seemingly unresponsive to external stimuli while sitting in, for example, the office chair, recovering after minutes to fractions of an hour, and not necessarily remembering the event. Factor analytic examinations of such patients' responses to questionnaires reveal the components of amnesia, absorption/imaginative involvement, and derealization/depersonalization.[94]

The view that dissociation has a role in the production of conversion symptoms has some empirical support. Patients with dissociative disorders often have conversion or other medically unexplained symptoms, and patients with conversion disorders often report symptoms of dissociation.[94] Dissociation occurs frequently when a person is exposed to life-threatening, traumatic events and becomes a symptom associated with post traumatic stress disorder (PTSD). In fact, dissociation occurring during the acute trauma is a predictor of the later development of PTSD[95] and conversion symptoms may occur in patients with PTSD. Dissociation may represent a state involving release of the neurotransmitter glutamate. Conversion symptoms tend to occur especially in socially disadvantaged individuals with poor verbal coping skills. Such individuals may have learning disabilities, mental retardation or personality disorders.

Patients with conversion disorder are rare in most psychiatric settings, with the exception perhaps of clinical services geared to treat patients with medical disorders who also have psychiatric symptoms. Conversion disorder is diagnosed more commonly in neurological settings, although concerns have been raised about over-diagnosis, and the validity of the diagnosis has been challenged.[96] The first author (R.G.J.) has participated in the treatment of a middle-aged female with a history of paralysis of her legs and part of one arm of several years' duration, which caused her to be wheelchair bound and develop contractures. Concomitantly, she had symptoms of severe depression as well as dissociative episodes. She was admitted to a psychiatric inpatient unit where she received electroshock therapy for her depression. The diagnosis of conversion paralysis was established with certainty only after the paralysis miraculously remitted with the electroshock therapy. The contractures subsequently resolved with intensive physical therapy.

The diagnostic criteria of conversion disorder are listed in Table 15.12. Conversion disorder is characterized by neurological symptoms involving either the sensory system or the motor system. In either case, the symptoms are not under the patients' voluntary control. Furthermore, the onset or exacerbation of the symptoms is thought to have a causal relationship with a preceding stressor or conflict. This criterion is one of the few remnants of 'psychogenic' causation in the DSM-IV (PTSD

being another example). Historically, the symptom choice was supposed to reflect the content of the underlying conflict and represent a (dysfunctional) solution to it (e.g. saddle anesthesia in response to sexual abuse). This 'primary gain' may explain why patients sometimes are seemingly cavalier about having the symptom (*la belle indifférence*). However, the qualitative type of relationship between content of the conflict and symptom choice is impossible to establish objectively.

The diagnosis of conversion disorder requires the exclusion of medical disorders. However, this can be difficult especially because conversion symptoms commonly occur in patients with comorbid medical disorders that also could explain their symptom (e.g. pseudoseizures in patients with epilepsy). The first author recently saw a patient with dramatic paralysis of her legs and an admission diagnosis of conversion disorder whose final diagnosis was encephalitis. The problem of such 'false positive' diagnoses of conversion disorder is demonstrated even in recent follow-up studies of patients with conversion symptoms. False-positive cases were particularly common in earlier studies, before modern imaging techniques were available. Among

Table 15.12 *The DSM-IV and ICD-10 criteria for conversion/dissociative motor disorder*[a]

DSM IV Conversion disorder	ICD-10 Dissociative (conversion) disorders
A. One or more symptoms or deficits affecting voluntary motor or sensory function that suggest a neurological or other general medical condition	
B. Psychological factors are judged to be associated with the symptom or deficit because conflicts or stressors precede the initiation or exacerbation of the symptoms and/or deficit	G2. There are convincing associations in time between the onset of symptoms of the disorder and stressful events, problems, or needs
C. The symptom is not intentionally produced or feigned	
D. The symptom or deficit cannot, after appropriate investigation, be fully explained by a general medical condition, by the direct effects of a substance, or as a culturally sanctioned behavior or experience	G1. There must be no evidence of a physical disorder that can explain the characteristic symptoms of this disorder (although physical disorders may be present that give rise to other symptoms)
E. The symptoms cause clinically significant distress or impairment in social, occupational or other important areas of functioning	
F. The symptom or deficit is not limited to pain or sexual dysfunction, does not occur exclusively during the course of somatization disorder, and is not better accounted for by another mental disorder	
Specify type of symptom or deficit	
With motor symptom or deficit	Dissociative motor disorders Either of the following must be present (1) Complete or partial loss of the ability to perform movements that are normally under voluntary control (including speech) (2) Various or variable degrees of incoordination or ataxia, or inability to stand unaided.
With sensory symptom or deficit	Dissociative anesthesia and sensory loss[b]
With seizures or convulsions	Dissociative convulsions[b]
With mixed presentation	Mixed dissociative (conversion) disorders[b]

[a]From the DSM-IV[9] (reprinted from the *Diagnostic and Statistical Manual of Mental Disorders*, 4th edn, text revision, Copyright 2000 American Psychiatric Association) and ICD-10 Diagnostic Research Criteria[12] with permission from the World Health Organization.
[b]Specific criteria not given here.

studies published in 1990 or later, the 'false positive rate' has ranged between 4 per cent and 15 per cent, [97] although one group of investigators reported zero per cent.[98] Table 15.13 represents a synopsis of recent studies of conversion disorder conducted in the emergency room setting.[97,99] A common source for the misdiagnosis was the fact that the patient demonstrated concomitant psychiatric symptoms, a reminder of the previously discussed possibility that psychiatric and medical disorders may coexist.

SPECIFIC DIZZINESS/IMBALANCE SYNDROMES SEEN IN NON–PSYCHIATRIC SETTINGS

In this section we discuss two conditions: psychogenic disorder of stance and gait, and phobic postural vertigo (PPV).

Conversion (psychogenic) disorder of stance and gait

Psychogenic disorder of stance and gait most likely is a conversion disorder; if so, the formal psychiatric diagnosis would be 'Conversion disorder with motor symptoms or deficit' (DSM-IV) or 'Dissociative motor disorder' (ICD-10). Therefore, in this discussion we will employ the term 'conversion' rather than 'psychogenic' as an etiologically more specific term. The importance of conversion disorder of stance and gait is not reflected in the recent literature and textbooks. For general descriptions, one needs to consult older textbooks or a few recent surveys.[100–105] Patients with conversion disorder of stance and gait exhibit an increased postural sway with stumbling, near tumbles, or outright falls. However, they rarely complain of dizziness. The patients display their disability in a bizarre, dramatic fashion. Mostly unable to work, they have poor social function. Even so, they tend to show little overt distress (i.e. they display *la belle indifférence*). The most common abnormal movements are tremor, dystonia[106] and gait disturbances, which account for more than 75 per cent of movements.[107]

In a unique case series, Lempert et al.[105] examined whether it would be possible to establish a diagnosis of 'conversion disorder of stance and gait' solely based on a patient's phenomenology or symptoms. Thirty-seven patients were examined and recorded on videotape (Figs 15.6–15.13). The characteristic features of these patients are listed in Table 15.14. Of these, six clinical features occurred alone or in combination in more than 90 per cent of the patients (these are marked with an asterisk in Table 15.14). Thus, if we were to employ a criterion of 'at least one of the six,' the sensitivity of identification would be 90 per cent of the sample from which the criterion was derived. Of course, the actual sensitivity and specificity of such a rule would need to be examined on a new series of patients before employment as a clinical tool.

1. Variability in performance (Fig. 15.6) occurred in more than half of the patients. Performance was considerably improved after encouragement or by distracting the patients with attention-deflecting tasks, such as finger–nose testing or walking on tiptoe (Figs 15.7 and 15.10). Variability in the degree of impairment may also occur in neurological disease

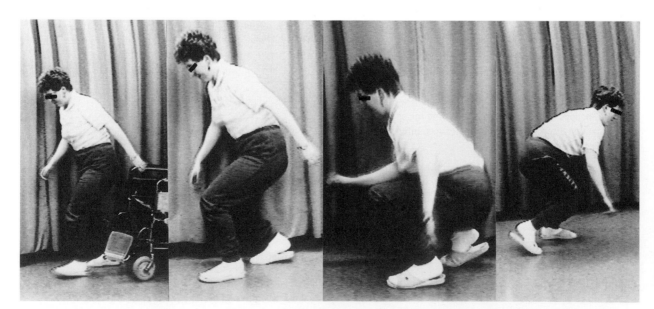

Figure 15.6 *Fluctuating gait disturbance with waste of muscular energy: patient starts walking upright, then goes slowly into a full knee bend and becomes erect again on her way back. (Reproduced from Lempert T, Brandt T, Dieterich M, Huppert D. How to identify psychogenic disorders of stance and gait. A video study in 37 patients. J Neurol 1991;238:140–6, © Springer-Verlag, with permission.)*

Table 15.13 *Ten patients misdiagnosed with conversion disorder in two recent studies*

Case[a]	Neurological symptoms	Stressors, indicators, psychiatric symptoms	Underlying lesion
G1	Inability to move legs and pain	Schizophrenia; rambling speech	Compression fracture with thoracic disk herniation
G2	Numbness and pain in leg, unable to get up	History of depression, age 82 years	Thoracic epidural abscess
G3	Right sided weakness	Jail inmate, pending court appearance	Cervical disc herniation with compression of the cervical cord
G4	Bilateral leg numbness, low back pain abdominal pain	Hostile affect; history of i.v. drug abuse	Spinal cord compression due to an abscess
G5	Numbness in legs and saddle area, lower leg weakness	7-months pregnant	Cauda equina syndrome due to herniated lumbar disc.
G6	Weakness in left arm, inconsistent physical signs, non-anatomical distribution of sensory loss.	Remote psychiatric problems and substance abuse, recently pregnant	Large right frontoparietal hematoma
M1	Involuntary movements and sensory disturbances in mouth and arm	Depression	Dyskinesia
M2	Paralysis of the legs, problematic arm movements and speech, incontinence	Depression	Amyotrophic lateral sclerosis
M3	Disturbed walking, balance, bladder dysfunction, dysarthria	Depression	Atrophy of brainstem and cerebellum
M4	Unusual walking pattern	Walking pattern improving with intense verbal guidance	Extrapyramidal syndrome
M5	Parkinson's disease with intense response fluctuations, pain and cramps in limbs	Patient convinced of psychogenicity	Parkinson's disease with response fluctuations
M6	Numbness in fingers, problem walking, disturbed micturition	Chronic headaches, anatomically incongruent sensory disturbance	Multiple sclerosis
M7	Sudden gait disturbance	Theatrical presentation	Dementia
M8	Trembling and pain	Unable to function for 22 h/day but functioning well for 2 h/day	Parkinson's disease with psychogenic aggravation
M9	Coordination problems with left extremities, lower back pain, headaches	Symptom presentation 'bizarre and attention seeking'	Lung cancer with metastatic space-occupying parietal–occipital lesion
M10	Lower back pain extending into left leg	Symptom presentation 'bizarre and attention seeking'	Radicular syndrome

[a] Abstracted from cases reported by Glick et al.[99] (cases G1–6) and Moene et al.[97] (cases M1–10).

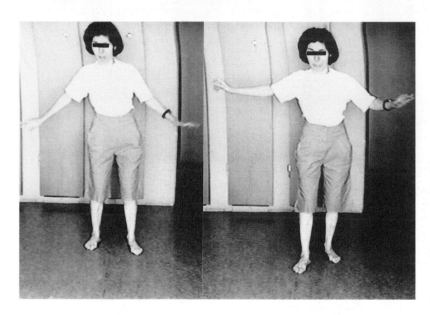

Figure 15.7 *Conversion instability of stance with 'non-neurological' stiff leaning to the side; this ceases once finger-nose testing distracts the patient. (Reproduced from Lempert T, Brandt T, Dieterich M, Huppert D. How to identify psychogenic disorders of stance and gait. A video study in 37 patients. J Neurol 1991;238:140–6, © Springer-Verlag,with permission.)*

Figure 15.8 *'Walking on ice': hesitant, slow gait with anxious balancing, stiff knees and ankles, and reduced step height and stride length. (Reproduced from Lempert T, Brandt T, Dieterich M, Huppert D. How to identify psychogenic disorders of stance and gait. A video study in 37 patients. J Neurol 1991;238:140–6, © Springer-Verlag,with permission.)*

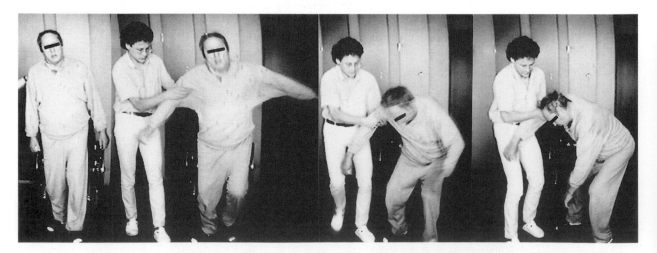

Figure 15.9 *Conversion knee buckling. Patient falls forward with sudden flexion of hips and knees and remains in a strained half-flexed posture. (Reproduced from Lempert T, Brandt T, Dieterich M, Huppert D. How to identify psychogenic disorders of stance and gait. A video study in 37 patients. J Neurol 1991;238:140–6, © Springer-Verlag, with permission.)*

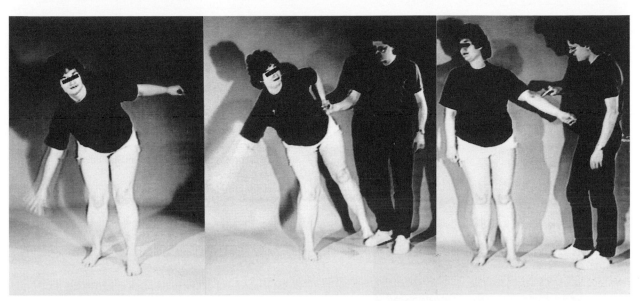

Figure 15.10 *Psychogenic pseudo-ataxic instability of stance and gait with wobbling of the trunk, bizarre balancing, and flailing of the arms, which ceases on distraction. (Reproduced from Lempert T, Brandt T, Dieterich M, Huppert D. How to identify psychogenic disorders of stance and gait. A video study in 37 patients.* J Neurol *1991;238:140–6, © Springer-Verlag, with permission.)*

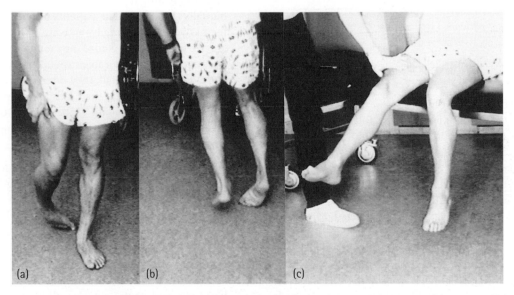

(a)   (b)   (c)

Figure 15.11 *Conversion monoparesis of the right leg: (a) dragging of the twisted leg, grasping the leg; (b) 'paralyzed' right leg supports the body during swing phase of the left leg; (c) resumption of function of the 'paralyzed' leg after encouragement. (Reproduced from Lempert T, Brandt T, Dieterich M, Huppert D. How to identify psychogenic disorders of stance and gait. A video study in 37 patients.* J Neurol *1991;238:140–6, © Springer-Verlag, with permission.)*

such as myasthenia gravis, dyskalemic paralysis, and extrapyramidal disorders. However, episodes of anterior–posterior or lateral sway suggest a conversion origin if their duration is brief.

2. Slow speed (Fig. 15.8) is usually brought about by simultaneous contraction of agonist/antagonist muscles. A related phenomenon is hesitation, such that initiation of intended movement is delayed or impossible. The patients engage in small forward and backward movements of their legs while their feet remain stuck on the ground. Hesitation also is

observed in Parkinson's disease; however, unlike Parkinson's patients, the conversion patients do not overcome the gait inhibition once they succeed in taking the first step. Rather, they show the hesitation at each and every step. Shuffling and freezing in a start and hesitation pattern has also been described in an organic syndrome of gait-ignition failure due to frontal lobe disorders.[108] Furthermore, in the elderly, higher level gait disorders, such as 'frontal or senile' disorders of gait[109] and gait 'apraxia' are relevant for the differential diagnosis (see Chapter 13).

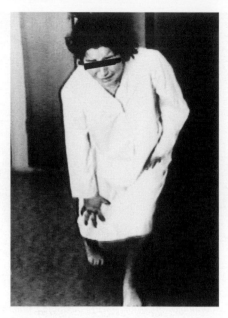

Figure 15.12 *Psychomotor symptoms of conversion gait disorder: suffering facial expression and grasping of the leg. (Reproduced from Lempert T, Brandt T, Dieterich M, Huppert D. How to identify psychogenic disorders of stance and gait. A video study in 37 patients.* J Neurol *1991;238:140–6, © Springer-Verlag, with permission.)*

Table 15.14 *Characteristic features of conversion disorder of stance and gait in 37 patients*

	n
Fluctuation of impairment*	19
Excessive slowness of movements*	13
Hesitation	6
'Psychogenic Romberg' test*	12
'Walking on ice' gait pattern*	11
Uneconomic postures with waste of muscle energy*	11
Sudden buckling*	10
without falls	8
with falls	2
Astasia	4
Vertical shaking tremor	3

Data from Lempert et al.[105]
Items belonging to the set of six main characteristics of conversion disorder of stance and gait are marked with an asterisk (see text).

3. The 'psychogenic' Romberg test is characterized by a silent latency over a few seconds, followed by body sway that builds up to a large magnitude. The patients repeatedly fall toward or away from the examiner (Figs 15.7 and 15.10) but they usually manage to abort the fall by clinging on to the examiner. The large-amplitude body sway build-up may improve when the patients are distracted, for example, by asking them to identify numbers written with a finger on the skin (Fig. 15.10).

4. 'Walking-on-ice,' is the gait pattern used by normals when walking on slippery ground. It is characterized by cautious, broad-based steps with decreased stride length and height, stiffening of the knees and ankles, antagonist stimulation and shuffling of feet (Fig. 15.8). The arms typically are kept abducted. The gait abnormality in normal-pressure hydrocephalus shares some of these features, including the abducted arms, but lacks the anxious balancing quality shown by the conversion patients.

5. Bizarre, strenuous postures. The patients adopt postures that waste muscle energy (e.g. eccentric displacement of the center of gravity, standing and walking with flexion of the hip and knees, or slowing or arresting a knee-bend halfway down; see Fig. 15.6). A related sign is camptocormia, or functional bent-back syndrome. It is characterized by a 30–90° anterior flexion of the trunk associated with back pain (Fig. 15.13).[110–112]

6. Sudden buckling of knees may occur with and without falls (Fig. 15.9). The patients usually prevent themselves from falling by activating the entire antigravity musculature before they touch the ground; this requires a considerable expenditure of strength. Should they actually fall, they often manage to avoid self-injury by directing their falls an optimal direction. This 'harm-avoidant' feature makes these falls easily distinguishable from those occurring in drop attacks (see Chapter 9).

Other features in addition to these six include vertical shaking tremor and astasia. Vertical shaking tremor is a rhythmical low-frequency, large-amplitude alternation of hip and knee flexion and extension, which can be easily distinguished from the 3 Hz fore/aft cerebellar tremor in alcoholics. Astasia is the inability to stand without support in the context of preserved function of the lower limb in the recumbent position.

In 73 per cent of the patients' additional symptoms, signs, or other characteristics were noted that might indicate a conversion disorder but their differentiation from a neurological dysfunction was less obvious (Table 15.15).

Pseudoataxia refers to instability of posture or gait associated with dramatic, 'exhibitionistic' balancing acts. Patients perform bizarre trunk excursions while flailing with their arms, with their legs remaining largely unaffected. In addition, patients may perform sudden sidesteps or tumble about, but the broad-based gait of neurological ataxia is rare.

In conversion monoparesis, the affected leg is often dragged behind or may be bizarrely twisted, usually in an equinovarus position (Fig. 15.11). At times, a temporary restoration of the function of the paralyzed leg may be observed. Furthermore, patients with otherwise normal

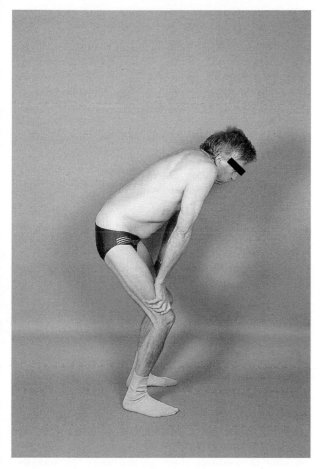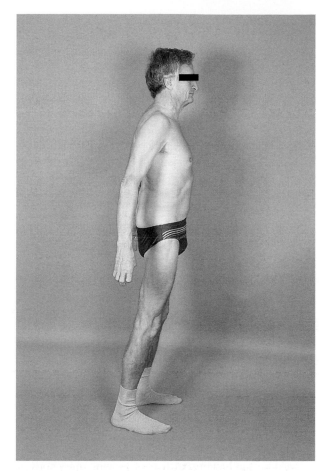

Figure 15.13 *Functional bent-back syndrome (camptocormia) in a 62-year-old patient presenting with about 30° anterior flexion of the trunk during stance and gait.*

Table 15.15 *Additional features suggestive of conversion disorder of stance*

	n
Motor symptoms (n = 22)	
Pseudoataxia	9
of the legs	3
of the trunk	6
Sudden sidesteps	6
Flailing of the arms	3
Dragging of the legs	4
Continuous flexion of the toes	2
Continuous extension of the toes	1
Bizarre tremors (hands, 7; legs, 3; trunk, 2; head, 1)	9
Expressive behavior (n = 19)	
Grasping the leg	6
Mannered posture of hands	6
Suffering or strained facial expression	15
Moaning	8
Hyperventilation	3

Data from Lempert et al.[105]

muscle tone may display a fixed flexion or extension of the toes.

Conversion tremors, which may be resting, postural, or kinetic, can be identified by their unusual distribution and their alleviation by distraction. In contrast to most organic tremors, the distal portions of the limbs may be spared and move limply in response to proximal muscle activity.

The prognosis of conversion disorder of stance and gait after treatment is guarded, but relatively more favorable for patients with short illness durations. In a follow-up study on 17 patients, three (18 per cent) became symptom free but nine (53 per cent) did not improve. There was a negative correlation of short-term improvement with symptom duration: the condition proved intractable in five patients in whom it had lasted longer than 2 years. We describe the actual treatment in a later section.

Phobic postural vertigo

THE CLINICAL SYNDROME

Phobic postural vertigo[113,114] is a syndrome characterized by a persistent sense of unsteadiness or postural imbalance, and recurrent dizziness attacks. Phobic avoidance is an associated symptom. The patients often have good and bad days. In clinical settings where the syndrome has been studied, the prevalence of PPV is quite high, amounting to 16 per cent among dizziness clinic patients[115] and is one of the most prevalent diagnosis in some clinical populations. The disorder often begins after a major stressor or after a physical illness[116] but it may also develop following a vestibular disorder (see next section).

In a group of PPV patients studied by Huppert et al.,[117] the age range was 18–70 years, with a clear peak for the fourth and fifth decades in both males and females. The sex distribution was about equal. The duration of the condition before definitive diagnosis ranged from 1 week to 30 years, with a mean of 38 months. The attacks recurred for months or even years, sometimes in cycles. On the basis of patient history and clinical examination, a proportion of patients were initially diagnosed to have an organic disorder of vestibular function that triggered the phobic condition.

The postural imbalance component involves feelings of weakness, reluctance or fear of moving one's body, or uncoordinated motion of the legs, head and trunk. Patients describe the dizziness attacks as feelings of unsteadiness combined with a fluctuation in alertness that they experience as frightening. Alternatively, they describe illusory motion of self or the environment, often lasting only fractions of seconds. Sometimes, however, the unsteadiness and dizziness can be more prolonged, in which case the patients often report that they are afraid of falling, losing consciousness, or of developing some other severe bodily calamity. The dizziness attacks occur at irregular intervals, sometimes several times a day. At times, the patient finds it necessary to secure physical support (for example, by finding a support on which they can lean).

In just over half of the patients, the dizziness attacks are accompanied by symptoms of anxiety. However, although the patient will readily complain about imbalance and dizziness attacks, they tend to be more secretive about their anxiety symptoms – admitting to having them only upon specific questioning. Overall, the patients often describe their condition as all-consuming, i.e. as 'dominating their lives.' Given this high degree of perceived impact, it is surprising that most PPV patients actually retain good social functioning and are able to continue their normal work.

The dizziness attacks sometimes occur spontaneously, but more often they are provoked either by certain bodily movements or when the patient is exposed to certain environments. The movement triggers are diverse, ranging from head movements to shifting one's weight from one foot to the other. Environmental triggers appear to follow the SMD pattern and include bridges, staircases, empty rooms, streets, department stores, crowds, restaurants, and concerts. After repeated attacks, any unexpected motion in the patient's normal everyday environment may also trigger them. Examples of the latter include: large-field slow movements of a curtain in the peripheral visual field (which would induce an physiologic optokinetic postural reaction); stepping on a soft surface (which would diminish somatosensory balance input); or mis-estimating the height of a stair step (which would require brief corrections in pre-calibrated sensorimotor programs subserving the regulation of posture).

As previously mentioned, the dizziness attacks in PPV are often accompanied by anxiety. With repeated attacks, the patients develop a fear of future attacks; this fear in turn paves the way for further attacks in an escalating cycle reminiscent of that observed in panic disorder. In addition, the patients begin to avoid the triggering situations; this avoidance is a major associated feature of PPV, and one that has particularly harmful effects on social functioning. As a result of the avoidance, patients become socially isolated and develop impairments in the performance of their vocational tasks. Given this high degree of perceived impact it is surprising that most PPV are able to continue their normal work. In addition, however, the avoidance behaviors contribute to perpetuating their condition, as the patients are deprived of exposures to the very environments that contribute to habituation or adaptation.

RELATIONSHIP TO VESTIBULAR DISORDERS

It has been debated whether PPV is a vestibular disorder or a psychiatric disorder. Perhaps the final answer will be 'both.' Among 32 of 154 PPV patients (21 per cent), the PPV symptoms began after an acute vestibular disorder.[117] Fourteen of these had histories of benign paroxysmal positional vertigo and 10 had histories of vestibular neuritis. In most of the 32, the transition from the original vestibular disorder to PPV occurred without a symptom-free interval, suggesting that a vestibular disorder may progress to become PPV. However, once started, the PPV appears to take a course that is seemingly independent from the recovery of the underlying vestibular disorder.

If PPV is a sequela of a vestibular disorder, the 21 per cent prevalence of preceding vestibular histories may seem low. However, the prevalence increases if patients with histories of head or whiplash trauma are included. Symptoms of post-traumatic dizziness often resemble those of otolith dysfunction (i.e. otolithic vertigo).[118-120] The impact of the trauma might dislodge otoconia, leading to unequal loads on the macular bed and consequent imbalance in tone between the two otolith organs. The symptoms of otolithic vertigo are similar to those of PPV, suggesting that the latter may evolve from an initial otolith dysfunction.

The neurological differential diagnosis of PPV includes central vestibular disorders, hereditary or acquired ataxias, senile gait disorders, bilateral vestibulopathy, peripheral or central vestibular paroxysmia, basilar migraine, familial periodic ataxia, perilymph fistulas, atypical Ménière's disease, and – most importantly – primary orthostatic tremor (see Chapter 7). Another differential diagnosis is primary orthostatic tremor, characterized by rhythmical antigravity muscle contractions with a high frequency of 12–16 Hz that causes unsteadiness while standing.[121-123]

BODY SWAY IN PPV PATIENTS

Clinical examination of balance function in patients with PPV essentially reveals normal clinical balance function. In fact, investigators of the condition tend to exclude those patients with PPV symptoms who have clinically abnormal vestibular or balance function. However, there may be more subtle differences. This question was pursued in a recent programmatic series of three studies.

In the first of these studies, Krafczyk et al.[124] analyzed parameters of body sway during experimental conditions that consisted of the patients with PPV keeping their eyes open or closed while standing on foam rubber under various head positions (upright, turned 20° right or left, or oscillating horizontally at a frequency of 1 Hz). The patients were examined on symptomatic days. The sway parameters examined included, among others, the power spectrum of sway in fore/aft and lateral directions. The results indicated that PPV patients had increased sway activity, particularly in the high-frequency band of 3.5–8 Hz. This concentration of the increase in sway to the high frequency band may reflect a change in postural control strategy. Unlike normal individuals, PPV patients, especially on symptomatic days, may be highly vigilant for perceived excesses in their own body sway excursions. Distrustful of their automatic balance reflexes, they engage in deliberate 'countercontrol.' In a sense, they 'try too hard' to remain stable. This countercontrol may employ a 'stiffening up' strategy by means of coactivation of antigravity muscles – the same strategy that normal subjects will employ when performing demanding balancing tasks.[125-127]

In the second study, Querner and co-workers[128] examined balance performance on foam rubber while the subjects kept their eyes open or closed, during either normal upright stance or tandem stance. During normal stance, patients showed an increase in body sway activity in both the low and high frequency bands and in sway path values for both the lateral and fore/aft directions. However, the difference between patients and controls was statistically significant only for the 'easier' experimental conditions. For the most difficult balance task (i.e. tandem stance with the eyes closed) body sway activity and sway path values did not differ between patients and controls (Fig. 15.14). Thus, the more difficult the balance task, the better was the balance performance of the PPV patients relative to the normals. This pattern seems to be the opposite of the expected results if the PPV patients had an active vestibular disorder. However, the lack of difference between PPV patients and controls in the more difficult conditions might have been because these conditions were 'too difficult' even for the normals, causing ceiling effects in both groups. Alternatively, the attentional demands of the more difficult conditions may, paradoxically, have reduced the patient's ability to excessively self-monitor their body-sway, thus eliminating the stimulus for their habitual over-control strategy. Since they are unable to 'try too hard' in the difficult conditions, their balance performance is relatively better. The clinical observation that these patients tend to have less symptoms when they are busy (i.e. have other things to attend to) seems to be consistent with this explanation.

In the third study, Querner et al.[129] examined the reactions of PPV patients to a stimulus that induces roll vection. Since the profile of triggering situations for PPV patients is similar to that of SMD, one might hypothesize that patients with PPV would be visually or proprioceptively dependent with respect to their control of balance (see earlier discussion of SMD). Therefore, one would expect patients with PPV symptoms to be particularly sensitive to optic flow stimuli.[70] Frommberger et al. examined body sway in response to visual motion stimulation from a rotating disk placed in front of the subject.[130] This stimulus induced a sensation of illusory body motion (roll vection) in all of the subjects.[130] In response to this stimulation, sway path increased by a multiple of two in the normal subjects and by a multiple of four in PPV patients. However, only the normals demonstrated the expected lateral shift of their center of pressure in the direction of the stimulus. Two explanations are conceivable for this pattern of increased body sway without an overall body deviation in patients with PPV: (1) when regulating upright stance, they rely more on proprioceptive and vestibular sensation rather than on visual cues, or at least disregard visual information in case of a mismatch between multisensory inputs; or (2) they have a lower threshold for initiating a compensatory body sway in the direction opposite to that of the perceived body deviation than do normal subjects. The latter explanation seems consistent with the over-control strategy discussed earlier.

RELATIONSHIP BETWEEN PPV AND DSM-IV OR ICD-10 PSYCHIATRIC DISORDERS

In the description of PPV above, we pointed out similarities with panic disorder. Several investigators have in

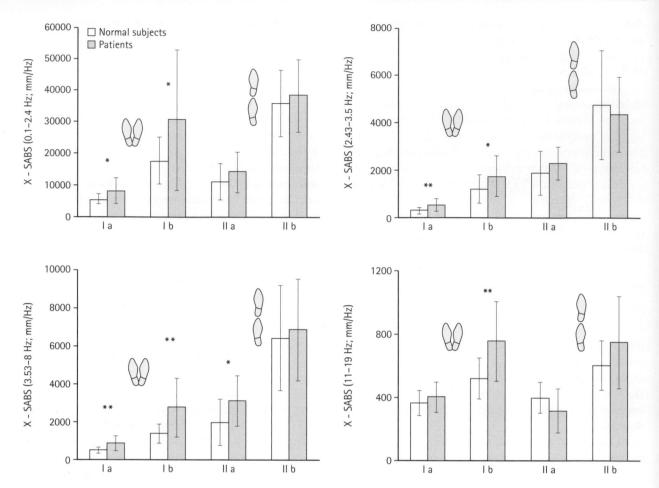

Figure 15.14 *Means and SD of lateral (X) sum activity of body sway (SABS) for four predefined frequency ranges (0.1–2.4, 2.43–3.5, 3.53–8, 11–19 Hz) in normal subjects (n = 15, white columns) and patients with phobic postural vertigo (n = 17, dark columns) standing with two different foot positions (feet splayed, I, or tandem stance, II) with the eyes open (a) or closed (b). With feet splayed (Ia, Ib) patients exhibited a significant increase (Student's t-test, *P < 0.05; **P < 0.01) in sum activity of body sway in the frequency range between 0.1 and 19 Hz (except for condition Ia, X-SABS 11–19 Hz). During tandem stance with the eyes open (IIa) the increase in sum activity of body sway in the patients was significant only between 3.53 and 8 Hz. In the most demanding balancing task (tandem stance with the eyes closed, IIb) sum activity of body sway did not differ between patients and normal subjects. (Reprinted from Querner V, Krafczyk S, Dieterich M, Brandt T. Patients with somatoform phobic postural vertigo: the more difficult the balance task the better the balance performance.* Neurosci Lett *2000;285:21–4, with permission from Elsevier.)*

fact argued that PPV is a subtype of panic disorder (i.e. one in which vertigo is the major complaint).[130,131] To address this question, Kapfhammer et al.[116] examined 42 patients with PPV using a structured psychiatric interview. The results are presented in Table 15.16. It shows that panic disorder was diagnosed only in one-third of the patients. If PPV is a homogeneous condition, it could not be panic disorder because two-thirds of the patients did not have panic disorder.

Another attribute of PPV patients is that they engage in phobic avoidance behaviors. Could it be that the PPV patients are agoraphobics? Table 15.16 shows that 27 of the patients, or 64 per cent, are listed as having agoraphobia with or without panic. These subjects, therefore, can be surmised to have ICD-10 agoraphobia (with or without panic). If PPV were a variant of a psychiatric

disorder, the most likely candidate would be ICD-10 agoraphobia. However, about one-third of the PPV patients did not have agoraphobia.

Thus, from a current psychiatric standpoint, PPV constitutes a diagnostically heterogeneous group. However, PPV has a high psychiatric comorbidity. Only three of 42 patients (7 per cent) did not have any psychiatric diagnosis.[132]. Of the 39 patients with psychiatric diagnoses, the great majority had an anxiety disorder (90 per cent). In addition, the patients also had a 100 per cent prevalence of dysfunctional personality traits or disorders. Of the different personality categories, obsessive–compulsive traits were by far the most common (48 per cent). (Recall that compulsive personality traits might be associated with a dysfunctional style of coping with illness.)

Table 15.16 *Diagnostic classification of the syndrome of phobic postural vertigo according to structured clinical interview (SCID) at onset of condition*

DSM-III-R diagnoses (axis I)	n	Personality features (axis II)	n
Major depressive episode	2	Compulsive	20
Dysthymic disorder	2	Narcissistic	7
		Dependent	3
Generalized anxiety disorder	6	Histrionic	2
Panic disorder	14	Avoidant	6
with agoraphobia (severe)	8	Passive-aggressive	4
with agoraphobia (mild–moderate)	4		
Phobic postural vertigo (monosymptomatic)	18		
with agoraphobia	15		
Total	42		42

Data from Kapfhammer et al.[132]

COMPARISON OF PPV WITH 'SPACE PHOBIA' AND 'MAL DE DÉBARQUEMENT SYNDROME'

The two conditions that most resemble PPV are 'space phobia'[76,77] and 'mal de débarquement syndrome'.[133,134] Space phobia, a pseudo-agoraphobic syndrome, describes a fear of absent visuospatial support (open spaces) for balance and of falling. Affected patients have various neurological or vestibular disorders. This special form of late-onset phobia is not necessarily accompanied by episodic unsteadiness and thus seems different from PPV.

Mal de débarquement (MDD) syndrome refers to the sensation of swinging, swaying, unsteadiness and disequilibrium that is commonly experienced immediately upon disembarking from sea travel and lasts a few hours.[135] In some individuals, MDD may persist for weeks to years after returning to land.[133,134,136] It can be an incapacitating condition. The degree of distress experienced by MDD patients can be appreciated by visiting a website specifically devoted to these patients.[137] Mal de débarquement is probably more common than is reflected in the literature and afflicts females more frequently than males.[138] The development of a persistent sensorimotor derangement in MDD resembles that of PPV; however, specific to MDD is the history of onset after motion exposure.

ETIOLOGICAL CONSIDERATIONS

Possibly representing the end result of several etiological mechanisms, PPV may not be a homogeneous condition. In some patients, the path toward PPV may start with space and motion discomfort (SMD). SMD can be expected in patients that have reweighted their multisensory balance inputs such that the information received via visual or somatosensory modalities becomes salient. Such reweighting might take place in the recovery phase from a vestibular disorder. The time of onset of PPV relative to an acute vestibular disorder or head trauma seems to be consistent with this hypothesis. In some PPV patients, SMD may have escalated to phobic levels, resulting in 'space and motion phobia.' Diagnostic criteria for this condition have been proposed[3] and are reproduced in Table 15.17.

Contributing to the development of space and motion phobia may be the amplifying symptom management style typical for patients with 'somatization,' a pattern to which anxiety-prone or compulsive individuals may be predisposed (see Fig. 15.5). The high prevalence of obses-

Table 15.17 *Criteria for space and motion phobia*

All of the following are required

(A) Marked and persistent fear that is excessive or unreasonable, cued by anticipation or presence of situations associated with intense vestibular stimulation, visual/vestibular/somatosensory mismatch or inadequate visual or somatosensory spatial cue
(B) The symptom-provoking stimuli are avoided or else endured with intense anxiety or distress
(C) The avoidance, anxious anticipation, or distress interferes significantly with the person's normal routine, occupational (or academic) functioning, or social activities or relationships, or there is marked distress about having the problem
(D) Duration of 6 months or more
(E) The pattern of distress is not better accounted for by an active or severe balance disorder (e.g., acute labyrinthitis, bilateral vestibular hypofunction), or by a mental disorder, such as obsessive-compulsive disorder or post-traumatic stress disorder

Reprinted from Furman JM, Jacob RG, A clinical taxonomy of dizziness and anxiety in the otoneurological setting, *J Anxiety Disord* 2001;15:9–26, with permission from Elsevier Science.

sive–compulsive personality traits observed in PPV patients also seems consistent with this theory.

Another mechanism that may be involved in PPV stems from the patient's constant and vigilant controlling and retrospective checking of balance that we have described as 'overcontrol' or 'trying too hard.' These efforts may interfere with the normal coupling of the efference copy signal. This would result in a disturbance of space constancy. Thanks to space constancy, we normally are able to perceive the environment as stationary despite the fact that automatic head movements during upright stance cause the retinal image of the environment to be shifted ('retinal slip'). Normally, space constancy is maintained because the impulse for initiating a movement is simultaneously accompanied by an appropriate efference-copy signal to make identification of self-motion possible (Fig. 15.15). The efference copy uses past experience to readjust the perceptual systems such that incoming sensory information is interpreted as movement of the self relative to a stationary environment rather than vice versa.[139] Transient decoupling of efference copy leading to a mismatch between antici-

pated and actual motion could lead to the sensation of vertigo described by PPV patients.[114,115]

TREATMENT CONSIDERATIONS

Treatment of psychiatric dizziness

The reader will recall that psychiatric dizziness is dizziness that is part of a symptom complex of a psychiatric disorder. Therefore, the treatment for psychiatric dizziness is the same as that of the underlying psychiatric disorder. For patients with panic disorder, specific practice guidelines have been published.[140] Treatment with one of the selective serotonin reuptake inhibitors (SSRIs) is the current standard. Among these, paroxetine and sertraline have been approved specifically for panic disorder by the US Food and Drug Administration. The older tricyclic agents, such as imipramine, are also effective but their use is associated with a greater incidence of side-effects. For generalized anxiety, paroxetine and vanlafaxine are specifically indicated.

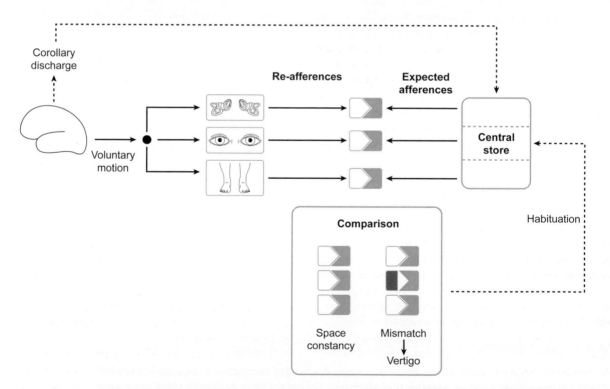

Figure 15.15 *Diagram of the sensorimotor derangement, or neural mismatch concept, of phobic postural vertigo caused by decoupling of the efference-copy signal. An active movement leads to sensory stimulation and this stimulation is then compared with a multisensory pattern of expectation calibrated by early experience of motions (central store). The pattern of expectation is prepared by the efference-copy signal, which is simultaneously emitted parallel to the motion impulse (efference) or by vestibular excitation during passive vehicular transportation. If concurrent sensory stimulation and the pattern of expectation are in agreement, self-motion is perceived while 'space constancy' is maintained. If the efference-copy signal (corollary discharge) is inappropriate, a sensorimotor mismatch occurs and a self-generated head motion or body sway may be erroneously perceived as external perturbations, causing the subjective postural vertigo. (Redrawn from ref. 115 with permission (© Springer Verlag).)*

The onset of SSRI treatment effect is usually delayed for 3–6 weeks and it is not uncommon for patients to experience increases in anxiety early in treatment. This problem may be ameliorated by choosing a more sedating type of SSRI (paroxetine or fluvoxamine), or by adding a serotonin type A receptor inhibitor (SARI), such as trazodone or mirtazapine, or a longer-acting type of benzodiazepine (e.g. clonazepam) to the regimen, on a time limited basis (about 4 weeks). Another side-effect of SSRI treatment is nausea. This problem tends to be dose-dependent. A common complication of SSRI treatment (or treatment with any other antidepressant except bupropion) is sexual dysfunction, mostly in the form of low sexual interest. Care should be taken not to withdraw from SSRIs abruptly, since this may cause a serotonin withdrawal syndrome that is associated with increased dizziness.[65]

Anxiety disorders can also be treated non-pharmacologically. Cognitive–behavioral treatment is the most widely accepted. Interestingly, there is much overlap between such therapy and vestibular rehabilitation therapy, including interoceptive exposure (i.e. exposure to the sensation of dizziness), management of anxiety (e.g. relaxation exercises) and encouragement of *in vivo* exposure to triggering situations.[16]

Treatment of psychiatric dizziness that is part of the integrated anxiety response in patients with phobias includes behavior therapeutic exposure to feared situations.[63] Such exposure treatment often requires prolonged sessions. Furthermore, it can be difficult physically to arrange for exposure to the actual phobic stimuli. Recently, a variant of such treatment employing phobic exposure in virtual environments offers an avenue of overcoming some of these restrictions.[141–144]

Treatment of conversion disorder

The treatment of conversion disorder is an unsettled matter in psychiatry, as indicated by the fact that even recent publications are mostly individual case reports. Hypnosis and narco-analysis have been advocated but their efficacy has not been convincingly established. Addressing comorbid conditions such as depression or PTSD may be of value, as in patients with comorbid depression who respond to electroshock therapy (discussed earlier). Treatment of conversion disorder requires a multidisciplinary approach that offers the patient the possibility of a face-saving retreat from the symptom. Physical therapy is one such avenue. Physical therapy may also be needed to prevent further disability, for example from contractures that may develop in patients with paralysis.

The approach to patients with conversion disorder of stance and gait is focused on the symptoms rather than on the inferred conflict. One type of treatment that has been advocated includes a short inpatient stay during which the patients are seen several times per day in an intensive treatment program. The treatment includes a careful examination by the consulting neurologist. One treatment consideration includes infusions of amitryptiline (10–25 mg qd) given for 3–5 days. During this time, patients are advised that they may experience temporary improvement with each of the infusions and that a long-term benefit also may occur. As mentioned earlier, it is important to begin treatment as early as possible. Complete symptom resolutions can be expected only in patients with illness durations of a few months or less.

Treatment of psychiatric complications of vestibular dysfunction

Patients with psychiatric or behavioral complications of syndromal or non-syndromal vestibular disorders are challenging to treat. They pose demands on the clinician's time that are incompatible with the clinician's schedule in a busy practice. Their treatment needs are best met using a multidisciplinary approach. Nevertheless, the patient's trajectory through the health system usually includes a consultation with an otoneurological clinician (i.e. otolaryngologist or neurologist) early in the clinical course.

OTONEUROLOGIST'S INITIAL APPROACH

Facing a patient with established symptoms of dizziness complicated by anxiety poses a high demand on the otoneurologist's interpersonal skills. If the wrong approach is used, these patients may become resentful or even angry. This problem may result from a set of behaviors on the part of the clinician that has been labeled 'clinician dismissive behaviors.'[145] These behaviors typically occur after the otoneurological work-up has not yielded any abnormalities or has resulted in findings deemed to be clinically insignificant. Table 15.18 shows typical patient reactions to such behaviors sampled from a website devoted to mal de débarquement syndrome.[137] Examples of clinician's dismissive behaviors include: not acknowledging that there is a problem; minimizing the impact of the problem; suggesting that the dizziness has a 'psychogenic' origin; and reducing the amount of time spent with the patient.

Alternate behaviors that can forestall these consequences have been called 'clinician's validating behaviors.' Their effect again can be appreciated in the MDD patients (Table 15.19).

These are the opposite of clinician's dismissive behaviors and include: acknowledging the limitations of medical knowledge, including the possibility that the otoneurological workup has left portions of the vestibular system unexamined; recognizing the impact of the patient's symptoms from the patient's perspective (e.g. businessman not being able to fly); providing expla-

Table 15.18 *Seven examples of the effect of clinician's dismissive behaviors as quoted from the autobiographical histories of patients with mal de débarquement (MDD)*[136]

Many of the doctors I had seen had told me 'common things occur commonly', the medical lingo for doubting that you might have a rare disorder, and instead placing it on that easy out called 'stress'
He just didn't know anything about MDD or just wasn't interested but I couldn't even get him to talk to me for 5 minutes on the phone about this
This doctor told me my symptoms were entirely age related and he offered no help
There I saw the Head of Neurology who had never heard of MDD and dismissed it immediately ...
The doctor in charge of my testing at the 'U' said, 'if it only happens when I fly, he suggests that I don't fly and even when I do at least I know it will eventually go away'. I have very few kind words to say about the University ... medical system!
I found the doctor there to be very indifferent and quite condescending. He suggested Paxil for my depression and swimming for my vertigo
He referred me to two different neurologists neither of whom had heard of MDD. Each of them suggested that I was depressed and needed psychiatric counseling. I knew in my heart they were wrong

Table 15.19 *Testimonials of beneficial effect of clinician's validating behaviors on mal de débarquement (MDD) patients, as quoted from the autobiographical histories of patients with MDD*[136]

After hearing my history and examining me I was correctly diagnosed with MDD. At least I now knew what I had
I was doing my own research on the internet and found the MDD website. OH! I was so excited to finally find my symptoms so clearly defined. I KNEW this was exactly what was wrong
I have found a wonderful doctor who understands MDD, unfortunately he is 225 miles away from me, and I see him only once or twice a year
After telling my story he didn't hesitate when he said, 'you have MDD'
I read the article in disbelief. It was the same thing I had been saying for years! I felt some relief in recognition of the syndrome
When I read some of the stories from others who suffer with this maddening problem, I sat and wept for hours. I believe that it was a relief just to know that I wasn't truly going crazy
I sat and cried with relief and amazement as I had found an exact description of everything I had been experiencing. Finding this information was a real turning point

nations for the dizziness anchored within vestibular physiology (e.g. uncoupling of efference copy, space and motion discomfort); increasing time spent with the patients by providing patient education, scheduling follow-up visits and arranging for further multidisciplinary evaluation.

REFERRAL TO PSYCHIATRIC OR PSYCHOLOGICAL CARE

Otoneurological clinicians outside of tertiary care settings do not always have access to the multidisciplinary approach advocated below. Thus, a question that needs to be considered is when to refer a patient to psychiatric care. The answer to this question depends, in part, upon whether or not the consulting psychiatrist has any special knowledge of the pathophysiology of vestibular disorders. Most will not. The following types of patients would benefit from referral to a 'general' psychiatrist:

- Patients that clearly have psychiatric dizziness (panic disorder other anxiety disorders), with no clinical or laboratory evidence to suspect a clinical or subclinical balance or vestibular disorder.

- Patients that develop severe depression as a consequence of long-term disability, as indicated by suicidal ideation, sleep disturbance, appetite disturbance with weight loss, or impaired concentration.
- Any patient with comorbid major psychiatric disorders that falls in the 'chance concurrence' category of the interface (see Table 15.1), for example, psychotic disorders and obsessive compulsive disorder.

Patients with complex issues involving somatopsychic, psychosomatic, or linkage relationships, perhaps further complicated by psychiatric potentiation or symptom amplification, may not benefit from the services of a general psychiatrist. Such professionals might create further complications by approaching the patient's vestibular-related symptoms with the already described clinician's dismissive behaviors. For example, one patient reported to one author (R.G.J.) 'The psychiatrist at my local mental health center does not believe in this vestibular stuff'. However, otolaryngologists could cultivate a relationship with a local psychiatrist or psychologist and inspire them to develop an expertise in the area of behavioral otoneurology as outlined in this chapter.

Some otoneurologists might prefer to refer such patients first to a vestibular therapist (e.g. a physical therapist with special expertise in balance), especially if this therapist has developed some psychiatric skills.

Also, not every patient needs a psychiatric referral. In our experience, patients with SMD without concomitant panic disorder, agoraphobia or generalized anxiety disorder are likely to respond to vestibular rehabilitation and or low-dose clonazepam (see below for further discussion of drug treatment) do not require psychiatric consultation. Similarly, patients with conversion disorder of stance and gait best receive their primary treatment in a neurological rather than a psychiatric setting.

MULTIDISCIPLINARY APPROACH

The multidisciplinary approach is employed in a number of tertiary centers and involves otoneurologists, vestibular rehabilitation therapists, and psychiatrists, psychologists, or other mental health providers. The specific components of the approach vary across centers.[145,146] The following discussion will reflect the approach used by the coauthors.

The interdisciplinary approach begins with a comprehensive assessment in the otoneurological, physical therapy and behavioral/psychiatric domains. If not done already, this includes a thorough neurological examination, vestibular testing and possibly brain imaging. In addition to being medically necessary, the otoneurological evaluation validates the patient's perceptions of their symptoms. This validation provides a basis for the patient's further cooperation.

The behavioral health clinician initially performs two tasks: a behavioral dizziness history and a psychiatric 'review of systems.' The latter identifies psychiatric conditions that may be present, with or without functional relationships with the vestibular disorder. For example, depression might be a consequence of the disability from the vestibular disorder. This part of the assessment will also identify conditions that may constitute vulnerability factors for increased symptom impact (anxiety proneness, somatization, compulsive personality traits). The psychiatric screening can be expedited by the use of structured interviews such as the Mini International Neuropsychiatric Interview (MINI)[147] and augmented by including questionnaire assessments. Anxiety and depression can be screened with a number of different instruments; the Hospital Anxiety and Depression scale was specifically developed for the screening for these states in patients with medical symptoms.[148] Compulsive personality traits can be quantified using the Frost Multidimensional Perfectionism scale.[84,149] Tendencies toward somatization can be examined by counting the number of 'yes' responses on the Cornell Medical Index.[150]

The behavioral dizziness history aims at providing a broader context for the dizziness complaint. Essentially, it is a behavioral analysis.[63] It includes information from previous interactions with healthcare providers, with a focus on exposure to clinician's dismissive behaviors. Other domains assessed include: (1) the dizziness symptom profile and its relationship to anxiety episodes; and (2) avoidance behaviors and their timing relative to the onset of the vestibular symptoms. Again, questionnaires are available to help with these tasks. The Symptom Questionnaire assesses vestibular and other autonomic symptoms separately for periods when a patient is, or is not, anxious or panicky.[66] Dizziness that occurs 'between' episodes of panic may be a form of non-psychiatric dizziness. The Chambless Mobility inventory provides an overview of agoraphobic behaviors.[151] The Situational Characteristics Questionnaire can be used to assess space and motion discomfort and the Cohen Acrophobia Scale can be used to quantify a patient's fear and avoidance of heights.[152]

Following the behavioral assessment, it is important to provide the patient with detailed explanations of symptoms and their genesis. Patients often derive therapeutic benefit while undergoing the behavioral assessment when they recognize the 'informed' nature of the questions and derive reassurance from the implication that their symptoms are not unusual. The explanations serve to influence the patients' beliefs about their condition. Pessimistic beliefs about the consequences of dizziness constitute a major predictor of future handicap (even after treatment).[153,154] The importance of providing a detailed explanation is also consistent with the clinical experience from treating patients with PPV symptoms.[115,145]

Patients are informed that vestibular imbalances are common and not necessarily dangerous. Patient education also includes an explanation that space and motion discomfort can be a consequence of vestibular dysfunction. They are educated about situational determinants of dizziness in ways that make the future occurrence of dizziness predictable or at least understandable. The patients should also be introduced to the notion of psychiatric potentiation, if appropriate. For example, if the patient shows a high degree of compulsiveness, it can be explained to the patient that their particular temperament will make them react more strongly to a symptom. They should be alerted to their risk of paradoxically increasing their awareness of dizziness by 'trying not to be dizzy' (i.e. engaging in the type of overcontrol that was discussed in the section on PPV).

Vestibular rehabilitation training is a major component in the multidisciplinary approach. This treatment modality has several advantages. First, the physical therapist, like the behavioral clinician, can devote longer periods of uninterrupted time to the patient than an otoneurologist. Second, the assessment by the vestibular rehabilitation therapist provides further details about the patient's functional limitations in a clinically validating context, thus augmenting previous efforts toward patient education. The physical therapist thus contributes to modifying those beliefs that contribute to handicap, an effect that was recently demonstrated by Yardley et al.[154] Third, the physical therapist instructs the patient to increase general physical activity and in performing specific bodily movements that have the effect of both increasing adaptation and, as a result of 'interoceptive exposure',[16] reducing anxiety about dizziness. Without being overly strenuous, regular physical activity to improve physical fitness is an important component of treatment. Finally and importantly, symptomatic improvement can be expected from the vestibular rehabilitation exercises.

Continued involvement with the behavioral clinician evolves along cognitive-behavior therapeutic and psychopharmacological lines. With respect to behavior therapy, one focus is on the patient's avoidance behaviors. The patient is encouraged to reduce avoidance by gradually entering more and more of the feared situations. Patients are instructed in a self-paced 'desensitization' by repeated exposure to situations that evoke the vertigo. Another focus is on modifying the patient's previously unsuccessful ways of coping with the symptom (e.g. 'trying too hard' not to be dizzy). Therapeutic interventions may involve efforts toward 'acceptance,' such as the principles found in Hayes et al.[155]

A final component of the psychiatric treatment is medication. One focus of drug treatment is the dizziness itself. Benzodiazepines are known to act as vestibular suppressants and dramatic improvements are sometimes seen with respect to both dizziness and anxiety. Clonazepam, in typical doses of 1.0–1.5 mg q.d. (range 0.25–3.00 mg q.d.), has become the treatment of choice and is often associated with dramatic improvement. If the symptoms are intermittent and predictable (e.g. planned travel), 'as needed' dosing may be sufficient. Benzodiazepines cause sedation and ataxia, and this is a particularly high risk with elderly patients. Furthermore, although many patients are able ultimately to discontinue the medication, a few develop prolonged rebound anxiety symptoms when the dose is reduced. Addiction remains a problem with benzodiazepines. Therefore, if at all possible, treatment should be time limited. However, this categorical statement needs to be tempered by the recognition that, even after years of treatment with low and constant doses, many patients derive therapeutic benefits that no other treatment can match.[156] Stopping treatment in these patients may constitute a form of undertreatment. Sometimes, fear of loss of prescription constitutes the major 'stressor' in the patient's life. It is important to remember that benzodiazepines are also used chronically to treat epilepsy, with many patients benefiting. The complexity surrounding chronic benzodiazepine treatment parallels that of the use of pain medication for chronic pain. One resolution often preferred by psychiatrists is to employ an antidepressant medication as the primary therapeutic modality (see below), limiting the use of benzodiazepines to the period before the antidepressant takes effect. In addition, by being cognizant of the known risk factors for a benzodiazepine withdrawal syndrome, the clinician can be selective. Thus, individuals with history of recreational alcohol or drug abuse, diagnosis of panic disorder or a high degree of personality pathology are at increased risk of problems with benzodiazepine treatment. Another set of risk factors for a withdrawal syndrome is drug variables, including high dose and short half-life. The duration of benzodiazepine treatment is also a risk factor. However, for patients that have already been treated for more than 1 month, extending the duration further does not increase risk.[156]

A second indication for drug treatment is depression, particularly if the patient has appetite disturbance, sleep disturbance, trouble concentrating, or suicidal ideation. Any of the antidepressants can be used for this purpose, but current practice favors the newer-generation antidepressants (SSRIs or vanlafaxine) because of their improved safety and side-effect profiles. A third indication for drug treatment is psychiatric conditions likely to cause symptom potentiation. Specifically, obsessive–compulsive personality traits may be amenable to SSRI treatment, which may involve higher doses than those typically prescribed for depression. Empirical data for this approach are scant, although data are currently being collected.[146]

The multidisciplinary approach has not been subject to controlled outcome research. Kapfhammer et al.,[116] in their follow-up study on 42 patients with PPV symptoms, found an improvement rate of 72 per cent, with 22 per cent of patients becoming symptom-free with patient education and behavioral instructions. The majority of patients experienced considerable improvement or complete remission, despite the fact that their symptoms had lasted between 1 year and 30 years prior to diagnosis.

The value of a multidisciplinary approach that included behavioral instructions and followed vestibular rehabilitation was tested in a small group of patients with agoraphobia that also had vestibular dysfunction. Combining behavioral treatment with vestibular rehabilitation, nine agoraphobics went through a 2-week no-treatment baseline phase, a 4-week behavioral phase focusing on self-directed exposure, and an 8- to 12-week period of weekly vestibular rehabilitation sessions.[34] After the initial behavioral treatment phase, four of the nine patients improved by at least one severity level (Fig. 15.16). After vestibular rehabilitation, four of the five previously unimproved patients improved, and one of the previously improved patients got worse. Overall, after completing both treatments seven of nine patients had improved. Furthermore the dizziness induced by head, eye or bodily movement described earlier also improved.

Even less empirical data exist about the effect of various components of the multidisciplinary approach.

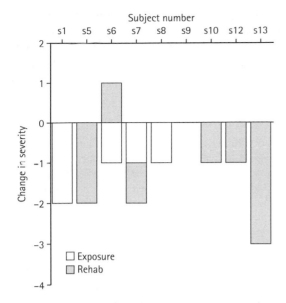

Figure 15.16 *Change in global impressions of severity (negative value = improvement) in patients with both agoraphobia and vestibular dysfunction after treatment with (a) 4 weeks of self-directed exposure to feared situations (open columns), followed by (b) 8–12 weeks of vestibular rehabilitation therapy (gray columns). Note that improvement after vestibular rehabilitation occurred particularly in those that had not responded to the behavioral treatment. (Reprinted from Jacob RG, Whitney SL, Detweiler-Shostak G, Furman JM. Vestibular rehabilitation for patients with agoraphobia and vestibular dysfunction: a pilot study. J Anxiety Disord 2001;15:131–46, © 2001, with permission from Elsevier.)*

However, the value of a brief patient education program combined with instructions in vestibular habituation exercises was recently tested by Yardley et al.[157] The treatment consisted of just two 30- to 40-minute sessions spaced 6 weeks apart, in which the patients were provided with verbal and written explanations of the workings of the balance system and a rationale for performing vestibular exercises. Patients were then instructed to perform the exercises twice a day. After 6 months, 60 per cent of the treated patients rated themselves as improved, compared with 37 per cent of the control group. On questionnaire assessments, the treated patients improved with respect to vertigo symptoms and anxiety/depression. In addition, there was improvement in their responses to provocative movements. After treatment, the patients agreed less with statements such as 'I will become very ill', 'I will be unable to behave normally in public' or 'I will faint or pass out.' Thus, the combination of instructions and performing the exercises was instrumental in changing the patient's beliefs. However, pretreatment negative beliefs still significantly predicted post-treatment handicap in both the treatment and the control groups. This pattern of results suggests that the treatment effect was not quite sufficient to overcome the effect of pretreatment negative beliefs on outcome.

CONCLUSION

This chapter discusses psychiatric aspects of dizziness and imbalance. Previously, and to some extent even now, this area of medicine has been dominated by the concept of 'psychogenic dizziness.' This concept has been used to explain conveniently all dizziness not judged to be due to a medical disorder. Unfortunately, the situation is not this simple. When studying the interface between psychiatry and neurotology, it is essential to remember that a unitary diagnosis such as 'psychogenic dizziness' may not be the most accurate categorization for a given patient. As we discuss in detail, many patients have both a psychiatric disorder and a neurotologic disorder. We identify six classes of relationship between psychiatric disorders and neurotologic disorders. Concepts that are of major importance include psychiatric dizziness, wherein dizziness is part of a recognized psychiatric symptom cluster, somatopsychic and psychosomatic interactions, and neurological linkage. The status of some syndromes with both psychiatric and vestibular symptoms remains unclear or controversial. For example, PPV may involve more than one type of interaction. Both the DSM-IV and ICD-10 diagnostic systems can be used to characterize patients with dizziness, imbalance, and psychiatric symptoms. Of particular interest are the anxiety disorders, for which dizziness is often a defining symptom. The interactions between anxiety disorders and vestibular disorders provide an especially convenient way to illustrate the complexities of the interface. For example, several studies have demonstrated that anxiety symptoms and disorders are common in patients with vestibular dysfunction. Patients with a vestibular disorder, a psychiatric disorder, or both may manifest SMD (i.e. discomfort in situations that may be disorienting even to some normal persons, such as heights).

Patients with a combination of a psychiatric disorder and dizziness or imbalance present a challenge to the healthcare system. Psychiatric potentiation (overlay) includes dysfunctional modes of coping with dizziness. For example, somatization refers to a pervasive tendency toward increased illness behaviors. A clinician's dismissive or validating behaviors may influence patient outcome. We discuss the issue of when to refer a patient for psychiatric or psychological care and how a multidisciplinary approach involves neurotologists, vestibular rehabilitation therapists and mental health professionals. Understanding the complexities of the interface between psychiatric disorders and neurotologic disorders will improve the quality of care for this patient population.

ACKNOWLEDGEMENT

The authors would like to acknowledge Emily Brown for her assistance with the preparation of the figures (15.1–15.5) and her editorial help.

REFERENCES

1. Hornsby J. Simple mindedness. *Defense of naïve naturalism in the philosophy of mind.* Cambridge: Harvard University Press.
2. Stahl SM. *Essential psychopharmacology: neuroscientific basis and practical applications.* New York: Cambridge University Press, 2000.
3. Furman JM, Jacob RG. A clinical taxonomy of dizziness and anxiety in the otoneurological setting. *J Anxiety Disord* 2001;15:9–26.
4. Breslau N, Schults LR, Stewart WF, et al. Headache types and panic disorder: directionality and specificity. *Neurology* 2001;56:350–4.
5. American Psychiatric Association. *Diagnostic and statistical manual of mental disorders,* 3rd edn. Washington, DC: American Psychiatric Association, 1980.
6. American Psychiatric Association. *Committee on nomenclature and statistics. diagnostic and statistical manual of mental disorders,* 2nd edn. Washington, DC: American Psychiatric Association, 1968.
7. American Psychiatric Association. *Committee on nomenclature and statistics. diagnostic and statistical manual: mental disorders.* Washington, DC: American Psychiatric Association, Mental Hospital Service, 1952.
8. American Psychiatric Association. *Diagnostic and statistical manual of mental disorders,* 3rd edn, revised. Washington, DC: American Psychiatric Association, 1987.
9. American Psychiatric Association. *Diagnostic and statistical manual of mental disorders,* 4th edn. Washington, DC: American Psychiatric Association, 1994.
10. American Psychiatric Association. *Diagnostic and statistical manual of mental disorders,* 4th edn, text revision. Washington, DC: American Psychiatric Association, 2000.
11. World Health Organization. *The ICD-10 classification of mental and behavioral disorders. Clinical descriptions and diagnostic guidelines.* Geneva: World Health Organization, 1992.
12. World Health Organization. *The ICD-10 classification of mental and behavioral disorders. diagnostic criteria for research.* Geneva: World Health Organization, 1993.
13. Jacob RG, Furman JM, Balaban CD, et al. In: Jacob RG, Furman JM, Balaban CD, et al., eds. *Psychiatric aspects of vestibular disorders.* New York: Oxford University Press, 1996;509–28.
14. Furman JM, Jacob RG. Psychiatric dizziness. *Neurology* 1997;48:1161–6.
15. Jacob RG, Furman JM, Durrant JD, Turner SM. Panic, agoraphobia and vestibular dysfunction: clinical test results. *Am J Psychiatry* 1996;153:503–12.
16. Beidel D, Horak F. Behavior therapy for vestibular rehabilitation. *J Anxiety Disord* 2001;15:121–30.
17. Crowe RR, Noyes R, Pauls DL: Slymen D. A family study of panic disorder. *Arch Gen Psychiatry* 1983;40:1065–9.
18. Kendler KS, Walters EE, Neale MC, et al. The structure of the genetic and environmental risk factors for six major psychiatric disorders in women. *Arch Gen Psychiatry* 1995;52:374–83.
19. Norton GR, Cox BJ, Malan J. Nonclinical panickers: A critical review. *Clin Psychol Rev* 1992;12:121–39.
20. Rachman S, Levitt K, Loptka C. Experimental analyses of panic –III: claustrophobic subjects. *Behav Ther* 1988;26:41–52.
21. Clark DB, Hirsch BE, Smith MG, et al. Panic in otolaryngology patients presenting with dizziness or hearing loss. *Am J Psychiatry* 1994;151:1223–5.
22. Clark D, Leslie MI, Jacob RG. Balance Complaints and Panic Disorder: A clinical study of panic symptoms in members of a selfhelp group for balance disorders. *J Anxiety Disord* 1992;6:47–53.
23. Eagger S, Luxon LM, Davies RA, et al. Psychiatric morbidity in patients with peripheral vestibular disorder: A clinical and neuro-otological study. *J Neurol Neurosurg Psychiatry* 1992;55:383–7.
24. Simpson RB, Nedzelski JM, Barber HO, Thomas MR. Psychiatric diagnoses in patients with psychogenic dizziness or severe tinnitus. *J Otolaryngol* 1988; 17:325–30.
25. Stein MB, Gordon J, Asmundson GJG, et al. Panic disorder in patients attending a clinic for vestibular disorders. *Am J Psychiatry* 1994;151:1697–700.
26. Hägnebo C, Andersson G, Melin L. Correlates of vertigo attacks in Meniere's disease. *Psychother Psychosom* 1998;67:311–16.
27. Asmundson GJG, Larsen DK, Stein MB. Panic disorder and vestibular disturbance: an overview of empirical findings and clinical implications. *J Psychosom Res* 1998; 44:107–20.
28. Afzelius L-E, Henriksson NG, Wahlgren L. Vertigo and dizziness of functional origin. *Laryngoscope* 1980;90:649–56.
29. Yardley L, Owen M, Nazareth I, Luxon L. Prevalence and presentation of dizziness in a general practice community sample of working age. *Br J Gen Pract* 1998;48:1131–5.
30. Jacob RG, Moller MB, Turner SM, Wall CWI. Otoneurological examination of panic disorder and agoraphobia with panic attacks: A pilot study. *Am J Psychiatry* 1985;142:715–20.
31. Sklare DA, Stein MB, Pikus AM, Uhde TW. Dysequilibrium and audiovestibular function in panic disorder: symptom profiles and test findings. *Am J Otol* 1990;11:338–41.
32. Hoffman DL, O'Leary DP, Munjack DJ. Autorotation test abnormalities of the horizontal and vertical vestibulo-ocular reflexes in panic disorder. *Otolaryngol Head Neck Surg* 1994;110:259–69.
33. Cadoret RJ, Widmer RB, Troughton EP. Somatic complaints: harbinger of depression in primary care. *J Affect Disord* 1980;2:61–70.
34. Yardley L, Britton J, Lear S, Bird J, Luxon LM. Relationship between balance system function and agoraphobic avoidance. *Behav Res Ther* 1995;33(4):435–9.
35. Perna G, Dario A, Caldirola D, Stefania B, Cesarani A, Bellodi L. Panic disorder: the role of the balance system. *J Psychiatr Res* 2001;35:279–86.
36. Jacob RG, Furman JM, Durrant JD, Turner SM. Surface dependence: a balance control strategy in panic disorder with agoraphobia. *Psychosom Med* 1997;59:323–30.
37. Weeks DJ, Ward K. Neuropsychological causes for agoraphobia? In: Weeks DJ ,Ward K, eds. *Developments in clinical and experimental neuropsychology.* New York: Plenum Press, 1989:305–13.
38. Kallai J, Koczan G, Szabo I, et al. An experimental study to operationally define and measure spatial orientation in panic agoraphobic subjects, generalized anxiety and healthy control groups. *Behav Cogn Psychother* 1995;23:145–52.
39. Jacob RG, Whitney SL, Detweiler-Shostak G, Furman JM.

Vestibular rehabilitation for patients with agoraphobia and vestibular dysfunction: a pilot study. *J Anxiety Disord* 2001;**15**:131–46.

40. Yardley L, Watson S, Britton J, et al. Effects of anxiety arousal and mental stress on the vestibulo-ocular reflex. *Acta Otolaryngol (Stockh)* 1995;**115**:597–602.

41. Viaud-Delmon I, Ivanenko YP, Berthoz A, Jouvent R. Adaptation as a sensorial profile in trait anxiety: a study with virtual reality. *J Anxiety Disord* 2000;**14**:583–601.

42. Viaud-Delmon I, Siegler I, Israel I, et al. Eye deviation during rotation in darkness in trait anxiety: an early expression of perceptual avoidance? *Biol Psychiatry* 2000;**47**:112–18.

43. Yardley L, Gardner M, Leadbetter A, Lavie N. Effect of articulatory and mental tasks on postural control. *NeuroReport* 1999;**10**:1–5.

44. Anderson G, Hägnebo C, Yardley L. Stress and symptoms of Ménière's disease: a time series analysis. *J Psychosom Res* 1997; **43**:585–603.

45. Anderson G, Yardley L. Time-series analysis of the relationship between dizziness and stress. *Scand J Psychol* 2000;**41**:41–54.

46. Sakellari V, Bronstein AM, Corna S, et al. The effects of hyperventilation on postural control mechanisms. *Brain* 1997;**120**:1659–73.

47. Minor LB, Haslwanter T, Straumann D, Zee D. Hyperventilation-induced nystagmus in patients with vestibular shwannoma. *Neurology* 1999;**53**:2158–68.

48. Melville Jones G. changing the pattern of eye–head coordination during six hours of reversed vision. *Exp Brain Res* 1988;**69**:531–4.

49. Siegler I, Israel I, Berthoz A. Shift of the beating field of vestibular nystagmus: an orientation strategy? *Neurosci Lett* 1998;**254**:93–6.

50. Yates BJ, Miller AD. Physiological evidence that the vestibular system participates in autonomic and respiratory control. *J Vestib Res* 1998;**8**:17–25.

51. Furman JM, Jacob RG, Redfern MS. Clinical evidence that the vestibular system participates in autonomic control. *J Vestib Res* 1998;**8**:27–34.

52. Jauregui-Renaud K, Yarrow K, Oliver R, et al. Effects of caloric stimulation on respiratory frequency and heart rate and blood pressure variability. *Brain Res Bull* 2000;**53**:17–23.

53. Jauregui-Renaud K, Gresty MA, Reynolds R, Bronstein AM. Respiratory responses of normal and vestibular defective human subjects to rotation in the yaw and pitch planes . *Neurosci Lett* 2001;**298**:17–20.

54. Yates B, Aoki M, Burchill P, Bronstein A, Gresty M. Cardiovascular responses elicited by linear acceleration in humans. *Exp Brain Res* 1999;**25**(4):476–84.

55. Radtke A, Popov K, Bronstein AM, Gresty MA. Evidence for a vestibulo-cardiac reflex in man . *Lancet* 2001;**356**:736–37.

56. Yardley L, Gardner M, Bronstein A, *et al.* Interference between postural control and mental performance in patients with vestibular disorder and healthy controls. *Neurol Neurosurg Psychiatry* 2001;**7**:48–52.

57. Lundin-Olsson L, Nyberg L, Gustafson Y. 'Stops walking when talking' as a predictor of falls in elderly people. *Lancet* 1997;**349**:617.

58. Jacob RG, Furman J, Cass SP. Psychiatric consequences of vestibular dysfunction. In: Luxon L, Martini A, Furman JM, eds. *Audiological medicine.* London: Martin Dunitz/Taylor & Francis, 2003;869–87.

59. Watson JB. *Behaviorism.* New York: People's Institute Publishing, 1925.

60. Lepicard EM, Venault P, Perez-Diaz F, et al. Balance control and posture differences in the anxious BALB/cByJ mice compared to the non anxious C57BL/6J mice. *Behav Brain Res* 2000;**17**:185–95.

61. Venault RLBJC. Balance control and posture in anxious mice improved by SSRI treatment. *NeuroReport* 2001;**121**:3091–4.

62. Maschke M, Drepper J, Kindsvater FEA. Fear-conditioned potentiation of the acoustic blink reflex in patients with cerebellar lesions. *J Neurol Neurosurg Psychiatry* 2000;**68**:358–64.

63. Jacob RG, Pelham B. Behavior therapy. In: Sadock BJ, Sadock VA, eds. *Kaplan & Sadock's comprehensive textbook of psychiatry.* Philadelphia: Lippincott, Williams & Wilkins, 1999;2080–128.

64. Neuhauser H, Leopold M, von Brevern M, et al. The interrelations of migraine, vertigo, and migrainous vertigo. *Neurology* 2001;**56**:436–41.

65. Balaban CD, Thayer JF. Neurological bases for balance-anxiety links. *J Anxiety Disord* 2001;**15**:53–79.

66. Jacob RG, Woody SR, Clark DB, et al. Discomfort with space and motion: A possible marker of vestibular dysfunction assessed by the Situational Characteristics Questionnaire. *J Psychopathol Behav Assess* 1993; 15:299–324.

67. Bronstein AM. Visual vertigo syndrome: Clinical and posturography findings. *J Neurol Neurosurg Psychiatry* 1995;**59**:472–6.

68. Jacob RG, Lilienfeld SO, Furman JMR, et al. Panic disorder with vestibular dysfunction: Further clinical observations and description of space and motion phobic stimuli. *J Anxiety Disord* 1989;**3**:117–30.

69. Redfern MS, Yardley L, Bronstein AM. Visual influences on balance. *J Anxiety Disord* 2001;**15**:81–94.

70. Jacob RG, Redfern MS, Furman JM. Optic flow-induced sway in anxiety disorders associated with space and motion discomfort. *J Anxiety Disord* 1995;9:411–25.

71. Guerraz M, Yardley L, Bertholon P, et al. Visual vertigo: symptom assessment, spatial orientation and postural control. *Brain* 2001;124:1646–56.

72. Ramos RT, Jacob RG, Lilienfeld SO. Space and motion discomfort in Brazilian versus American patients with anxiety disorders. *J Anxiety Disord* 1997;**11**:131–9.

73. Jones RB, Humphris G, Lewis T. Do agrophobics interpret the environment in large shops and supermarkets differently? *Br J Clin Psychol* 1996;**35**:635–7.

74. McCabe BF. Disease of the end organ and vestibular nerve (Abstract). In: Naunton RF, ed. *The vestibular system.* New York: Academic Press, 1975.

75. Page NGR, Gresty MA. Motorist's vestibular disorientation syndrome. *J Neurol Neurosurg Psychiatry* 1985;**48**:729–35.

76. Marks I. Space 'phobia': A pseudo-agoraphobic syndrome. *J Neurol Neurosurg Psychiatry* 1981;**44**:387–91.

77. Marks I, Bebbington P. Space phobia: Syndrome or agoraphobic variant? *BMJ* 1976;**2**:345–7.

78. Balaban CD, Jacob RG. Background and history of the interface between anxiety and vertigo. *J Anxiety Disord* 2001;**15**:27–51.

79. Holgers KM, Erlandsson SI, Barrenas ML. Predictive factors for the severity of tinnitus. *Audiology* 2000;**39**:284–91.

80. Jager B, Lamprecht F. Subgroups of styles of coping with

chronic tinnitus: a cluster-analytic taxonomy . *Z Klinische Psychol Psychother* 2001;**30**:1–9.

81. Robinson M, Riley J. The role of emotion in pain. In: Anonymous, ed. *Psychosocial factors in pain; critical perspectives.* New York: The Guilford Press, 1999;3–17.

82. Lewis J, Stephens S, McKenna L. Tinnitus and suicide. *Clin Otoloaryngol* 1994;**19**:50–4.

83. Johnston M, Walker M. Suicide in the elderly – recognizing the signs. *Gen Hosp Psychiatry* 1996;**18**:257–60.

84. Frost RO, Marten P, Lahart C, Rosenblate R. The dimensions of perfectionism. *Cogn Ther Res* 1990;**14**:449–68.

85. Frost RO, Heimberg RG, Holt CS, et al. A comparison of two measures of perfectionism. *Person Individ Diff* 1993;**14**:119–26.

86. Frost RO, Steketee G, Cohn L, Griess K. Personality traits in subclinical and non-obsessive-compulsive volunteers and their parents. *Behav Res Ther* 1994;**32**:47–56.

87. Turner SM, Jacob RG, Morrison R. Somatoform disorders. In: Adams HE, Suther P, eds. *Handbook of psychopathology.* New York: Plenum, 1984;307–28.

88. Jacob RG, Turner SM. Somatoform disorders. In: Turner SM, Hersen M, eds. *Adult psychopathology.* New York: John Wiley, 1984;304–28.

89. Barsky AJ. Amplification, somatization, and the somatoform disorders. *Psychosomatics* 1992;**33**(1):28–34.

90. Barsky AJ Wyshak G, Kleman GL. The somatosensory amplification scale and its relationship to hypochondriasis. *J Psychiatr Res* 1990;**24**:323–34.

91. Barsky AJ. Patients who amplify bodily sensations. *Ann Intern Med* 1979;**91**:63–70.

92. Yardley L, Gresty M, Bronstein A, Beyts J. Changes in heart rate and respiration rate in patients with vestibular dysfunction following head movements which provoke dizziness. *Biol Psychol* 1998;**49**:95–108.

93. Martin RL. Conversion disorder, proposed autonomic arousal disorder and pseudocyesis. In: *DSM-IV sourcebook.* Washington DC: American Psychiatric Association, 1996:893.

94. Spitzer C, Spelzberg B, Hans-Joergen G, et al. Dissociative experiences and psychopathology in conversion disorders. *J Psychosom Res* 1999;**46**:291–4.

95. Chambers RA, Bremner JD, Moghaddam B, et al. Glutamate and post-traumatic stress disorder: toward a psychobiology of dissociation. *Semin Clin Neuropsychiatry* 1999;**4**:274–81.

96. Mace CJ. Hysterical conversion. II: A critique. *Br J Psychiatry* 1992;**161**:378–89.

97. Moene F, Landberg E, Kees A, et al. Organic syndromes diagnosed as conversion disorder; identification and frequency in a study of 85 patients. *J Psychosom Res* 2000;**49**:7–12.

98. Binzer M, Kullgren G. Motor conversion disorder: a prospective 2- to 5-year follow-up study. *Psychosomatics* 1998;**39**:519–27.

99. Glick TH, Workman TP, Gaufberg SV . Suspected conversion disorder: foreseeable risks and avoidable errors. *Acad Emerg Med* 2000;**7**:1272–7.

100. Strumpell A, ed. *Lehrbuch der speziellen Pathologie und Therapie der inneren Krankheiten*, 12 edn, Vol. 3. Leipzig: Vogel1899;614–16.

101. Dejerine J. In: *Semiologie des affections du systeme nerveux.* Paris: Masson, 1914;541–9.

102. Janet P. *The major symptoms of hysteria*, 2nd edn. New York: MacMillan, 1920.

103. Bing R. *Lehrbuch der Nervenkrankheiten* Vol 3. Berlin: Urban & Schwarzenberg, 1924;663–7.

104. Keane J. Hysterical gait disorders: 60 cases. *Neurology* 1989;**39**:586–9.

105. Lempert T, Brandt T, Dieterich M, Huppert D. How to identify psychogenic disorders of stance and gait. A video study in 37 patients. *J Neurol* 1991;**238**:140–6.

106. Marsden C. Psychogenic problems associated with dystonia. In: *Behavioral neurology movement disorders.* New York: Raven Press, 1995:387–91.

107. Williams D, Ford B, Fahn S. Phenomonology and psychopathology related to psychogenic movement disorders. In: *Behavioral neurology movement disorders.* New York: Raven Press, 1995:231–57.

108. Atchinson P, Thompson P, Frackowiak R, Marsden C. The syndrome of gait ignition failure: a report of six cases. *Mov Disord* 1993;**8**:285–92.

109 Nutt JD, Marsden CD, Thompson PD. Human walking and higher-level gait disorders, particularly in the elderly. *Neurology* 1993;**43**:268–79.

110. Rockwood C, Eilert RE. Camptocormia. *J Bone Joint Surg* 1969;**51**:553–6.

111. Soreff H. Camptocormia. *Arch Orthop Trauma Surg* 1983;**101**:151–2.

112. Sinel M, Eisenberg M. Two unusual gait disturbances: astasia, abasia, and camptocormai. *Arch Phys Med Rehabil* 1990;**71**:1078–80.

113. Brandt T. Phobic postural vertigo. *Neurology* 1996;**46**:1515–19.

114. Brandt T, Dieterich M. Phobischer Attacken-Shwankschwindel. Ein neues Syndrom. *Münch Med Wochenschr* 1986;**128**:247–50.

115. Brandt T. *Vertigo; its multisensory syndromes*, 2nd edn. London: Springer, 1999.

116. Kapfhammer HP, Mayer C, Hock U, et al. Course of illness in phobic postural vertigo. *Acta Neurol Scand* 1997;**95**:23–8.

117. Huppert D, Brandt T, Dieterich M, Strupp M. Phobischer Schwankschwindel: Zweithäufigste Diagnose in einer Spezialambulanz. *Nervenarzt* 1994;**65**:421–3.

118. Brandt T. Phobic postural vertigo. *Neurology* 1997;**49**:1480–1.

119. Brandt T, Daroff RB. The multisensory physiological and pathological vertigo syndromes. *Ann Neurol* 1980;**7**:195–203.

120. Gresty MA, Bronstein AM. Testing otolith function. *Br J Audiol* 1992;**26**:125–36.

121. Boroojerdi B, Ferbert A, Foltys H. Evidence for a non-orthostatic origin of orthostatic tremor. *J Neurol Neurosurg Psychiatry* 1999;**66**:284–8.

122. Yarrow K, Brown P, Gretsy M, Bronstein A. Force platform recordings in the diagnosis of primary orthostatic tremor. *Gait Posture* 2001;**13**:27–34.

123. Fung V, Sauner D, Day B. A dissociation between subjective and objective unsteadiness in primary orthostatic tremor. *Brain* 2001;**124**:322–30.

124. Krafczyk S, Schlamp V, Dieterich M, et al. Increased body sway at 3.5–8 Hz in patients with phobic postural vertigo. *Neurosci Lett* 1999;**259**:149–52.

125. De Luca C, Mambrito B. Voluntary control of motor units in

human antagonist muscles: coactivation and reciprocal activation. *J Neurophysiol* 1987;**58**:525–42.

126. Hoehn-Saric R, Merchant AF, Keyser ML, Smith VK. Effects of clonidine on anxiety disorders. *Arch Gen Psychiatry* 1981;38:1278–82.

127. Smith A. The coactivation of muscles. *Can J Physiol Pharmacol* 1981;59:733–47.

128. Querner V, Krafczyk S, Dieterich M, Brandt T. Patients with somatoform phobic postural vertigo: the more difficult the balance task the better the balance performance. *Neurosci Lett* 2000;**285**:21–4.

129. Querner V, Krafczyk S, Dieterich M, Brandt T. Phobic postural vertigo: body sway during visually induced fall vection. *Exp Brain Res* 2002;**143**:269–75.

130. Frommberger U, Hurth-Schmidt S, Dieringer H, et al. Panic disorder and dizziness. Aids for the differentiation between neurological and psychiatric illness. *Nervenarzt* 1993;**64**:377–83.

131. Stahl S, Soefje S. Panic attacks and panic disorder: the great neurologic imposters. *Semin Neurol* 199515:126–32.

132. Kapfhammer HP, Mayer C, Hock U, et al. Phobic postural vertigo, a panic disorder? *Nervenarzt* 1995;**66**:308–10.

133. Brown JJ, Baloh RW. Persistent mal de debarquement syndrome: a motion-induced subjective disorder of balance. *Am J Otolaryngol* 1987;**8**:219–22.

134. Murphy TP. Mal de debarquement syndrome: a forgotten entity? *Otoloaryngol Head Neck Surg* 1993;**109**:10–13.

135. Gordon CR, Spitzer O, Doweck I, et al. The vestibulo-ocular reflex and seasickness susceptibility. *J Vestib Res* 1996;**6**:229–33.

136. Hain T, Hanna P, Rheinberger M. Mal de Debarquement. *Arch Otolaryngol Head Neck Surg* 1999;**125**:615–20.

137. Torrie, Evan. *Mal de Debarquement: support page for people with MDD.* http://www.etete.com/mdd/

138. Mair W. The mal de debarquement syndrome. *J Audiol Med* 1996;**5**:21–25.

139. von Holst E, Mittelstaedt H. Das Reafferenzprincip (Wechselwirkung zwischen Zentralnervensystem und Peripherie). *Naturwissenschaften* 1950;**37**:464–76.

140. Work group on panic disorder. Practice guideline for the treatment of patients with panic disorder. *Am J Psychiatry* 1998;**155**:1–28.

141. Vincelli F, Choi YH, Molinari E, et al. A VR multicomponent treatment for panic disorders with agoraphobia. In: Westwood JD, ed. *Medicine meets virtual reality.* Amsterdam: IOS Press, 2001;544–50.

142. Pertaub D-P, Slater M, Barker C. An experiment on fear of public speaking in virtual reality. In: Westwood JD, ed. *Medicine meets virtual reality.* Amsterdam: IOS Press, 2001;372–78.

143. Olasov Rothbaum B, Hodges L. The use of virtual reality exposure in the treatment of anxiety disorders. *Behav Mod* 1999;**23**:507–25.

144. North M. Virtual reality therapy for fear of flying. *Am J Psychiatry* 1997;**154**:130.

145. Jacob RG, Furman JM, Cass SP. Psychiatric consequences of vestibular dysfunction. In: Luxon L, Martini A, Furman J, Stephens D, eds. *Audiological medicine.* London: Martin Dunitz/Taylor & Francis, 2003;869–87.

146. Clark MR, Swartz KL. A conceptual structure and methodology for the systematic approach to the evaluation and treatment of patients with chronic dizziness. *J Anxiety Disord* 2001;**15**:95–106.

147. Sheehan D, Janavs J, Baker R, et al. MINI: Mini International Neuropsychiatric Interview. English version 5.0.0 – DSM-IV. Tampa: DV Sheehan & Y Lecrugier, 1998.

148. Zigmond A, Snaith R. The Hospital Anxiety and Depression Scale. *Acta Psychiatr Scand* 1983;**67**:361–70.

149. Antony MM, Purdon CL, Swinson RP. Psychometric properties of the Frost Multidimensional Perfection Scale in a clinical anxiety disorders sample. *J Clin Psychol* 1999;**55**:1271–86.

150. Anonymous. *Cornell Medical Index Health Questionnaire.* New York NY: Cornell University Medical College, 1949.

151. Chambless DL, Caputo C, Jason SE, et al. The mobility inventory for agoraphobia. *Bchav Res Ther* 1985;**23**:35–44.

152. Cohen DC. Comparison of self-report and overt-behavioral procedures for assessing acrophobia. *Behav Ther* 1977;**8**:17–23.

153. Yardley L. Contribution of symptoms and beliefs to handicap in people with vertigo: a longitudinal study. *Br J Clin Psychol* 1994;**33**:101–13.

154. Yardley L, Beech S, Weinman J. Influence of beliefs about the consequences of dizziness on handicap in people with dizziness, and the effect of therapy on beliefs. *J Psychosom Res* 2001;**50**:1–6.

155. Hayes S, Strosahl K, Wilson K. *Acceptance and commitment therapy: an experiential approach to behavior change.* New York: Guilford Press, 1999.

156. Schweizer E, Rickels K. Benzodiazepine dependence and withdrawal: a review of the syndrome and its clinical management. *Acta Psychiatrica Scand* 1998;**98**:95–101.

157. Yardley L, Beech S, Zander L, et al. A randomised controlled trial of exercise therapy for dizziness and vertigo in primary care. *Br J Gen Pract* 1998;**48**:1136–40.

16

Syncopal falls, drop attacks and their mimics

BASTIAAN R. BLOEM, SEBASTIAAN OVEREEM AND J. GERT VAN DIJK

SCOPE AND AIMS

In this chapter we outline the clinical approach to patients who fall because of an impairment or loss of consciousness. Following a set of definitions, we first describe the salient clinical features of disorders leading to such falls. Particular emphasis will be laid upon the distinction between falls caused by a true or an apparent loss of consciousness. Among falls caused by true loss of consciousness, we separate the clinical characteristics of syncopal falls (due to reflex syncope, orthostatic hypotension or cardiac syncope) from falls due to other causes of transient unconsciousness, such as seizures. With respect to the falls caused by an apparent loss of consciousness, we discuss the presentation of cataplexy, drop attacks, hyperekplexia and psychogenic falls. Each section contains practical recommendations for the treatment of these conditions. We underscore the clinical importance of a proper diagnosis, not only to minimize recurrent falls and injuries, but also to prevent further morbidity and mortality from the underlying disorder. We conclude by presenting some advice for the diagnostic work-up, in particular regarding history taking and the physical examination. We also touch upon several useful ancillary studies.

INTRODUCTION

In the diagnostic work-up and therapeutic approach, it is important to realize that 'transient loss of consciousness (TLC)' and 'falling' are not synonymous (Fig. 16.1). First, TLC usually leads to a loss of postural control, but this will not cause a fall when subjects are seated or lying down, as may occur due to vasovagal syncope during venapuncture.[1] In rare instances, even standing patients may not fall despite being unconscious, but stumble or stare without responding to the environment.[2] Second, a substantial proportion of falls are not caused by TLC. Many falls can be attributed to an obvious environmental cause such as accidental collisions, slips or trips. These 'extrinsic' falls require a very different approach than falls associated with TLC. Other falls are caused by an underlying balance disorder. Such 'intrinsic' falls typically occur during weight shifts or turning movements.[3] In some patients, the balance deficit can be sufficiently severe to cause seemingly spontaneous falls. This happens for example in patients with progressive supranuclear palsy, as outlined in Chapter 11. These spontaneous falls are easily mistaken for those being caused by TLC. The group of intrinsic falls also includes a number of disorders that are characterized by features that merely mimic TLC, but in fact lead to falls via very different mechanisms. Examples are drop attacks, cataplexy and hyperekplexia. To complicate matters further, different types of falls may occur in the same patient. For example, disorders such as multiple system atrophy (MSA) lead to both syncopal falls (caused by autonomic failure) and falls due to the underlying balance deficit (parkinsonism or cerebellar ataxia).

In this chapter, we concentrate on falls that were preceded by a true or apparent TLC. For this purpose, we will consider three main categories: (1) falls caused by syncope; (2) falls caused by TLC other than syncope; and (3) conditions that merely mimic TLC. The diagnostic work-up and management of extrinsic falls and intrinsic falls without TLC are discussed in Chapter 21.

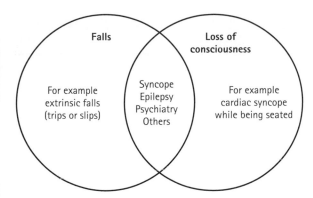

Figure 16.1 *A transient loss of consciousness is not synonymous to falls, and vice versa.*

regarded as denoting any form of TLC, or even any attack with an apparent loss of consciousness. Since this may include epilepsy, brain concussion or psychogenic attacks, the extent of possible confusion is considerable. Note that epidemiological studies may also be hampered by a lack of consistency; readers should always ask themselves what authors mean by 'syncope'. Here, syncope is defined as 'a transient, self-limited loss of consciousness, with a rapid onset, spontaneous and prompt recovery, and that is caused by global cerebral hypoperfusion'.[4] A practical consequence is that falls associated with TLC must not be called syncopal until that specific cause has been made at least probable.

DEFINITIONS

For many clinicians, falls associated with TLC can be a source of considerable confusion. One important reason for misunderstandings relates to the use of inconsistent terminology and conflicting definitions in the literature. Indeed, there is no internationally accepted 'Classification of Faints, Fits and Funny Turns'. For practical purposes, we will use the definitions shown in Table 16. 1.

One item must be discussed in more detail here, and that is syncope. In the past, syncope has sometimes been

EPIDEMIOLOGY

Falls caused by TLC appear to be common. At least, that is certainly the impression of clinicians who have worked for some time in an accident and emergency unit or an outpatient clinic of a neurology, cardiology or geriatrics department. It is certainly true that a TLC is often considered to be the cause for unexpected falls. Whether this was actually the case often remains unclear for various reasons that will be outlined later. Because of the many difficulties involved in establishing a causal relationship between falls and TLC, epidemiological figures are prob-

Table 16.1 *An alphabetical list of definitions used in this chapter, largely according to recent recommendations[4]*

Autonomic failure	Any type of pathologically reduced function of the autonomic nervous system (sympathetic, parasympathetic, or both)
Epileptic seizures	(Usually) transient and (usually) short-lived attacks of a (usually) self-limited nature, caused by hyperactivity of cortical neuronal networks
Extrinsic falls	Any fall caused by an environmental cause, such as accidental slips, trips or collisions; this group does *not* include falls caused by loss of consciousness, but can include falls that led to secondary loss of consciousness, for example due to traumatic brain injury
Intrinsic falls	Any fall caused by mobility or balance disorders, misperception of the environment or preceding loss of consciousness
Orthostatic intolerance	Subjective complaints (symptoms) associated with the upright position
Orthostatic hypotension	A drop in systolic blood pressure by more than 20 mmHg, a drop in systolic blood pressure to less than 90 mmHg, or a drop in diastolic blood pressure by more than 10 mmHg, within 3 min after rising
Postprandial hypotension	A decrease in systolic blood pressure of 20 mmHg or more, occurring within 3 h after the start of a meal
Presyncope	All sensations directly preceding syncope, including symptoms due to diminished cortical blood flow (for example blurring of vision or visual field constriction) and symptoms related to the mechanism causing syncope (for example nausea in reflex syncope)
Psychogenic pseudosyncope	Apparent loss of consciousness caused by psychiatric disease or other psychogenic factors
Syncope	A transient, self-limited loss of consciousness, with a rapid onset, spontaneous and prompt recovery, caused by global cerebral hypoperfusion due to failure of the *systemic* blood circulation, often (but not always) leading to falls
Transient loss of consciousness	A transient, short-lived and self-limited loss of consciousness, not due to a traumatic brain injury. Note that this definition includes the different forms of syncope, as well as non-syncopal disorders such as epilepsy
Vasovagal syncope	A form of reflex syncope which emphasizes both the sympathetic ('vaso') and parasympathetic ('vagal') components of the pathophysiology

ably unreliable. Epidemiological information about mere TLC is not informative, because whether falls actually occur depends on the position in which consciousness is lost. Just to give an impression, one study suggested that up to 5 per cent of emergency room visits are related to syncope,[5] but this does not imply that all these events resulted in falls.

CLINICAL IMPACT

The clinical impact of falls caused by TLC is considerable. Depending on the underlying disorder, mortality rates are increased, most notably as a result of concurrent cardiovascular disease. Irrespective of the underlying disorder, patients may sustain major or minor physical injuries.[6] For example, recurrent syncopal falls are associated with soft-tissue injuries and fractures in at least 10 per cent of patients.[7] This high rate of injuries can perhaps be attributed to the absence of premonitory symptoms for many falls caused by TLC, such as the carotid sinus syndrome and cardiac syncope. Indeed, among patients with syncopal falls due to the carotid sinus syndrome, up to one-quarter of patients sustained a fracture with their falls.[8,9]

Even in the absence of physical injury, patients with recurrent falls may encounter employment and lifestyle restrictions because of fear or shame of falls in public. Not surprisingly, these falls negatively affect the quality of life, to a similar extent as for example rheumatoid arthritis.[10]

FALLS PRECEDED BY TRANSIENT LOSS OF CONSCIOUSNESS

A wide range of different disorders can lead to falls that were preceded by TLC (Table 16.2). The underlying mechanism leading to TLC is very different for each of these disorders. One major category involves syncope, that is, a TLC due to failure of the systemic blood circulation. The second category includes disorders that impair consciousness through mechanisms other than impaired blood flow. In the following sections, we will summarize the salient clinical features for both these main groups of disorders. Furthermore, we will distinguish between these two groups based upon triggering events, premonitory symptoms, accompanying features and postictal phenomena.

Falls caused by to syncope

GENERAL FEATURES OF SYNCOPE

The clinical presentations of the different types of syncope share several common features, irrespective of the original mechanism that hampered the systemic blood circulation and led to diminished cortical and retinal functioning. Early presyncopal features include: blurred vision and loss of color vision ('graying out') due to retinal ischemia, loss of control over eye and other movements, constriction of the field of vision, and hearing loss. Falls are a key feature of syncope. About half of the patients slump flaccidly to the floor, whereas

Table 16.2 *Diso associated with falls caused by a transient loss of consciousness (TLC)*

Syncopal TLC	
1. Reflex syncope	Vasovagal syncope
	Situational faint
	Carotid sinus syncope
2. Orthostatic syncope	Autonomic failure
	primary autonomic failure
	secondary autonomic failure
	drugs
	alcohol
	Hypovolemia
3. Cardiac or cardiopulmonary syncope	Cardiac arrhythmias
	Structural abnormalities
4. Postprandial hypotension	
Non-syncopal TLC	
1. Vascular steal syndromes	
2. Epileptic seizures	
3. Metabolic disorders	Hypoxia
	Hypoglycemia
	Hyperventilation?
4. Intoxications	
5. Cerebrovascular disorders	
6. Migraine	

others fall in a more stiff fashion.[2] Most falls are backwards, although initial forward or lateral drifts may precede the fall. The duration of unconsciousness is usually brief and rarely lasts longer than 20 s. However, occasionally, patients may be unconscious for several minutes. Involuntary, non-rhythmic and multifocal jerking movements of the limbs (myoclonus) are very common, and this may lead to confusion with epileptic seizures. The nature of the jerking movements helps to separate syncope from seizures. In both conditions, the myoclonic jerks occur in both proximal and distal muscle groups, but in syncope, these are not synchronous over various parts of the body, unlike epileptic seizures. Brief tonic stiffening may precede the period of myoclonic jerks. Urinary incontinence frequently accompanies syncope.[11] Tongue bite is very rarely seen and, if it occurs, affects the tip of the tongue, not the lateral side as in epilepsy.[12] The eyes are usually open during syncope, and tonic upward deviation is common.[2,13] Recovery occurs spontaneously and is typically prompt. In the postictal phase, patients may feel fatigued, but behavior and orientation are usually appropriate within 30 s. Retrograde amnesia can occur, particularly in older individuals. Recurrences are common for all types of syncope.[7]

REFLEX SYNCOPE

The most common form is vasovagal syncope. The name of this condition helps one to understand the underlying pathophysiology, which is essentially a rather odd cardiovascular reflex exerted by an otherwise normal autonomic nervous system (Fig. 16.2). Triggered by a variety of events, the systemic blood pressure drops because of a lack of sympathetic vasoconstriction in the legs and abdomen ('vaso-'), while at the same time a vagal nerve-mediated bradycardia occurs ('-vagal'). The two mechanisms usually concur to a varying extent in individual patients, but predominantly sympathetic and parasympathetic forms exist as well. The vasodepressor variant is more common than the cardio-inhibitory variant.[14] Recognition of these variants has important therapeutic implications, in particular with respect to cardiac pacing, as the drop in blood pressure is often more important in causing TLC than a coexistent bradycardia. Indeed, attempts to prevent vasovagal syncope by blocking the vagal nerve have largely failed.[15,16]

Table 16.3 *Features supporting a diagnosis of vasovagal syncope*

Young age
Precipitating events
Typical prodromal symptoms ('autonomic activation')
Absence of competing cause of syncope
   Reproduction of vasovagal syncope after prolonged
   upright tilting

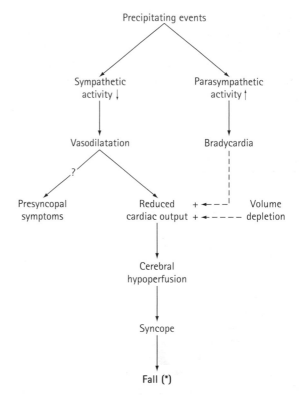

Figure 16.2 *Pathophysiology of vasovagal syncope. Bradycardia, if present, contributes via a diminished cardiac output to the systemic hypotension, which chiefly results from sympathetic-derived vasodilatation. Volume depletion, if present, aggravates the tendency to develop systemic hypotension. The mechanism leading to the presyncopal symptoms, which are characteristic for this type of syncope, is not precisely known but appears related to the autonomic hyperactivity ('autonomic activation'). *, Falls only develop if syncope occurs in upright, standing persons.*

Falls occur when vasovagal syncope develops in upright standing persons. Vasovagal syncope may also lead to injurious falls in young persons when it develops during or shortly after exercise.[17,18] Several features may help in reaching the proper diagnosis of falls caused by vasovagal syncope (Table 16.3). It is essential to ask for a triggering factor. Usual precipitants of vasovagal syncope include fear, pain, emotional distress, or their anticipation. Gastrointestinal stimulation, for example induced by visceral pain, is also a frequent precipitant, but this rarely causes falls. Prolonged standing is another common precipitating event, particularly when subjects are dehydrated and concurrent volume depletion compounds the systemic hypotension. This occurs, for example, in persons watching a parade while standing in the blazing sun, or in guards instructed to stand motionless in a tight harness. This occurrence of vasovagal syncope with prolonged standing formed the basis for using head-up tilt table tests as a diagnostic tool for vasovagal syncope.[19,20] These tilt tests, which are explained in more detail under 'Ancillary studies' (page 308), are becoming the 'gold standard' to reproduce the vasodepressor and cardio-inhibitory events of vasovagal syncope under controlled experimental conditions and thus assist clinicians in reaching a diagnosis. An example of a vasovagal syncope during tilt testing is shown in Fig. 16.3. It is also essential to ask for vegetative symptoms, as these are typical for vasovagal syncope. This 'autonomic activation' consists of nausea, diaphoresis, pallor or pupillary dilation; the last two features are invisible to the patient, but may have been noted by alert bystanders. Patients may also report early presyncopal features prior to the fall, but these are not unique for vasovagal syncope.

The term 'situational syncope' has been coined for forms of reflex syncope occurring under a variety of specific circumstances (Table 16.4); examples include urination, defecation, cough or swallowing. Micturition syncope

Table 16.4 *Forms of situational syncope*

Related to bleedings
Cough, sneeze
Gastrointestinal stimulation
Post-micturition or defecation
Post-exercise
Others

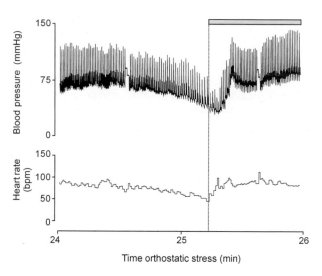

Figure 16.3 *Example of a typical vasovagal syncope in a 24-year-old man with recurrent syncope, demonstrated during orthostatic stress testing on a tilt table. Finger arterial pressure was monitored continuously with a Finapres device. Note the progressive fall in both the blood pressure and the heart rate that develops after more than 24 min of orthostatic stress (passive upright tilting). This vasovagal syncope thus has both a vasodepressor and a cardio-inhibitory element. The vertical line indicates the onset of leg crossing and tensing of leg and abdominal muscles; this was continued throughout the period indicated by the gray horizontal bar. Following these maneuvers, the blood pressure and heart rate recover quickly. (This figure was revised after ref. 21, with permission from the authors and the publisher.)*

is a rather common cause of falls in men, perhaps because the act of micturition prevents subjects from quickly sitting down when premonitory symptoms emerge.

Carotid sinus syncope is a particular form of reflex syncope that mainly occurs in elderly persons, and rarely before 40 years of age. This syndrome is increasingly recognized as a common cause of falls in the elderly.[22] Syncopal falls are typically provoked by turning movements of the head or neck compression, such as the knotting of a tie. It can be provoked during physical examination by carotid sinus massage (see the section on 'Physical examination', page 306). Carotid sinus syncope is considered in more detail in Chapter 22.

ORTHOSTATIC SYNCOPE

Orthostatic syncope is not the same as syncope in the upright position, because reflex syncope may also occur while standing up. The primary difference is that in orthostatic syncope the autonomic nervous system attempts to keep blood pressure adequate, but fails to do so. This may be because the autonomic nervous system does not function well (autonomic failure) or because of a lack of circulating volume. Blood pressure drops while standing, but there is no associated bradycardia. In fact, patients may be able to generate a normal compensatory tachycardia. Significantly, the characteristic set of premonitory vegetative symptoms seen in reflex syncope is distinctly absent in orthostatic hypotension, an important feature for the differential diagnosis. Note that patients with orthostatic hypotension do report visual impairment, 'graying out' and hearing loss, as these are manifestations of cerebral or retinal hypoperfusion. Patients may also report pain in the shoulders or neck at the onset of the attack ('coat hanger pain'); this is caused by ischemia of local muscles. Unlike reflex syncope, falls occur after standing up or after prolonged standing unless the patient manages to sit down in time.

Autonomic failure can be primary, secondary or medication-induced. Examples of primary autonomic failure include pure autonomic failure and MSA. When autonomic symptoms concur with parkinsonism, MSA is much more likely than idiopathic Parkinson's disease. This is particularly true for syncopal falls, which are distinctly rare in idiopathic parkinson's disease,[3] but which are present in some 15–20 per cent of MSA patients.[23,24] Orthostatic symptoms such as light-headedness are even more common and occur in up to 70 per cent of MSA patients. Other parkinsonian patients with syncopal falls may have dementia with Lewy bodies, owing to spread of pathology to the brainstem and autonomic nervous system.[25] If symptomatic orthostatic hypotension does occur in Parkinson's disease, it can usually be ascribed to excessive dopaminergic therapy.[26] Secondary autonomic failure refers to autonomic failure due to diseases that primarily affect organs other than the autonomic nervous system. Numerically relevant causes are diabetic neuropathy and

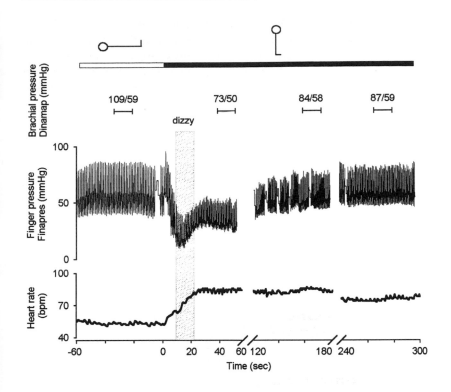

Figure 16.4 *Initial orthostatic hypotension in a 60-year-old man with recurrent syncope, demonstrated during orthostatic stress testing on a tilt table. Arterial pressure was monitored continuously from the fingers with a Finapres device, and intermittently from the arms with a Dinamap device. Note the transient and symptomatic decrease in blood pressure, almost immediately after standing up. An essential difference with vasovagal syncope (cf. Fig. 16.3) is the compensatory tachycardia that also comes on instantaneously after standing up. Note also the spontaneous and gradual recovery of the blood pressure. Although a mild initial hypotension is physiological in nature, it was pathological in this patient where it was compounded by multiple vasoactive drugs. (This figure was reproduced from ref. 28, with permission from the authors and the publisher.)*

amyloid neuropathy. Alcohol and a variety of drugs (antidepressants in particular, often in a polypharmacy setting) can also lead to symptomatic orthostatic hypotension.

It is important to separate initial orthostatic hypotension (immediately or shortly after rising) from late orthostatic hypotension. Initial orthostatic hypotension is illustrated in Fig. 16.4. The common finding of temporary light-headedness or a 'black-out' just after standing up does not point to autonomic failure. Instead, this results from a physiological drop in blood pressure which, in healthy subjects, is temporary and usually counteracted within 1 min of standing. The initial orthostatic hypotension results from vasodilatation in active muscles and is therefore absent when subjects are passively tilted to the upright position.[27] The drop in blood pressure is usually accompanied by a compensatory tachycardia (Fig. 16.4), and this clearly separates initial orthostatic syncope from reflex syncope where a vagal nerve-mediated bradycardia occurs (Fig. 16.3). The symptoms associated with initial orthostatic hypotension usually disappear within seconds. This initial physiological hypotension is universally present, but the magnitude varies across subjects. It is most pronounced among young, lean persons and is certainly not 'innocent', as it may underlie some 5 per cent of their falls. Symptomatic initial orthostatic hypotension also occurs among elderly persons with the carotid sinus syndrome (see Chapter 22) or as a result of vasoactive medication.[28] Culprit medication is

discussed in the section 'Diagnostic work-up' (page 301). Initial orthostatic hypotension might be a frequently missed cause of falls in the elderly, because standard teaching emphasizes the drops in blood pressure that may occur minutes after standing up.

Late orthostatic hypotension is not a physiological phenomenon, but results from autonomic failure, causing inability to spontaneously restore the blood pressure while patients remain standing. Instead, the initially reduced blood pressure stabilizes at a lower level or continues to drop even further. The compensatory tachycardia may be preserved. Thus, patients with autonomic failure are unable to stand upright for longer periods of time. The severity of autonomic failure is therefore best expressed as the maximal duration of standing before a person starts to experience orthostatic symptoms. It can be very informative to ask whether patients are still able to do common jobs in and around the house, such as washing dishes. Taking a hot shower causes particular difficulties, because redistribution of the circulating volume to the skin further promotes development of orthostatic hypotension. Patients have typically resorted to taking seated showers. The tendency to develop orthostatic hypotension is greatest after a period of prolonged recumbence, hence falls occur mostly at night (during micturition in men with nocturia) or in the morning (when medication taken with breakfast compounds the orthostasis).

One particular form of orthostatic hypotension deserves separate mention. Some syncopal falls may occur following prolonged exercise. This post-exercise hypotension results from a drop in blood pressure that normally occurs after exercise; patients with autonomic failure have difficulty in increasing their blood pressure during exercise, but unfortunately the physiological drop afterwards does take place. This is compounded by a reduced capability for vasoconstriction, owing to presence of hypothermia and lactic acidosis in laboring muscles. Post-exercise hypotension commonly leads to falls, for example when patients take a rest after they have reached the top of a staircase. This form of syncope may occasionally occur during exercise, but such patients more likely have a cardiac syncope (see below). Post-exercise hypotension leading to injurious falls has also been described in young persons as a result of vasovagal syncope.[17,18]

CARDIAC OR CARDIOPULMONARY DISEASE

The potential presence of severe underlying cardiac disease is perhaps the greatest concern when patients present with syncopal falls. Cardiac causes of syncope can be separated into arrhythmias and structural abnormalities (Table 16.5). The cardiac arrhythmias mostly include examples of bradycardia; syncope less commonly results from tachycardia, usually when the atrial firing frequency exceeds 300/min. Note that there are no 'absolutely unsafe' limits because the consequences for blood pressure also depend upon the subject's posture and for how long the cardiac arrhythmia had been present; chronic arrhythmia is tolerated better than acute changes in heart rhythm.

Suspicion of an underlying cardiac cause should be particularly high when syncopal falls occur in elderly subjects or patients with prior cardiac disease. Patients with a prior myocardial infarction have a high risk of developing arrhythmias. However, several cardiac causes of syncope occur in young subjects, including the long QT syndrome and hypertrophic cardiomyopathy. Cardiac arrhythmias should also be suspected in patients taking pro-arrhythmic drugs, such as antihistamines, antibiotics and neuroleptics. The presence of a cardiac pacemaker or implanted cardioverter defibrillator does not entirely exclude cardiac syncope, because such devices can fail.

Cardiac disease often causes spontaneous and abrupt loss of consciousness, without any specific precipitating event. One exception is syncope that occurs during exercise, and this form of cardiac syncope commonly leads to falls. Syncope during exercise mostly occurs with obstructive outflow disease of the heart (e.g. valvular stenosis or obstructive cardiomyopathy), but some arrhythmias (most notably the long QT syndrome) also emerge during exercise. In this respect, cardiac causes differ from orthostatic hypotension, which typically leads to syncope after cessation of exercise. Another exception is cardiac syncope triggered by emotional stimuli such as startle, fear or loud sounds; this occurs in patients with the long QT syndrome. Premonitory vegetative symptoms are absent, in contrast to reflex syncope. Injuries are frequent, possibly because there is no warning of an impending attack. Palpitations may occur, usually with a brief pause prior to the actual syncope. During syncope, patients are initially pale, but this is followed by a characteristic flushing of the face when consciousness is regained.

Timely detection of cardiac syncope with underlying structural heart disease is important, because these persons are at risk for sudden death. Structural disorders that are particularly associated with increased mortality include aortic valve stenosis, hypertrophic cardiomyopathy, right ventricular dysplasia and ventricular tachyarrhythmias.[29] Patients with the long QT syndrome are also at risk for sudden death. Mortality does not seem to be increased for most types of supraventricular tachycardia, atrioventricular conduction abnormalities and sick

Table 16.5 *Cardiac and cardiopulmonary causes of syncopal falls*[4]

Arrhythmias	Sinus node dysfunction
	Atrioventricular conduction system disease
	Paroxysmal supraventricular and ventricular tachycardias
	Inherited syndromes (e.g. long QT syndrome)
	Drug-induced
Structural abnormalities	Cardiomyopathy
	myocardial ischemia
	obstructive cardiomyopathy
	atrial myxoma
	Outflow obstruction
	valvular disease
	acute aortic dissection
	pulmonary hypertension
Pericardial disease	

sinus syndrome. Morbidity and mortality are also increased for the occasional patients with unexplained syncope who suffer from underlying pulmonary thromboembolism.[30]

VOLUME DEPLETION

Volume depletion usually acts as a supportive factor in falls caused by vasovagal syncope or orthostatic hypotension. If sufficiently severe, hypovolemia alone could also lead to syncope with falls. Such severe volume depletion can be caused by massive hemorrhage or diarrhea. It may be exacerbated by drugs or heat, which causes additional volume depletion and vasodilatation; mostly young persons seem to be affected. A low sodium excretion in the urine can index hypovolemia; such persons may benefit from oral salt supplements.[31]

POSTPRANDIAL HYPOTENSION

Postprandial hypotension is defined as decreases in systolic blood pressure of 20 mmHg or more, occurring within 2 h after the start of a meal.[32] This disorder is a separate form of syncope with its own pathophysiology. Following meals, a considerable part of the circulating blood volume is drawn to the gastrointestinal (splanchnic) system. Healthy subjects compensate for this normal and physiological redistribution of circulating blood with an increase in cardiac output. However, if compensatory mechanisms fail, the remaining volume of circulating blood becomes inadequate to supply the cerebrovascular system, and this leads to syncope. Such faulty compensatory mechanisms include autonomic failure and cardiac disease, leading to an inadequate cardiac output. Medication taken at mealtimes may aggravate the drop in systemic blood pressure.

Mild and asymptomatic postprandial hypotension is common among elderly subjects. However, if postprandial declines in blood pressure are severe enough, a TLC can occur, even while subjects are seated. Postprandial hypotension also appears to be a risk factor for recurrent falls.[33] Such symptomatic forms of postprandial hypotension are mainly seen in high-risk groups, including patients with hypertension, autonomic failure or Parkinson's disease.[34,35] In one study, no less than 80 per cent of patients with parkinsonism, including a few with atypical syndromes, had postprandial hypotension.[36]

Note that postprandial hypotension and orthostatic hypotension may be concurrent in individual subjects with autonomic failure, but this is not always the case because the pathophysiology overlaps only partly. Among a group of 16 elderly patients with unexplained syncope, none had orthostatic hypotension, whereas half had postprandial hypotension.[37] Further enquiry revealed that all syncopal episodes occurred shortly after meals.

SYMPTOMATIC TREATMENT OF SYNCOPAL FALLS

Non-pharmacological

Patients with vasovagal syncope should be primarily reassured by informing them about the benign nature and good prognosis of their condition. The non-pharmacological management further consists of advice that was developed primarily for patients with orthostatic hypotension, but also helps patients with reflex syncope (Table 16.6). Behaviors to be avoided include rapid changes in posture, prolonged episodes of quiet stance, and prolonged recumbence. Patients with postprandial hypotension should replace large meals with a high carbohydrate content by more frequent and smaller meals.[38] Behaviors that should be encouraged include an adequate intake of salt and fluids; patients should strive for an average increase in body weight by some 2–3 kg. Use of sodium chloride tablets is sometimes required to achieve this.[39] Raising the cranial end of the bed helps to reduce the recumbent blood pressure in individual patients, leading to a smaller drop when standing up. It also helps to reduce nocturia, thereby restricting further volume depletion. Furthermore, this may help to prevent night time falls associated with urination.

There are several measures to reduce venous pooling in the legs and abdomen. One option is to use specific anti-orthostatic maneuvers, such as standing with crossed legs or squatting.[21,40] This is illustrated in Fig. 16.5. Squatting is most effective, but standing with

Table 16.6 *Treatment of syncope*

Non-pharmacological	Education about underlying disorder
	Avoid/remove triggering events
	Anti-orthostatic maneuvers (Fig. 16.5)
	Moderate exercise training
	Tilt training
	Volume expansion
	adequate fluid intake
	increased dietary salt
	Compression stockings
	Compressive abdominal band
	Raising cranial end of the bed
	Lightweight portable chairs
	Frequent and small meals
Pharmacological	Reduce or discontinue hypotensive drugs
	Fludrocortisone
	Midodrine
	L-Threo-dihydroxyphenylserine
	Octreotide (for postprandial hypotension)
	Desmopressin (for nocturia)
	Erythropoietin (for anemia)
Pacemakers	Single chamber
	Dual chamber

crossed legs is more comfortable for patients. The beneficial effect on standing blood pressure is most pronounced when patients co-contract their leg muscles. Such effects are evident not only in a controlled laboratory setting, but also are translated into fewer complaints in daily life.[21] A drawback is that these maneuvers can be too demanding for patients with neurological deficits, for example those with MSA. Such patients may benefit from graduated pressure supplied by elastic compression stockings applied to the lower limbs or, preferably, the entire leg, or a compressive abdominal band. The individual response varies and compliance is suboptimal because of hygiene problems and discomfort.[14] An alternative is the use of lightweight portable chairs, which permit the patient to sit down in case of presyncope.

Head-up tilt table tests can sometimes be used to teach patients with syncope how to recognize their own premonitory symptoms. This may help them to prevent actual syncopal falls in daily life by sitting down before consciousness is lost. More recent studies advocate 'tilt training' in vasovagal syncope:[42,43] through an unknown mechanism, the tendency to develop syncope diminishes by instructing patients to stand quietly upright in the morning for increasing periods of time (45–90 min). Patients must be highly motivated to follow this training program.

Pharmacological

Various pharmacological agents have been tested to prevent the recurrence of reflex syncope, but none of them was unequivocally effective.[44] One study suggested that paroxetine can be helpful,[45] but this needs to be confirmed by additional studies.

For patients with orthostatic hypotension, drug treatment should be withheld until the above conservative

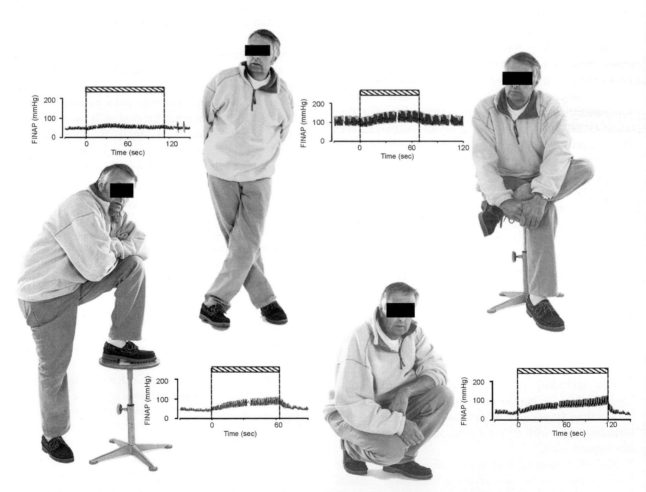

Figure 16.5 *Physical counter-maneuvers in a 54-year-old man with pure autonomic failure and incapacitating orthostatic hypotension. The photographs are shown with permission of the patient. Finger arterial pressure was monitored continuously with a Finapres device. The four different counter maneuvers consist of various isometric contractions of the lower limbs and abdominal compression: leg crossing in a standing and sitting position (top row), placing a foot on a chair, and squatting. The patient was standing or sitting quietly prior to these maneuvers. The horizontal bars indicate the duration of the maneuvers. Note the increase in blood pressure and pulse pressure during the maneuvers. (This figure was reproduced from ref. 41, with permission from the authors and Elsevier.)*

measures have failed. Withdrawing any offending drugs is often more helpful than introducing new ones. Pharmacological intervention for orthostatic hypotension has several practical drawbacks.[46] First, it may lead to an increase in recumbent blood pressure. Second, post-exercise hypotension and syncope in warm environments usually do not improve. If drug treatment is deemed necessary, fludrocortisone is a first choice option to expand the volume of extravascular and intravascular body water. It should be combined with an adequate salt intake. Another option is the use of sympathomimetics such as midodrine.[39] Patients receiving this treatment must be monitored for development or worsening of supine hypertension. The compound (D)L-threo-dihydroxyphenylserine (DOPS), a synthetic precursor of norepinephrine, has been used to restore plasma norepinephrine levels (and thus reduce orthostatic hypotension) in patients with Parkinson's disease, MSA and pure autonomic failure. Therapeutic effects ranging from subjective improvement to complete remission have been observed in patients with orthostatic hypotension due to autonomic failure and in patients with postprandial hypotension.[47–49] One preliminary report mentioned a significant increase in standing blood pressure in Parkinson's patients, along with fewer subjective complaints of orthostatic hypotension.[50] DOPS was also found to increase the upright blood pressure in one small study of four patients with MSA.[51] Octreotide is an effective treatment for postprandial hypotension, but it is expensive and must be given parenterally.[52]

Pacemakers

The role of pacemakers in the treatment of reflex syncope remains a matter of debate. Cardiac pacing appears to provide benefit for only a subgroup of patients with vasovagal syncope, while for the majority of patients the effects were small and inconsistent.[15,16] One controlled study in patients with vasovagal syncope was terminated early because the risk of recurrent syncope was considerably lower in patients assigned to the cardiac pacemaker group, compared with controls.[53] These patients all had bradycardia during tilt-table testing. However, it remains to be demonstrated what kind of patient responds best to cardiac pacing, in particular when prominent bradycardia is absent (as appears to be the case for many patients). Furthermore, the magnitude and duration of the clinical effects are still largely unclear. Patients with carotid sinus syncope are perhaps the best candidates for cardiac pacing because bradycardia is usually present in this condition. The results of a recent randomized controlled trial of cardiac pacing in this disorder were encouraging, with a marked reduction of falls (both syncopal and non-syncopal) and injuries in the treated group.[54] However, feelings of presyncope persisted in a significant number of patients, particularly those with single chamber system. Dual chamber pacemakers are perhaps more effective, but are also more expensive.

Falls caused by non-syncopal forms of transient loss of consciousness

Various disorders may lead to falls that were preceded by TLC, but here the underlying mechanism is not related to a failing systemic blood circulation. Distinguishing these disorders from syncope and recognition of the underlying pathophysiology has important implications for treatment and prevention of further falls.

VASCULAR STEAL SYNDROMES

The most common example in this category is a stenosis of the subclavian artery, where the post-stenotic artery draws blood away from ipsilateral 'donating' arteries that normally supply the brain.[55] Although this condition may be grouped under syncope,[4] this is not strictly correct as the hypoperfusion of part of the brain is not due to a problem of the systemic circulation. We therefore prefer to list vascular steal syndromes as a non-syncopal cause of TLC and falls. The left arm is more often involved than the right arm. Steal syndromes can lead to falls, but only when there is steal of the vertebrobasilar arteries, leading to ischemia of the brainstem and TLC. Several features help in reaching this diagnosis. First, vascular steal rarely leads to an isolated TLC.[56] Instead, there is typically an associated range of tell-tale symptoms and signs of vertebrobasilar ischemia. These include diplopia, vertigo, dysarthria, dysphagia and ataxia (brainstem ischemia), as well as a blurred vision (ischemia of the occipital lobes). For all practical purposes, it is safe to assume that TLC without accompanying neurological deficits is not caused by vertebrobasilar ischemia, whether due to vascular steal or cerebrovascular disease (see below). Second, patients with vascular steal may report that the episodes are provoked by exercise of one arm, owing to an increased vascular demand. Transient loss of consciousness and falls are particularly linked to upper arm exercise. This can be associated with intermittent claudication of the affected arm. Third, when physical examination reveals a marked blood pressure difference between both arms, this is indicative of a steal phenomenon. Vascular steal syndromes can usually be treated with corrective angioplasty.

CEREBROVASCULAR DISORDERS

Cerebrovascular disorders can directly hamper blood flow to parts of the brain. Strokes affecting a part of one hemisphere do not impair consciousness, unless there is considerable mass effect with horizontal shift, leading to compression of the other hemisphere, or vertical shift, leading to compression of the brainstem. Primary involvement of the brainstem can affect consciousness and lead to falls when it occurs in a standing person, but there is rarely isolated TLC.[56] Just as with vascular steal syndromes, there is nearly always additional evidence for ischemia of the brainstem or occipital lobes. Most patients have a bilateral paresis, usually affecting the legs and arms to a similar extent. ischemia extending to the lower brainstem may also affect respiration. This loss of brainstem functions comes on rapidly and simultaneously, unlike the migrainous auras or the marching symptoms of epilepsy (Jacksonian fits). Vertebrobasilar strokes nearly always lead to a marked reactive hypertension, hence a normal blood pressure during or shortly after the attack strongly argues against stroke as cause of the fall.

EPILEPSY

Epilepsy is a common neurological cause of falls, both with and without TLC. Only primary and secondary generalized epileptic seizures are associated with falls caused by TLC. Falls are not a feature of partial complex seizures, but 'automatisms' such as wandering and purposeless behavior sometimes cause diagnostic confusion because of resemblance to presyncope.

The associated movements help to classify the type of seizure. If there is a tonic phase to the generalized seizure, patients keel over like a falling log. The ensuing clonic phase with massive and synchronous jerking movements of the face and limbs usually takes place when the patient is already on the floor. Some seizures are associated with only brief (1–2 s) tonic contractions of axial muscles; this has been termed positive myoclonus or 'epileptic spasms'. These are a common form of epileptic falls in adults.[57]

Other seizures are not accompanied by excessive movements, but rather by transient loss of tone in postural muscles: negative myoclonus, atonic seizures or drop seizures. Such seizures cause patients to fall limply to the floor, with flaccid muscles. Partial atonic seizures can be restricted to a sagging of the knees or a mere head drop. The attacks are often so brief that consciousness appears to remain preserved; this may cause confusion with idiopathic drop attacks (see below). These atonic seizures usually occur in children as part of specific epileptic syndromes, such as the Lennox–Gastaut syndrome and juvenile myoclonic epilepsy.[58,59] However, adults can also be affected, for example in survivors of a severe post-anoxic encephalopathy who fall due to negative myoclonus.[60] In these patients, the negative myoclonus appears to result from inactivation of reticulospinal pathways. Atonic seizures can also occur in adult patients with temporal lobe epilepsy.[61] Such atonic seizures can be very resistant to anti-epileptic drug treatment, and corpus callosotomy may be required for some patients.[62] Sodium valproate is the drug of first choice in juvenile myoclonic epilepsy.[59] In other myoclonic epilepsies, conventional drugs against myoclonus, benzodiazepines in particular, may alleviate the falling episodes.

Several clinical features help to recognize epilepsy as the underlying cause of falls. Age is one of them. Seizures occur predominantly in childhood (specific epileptic syndromes such as juvenile myoclonic epilepsy) and become increasingly common again with advancing age due to development of symptomatic seizures. As a general rule, being younger than 45 years of age suggests epilepsy, rather than other causes of TLC such as cardiac syncope.[11] Epileptic seizures usually occur without a clear trigger, although fatigue or alcohol withdrawal may act as such. An exception is reflex epilepsy, where seizures are precipitated by particular triggers. The most common form is photosensitive epilepsy where repeated visual stimuli can trigger attacks, but variants are provoked by, for example, kinesthetic stimuli, music or startling sounds.[63] Note that the high prevalence of such 'triggers' during everyday activities may lead to pseudo-causal relationships with epileptic seizures. Most of these epileptic triggers do not evoke any other type of TLC, hence the distinction is usually not difficult.

Premonitory symptoms are often absent. A classical 'textbook' aura with a rising epigastric sensation, unprovoked fear or strange olfactory sensations obviously suggests epilepsy, but such auras are often absent.[64] Less specific premonitory symptoms are difficult to interpret, even for experienced neurologists. Sometimes a given individual may present with a specific pattern of premonitory symptoms that remains consistent over recurrent attacks. When these symptoms cannot be classified in any way, they may suggest the presence of an epileptic aura. Some patients with generalized seizures utter a cry at the onset of their epileptic attacks.

The duration of actual seizures is usually brief, often only several minutes. Falls caused by TLC without any tonic or clonic muscle contraction are unlikely to be caused by epilepsy. (Absence seizures are an exception to this rule of thumb, but these do not lead to falls.) Tongue bite is virtually specific for primary or secondary generalized epileptic seizures that have a clonic phase. Tonic seizures or partial seizures rarely produce tongue bite. The laceration is typically situated on the lateral side of the anterior third part of the tongue.[12] Although tongue bite is not a consistent feature of epilepsy (it occurs in less than half of all generalized tonic–clonic seizures), its presence renders syncope and psychogenic causes for falls considerably less likely. Muscle jerks and urinary incontinence are often deemed to be typical manifestations of epilepsy but, as noted before, can also be present in different forms of syncope.

Seizures are typically associated with postictal confusion and anterograde amnesia. However, this can be mild if the seizure was brief, and may be absent in focal seizures. Furthermore, it can be difficult to distinguish between ictal and postictal features. A practical rule of thumb is that complete absence of postictal confusion following a major episode strongly argues against epilepsy as the underlying cause of falls. Many epileptic patients complain of headache, either as manifestation of the actual seizure or during the postictal phase.[65,66] Finally, generalized seizures often cause muscle aches which can persist for days.

As mentioned earlier, care must be taken not to miss seizures that were the result, rather than the cause of the fall. Patients may fall, for whatever reason, on the head, leading to a brain concussion and secondary seizures. A traumatic concussion may also lead to several brief muscle jerks, without a real seizure; this has been termed 'concussional convulsion'.

The diagnosis of epilepsy largely relies upon the interview. The role of electroencephalograph (EEG) is discussed in the section 'Ancillary studies' (page 308).

The disappearance of falls following start of antiepileptic treatment does not prove that the falls were caused by epilepsy, as spontaneous remission may have occurred. Furthermore, several anti-epileptic drugs are also effective against other conditions such as myoclonus. As with any other diagnosis, absence of a clear therapeutic response should not automatically lead to trials of different drugs, but warrants reconsideration of the original diagnosis.

METABOLIC DISORDERS AND INTOXICATIONS

This category rarely leads to diagnostic confusion for patients who present with unexplained falls. Most metabolic disorders and intoxications do not remit spontaneously, and therefore impair consciousness for longer periods of time. Examples include hypoxia and hypoglycemia. Most of these disorders can be fatal, if left untreated. Other disorders cause secondary brain damage, which continues to impair consciousness even if the underlying disorder has been treated. A common example is laminar cortical necrosis secondary to hypoxia or hypoglycemia.

The only disorder which may perhaps cause falls due to TLC is hyperventilation. Symptoms include feelings of anxiety or even panic, lightheadedness, tingling fingers and toes, a dry mouth, dyspnea and chest pain. It is unknown whether hyperventilation can actually cause TLC, but, if so, this seems to be rare. In the consultation room, it is sometimes possible to provoke the characteristic symptoms by forced ventilation, but the diagnostic yield of this test appears low.[67,68] Simply asking patients about episodes of breathlessness produces a similar diagnostic gain.

Hyperventilation was long thought to result from stress-induced excessive breathing, leading to hypocapnia and subsequent reductions in cerebral blood flow through vasoconstriction. However, more recent studies have challenged this assumption and suggested that hypocapnia was not strongly linked to the symptoms.[69] However, this matter has not been laid to rest because of methodological shortcomings: the sensor used in the latter study might have missed relevant hypocapnia. It is possible that anxiety during a panic attack produces both hyperventilation and vasovagal syncope.

MIGRAINE

Episodes of basilar migraine may lead to a decreased level of consciousness.[70] For this reason, the term syncopal migraine has sometimes been used to describe this condition. However, that term should be avoided because TLC is not an essential feature of basilar migraine, and because regional cerebral hypoperfusion does not fit in the definition of syncope. Basilar migraine is a form of migraine with aura, and in this particular condition the aura consists of two or more brainstem signs (e.g. dysarthria, vertigo, tinnitus, diplopia and sometimes a reduced consciousness). When consciousness is impaired, this should not last more than 60 min. The disorder mostly occurs in young adults, many of whom will also have migraine attacks with typical aura.

Note also that common migraine appears to be associated with syncope, both during and outside attacks.[71] Just how often this combination occurs remains unknown.

MIMICS OF LOSS OF CONSCIOUSNESS

Various conditions pose particular diagnostic difficulty because they may, even after careful enquiry, resemble falls caused by TLC (Table 16.7). Such 'look-alike' conditions include disorders where consciousness is altered rather than lost. Psychiatric disorders are part of this category because they may impose as a TLC and lead to falls. In other disorders, consciousness is only seemingly lost. This category includes drop attacks, cataplexy and forms of positive or negative myoclonus, including hyperekplexia (myoclonic epilepsy was dealt with in the section on epileptic falls).

Table 16.7 *Disorders resembling falls caused by transient loss of consciousness ('mimics'). These include conditions where consciousness is altered, rather than lost (e.g. psychogenic pseudosyncope), and conditions where consciousness is only apparently lost*

Altered consciousness	Partial epilepsy with amnesia
	Psychogenic pseudosyncope
	somatization disorders
	– hysteria
	– conversion reaction
	– simulation
Apparent loss of consciousness	Drop attacks
	Cataplexy
	Myoclonus
	hyperekplexia
	myoclonic epilepsy

Cataplexy

In contrast to widespread belief, cataplexy is not rare. It consists of a sudden and bilateral loss of muscle tone in response to emotional stimuli.[72,73] All striated muscles may be involved, but ocular movements and respiration remain possible. During a complete attack, patients slump to the ground with a complete paralysis, being fully conscious but unable to respond. This is often mistaken for TLC, but the absence of amnesia proves that consciousness was in fact preserved during the cataplectic attack. Curiously, injuries are uncommon during cataplectic attacks.[72] Actual falls can sometimes be prevented if the attacks develop slowly enough to allow the patient to stagger and grasp for support. Not all attacks are complete, and partial attacks frequently occur with buckling of the knees, nodding of the head or dropping of the jaw. Laughter is the most typical trigger for cataplexy, so the patients literally become 'weak with laughter'.[74] Additional emotions that may elicit a cataplectic attack include anger, surprise or startle. Cataplexy provoked by startle may occasionally cause confusion with hyperekplexia, but startle is never the only or most common trigger over a series of cataplectic attacks. Furthermore, unlike cataplexy, hyperekplexia leads to stiff falls (see below). Pain, fear and anxiety are not strong triggers, in contrast to reflex syncope.

Isolated cataplexy has been described in a few families.[75] However, cataplexy is almost always part of the narcoleptic syndrome. In fact, cataplexy in combination with excessive daytime sleepiness is pathognomonic for narcolepsy. In rare cases, symptomatic cataplexy has been reported with lesions of the diencephalons and upper brainstem.[76]

It is important to reliably identify cataplexy, but this proves difficult. History taking is not always conclusive and, curiously, patients rarely manifest cataplexy when they visit their clinician, even when confronted with emotionally provoking stimuli.[73] Apparently, the occurrence of cataplexy requires patients to be relaxed. Furthermore, patients are sometimes able to suppress temporarily the occurrence of cataplexy.

It is currently thought that cataplexy is a dissociated expression of the muscle weakness that normally only occurs during rapid eye-movement (REM) sleep,[77] although this hypothesis has been questioned.[78] Nuclei in the pontine brainstem form the final common pathway in the suppression of muscle tone during both cataplexy and REM sleep.[79] However, the brain areas responsible for the triggering of these brainstem nuclei remain unknown.

Tricyclic antidepressants (relatively low-dosed) are the most effective treatment for cataplexy.[73] The most commonly used ones are imipramine (10–100 mg), protryptiline (2.5–40 mg) and clomipramine (10–150 mg). Most authors consider clomipramine the treatment of first choice. Several alternatives to the tricyclic antidepressants have been studied, especially selective serotonin reuptake inhibitors. Gammahydroxybutyrate, given orally at night divided into two doses of 30 mg/kg each, can also improve cataplexy.[80,81]

Drop attacks

The term 'drop attack' has been widely used to indicate all kinds of possible falls, with or without TLC and regardless of the cause. This includes falls caused by vestibular disease, by tonic spasms or by atonic epileptic seizures.[62,82,83] As such, this term has caused more confusion than understanding. If used at all, it is best to reserve the term drop attacks to denote a particular and benign syndrome of sudden, unexpected falls onto the knees without TLC and without prodromal or postictal symptoms, that occurs in women over 40 years of age.[84] Men are very rarely affected. The majority of these drop attacks, more than 60 per cent, remain cryptogenic. The frequency of drop attacks ranges from a single fall to more than 12 falls a year. Falls occur suddenly as a result of buckling of the legs, without subjective sensations of vertigo or any other prior warning. Indeed, patients nearly always remember hitting the floor, hence any possible loss of consciousness would have to be extremely short. The drop attacks nearly always occur during walking, and only rarely during standing.[84] Other than that, there is no relation to changes in posture, head movements or any other specific precipitating event. Unlike syncope and epilepsy, there are no associated involuntary movements. Usually patients can get up immediately after the fall and resume their normal activities, unless injuries are present. Patients typically fall straight down or forward onto their knees, often leading to hematomas in the patella region; hence the French term 'maladie des genoux bleus'. This type of injury is rather characteristic and, in our experience, extremely rare in other causes of falls. Other major injuries are relatively rare,[85] although one report mentioned drop attacks as one of the most common causes of hip fractures in the elderly.[86] Another report mentioned wrist fractures, suggesting that patients have enough time (and awareness) to stretch out their arm for protection.[84] The interictal examination does not reveal signs of an underlying balance disorder.

Some clinicians feel that idiopathic drop attacks might represent a form of vertebrobasilar ischemia. However, if this mechanism applied to the majority of patients with drop attacks, then such persons should have an increased overall risk of cerebrovascular and, presumably, other forms of cardiovascular morbidity and mortality. This does not seem to be the case.[84,85] It is also unlikely that drop attacks are related to external compression of vertebral arteries, for example caused by osteophytic spurs in the cervical spine. Such degenerative abnormalities are very common and their presence in patients with drop attacks is probably due to chance. Patients who suddenly fall after neck rotation are much more likely to have reflex syncope due to the carotid sinus syndrome, and radiographic studies of the cervical spine are not indicated. There is no specific treatment for idiopathic drop attacks, but patients can be informed that some 80 per cent will enjoy spontaneous remission after several years.[85] In other patients, the disorder can exist unaltered for many years. We usually recommend the use of wheeled rollators, but many patients fail to benefit, apparently because they have insufficient time to grasp for support.

A small proportion of what appear to be 'drop attacks' are symptomatic, that is, the falls are seemingly caused by an identifiably underlying neurological disorder. One large series observed an associated medical condition in about 36 per cent of patients with otherwise typical drop attacks, but whether these conditions were causally related to the occurrence of drop attacks remained unclear.[85] It is actually more likely that these medical conditions were fortuitous bystanders, as their treatment did not affect the overall remission rate of drop attacks compared with idiopathic cases. Examples include a colloid cyst in the third ventricle or a structural central nervous system lesion located around the foramen magnum (Table 16.8). Sudden falls are sometimes the only symptom of a type 1 Chiari malformation or an arachnoid cyst

in the fossa posterior. Myasthenia gravis rarely can lead to sudden leg weakness and cause what appears to be a drop attack. Patients with a myopathy can also fall rather abruptly as a result of proximal leg weakness. The diagnosis is not so difficult in patients with clear muscle wasting and paresis during physical examination, but falls can sometimes precede other symptoms by months or years.[87] We have occasionally seen patients with Parkinson's disease who presented with otherwise typical drop attacks, including blue knees, along with the usual external falls due to the balance deficit. However, this may have been due to mere chance, because drop attacks were distinctly absent in large series of Parkinson's disease patients whose falls were monitored prospectively.[3,88,89]

Symptomatic forms of sudden falls should not be labeled as drop attacks to avoid confusion. It is usually not difficult to distinguish the symptomatic falls from idiopathic drop attacks, both by unusual features of the fall and by the presence of an abnormal interictal neurological examination. For example, structural lesions located around the foramen magnum may cause sudden falls, but are usually accompanied by neurological signs such as a paraparesis.[90] Similarly, atonic seizures nearly always occur in young children with myoclonic jerks and a prior history of years with other seizure types.[61] These atonic seizures

Table 16.8 *Examples of falls that mimic drop attacks. The second column lists some atypical features that help in the distinction between idiopathic drop attacks and symptomatic forms of sudden falls*

Underlying disorder	Atypical feature
Colloid cyst in the third ventricle	Interictal neurological signs
Space-occupying process in fossa posterior	Interictal neurological signs
Atonic seizures	Young children
	Myoclonic jerks
	Preceded by other seizure types
	Consciousness lost for minutes
	Postictal confusion
	Specific electroencephalogram (EEG) abnormalities
Startle epilepsy	Preceded by specific trigger
	EEG abnormalities
Peripheral vestibular disease	Feels as being pushed to one side
	Association with vertigo
	Interictal ear, nose and throat (ENT) abnormalities
Leg weakness (e.g. myopathy, myasthenia gravis)	Interictal neurological signs
	Abnormal electromyograph studies
Neurodegenerative disorders (e.g. Parkinson's disease, normal pressure hydrocephalus)	Interictal neurological signs
	Additional fall types (e.g. trips or slips)
Carotid sinus syndrome	Loss of consciousness
	Provoked by head movements or neck compression
Vertebrobasilar ischemia	Additional brainstem signs
	Increased cerebrovascular and cardiovascular morbidity/mortality
Cataplexy	Triggered by emotional stimuli (laughter, anger, surprise or startle)
	Almost always part of the narcoleptic syndrome

also last longer and are usually followed by postictal confusion. 'Drop attacks' have also been described in patients with hydrocephalus or periventricular white matter abnormalities, but these subjects always have additional neurological signs such as cognitive impairment, incontinence, spasticity and gait impairment. Grasp reflexes of the feet are particularly common in these patients.[91] Falls referred to as 'drop attacks' can occur in patients with otological disease, but such patients report a subjective sensation of being pushed to one side.[83] These patients also complain of recurrent episodic vertigo. Finally, startle epilepsy can sometimes present with remarkable resemblance to drop attacks, but the presence of a preceding trigger provides a clue to the diagnosis. Proper identification of symptomatic sudden falls is important, as the underlying disorder negatively affects the overall prognosis. Mortality is particularly increased for patients with associated cardiac disease or an abnormal neurological examination.[85]

Falls caused by the carotid sinus syndrome are sometimes mislabeled as drop attacks, because elderly patients in particular may have an amnesia for the TLC that accompanied the fall.[92] However, careful history taking usually reveals a preceding trigger, mostly turning movements of the head or neck compression.

Hyperekplexia (startle disease)

Hyperekplexia consists of excessive startle reactions induced by sudden sounds or other unexpected stimuli (touch or visual cues). Even the expectation of being frightened can provoke the startle reactions. The pattern of the startle reactions is normal, but the threshold for their occurrence is abnormally low. Furthermore, startle reactions habituate less than in healthy subjects. Another abnormal feature is the spread of the startle reaction to the legs, which is rare in healthy subjects.[93] What bothers patients most is the presence of generalized stiffening due to tonic spasms with a longer latency than the startle reflex, again caused by unexpected (mainly acoustic) stimuli. Voluntary movements are impossible during such stiffening episodes, which commonly leads to falls and, because patients cannot break their fall, injuries. However, consciousness is completely preserved during these falls.

Hyperekplexia can be genetically determined or occur sporadically. Some of the latter group are symptomatic cases. Symptomatic hyperekplexia has been described in postanoxic encephalopathy, post-traumatic encephalopathy, viral encephalitis, multiple sclerosis and as part of a paraneoplastic syndrome. Familial forms are usually autosomal dominant and are related to missense mutations in a gene that encodes for a subunit of the glycine receptor. Hereditary hyperekplexia or familial startle disease appears in two different forms: a major and a minor form. Patients with the major form of hereditary hyperekplexia have generalized stiffness immediately after birth, but this disappears during the first one to two years of life.[94] Furthermore, life-long exaggerated startle responses accompanied by brief (1–2 s) periods of general muscle stiffness with startle occur in the major form of hereditary hyperekplexia, but not in the minor form, which is characterized by excessive startle responses alone.[94] Adult patients with the major form of hyperekplexia can have a stiff-legged and slightly wide-based gait, without signs of ataxia or spasticity; this appears especially while walking on uneven ground. Hereditary hyperekplexia tends to improve spontaneously after the first two decades of life. Imaging of the brain is unremarkable. Clonazepam can help prevent falls by reducing stiffness and, to a lesser extent, the excessive startle reactions.[95]

Psychogenic attacks

Psychiatric disorders were long thought to be a rare source of falls associated with a real or apparent TLC. However, more recent studies suggested a higher prevalence of psychiatric disorders among fallers suspected of having TLC.[3,96] A major problem here relates to how the psychogenic attacks were defined. Some studies used positive criteria to identify psychiatric disorders, but others merely defined psychogenic attacks *per exclusionem*, that is by taking the rest group after excluding other possible causes for the falls. The prevalence figures must therefore be interpreted with caution.

Complete falls to the ground are part of the spectrum of psychogenic attacks. In rare cases, psychogenic attacks may take the form of drop attacks. Even physical injury can occur, so injuries do not exclude psychogenic attacks as a possible cause of the falls.

Several arguments support a diagnosis of psychogenic attacks (Table 16.9). This is particularly true for young patients with very frequent episodes and a range of additional, non-specific symptoms. A prior history of psychiatric disease or presence of psychiatric signs during the examination, in particular depression or anxiety, are also suggestive. A state of psychogenic TLC usually lasts much longer than true syncope and therefore better resembles coma. This long duration of unresponsiveness provides physicians sufficient time to perform a physical examination during the attack. This may reveal hints that consciousness is only apparently lost (e.g. when the eyes are actively shut during attempts to open them passively). Furthermore, falls that merely occur in the presence of bystanders are possibly psychogenic in origin. A final supportive argument is a reduction of falls following psychotherapy.

Falls with TLC in a psychiatric patient are most likely caused by the medication prescribed to treat the underlying disorder. Indeed, various types of drug treatment for psychiatric disorders have been associated with falls.[28,97,98] Antidepressants are the greatest cause of concern, as these commonly lead to orthostatic hypotension

Table 16.9 *Arguments in favor of psychogenic pseudosyncope as the cause of unexplained falls. Note that patients may also have psychogenic falls without an apparent transient loss of consciousness*

Young age
Multiple premonitory symptoms
Very frequent episodes
Long duration of unresponsiveness
Prior history of psychiatric disease
Abnormal interictal psychiatric examination
Severe psychosocial consequences
Falls merely in presence of bystanders
Falls precipitated by psychosocial stressors
Fall reduction following psychotherapy
Suggestive features *during* the attack:
 Absence of neurological signs[a]
 Non-flaccid posturing of the limbs
 Eyes actively shut during passive opening
 Eyes consistently turned away from investigator
 Hand dropped above patient's head just misses the head
 Reflexive gaze movements
 Ice-water irrigation of the ears produces lively nystagmus[b]

[a]Except for a lack of responsiveness.
[b]As opposed to the tonic eye deviation towards the cold ear in comatose patients.

and syncopal falls. Benzodiazepines are an important risk factor for hip fractures, particularly when multiple compounds are used concurrently.[99,100] The risk of falls is also increased for patients taking neuroleptics, which can lead to drug-induced parkinsonism or tardive dyskinesias. Care must be taken not to falsely incriminate the underlying disorder and further increase the medication, when it is a dose reduction that is required.

If medication is not the culprit, one must consider whether the psychiatric disorder itself led to psychogenic pseudosyncope and falls. This occurs with several psychiatric disorders. Hyperventilation was mentioned earlier. Note that hyperventilation typically occurs under circumstances associated with feelings of panic. For this reason, the symptoms usually attributed to hyperventilation are classified under the heading 'panic attacks' in the psychiatric diagnostic classification system (DSM-IV). Panic disorders often coincide with depression. Conversion reactions are rare, but they may cause falls. The pattern of falls is often theatrical, for example slow sagging to the knees, and rather stereotypical for individual patients. Note, however, that cataplexy may also lead to slow and prolonged falls. The falls can be associated with an apparent TLC and incontinence, but tongue bite is absent.[12] Other possible psychiatric causes of falls include somatization disorders, hysteria, factitious disorders and simulation (malingering).

Tilt table tests can sometimes assist in the diagnostic work-up of patients with unexplained falls that were possibly caused by psychogenic pseudosyncope. Thus, a

psychiatric cause is likely in patients that become unresponsive when they are passively tilted upright, in the absence of concurrent changes in heart rhythm or blood pressure.[101,102] Ideally, such studies should be combined with a concurrent EEG registration to ascertain the absence of functional cerebral disturbances during the attack.

DIAGNOSTIC WORK-UP: PROBLEMS AND PRACTICAL SOLUTIONS

Clinicians confronted with patients whose falls were possibly caused by TLC face a formidable challenge. Difficulties may be encountered during history taking, during physical examination and in the interpretation of ancillary studies. Some of these practical problems are listed in Table 16.10. In the following sections, we will systematically review the diagnostic work-up and, whenever possible, provide practical solutions for the most common difficulties.

History taking

SOME PROBLEMS

Generally speaking, history taking is difficult in subjects that have fallen. This is particularly true for patients that have sustained a possible TLC, either before or after the fall. Many falls are forgotten or simply not volunteered (see Chapter 11) and therefore never come to medical attention. Other patients may present with their first episode; hence no pattern is yet discernible. Sudden falls can be a startling experience to patients and bystanders alike. The resulting anxiety often hampers accurate recollection of important details. The circumstances of the fall thus remain unclear and most patients find it difficult to indicate whether any symptoms preceded the fall. Particularly elderly patients often deny a TLC, even when eyewitnesses are convinced it had occurred.[22,92,103] Some patients claim to remember the entire event, but merely report an unexpected fall or some form of 'dizziness'.[8] Several questions can help in deciding whether a TLC preceded the fall. First, barring rare exceptions,[2] true TLC is incompatible with staying upright. Hence, if patients wandered about, consciousness was not lost. In case of a fall to the floor, it may be helpful to ask whether the person recalls hitting the ground. Second, there must be an associated amnesia for the event in case of TLC. If patients convincingly remember every moment of the fall, true unconsciousness is unlikely. Note that amnesia *per se* does not prove that the patient has fallen. For example, patients with partial complex epilepsy have an amnesia for their seizures, but do not fall.

Different problems arise when patients do mention symptoms that possibly point to a preceding TLC. In many cases, consciousness only appeared to be lost. This

Table 16.10 *Some practical problems that are commonly encountered in the clinical approach to fallers with a possible transient loss of consciousness (TLC)*

Was there a loss of consciousness?	Amnesia for falls, TLC, or both
	Brief TLC easily missed
	Other funny turns (e.g. vertigo) mistaken for TLC
	Mimics of impaired consciousness (Table 16.7)
If there was a loss of consciousness	Preceding the fall? →Cause (e.g. syncope)
	After the fall? →Consequence (e.g. concussion)
Precipitants and associated symptoms	Details of falls often forgotten
	Inaccurate eyewitness report due to anxiety
	Overlap between different conditions
	Single fall, hence no pattern
Physical examination and ancillary studies	False-positive results (background incidence in population)
	False-negative results (normal interictal findings)
Worries about consequences	Recurrence of falls
	Injurious falls
	Secondary morbidity/mortality
	Psychosocial impact

occurs with 'lookalike' conditions such as drop attacks, cataplexy and hyperekplexia. The amnesia associated with traumatic temporal lobe lesions can be mistaken for a TLC. Also, seemingly spontaneous falls due to severe balance deficits are easily misinterpreted as TLC. Furthermore, many patients merely indicate that 'a funny turn' of some kind had preceded the fall. It can be difficult to decide whether this actually represented a true TLC. Surprisingly many patients mistake symptoms of vertigo for unconsciousness. Useful clues are that peripheral vertigo is typically evoked or aggravated by sudden movements, and is often associated with nausea and vomiting. Patients also commonly mislabel feelings of anxiety, visual symptoms, nausea and palpitations as being unconscious. (Note that some of these symptoms could actually represent presyncopal features.) Specifically directed questions, for example about spinning sensations in the head or changes of color in the visual field ('graying out') can help to identify true TLC.

If a true TLC seems likely, one must distinguish between falls that were preceded by unconsciousness versus falls that led to secondary unconsciousness. This distinction is not always straightforward. Examples of a reduced consciousness directly after the fall include brain injuries because the patient fell onto the head (concussion and intracranial hemorrhage). Another possibility is a post-fall vasovagal syncope induced by pain or seeing blood. Also, the anxiety associated with falls could induce hyperventilation and thus blur the subject's consciousness. Traumatic brain injuries may also lead to post-fall epileptic seizures, making it difficult to decide whether the patient fell because of an epileptic seizure, or whether they fell on the head, for some other reason, leading to a concussion and acutely symptomatic secondary seizures. Even when it is clear that a TLC preceded the fall, one must be certain that this could not be attributed to an external cause, such as bumping the head against a shelf.

Assuming that the TLC preceded the fall and that this did not have an external cause, the next logical step is to ask for accompanying symptoms. Few bystanders have the presence of mind to monitor the patient's pulse, to note the color of the skin or to look for involuntary movements. Even when such features were passively observed, it is difficult to retrieve the information from bystanders later. Bystanders commonly considerably overestimate the duration of an episode.

A final problem is that for many patients with falls or a TLC, multiple contributing factors can be identified.[104] This is often the case in elderly patients. Some of these factors may be causally linked to the falls, others may be predictive of an increased morbidity or mortality, while still others can be innocent bystanders.

POSSIBLE SOLUTIONS

It is helpful to gather specific information about the following elements: the individual characteristics of the faller (e.g. age, gender, prior history or medication); frequency and duration of unexplained falls; presence of any specific precipitants or provoking circumstances; presence and nature of any premonitory symptoms; in the case of syncope, presence and nature of any associated features (skin color, pulse, involuntary movements, etc.); speed of recovery and nature of postictal symptoms; and effects of any attempted therapeutic interventions (Table 16.11). Several important elements are discussed in more detail below.

Patient characteristics

A greater age suggests underlying cardiovascular disease. Cardiac syncope typically occurs from middle-age onwards, but one notable exception is the long QT syndrome which may occur in younger persons. Being younger than 45 years of age increases the possibility of reflex syncope or a seizure.[11]

Table 16.11 *Helpful elements of the medical interview*

Feature	Reflex syncope	Orthostatic syncope	Cardiac syncope	Seizures	Other diagnoses
Patients					
Age (years)	< 45	> 45	> 45	<20; > 45	See text
Medication	–	++	+	±	–
Prior history					
Cardiac	–	–	++	–	–
Psychiatric	–	–	–	–	PP
Autonomic	–	++	–	–	PH
Parkinsonism	–	++	–	–	PH
Ataxia	–	++	–	–	–
Family history					
Long QT syndrome	–	–	++	–	–
Sudden death	–	–	++	±	–
Pattern of attacks					
Frequency	Low	High	Low	Low	PP: high
Precipitants					
Pain, emotions	++	–	–	–	
Coughing, swallowing	++	–	–	–	–
Urination, defecation	+	±			
Heat	+	+	–	–	–
Laughter, anger, surprise	–	–	–	–	CA
Usually in the morning	–	+	–	–	–
< 2 h after a meal	–	+	–	–	PH
Standing up	–	+[a]	–	–	VE
Prolonged stance	+	++	–	–	–
Regular walking	–	–	±	–	DA
While lying or sitting	±	±	+	+	CA,HY,PH,PP,RE,VI
Head movements	+	–	–	–	VE
Pressure on the neck	++	–	–	–	–
Startle	+	–	+[b]	RE	HY
Flashing light	–	–	–	RE	
Sleep deprivation	–	–	–	+	–
Hypovolemia	+	++	–	–	–
Merely in company	–	–	–	–	PP
None (random pattern)	–	–	+	+	–
Premonitory phase					
Vegetative symptoms	++	–	–	–	Panic attacks
Presyncope	+	+	+	–	–
Palpitations	–	–	+	–	Panic attacks
'Coat hanger pain'	–	+	–	–	–
Aura	–	–	–	±	–
Shout	–	–	–	+	–
Panic, dyspnea, dry mouth, perioral tingling	–	–	–	–	Panic attacks
Brainstem symptoms	–	–	–	–	VI
Ictal phase					
Typical duration	< 20 s	< 20 s	< 20 s	> 5 min	See text
Keeling over, stiff	±	±	±	Tonic fit	HY
Flaccid fall	+	+	+	Atonic fit	CA, DA
Abrupt loss of consciousness	+	+	+	–	–
Involuntary movements					
Absent	+	+	+	Atonic fit	CA, DA, HY
Present before fall	–	–	–	+	–
Present after fall	+	+	+	+	–
Symmetric, synchronous	–[c]	–[c]	–[c]	+	–
Strictly unilateral	–	–	–	+	–
Duration < 15 s	+	+	+	–	–
Duration > 30 s	–	–	–	+	–
Incontinence	+	+	I	+	–

Table 16.11 – continued

Feature	Reflex syncope	Orthostatic syncope	Cardiac syncope	Seizures	Other diagnoses
Lateral tongue bite	–	–	–	++	–
Cyanotic face	–	–	–	+	–
Snoring	–	–	–	+	–
Eyes open	+	+	+	+	CA,DA,HY,VE
Postictal phase					
Rapid recovery	+	+	++	–	DA, HY
Vegetative symptoms	++	–	–	–	Panic attacks
Fatigue	±	±	±	++	–
Confusion	±	±	–	++	–
Retrograde amnesia	+	+	+	+	PP
Anterograde amnesia	±	±	–	++	PP
Aching muscles	–	–	–	++	–
Headache	–	–	–	++	–
Palpitations, chest pain	–	–	++	–	–
Injured patellae	–	–	–	–	DA
Disproportional psychosocial impact	–	–	–	–	PP

Abbreviations: CA, cataplexy; DA, drop attacks; HY, hyperekplexia; PH, postprandial hypotension; PP, psychogenic pseudosyncope; RE, reflex epilepsy; VE, vertigo; VI, vertebrobasilar ischemia.
[a]In this case related to duration of standing, not the act of rising itself.
[b]Arrhythmias in patients with the long QT syndrome may be provoked by startling loud noises.
[c]Conversely, asymmetric and asynchronous jerks suggest syncope.

Use of medication is exceptionally important, certainly when multiple drugs are being taken by older persons.[105] Recent changes in the type or dose of medication should alert the clinician to the possibility of iatrogenic falls. Medication is a common cause or supportive factor for the development of orthostatic hypotension. Commonly implicated drugs include tricyclic antidepressants, phenothiazines, antihistamines, dopaminergic drugs (levodopa and receptor agonists), antihypertensive medication and monoamine oxidase (MAO) inhibitors. A less well recognized drug category in elderly men includes prostate medication (W. Wieling, personal communication). Furthermore, many different drugs have been associated with an increased risk of developing cardiac arrhythmias.[4] Psychoactive drugs form a major category, and prolonged QT intervals can occur with the commonly prescribed drug cisapride. Finally, various drugs may increase the risk of developing seizures.[106]

When looking symptoms of autonomic failure, it should be remembered that the main early features are erectile dysfunction for men and urinary incontinence for women.

Pattern and frequency of unexplained falls

The diagnosis often rests on a consistent pattern in the falls, as this may reveal the underlying pathophysiology. Thus, patients suspected of having orthostatic hypotension will typically report a consistent pattern of falls that occur shortly after rising or following prolonged upright stance. However, when such patients also begin to develop syncope while seated or even recumbent, the original diagnosis must be reconsidered. (Another possibility is further progression of autonomic failure, such that even sitting can provoke syncope; we have occasionally seen this in patients with, for example, severe MSA.) Also bear in mind that individual patients may manifest different types of falls, and each pattern must be addressed separately. This is certainly not rare.

The frequency of falls is another helpful feature. Vasovagal syncope leading to falls is usually a relatively rare event, although occasional patients may sustain weekly or even daily episodes. Cardiac syncope and seizures are also infrequent causes of falls for most patients. Conversely, patients with orthostatic hypotension frequently sustain falls, because the precipitants (rising and standing) are so ubiquitous. The falling frequency also tends to be high for patients with psychogenic attacks, where weekly or daily falls can occur.

Precipitants and circumstances

Items that need to be addressed include the position from which consciousness was lost (supine, sitting or standing), the activity at the time of the fall (rest, change in posture, during or after exercise, neck movement), the specific circumstances (such as crowded or warm places) and any other predisposing factors. One should ask specifically about the relation between falls and preceding meals, because patients often fail to see this link because of the long time interval (it can be as long as 2 h after the start of a meal). The presence of specific precipitants such as fear or pain is required to establish a diagnosis of reflex syncope.

Several precipitants may lead to diagnostic confusion. For example, falls associated with sudden startle may be caused by vasovagal syncope, the long QT syndrome (via cardiac syncope), hyperekplexia (leading to stiff falls with preserved consciousness) or reflex epilepsy. Falls related to exercise can also point to various underlying disorders (Table 16.12). Falls that occur with prolonged standing should point to late orthostatic syncope, but may also suggest vasovagal syncope, particularly when there is concurrent volume depletion. Tilt testing can help make the distinction if history taking is unreliable (cf. Figs 16.3 and 16.4). Falls during or right after a transfer from a seated or recumbent position may be caused by initial orthostatic hypotension, but could also be caused by an underlying balance deficit, such as vestibular disease or Parkinson's disease. Falls that happen shortly after or during micturition may suggest reflex syncope, particularly when this occurs in young healthy men.[107] However, another possibility is orthostatic hypotension, which often leads to falls at night while men urinate in a standing position. This second group mainly includes older patients with medication-induced autonomic failure. Falls related to neck movements can also be confusing. Despite common belief, such falls are hardly ever caused by impaired blood flow in the vertebrobasilar system. The carotid sinus syndrome is far more likely, and it may be helpful to ask whether these patients also sustained falls in relation to neck compression, for example by a tight collar. Vestibular disorders may also cause falls in relation to neck movements. Such patients usually report vertigo and nausea, and state that balance is consistently lost sideways in the same direction.

Premonitory symptoms

These symptoms directly precede the fall caused by TLC. One class of premonitory symptoms relates to impairment of cerebral perfusion and has been termed 'presyncope'. A second class of symptoms is related to the mechanism causing TLC. This includes, for example, the vegetative symptoms that specifically precede reflex syncope (autonomic activation). Recognition thereof is important as these symptoms are distinctly absent in other causes of syncope. Presence of presyncopal symptoms such as nausea or sweating also argues against epileptic seizures.[11] Further examples include pain in the head and shoulder region in autonomic failure, palpitations or chest pain in cardiac syncope, tingling in hyperventilation and auras in epilepsy.

Table 16.12 *Falls related to physical exercise*

During exercise	External falls (trips, slips)
	Cardiac syncope
	Young persons with vasovagal syncope
During exercise of one arm	Vascular steal syndrome
Following exercise	Orthostatic hypotension
	Young persons with vasovagal syncope

Ictal phase

The way in which patients have fallen needs to be determined. Flaccid falls ('sinking to the floor') occur in drop attacks, cataplexy or atonic seizures, whereas stiff falls (keeling over) occur in tonic seizures or hyperekplexia. Both fall types have been described in syncope. Prolonged 'theatrical' falls suggest a psychogenic origin, but can also occur with cataplexy. Lateral falls into one direction, as if being pushed, suggest a vestibular cause.

The duration of unconsciousness is a helpful feature in the differential diagnosis. Transient loss of consciousness is absent or hardly noticeable in drop attacks, brief in the various forms of syncope (usually less than 20 s, but can be up to several minutes) and longer with epileptic seizures. A TLC of more than 5 min is suggestive of a seizure.[11] However, some forms of epilepsy can be brief, such as partial seizures and epileptic tonic or atonic falls. Intoxications and metabolic disorders will usually cause long-lasting impairment of unconsciousness (coma).

It is mandatory to enquire about features that were associated with the actual fall and TLC. Involuntary jerking movements of the limbs can occur in syncope of any cause, and this may obscure the distinction between epilepsy and syncope ('not all that moves is epilepsy'). Involuntary movements are particularly common for the extreme situation where syncope is provoked by the 'mess trick', that is, in the laboratory by a rather artificial combination of squatting, hyperventilation and a Valsalva maneuver.[2] However, observations in patients with vasovagal syncope induced by venepuncture suggest that myoclonus may be less common in more everyday forms of syncope. Syncope associated with involuntary movements can be misdiagnosed as epilepsy, and it is only when the 'seizures' prove resistant to antiepileptic treatment that the original diagnosis is reconsidered.[108] Hence, presence of involuntary movements does not reliably separate epilepsy from syncope. However, the absence of such involuntary movements argues against the presence of epilepsy. It is helpful to ask about the nature of the involuntary movements, as several features help to differentiate between the myoclonic jerks in seizures and syncope.[2] In syncope, the involuntary jerking movements are non-rhythmic and multifocal, whereas in generalized epilepsy they are symmetrical and synchronous over various parts of the body. The movements are also smaller in syncope compared with seizures. Furthermore, if the jerks are strictly unilateral at any moment during the attack, or if they start before consciousness is lost, epilepsy is more likely than syncope. Jerks always follow the fall in syncope, whereas they may precede the fall in some epileptic seizures. Note that tonic stiffening may precede the period of myoclonic jerks in both conditions, but tends to be briefer (several seconds only) in syncope. Eyewitnesses may find it difficult to verbalize their observations, but can usually make a choice when the physician mimics the different types of involuntary movements.

Urinary incontinence is not a helpful distinguishing feature, as this occurs in 17 per cent of generalized tonic–clonic seizures and in 26 per cent of syncopal events.[11,12] The presence of tongue bite is highly suggestive of epilepsy (occurs in 24–41 per cent of generalized tonic–clonic seizures), although it may occasionally occur in syncope (2–6 per cent of syncopal events). The site of the laceration should be noted, as it is typically lateral in epilepsy, but at the tip of the tongue in syncope. Asking whether the patient kept their eyes open during the attack does not help to distinguish between syncope, epilepsy and disorders with only apparent TLC. An exception is psychiatric pseudosyncope, where the eyes are often closed;[109] attempts to open the eyes are actively resisted. Tonic gaze deviations occur in both syncope and epilepsy, but usually persist longer during seizures. Being pale during the attack renders a seizure less likely, while a blue face supports a diagnosis of epilepsy.[11]

Postictal symptoms

These are particularly helpful to separate syncope from epilepsy. Cardiac syncope is at the one end of the spectrum, where recovery is usually abrupt, with almost immediate restoration of appropriate behavior and orientation. For obvious reasons, mimics of impaired consciousness also have little, if any, postictal manifestations, except perhaps psychogenic attacks and cataplexy, which can proceed to a sleep state after the fall. Epilepsy is at the other end of the spectrum where, depending on the duration and features of the seizure, postictal confusion is the rule. This is more pronounced for generalized convulsive seizures than for partial complex seizures. Reflex syncope is somewhere in between these two extremes, and confusion or fatigue may be present briefly (less than 30 s) during the recovery period. A global rule of thumb is that prolonged postictal confusion (more than 2 min) after the fall suggests epilepsy, unless secondary head injury is present.[11,109] Aching muscles and headache after the attack, assuming that these are not caused by bruises or other fall-related injuries, also suggest epilepsy, but these features have less than perfect discriminatory power with respect to syncope. Note that headache can also be a premonitory or ictal manifestation of epileptic seizures.

The nature of any resultant injuries is sometimes informative. Injured 'blue' patellae suggest drop attacks. Wrist fractures are typically caused by a fall on the outstretched hand.[110] and suggest that consciousness was preserved during the attack. Hip fractures are less helpful for the differential diagnosis; although commonly stated to result from lateral falls onto the trochanter, hip fractures can also be caused by more vertical falls, as in drop attacks.

Effects of treatment

Falls may disappear after initiation of treatment for an associated medical condition, but this does not necessarily imply that this medical condition was causally related to the occurrence of falls. For example, falls may remit after prescription of an anti-epileptic drug, but this does not prove that seizures led to the falls because spontaneous remission of the underlying condition may have occurred. Prescription of medication for an incorrect diagnosis is actually not rare in light of the high rate of false-positive findings that hampers both the physical examination and all ancillary studies. This creates a considerable risk of 'treating' an abnormal test result rather than the actual patient. The opposite situation (when falls continue despite treatment) is perhaps more informative because this should force the clinician to reconsider the original diagnosis. Inadequate treatment compliance must also be considered, particularly in elderly persons.

Physical examination

Following the interview, a proper physical examination is mandatory. Table 16.13 lists several important elements that help to distinguish between different types of falls caused by TLC and its mimics.

Ideally, physicians should be in a position to examine the patient directly after a fall, but this is rarely possible. A problem with interictal examinations is that the observed abnormalities may not bear a causal relationship to the falls. For example, finding a cardiac arrhythmia during auscultation does not necessarily imply that this was causally related to the falls suffered by the patient. An even greater problem is that most patients have a normal physical examination between fall episodes.

One key facet of the physical examination is measurement of blood pressure in both the recumbent and standing positions, in order to detect orthostatic hypotension. Unfortunately, there is a great deal of variation in how physicians perform and interpret this test. Several consensus statements have provided recommendations for proper assessment of orthostatic hypotension.[111,112] Measurements are best performed in the morning when the tendency to develop orthostasis is greatest; this produces fewer false-negative results.[113] The first blood pressure measurement is in the recumbent position and should be taken after 5 min of supine position. Blood pressure should be then checked repeatedly at least each minute, or more often, while standing up for 3 min. Care must be taken not to miss the initial orthostatic hypotension within the first minute of rising (Fig. 16.4). The value of the standard cuff sphygmomanometer is questionable for this reason, and continuous non-invasive blood pressure measurements should be used when possible.[28,114] Active standing is equally diagnostic as passive head-up tilting; the latter is only required if patients have difficulty standing unaided. Measurements could be continued if the blood pressure is still falling at 3 min. If the patient does not tolerate standing for this period, the lowest systolic blood pressure during the

Table 16.13 *Physical examination*

Feature	Reflex syncope	Orthostatic syncope	Cardiac syncope	Seizures	Other diagnoses
Ictal examination					
Bradycardia[a]	++	–	+	±[b]	–
Other vegetative signs[c]	++	–	–	–	–
Pale throughout	+	+	±	–	–
First pale, then red	–	–	+	–	–
Marked hypertension	–	–	–	–	VI
Bizarre presentation	–	–	–	–	PP
Interictal examination					
General physical					
Supine hypertension	–	+	+	–	VI
Orthostatic hypotension	–	++	–	–	–
Carotid sinus massage	+	–	–	–	–
Lateral tongue bite	–	–	–	++	
Neurological					
Parkinsonism	–	+[d]	–	–	–
Cerebellar ataxia	–	+[d]	–	–	–
Pyramidal signs	–	+[d]	–	–	–
Other balance deficit	–	–	–	–	See text
Brainstem signs	–	–	–	–	VI
Cardiopulmonary signs[e]					
Cardiac	–	–	++	–	–
Psychiatric	–	–	–	–	PP

Abbreviations: CA, cataplexy; DA, drop attacks; HY, hyperekplexia; PH, postprandial hypotension; PP, psychogenic pseudosyncope; RE, reflex epilepsy; VE, vertigo; VI, vertebrobasilar ischemia.

[a]If felt by non-medically trained bystanders, this is often unreliable because of inexperience in taking a pulse and the concurrent anxiety; it may be helpful to invite the bystander, if present during the medical consultation, to rapidly evaluate someone's pulse in the examination room and check for reliability.

[b]Most convulsive seizures lead to tachycardias because of increased energy expenditure; some temporal lobe seizures occasionally cause secondary bradycardia or even asystole.

[c]Most notably sweating and pupillary dilation.

[d]Orthostatic hypotension, along with a varying combination of parkinsonism, cerebellar ataxia or pyramidal signs, suggests the presence of multiple system atrophy.

[e]This includes signs of heart failure and presence of a cardiac bruit; hypertrophic cardiomyopathy is likely if the cardiac bruit can be provoked by a Valsalva maneuver.

upright posture should be recorded. Repeated measurements may be required because false-negative results are not uncommon, particularly in elderly persons or subjects with drug-induced orthostatic hypotension.[113] Occasionally 24-h ambulatory blood pressure recordings are needed, particularly in patients with postprandial hypotension where abnormalities can be missed with routine blood pressure measurements.[115] The presence of orthostatic hypotension is arbitrarily defined as a drop in systolic blood pressure by more than 20 mmHg, a drop in systolic blood pressure to less than 90 mmHg, or a drop in diastolic blood pressure by more than 10 mmHg, within 3 min after rising.[111,112] This definition does not include the absence or presence of subjective complaints. Therefore, some persons can have a very pronounced drop in blood pressure within the first three minutes (sufficient to diagnose orthostatic hypotension), yet not sustain presyncope during this period. Conversely, many subjects report 'dizziness' directly after standing up, but

this early physiological drop in blood pressure may be missed with a conventional sphygmomanometer. During the assessment, it may be helpful to inspect the patient for vegetative manifestations such as pallor or sweating.

Carotid sinus massage is recommended in patients over age 40 years with syncopal falls of unknown etiology.[116] For this purpose, one of the carotid arteries is firmly massaged for 5–10 s at the anterior margin of the sternocleidomastoid muscle at the level of the cricoid cartilage (this is the site where the common carotid artery bifurcates). This should be performed with the patient both supine and erect because, for unknown reasons, up to one-third of elderly patients only show abnormalities in the upright position. Electrocardiographic monitoring (ECG) and blood pressure measurement during carotid massage is mandatory. A positive response is defined by appearance of syncope during or immediately after the massage, in presence of asystolia for <3 s (cardio-inhibitory type of the carotid sinus syndrome), a fall in systolic blood pressure of >50 mmHg (vasodepressor type), or both (mixed type). The test–retest reliability of carotid sinus massage is excellent.[4] A positive response is diagnostic only in the absence of other competing diagnoses. Note that carotid massage should be avoided if there is a risk of stroke because of carotid artery disease. If there is no underlying cardiovascular disease, the risk of fatal arrhythmias or other complications is very rare.

Ancillary studies

Most clinicians will order ancillary studies, at the least an ECG, but often also blood tests, an EEG or other investigations. A problem that arises here relates to the high proportion of false-positive and false-negative findings. All ancillary studies have their own background prevalence of abnormalities in the general population. And even when significant abnormalities are found, it may remain unclear where this finding belongs in the chain of events that eventually caused the fall. For example, neurological disorders such as epilepsy or raised intracranial pressure can lead to secondary ECG abnormalities (for example prolonged long QT intervals), whereas primary cardiac disease can lead to secondary neurological dysfunction (for example post-anoxic seizures). What does one do when more than one 'abnormality' is found, as is common in elderly patients? These can be challenging issues.

False-positive findings are not the only problem. Patients are typically asymptomatic at the time of evaluation because falls and TLC are transient phenomena. Objective evidence of the underlying cause is therefore often not captured during diagnostic testing, leading to false-negative findings. Thus, patients whose falls were caused by a cardiac arrhythmia or an epileptic seizure may show a perfectly normal interictal ECG or EEG. Only rarely are we fortunate enough to perform an ancillary study just at the same time when a patient manifests the transient symptoms or signs. This is a major problem inherent to any paroxysmal disorder. Such drawbacks further underscore the importance of a careful and thorough medical interview.

BASIC LABORATORY TESTS

Blood counts, electrolytes, glucose, renal or hepatic function tests are generally not indicated in patients with falls, irrespective of any preceding TLC.[11,116,117] The only indication is suspicion of a reduced circulating volume or a specific metabolic disorder, such as diabetes. A low sodium excretion in urine suggests the presence of volume depletion, and possibly predicts a therapeutic response to oral salt supplementation.[31] Prolactin and creatine kinase levels are increased shortly after generalized tonic–clonic seizures, but not after syncope or psychiatric pseudoseizures.[118,119] However, false-negative results may occur and blood samples need to be drawn shortly after the episode.

ELECTROCARDIOGRAPHY

A 'cardiac work-up' is indicated in patients with falls associated with TLC and palpitations, chest pain or a prior cardiac history. Ideally, one would like to have a 'smoking gun' in the form of an abnormal ECG, but for paroxysmal arrhythmias the ECG can be entirely normal in the interictal period. A simple 12-lead ECG is informative in less than 10 per cent of patients, due to the transient nature of most cardiac causes of syncope. However, a prolonged QT time can usually be found interictally in patients with the long QT syndrome. The diagnostic yield is somewhat better for 24-h Holter recordings, although this technique continues to be plagued by false-negative results in patients with rare episodes.[120] In addition, there is a substantial risk of finding incidental arrhythmias that are unrelated to the syncopal falls. Note, however, that even incidentally observed ECG abnormalities do have predictive value with respect to mortality. A promising new approach is the loop recorder, which allows for prolonged ECG monitoring during weeks or months.[121] The patients can trigger the recording when they experience symptoms, and back-averaging techniques assure that the entire (pre-)syncopal episode is captured. The recording electrodes can be attached onto the skin or, if this is inconvenient for very long periods, be implanted subcutaneously. Loop recordings are indicated in patients with recurrent unexplained syncope and a high pretest suspicion of underlying cardiac arrhythmia. Syncopal falls related to exercise call for an ECG recording with blood pressure monitoring during and immediately after controlled exercise, but it proves difficult to detect exercise-induced cardiac arrhythmias.[10] Exercise testing can also be used to detect post-exercise orthostatic hypotension.

Additional diagnostic techniques include echocardiography, electrocardiographic monitoring (non-invasive and invasive) and electrophysiological testing. Recommendations for their use can be found in a recent consensus statement.[4]

ELECTROENCEPHALOGRAPHY

The use of EEG should be restricted to the evaluation of patients that are thought to have sustained epileptic falls. It is not helpful in the diagnostic work-up of patients with syncopal falls, where the EEG shows non-specific slowing of background rhythms, irrespective of the pathophysiological mechanism that led to syncope.[122] An EEG is not indicated for patients with 'funny turns', where it may produce potentially misleading information.[123] For patients suspected of having epilepsy, the EEG helps to confirm the diagnosis of a seizure, to classify the seizure type and to assist in predicting the risk of recurrent seizures. Thus, patients that do present with epileptiform abnormalities, even in the absence of concurrent clinical manifestations, have a higher risk of recurrent seizures than patients with a normal interictal recording.[124,125] However, a normal interictal examination does not exclude epilepsy.[11] The diagnostic yield is improved by using provoking stimuli, including hyperventilation, photic stimulation and sleep deprivation.

An example of an EEG registration in a patient with atonic seizures is given in Fig. 16.6. This figure also shows the added value of simultaneously recording multiple electromyographic signals.

One problem in the interpretation of EEG findings is the background incidence of epileptiform abnormalities in the general population of non-epileptic subjects, which can be as high as 2–6 per cent.[66,127] This leads to false-positive results in patients that have never sustained a seizure, let alone in relation to falls. Another problem is that seizures may lead to secondary ECG abnormalities, including supraventricular tachycardias, bradycardia and even asystolia; this may falsely create the impression that the TLC was cardiac in origin, rather than epileptic.[119,128] Co-registration of EEG and ECG is required to unravel this complex sequence of events and help to determine what came first: cardiac arrhythmia or epileptic discharges.

TILT TABLE TESTING

Tilt table testing aims to provoke syncope under controlled conditions.[19,20] Various testing protocols are around, but recent recommendations suggest that patients are first placed in a supine position for at least 25 min.[4] The beat-to-beat blood pressure is monitored non-invasively and in some instances venous cannulation is performed. An ECG with at least three leads is also recorded continuously. The patients are then passively tilted to an upright position (60–70°) for 20–45 min; a foot-board support prevents the subject from sliding down and obviates the need for active muscle contraction to remain in the upright position. Positive responses to tilt testing include a cardioinhibitory response (bradycardia, sometimes even asystole), a vasodepressor response (hypotension) or a mixed response. Some centers recommend that patients who remain without abnormalities during this period receive intravenous isoproterenol or sublingual nitroglycerin to provoke syncope. The sensitivity and specificity of tilt testing are insufficiently known, given the lack of a gold standard. A practical drawback is the generally moderate test–retest reliability.

Tilt testing can be used in the diagnostic work-up of patients with unexplained syncope that is presumed to be vasovagal in origin. A typical vasovagal response to upright tilting is shown in Fig. 16.3 (page 290). Organic heart disease should be absent or, if present, cardiac causes of syncope must have been excluded to facilitate interpretation of an abnormal test result. Tilt testing can also be used to search for bradycardia, because this could have therapeutic consequences in the form of cardiac pacing. Tilt testing can be potentially useful for several other diagnostic purposes, including the differentiation of syncope with jerking movements from epilepsy, and the evaluation of patients with recurrent unexplained falls, syncope or dizziness.

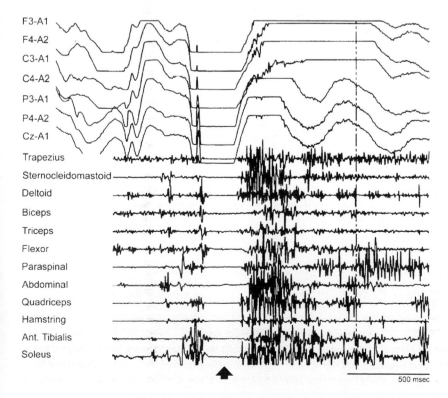

Figure 16.6 *An atonic seizure recorded by a video-polygraph. The patient was a 3-year-old boy who suddenly collapsed down onto his buttocks. This fall corresponded to an electromyograph silent area in all muscles recorded on the polygraph, as well as concurrent electroencephalogram (EEG) changes in the form of a positive–negative–deep positive spike wave, followed by a large, negative slow wave. Note that the second positive spike component was not fully recorded because a large positive EEG potential prevented the pen from going down. (This figure was revised after ref. 126, with permission from the authors and the publisher.)*

F3-A1
F4-A2
C3-A1
C4-A2
P3-A1
P4-A2
Cz-A1
Trapezius
Sternocleidomastoid
Deltoid
Biceps
Triceps
Flexor
Paraspinal
Abdominal
Quadriceps
Hamstring
Ant. Tibialis
Soleus

500 msec

OTHER TESTS

Neuroimaging studies such as computed tomography or magnetic resonance imaging are rarely needed and should be reserved for patients with an abnormal inter-ictal neurological examination. Neuroimaging can be used to detect underlying structural deficits, such as colloid cysts in the third ventricle or Chiari malformations. The diagnostic work-up for patients with MSA or other hypokinetic–rigid syndromes is discussed in Chapter 11. The Multiple Sleep Latency test is the diagnostic standard for narcolepsy. Most patients with narcolepsy also have low or absent levels of hypocretin in their cerebrospinal fluid,[129] but this requires invasive testing. Low catecholamine levels in serum are suggestive of so-called pure autonomic failure,[130] but further discussion of this disorder is beyond the scope of this chapter.

A decision tree

The decision tree outlined in Fig. 16.7 summarizes some of the key steps in the diagnostic work-up of patients with falls and possible TLC. As a first step, one can evaluate whether any environmental factors were obviously responsible for the falling incidents. Examples include so-called 'base of support falls', such as trips over objects on the floor or slips on a slippery surface, and externally applied 'center of mass falls' (e.g. a collision with another person).[131] This group also includes accidents leading to traumatic brain injury and subsequent TLC. When there is no debate that such environmental factors were causally involved, the fall can be classified as 'external' and managed as such.[132] When the role of environmental factors is unclear or frankly denied, a next step is to enquire whether any TLC was associated with the fall. If this was not the case, the fall can be classified as 'intrinsic' (usually defined as a fall that was caused by mobility or balance disorders or misperception of the environment).[133]

Part of the remaining group includes falls that were apparently associated with TLC. Note that falls preceded by TLC are also formally included in the definition of intrinsic falls,[133] but one must be certain that the patient did not faint after the fall. Therefore, care must be taken to distinguish between TLC before or after the fall. Clinicians should be aware that the cause of falls still requires clarification in patients with secondary unconsciousness.

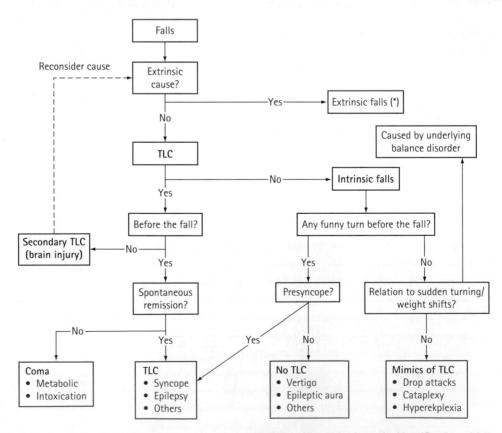

Figure 16.7 *Decision tree in the diagnostic work-up of patients with falls, with emphasis on the identification of falls caused by preceding loss of consciousness. *, The subsequent approach of external falls depends largely upon their frequency and pattern; for more details, see Bloem et al.[117]*

When a TLC appeared to be the cause of the fall, the next step is to determine its duration. Most disorders discussed in this chapter lead to a short-lived and self-limited TLC, either real or apparent. However, metabolic disorders such as hypoglycemia and hypoxia rarely resolve spontaneously, and therefore lead to persistent somnolence or even coma. The same holds true for intoxications of the central nervous system. This category will rarely lead to diagnostic confusion with syncope or other forms of TLC.

The remaining group includes patients with TLC, usually only for several minutes, prior to the fall. This group includes patients with syncope and partial complex or generalized seizures. Several psychogenic and psychiatric disorders can also lead to TLC, even resulting in falls. These include, among others, hyperventilation, but also simulation.

If patients deny a TLC, it is helpful to ask patients whether any other 'funny turns' preceded the fall. It is possible that patients do report symptoms suggestive of presyncope, such as nausea or graying out, but fail to remember whether they had subsequently fainted. Presyncopal symptoms strongly support the presence of syncope, while arguing against a cardiac cause and orthostatic hypotension. Surprisingly many patients report that some form of 'dizziness' preceded the fall. It can be very difficult to clarify whether the patient actually referred to an impending TLC (could be presyncope), spinning sensations (could be vertigo), visual symptoms (could be presyncope), feelings of derealization, or something else. In patients with 'funny turns', it is also important to ask for symptoms that could point to the presence of an epileptic aura.

When the fall was not preceded by any kind of 'funny turn', there is possibly involvement of an underlying balance deficit. This will become evident during physical examination in between falling episodes. Patients with a wide range of balance disorders sustain intrinsic falls in association with shifts of the center of mass. Common fall circumstances include bending, reaching or turning movements, in particular when these are executed abruptly.[3] If the balance disorder is severe enough, even small movements can be destabilizing and the patient starts to fall almost spontaneously. In such patients with apparently unprovoked falls, care must be taken not to attribute everything automatically to the balance deficit and thus miss a possible preceding TLC.

Some fallers do not experience any premonitory symptoms, and their interictal neurological examination does not reveal a balance disorder. In addition, their falls do not seem to be associated with abrupt self-initiated movements, and environmental causes are distinctly absent. Pending a better explanation, both clinicians and patients attribute many of these 'unexplained falls' to a very brief TLC that seemed to have escaped the patient's attention. However, in such patients it is important to consider the disorders with features that mimic a TLC (Table 16.7, page 297).

PROGNOSIS

Despite a complete work-up, up to one-third of the fall types described in this chapter remain unexplained.[4] What to do next? A primary concern is to weigh the potential health risks of the unknown underlying disorder, which can range from rather benign (for example vasovagal syncope) to life-threatening (for example some cardiac arrhythmias). Emphasis is therefore on risk stratification and detection of underlying disorders with an increased mortality risk, and this largely determines the need for ancillary studies or even hospitalization (Fig. 16.8). A detailed medical interview, together with eyewitness reports, a physical examination and an ECG (usually interictal) play a cardinal role in this process.

Table 16.14 summarizes the prognosis for patients with falls caused by syncope. Mortality rates are very low for persons with reflex syncope (including the carotid sinus syndrome) and for young (< 45 years) healthy individuals without prior heart disease and a normal ECG.[134] Note that these subjects do have an increased risk of sustaining injurious falls. The mortality rates among patients with orthostatic hypotension depend on the underlying disorder. For example, prognosis is excellent for syncope caused by volume depletion, but much worse for patients with MSA who have, on average, a markedly reduced survival.[73] The mortality rate among patients with cardiac syncope is increased compared with persons with non-cardiac or unknown causes, mainly because of underlying structural heart disease.[135] Therefore, if there is any possibility of an underling dangerous arrhythmia, the patient should be admitted and

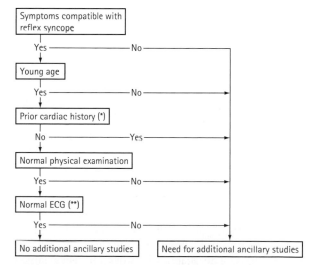

Figure 16.8 *Factors that determine the need for ancillary studies in patients with falls caused by preceding loss of consciousness. *, This includes a family history of sudden death. **, Preferably an ictal recording, but usually the electrocardiogram will have been recorded between episodes.*

Table 16.14 *Prognosis (in terms of mortality rates) among patients with syncope*

Excellent prognosis	Young healthy individuals without heart disease and normal electrocardiogram[a]
	Reflex syncope
Good prognosis	Orthostatic hypotension[b]
	Unexplained syncope[b]
	Cardiac syncope without increased mortality rate
	supraventricular tachycardias (most types)
	atrio-ventricular conduction disturbances
	sick sinus syndrome
Increased mortality rate	Cardiac syncope with underlying structural heart disease
	aortic valve stenosis
	hypertrophic cardiomyopathy
	right ventricular dysplasia
	ventricular tachyarrhythmias
	Pulmonary thromboembolism

[a]Usually reflex syncope or unexplained syncope.
[b]Prognosis depends on severity of underlying disorder, and possible occurrence of injuries.

monitored while waiting for further investigations. Finally, among patients in whom the nature of their syncope remains unknown, the 1-year mortality rate approximates 5 per cent, largely owing to underlying co-morbid illnesses.[136–138] Clinicians must therefore face the reality that among those patients that remain without a definitive diagnosis, even after a careful diagnostic work-up, some will have a potentially life-threatening underlying condition.

CONCLUSIONS

Falls associated with a true or apparent TLC are common, but it is important to bear in mind that a TLC is not synonymous with falls. The clinical approach is strewn with various obstacles, and important decisions often have to be based on initially incomplete histories and physical findings between falls, when many patients are asymptomatic. However, we have indicated that the correct diagnosis can often be made using careful and systematic history taking, preferably including an eye-witness report, and sometimes supplied by relevant physical signs. The diagnostic work-up relies largely upon recognition of particular symptom patterns, in concert with pathophysiological considerations. The complexity of the problem calls for a structured approach where clinicians systematically ask for the indi-

vidual characteristics of the faller, the precipitating events, the premonitory symptoms, the associated features, the postictal manifestations and the effects of treatment. The diagnostic work-up can be supplemented by individually tailored ancillary studies, but physicians ordering these tests must be aware of false-positive and false-negative results. Care must be taken not to mislabel disorders with only an apparent TLC, such as drop attacks or cataplexy. The diagnostic approach revolves around two central themes, the first one being prevention of recurrent falls and the associated injuries, the second one being prevention of secondary morbidity and mortality due to the underlying disease. We conclude this chapter with a brief list of 'rules of thumb' that clinicians may find helpful to memorize for use in daily practice (Table 16.15).

ACKNOWLEDGEMENTS

We thank Dr D. J. Beckley and Dr P. Blijham for their critical comments. Dr W. Wieling is gratefully acknowledged for his advice and assistance in the preparation of several figures. Dr B. R. Bloem was supported by a research grant of the Prinses Beatrix Fonds.

Table 16.15 *Rules of thumb. Nuances and exceptions to the general rule can be found in the text*

Transient loss of consciousness (TLC) is not synonymous to falls

Syncope does not equal TLC

Not all that moves is epilepsy

Syncope is commonly triggered, epilepsy usually is not

Vasovagal syncope is an odd reflex by a normal autonomic nervous system; orthostatic syncope is caused by autonomic failure

Vegetative symptoms (nausea, diaphoresis, pallor or pupillary dilation) prior to the fall suggest autonomic activation in reflex syncope, and argue against orthostatic or cardiac syncope

Falls preceded by isolated TLC are not caused by cerebrovascular disease

Falls in psychiatric patients are usually caused by medication

Drop attacks form a specific idiopathic syndrome; they are not synonymous to 'unexplained falls'

Postictal confusion for > 2 min after the fall suggests epilepsy; postictal confusion < 30 s suggest syncope; absence of postictal confusion following a major episode argues against epilepsy as the underlying cause of falls

Falls due to TLC without any tonic or clonic muscle contraction are unlikely to be caused by epilepsy

A lateral tongue bite strongly suggests epilepsy as cause of the fall; urinary incontinence does not separate epilepsy from syncope

When persons recall hitting the ground, it is unlikely that TLC preceded the fall

REFERENCES

1. Verrill PJ, Aellig WH. 1970. Vasovagal faint in the supine position. *BMJ* 1993;**4**:348.
2. Lempert T, Bauer M, Schmidt D. Syncope: a videometric analysis of 56 episodes of transient cerebral hypoxia. *Ann Neurol* 1994;**36**:233–7.
3. Bloem BR, Grimbergen YAM, Cramer M, et al. Prospective assessment of falls in Parkinson's disease. *J Neurol* 2001;**248**:950–8.
4. Brignole M, Alboni P, Benditt D, et al. Guidelines on management (diagnosis and treatment) of syncope. *Eur Heart J* 2001;**22**:1256–306.
5. Day SC, Cook EF, Funkenstein H, Goldman L. Evaluation and outcome of emergency room patients with transient loss of consciousness. *Am J Med* 1982;**73**: 15–23.
6. Linzer M, Yang EH, Estes NA III, et al. Diagnosing syncope. Part 2: unexplained syncope. Clinical Efficacy Assessment Project of the American College of Physicians. *Ann Intern Med* 1997;**127**:76–86.
7. Kapoor WN, Peterson J, Wieand HS, Karpf M. Diagnostic and prognostic implications of recurrences in patients with syncope. *Am J Med* 1987;**83**:700–8.
8. McIntosh SJ, Lawson J, Kenny RA. Clinical characteristics of vasodepressor, cardioinhibitory, and mixed carotid sinus syndrome in the elderly. *Am J Med* 1993;**95**:203–8.
9. Kenny RA, Richardson DA. Carotid sinus syndrome and falls in older adults. *Am J Geriatr Cardiol* 2001;**10**:97–9.
10. Linzer M, Pontinen M, Gold DT, et al. Impairment of physical and psychosocial function in recurrent syncope. *J Clin Epidemiol* 1991;**44**:1037–43.
11. Hoefnagels WA, Padberg GW, Overweg J, et al. Transient loss of consciousness: the value of the history for distinguishing seizure from syncope. *J Neurol* 1991;**238**:39–43.
12. Benbadis SR, Wolgamuth BR, Goren H, et al. Value of tongue biting in the diagnosis of seizures. *Arch Intern Med* 1995;**155**:2346–9.
13. Lempert T, von Brevern M. The eye movements of syncope. *Neurology* 1996;**46**:1086–8.
14. van Lieshout JJ, Wieling W, Karemaker JM. Vasovagal reaction. *Ned Tijdschrift voor Geneeskunde* 1993;**137**:989–95.
15. Almquist A, Gornick C, Benson W Jr, Dunnigan A, Benditt DG. Carotid sinus hypersensitivity: evaluation of the vasodepressor component. *Circulation* 1985;**71**:927–36.
16. Benditt DG, Petersen M, Lurie KG, et al. Cardiac pacing for prevention of recurrent vasovagal syncope *Ann Intern Med* 1995;**122**:204–9.
17. Kapoor WN. Syncope with abrupt termination of exercise. *Am J Med* 1989;**87**:597–9.
18. Sakaguchi S, Shultz JJ, Remole SC, et al. Syncope associated with exercise, a manifestation of neurally mediated syncope. *Am J Cardiol* 1995;**75**:476–81.
19. Kenny RA, Ingram A, Bayliss J, Sutton R. Head-up tilt: a useful test for investigating unexplained syncope. *Lancet* 1986;**i**:1352–5.
20. Benditt DG, Ferguson DW, Grubb BP, et al. Tilt table testing for assessing syncope. American College of Cardiology. *J Am Coll Cardiol* 1996;**28**:263–75.
21. Krediet CTP, van Dijk N, Linzer M, et al. Management of vasovagal syncope: controlling or aborting faints by leg crossing and muscle tensing. *Circulation* 2002;**106**:1684–9.
22. Davies AJ, Steen N, Kenny RA. Carotid sinus hypersensitivity is common in older patients presenting to an accident and emergency department with unexplained falls. *Age Ageing* 2001;**30**:289–293.
23. Wenning GK, Ben-Shlomo Y, Magalhaes M, et al. Clinical features and natural history of multiple system atrophy. An analysis of 100 cases. *Brain* 1994;**117**:835–45.
24. Wenning GK, Ben Shlomo Y, Magalhaes M, et al. Clinicopathological study of 35 cases of multiple system atrophy. *J Neurol Neurosurg Psychiatry* 1995;**58**:160–6.
25. McKeith IG, Galasko D, Kosaka K, et al. Consensus guidelines for the clinical and pathologic diagnosis of dementia with Lewy bodies (DLB): report of the consortium on DLB international workshop. *Neurology* 1996;**47**:1113–24.
26. van Dijk JG, Haan J, Zwinderman K, et al. Autonomic nervous system dysfunction in Parkinson's disease: relationships with age, medication, duration, and severity. *J Neurol Neurosurg Psychiatry* 1993;**56**:1090–5.
27. van Dijk N, Harms MP, Wieling W. Three patients with unrecognized orthostatic intolerance. *Ned Tijdschr Geneeskd* 2000;**144**:249–54.
28. Wieling W, Harms MP, Kortz RA, Linzer M. Initial orthostatic hypotension as a cause of recurrent syncope: a case report. *Clin Auton Res* 2001;**11**:269–70.
29. The Multicentre Postinfarction Research Group. Risk stratification and survival after myocardial infarction. *N Engl J Med* 1983;**309**:331–6.
30. Wilk JS, Nardone AL, Jennings CA, Crausman RS. Unexplained syncope: when to suspect pulmonary thromboembolism. *Geriatrics* 1995;**50**:46–50.
31. el Sayed H, Hainsworth R. Salt supplement increases plasma volume and orthostatic tolerance in patients with unexplained syncope. *Heart* 1996;**75**:134–40.
32. Jansen RW, Lipsitz LA. Postprandial hypotension: epidemiology, pathophysiology, and clinical management. *Ann Intern Med* 1995;**122**:286–95.
33. Jonsson PV, Lipsitz LA, Kelley M, Koestner J. Hypotensive responses to common daily activities in institutionalized elderly. A potential risk for recurrent falls. *Arch Intern Med* 1990;**150**:1518–24.
34. Lipsitz LA, Fullerton KJ. Postprandial blood pressure reduction in healthy elderly. *J Am Geriatr Soc* 1986;**34**:267–70.
35. Micieli G, Martignoni E, Cavallini A, et al. Postprandial and orthostatic hypotension in Parkinson's disease. *Neurology* 1987;**37**:386–93.
36. Mehagnoul-Schipper DJ, Boerman RH, Hoefnagels WH, Jansen RW. Effect of levodopa on orthostatic and postprandial hypotension in elderly Parkinsonian patients. *J Gerontol A Biol Sci Med Sci* 2001;**56**:M749–55.
37. Jansen RW, Connelly CM, Kelley-Gagnon MM, et al. Postprandial hypotension in elderly patients with unexplained syncope. *Arch Intern Med* 1995;**155**:945–52.
38. Vloet LC, Mehagnoul-Schipper DJ, Hoefnagels WH, Jansen RW. The influence of low-, normal-, and high-carbohydrate meals on blood pressure in elderly patients with postprandial hypotension. *J Gerontol A Biol Sci Med Sci* 2001;**56**:M744–8.
39. Mathias CJ, Kimber JR. Treatment of postural hypotension. *J Neurol Neurosurg Psychiatry* 1998;**65**: 285–9.

40. van Lieshout JJ, ten Harkel AD, Wieling W. Physical manoeuvres for combating orthostatic dizziness in autonomic failure. *Lancet* 1992;**339**: 897–8.

41. Wieling W. Physical measures. In: Robertson D,Low PA, Burnstock G, Biaggioni I, eds. *Primer on the autonomic nervous system*, 2nd edn. New York: Academic Press, 2003;in press.

42. Ector H, Reybrouck T, Heidbuchel H, et al. Tilt training: a new treatment for recurrent neurocardiogenic syncope and severe orthostatic intolerance. *Pacing Clin Electrophysiol* 1998;**21**:193–6.

43. Di Girolamo E, Di Iorio C, Leonzio L, et al. Usefulness of a tilt training program for the prevention of refractory neurocardiogenic syncope in adolescents: a controlled study. *Circulation* 1999;**100**: 1798–801.

44. Benditt DG, Fahy GJ, Lurie KG, et al. Pharmacotherapy of neurally mediated syncope. *Circulation* 1999;**100**:1242–8.

45. Di Girolamo E, Di Iorio C, Sabatini P, et al. Effects of paroxetine hydrochloride, a selective serotonin reuptake inhibitor, on refractory vasovagal syncope: a randomized, double-blind, placebo-controlled study. *J Am Coll Cardiol* 1999;**33**: 1227–30.

46. Wieling W, Cortelli P, Mathias CJ. Treating neurogenic orthostatic hypotension. In: Appenzeller O, ed. *Handbook of clinical neurology, vol 75(31): the autonomic nervous system part ii dysfunctions*. Amsterdam: Elsevier, 2000;713–29.

47. Freeman R, Landsberg L. The treatment of orthostatic hypotension with dihydroxyphenylserine. *Clin Neuropharmacol* 1991;**14**:296–304.

48. Freeman R, Young J, Landsberg L, Lipsitz L. The treatment of postprandial hypotension in autonomic failure with 3 4-DL-threo-dihydroxyphenylserine. *Neurology* 1996;**47**:1414–20.

49. Mathias CJ, Senard JM, Braune S, et al. L-threo-dihydroxyphenylserine (L-threo-DOPS; droxidopa) in the management of neurogenic orthostatic hypotension: a multi-national, multi-center, dose-ranging study in multiple system atrophy and pure autonomic failure. *Clin Auton Res* 2001;**11**:235–42.

50. Hasegawa Y, Mukai E, Matsusoka Y, et al. Effect of oral L-threo-3 4-dihydroxyphenylserine (L-DOPS) on orthostatic hypotension in Parkinson's disease. *Mov Disord* 1997;**12**(Suppl 1):88.

51. Kaufmann H, Oribe E, Yahr MD. Differential effect of L-threo-3,4-dihydroxyphenylserine in pure autonomic failure and multiple system atrophy with autonomic failure. *J Neural Transm Park Dis Dement Sect* 1991;**3**:143–8.

52. Jansen RW, Peeters TL, Lenders JW, et al. Somatostatin analog octreotide (SMS 201–995) prevents the decrease in blood pressure after oral glucose loading in the elderly. *J Clin Endocrinol Metab* 1989;**68**: 752–6.

53. Connolly SJ, Sheldon R, Roberts RS, Gent M. The North American Vasovagal Pacemaker Study (VPS). A randomized trial of permanent cardiac pacing for the prevention of vasovagal syncope. *J Am Coll Cardiol* 1999;**33**:16–20.

54. Kenny RA, Richardson DA, Steen N, et al. Carotid sinus syndrome: a modifiable risk factor for nonaccidental falls in older adults (SAFE PACE). *J Am Coll Cardiol* 2001;**38**:1491–6.

55. Gosselin C, Walker PM. 1996. Subclavian steal syndrome: existence, clinical features, diagnosis and management. *Semin Vasc Surg* **9**: 93–97.

56. Warlow CP, Dennis MS, van Gijn J, et al. *Stroke: a practical guide to management*. Oxford: Blackwell Science, 1996.

57. Ikeno T, Shigematsu H, Miyakoshi M, et al. An analytic study of epileptic falls. *Epilepsia* 1985;**26**:612–21.

58. Aicardi J. *Diseases of the nervous system in childhood*. Oxford: Blackwell Scientific Publications Ltd, 1992.

59. Wolf P. Juvenile myoclonic epilepsy. In: Roger J, Bureau M, Dravet C, Dreifuss FE, et al, eds. *Epileptic syndromes in infancy, childhood and adolescence*. London: John Libbey & Company, 2002;313–27.

60. Lance JW. Myoclonic jerks and falls: aetiology, classification and treatment. *Med J Aust* 1968;**1**:113–19.

61. Gambardella A, Reutens DC, Andermann F, et al. Late-onset drop attacks in temporal lobe epilepsy: a reevaluation of the concept of temporal lobe syncope. *Neurology* 1994;**44**: 1074–8.

62. Maehara T, Shimizu H. Surgical outcome of corpus callosotomy in patients with drop attacks. *Epilepsia* 2001;**42**:67–71.

63. Roos RA, van Dijk JG. Reflex-epilepsy induced by immersion in hot water. Case report and review of the literature. *Eur Neurol* 1988;**28**:6–10.

64. van Donselaar CA, Geerts AT, Schimsheimer RJ. Usefulness of an aura for classification of a first generalized seizure. *Epilepsia* 1990;**31**:529–35.

65. Schon F, Blau JN. Epilepsy and headache. *Lancet* 1988;**1**:187–8.

66. Leniger T, Isbruch K, von den Driesch DS, et al. Seizure-associated headache in epilepsy. *Epilepsia* 2001;**42**:1176–9.

67. Hoefnagels WA, Padberg GW, Overweg J, Roos RA, et al. Syncope or seizure? The diagnostic value of the EEG and hyperventilation test in transient loss of consciousness. *J Neurol Neurosurg Psychiatry* 1991;**54**:953–6.

68. Hornsveld H, Garssen B. The low specificity of the Hyperventilation Provocation Test. *J Psychosom Res* 1996;**41**:435–49.

69. Hornsveld HK, Garssen B, Dop MJ, et al. Double-blind placebo-controlled study of the hyperventilation provocation test and the validity of the hyperventilation syndrome. *Lancet* 1996;**348**:154–8.

70. Headache Classification Committee of the International Headache Society. Classification and diagnostic criteria for headache disorders, cranial neuralgias and facial pain. *Cephalalgia* 1988;**8**(Suppl 7):1–96.

71. Markush RE, Karp HR, Heyman A, O'Fallon WM. Epidemiologic study of migraine symptoms in young women. *Neurology* 1975;**25**:430–5.

72. Lammers GJ. Narcolepsy. Thesis. Delft, Eburon, 1999.

73. Overeem S, Mignot E, van Dijk JG, Lammers GJ. Narcolepsy: clinical features, new pathophysiologic insights, and future perspectives. *J Clin Neurophysiol* 2001;**18**:78–105.

74. Overeem S, Lammers GJ, van Dijk JG. Weak with laughter. *Lancet* 1999;**354**:838.

75. Hartse KM, Zorick FJ, Sicklesteel JM, Roth T. Isolated cataplexy: a familial study. *Henry Ford Hosp Med J* 1988;**36**:24–7.

76. Autret A, Lucas B, Henry-Lebras F, de Toffol B. Symptomatic narcolepsies. *Sleep* 1994;**17**:S21–4.

77. Guilleminault C, Gelb M. Clinical aspects and features of cataplexy. *Adv Neurol* 1995;**67**:65–77.

78. Overeem S, Lammers GJ, van Dijk JG. Cataplexy: 'tonic immobility' rather than 'REM sleep atonia? *Sleep Med* 2002;**3**:471–377.

79. Siegel JM, Nienhuis R, Fahringer HM, et al. Neuronal activity in narcolepsy: identification of cataplexy-related cells in the medial medulla. *Science* 1991;**252**:1315–18.

80. Lammers GJ, Arends J, Declerck AC, et al. Gammahydroxybutyrate and narcolepsy: a double-blind placebo-controlled study. *Sleep* 1993;**16**:216–20.

81. The US Xyrem Multicenter Study Group. A randomized, double blind, placebo-controlled multicenter trial comparing the effects of three doses of orally administered sodium oxybate with placebo for the treatment of narcolepsy. *Sleep* 2002;**25**:42–49.

82. Lipsitz LA. The drop attack: a common geriatric symptom. *J Am Geriatr Soc* 1983;**31**:617–20.

83. Ishiyama G, Ishiyama A, Jacobson K, Baloh RW. Drop attacks in older patients secondary to an otologic cause. *Neurology* 2001;**57**:1103–6.

84. Stevens DL, Matthews WB. Cryptogenic drop attacks: an affliction of women. *BMJ* 1973;**1**:439–42.

85. Meissner I, Wiebers DO, Swanson JW, O'Fallon WM. The natural history of drop attacks. *Neurology* 1986;**36**:1029–34.

86. Brocklehurst JC, Exton-Smith AN, Lempert Barber SM, et al. Fracture of the femur in old age: a two-centre study of associated clinical factors and the cause of the fall. *Age Ageing* 1978;**7**:2–15.

87. Boddie HG, Stewart-Wynne EG. Quadriceps myopathy – entity or syndrome? *Arch Neurol* 1974;**31**:60–2.

88. Gray P, Hildebrand K. Fall risk factors in Parkinson's disease. *J Neurosci Nursing* 2000;**32**:222–8.

89. Ashburn A, Stack E, Pickering R, Ward C. Predicting fallers in a community-based sample of people with Parkinson's disease. *Gerontology* 2001;**47**:277–81.

90. Kremer M. Sitting, standing and walking. *BMJ* 1958;**2**:63–8.

91. Botez MI. Drop attacks, chalastic fits, and occult hydrocephalus. *Neurology* 1979;**29**:1555–6.

92. Dey AB, Stout NR, Kenny RA. Cardiovascular syncope is the most common cause of drop attacks in the elderly. *Pacing Clin Electrophysiol* 1997;**20**:818–19.

93. Brown P. The startle syndrome. *Mov Disord* 2002;**17**(Suppl 2):S79–82.

94. Tijssen MA. Hyperekplexia. Thesis. Delft: Eburon, 1997.

95. Tijssen MA, Schoemaker HC, Edelbroek PJ, et al. The effects of clonazepam and vigabatrin in hyperekplexia. *J Neurol Sci* 1997;**149**:63–7.

96. Kapoor WN, Peterson JR, Karpf M. Micturition syncope. A reappraisal. *JAMA* 1985;**253**:796–8.

97. Cumming RG. Epidemiology of medication-related falls and fractures in the elderly. *Drugs Aging* 1998,**12**:43–53.

98. Leipzig RM, Cumming RG, Tinetti ME. Drugs and falls in older people: a systemic review and meta-analysis: 1. psychotropic drugs. *J Am Geriatr Soc* 1999;**47**:30–9.

99. Grisso JA, Kelsey JL, Strom BL, et al. Risk factors for falls as a cause of hip fracture in women. *N Engl J Med* 1991;**324**:1326–31.

100. Caramel VMB, Remarque EJ, Knook DL, et al. Use of medications related to function and falls in the 85-plus population of Leiden the Netherlands. *J Am Geriatr Soc* 1998;**46**:1178–9.

101. Grubb BP, Gerard G, Wolfe DA, et al. Syncope and seizures of psychogenic origin: identification with head- upright tilt table testing. *Clin Cardiol* 1992;**15**:839–42.

102. Mathias CJ, Deguchi K, Schatz I. Observations on recurrent syncope and presyncope in 641 patients. *Lancet* 2001;**357**:348–53.

103. Shaw FE, Kenny RA. The overlap between syncope and falls in the elderly. *Postgrad Med* 1997;**73**:635–9.

104. O'Mahony D, Foote C. Prospective evaluation of unexplained syncope, dizziness, and falls among community-dwelling elderly adults. *J Gerontol Med Sci* 1998;**53**(A):M435–40.

105. Hanlon JT, Linzer M, MacMillan JP, et al. Syncope and presyncope associated with probable adverse drug reactions. *Arch Intern Med* 1990;**150**:2309–12.

106. Stephen LJ, Brodie MJ. Epilepsy in elderly people. *Lancet* 2000;**355**:1441–6.

107. Kapoor WN, Fortunato M, Hanusa BH, Schulberg HC. Psychiatric illnesses in patients with syncope. *Am J Med* 1995;**99**:505–12.

108. Zaidi A, Clough P, Scheepers B, Fitzpatrick A. Treatment resistant epilepsy or convulsive syncope. *BMJ* 1998;**317**:869–70.

109. Lempert T. Recognizing syncope: pitfalls and surprises. *J R Soc Med* 1996;**89**: 372–5.

110. Allum JH, Carpenter MG, Honegger F, et al. Age-dependent variations in the directional sensitivity of balance corrections and compensatory arm movements. *J Physiol (Lond)* 2002;**542**:643–63.

111. The Consensus Committee of the American Autonomic Society and the American Academy of Neurology. Consensus statement on the definition of orthostatic hypotension, pure autonomic failure, and multiple system atrophy. *Neurology* 1996;**46**:1470.

112. Brignole M, Alboni P, Benditt D, et al. Task force on syncope European Society of Cardiology. Part 1. The initial evaluation of patients with syncope. *Europace* 2001;**3**:253–60.

113. Ward C, Kenny RA. Reproducibility of orthostatic hypotension in symptomatic elderly. *Am J Med* 1996;**100**:418–22.

114. Harbison J, Newton JL, Seifer C, Kenny RA. Stokes Adams attacks and cardiovascular syncope. *Lancet* 2002;**359**:158–60.

115. Puisieux F, Bulckaen H, Fauchais AL, et al. Ambulatory blood pressure monitoring and postprandial hypotension in elderly persons with falls or syncopes. *J Gerontol A Biol Sci Med Sci* 2000;**55**:M535–40.

116. Brignole M, Alboni P, Benditt D, et al. Task force on syncope European Society of Cardiology. Part 2. Diagnostic tests and treatment: summary of recommendations. *Europace* 2001;**3**:261–8.

117. Bloem BR, Boers I, Cramer M, et al. Falls in the elderly. I. Identification of risk factors. *Wien Klin Wochenschr* 2001;**113**:352–62.

118. Libman MD, Potvin L, Coupal L, Grover SA. Seizure vs. syncope: measuring serum creatine kinase in the emergency department. *J Gen Intern Med* 1991;**6**:408–12.

119. Anzola GP. Predictivity of plasma prolactin levels in differentiating epilepsy from pseudoseizures: a prospective study. *Epilepsia* 1993;**34**:1044–8.

120. Gordon M, Huang M, Gryfe CI. An evaluation of falls, syncope, and dizziness by prolonged ambulatory cardiographic monitoring in a geriatric institutional setting. *J Am Geriatr Soc* 1982;**30**:6–12.

121. Kapoor WN. Syncope. *N Engl J Med* 2000;**343**:1856–62.

122. Brenner RP. Electroencephalography in syncope. *J Clin Neurophysiol* 1997;**14**:197–209.

123. Smith D, Bartolo R, Pickles RM, Tedman BM. Requests for electroencephalography in a district general hospital: retrospective and prospective audit. *BMJ* 2001;**322**:954–7.

124. Berg AT, Shinnar S. The risk of seizure recurrence following a first unprovoked seizure: a quantitative review. *Neurology* 1991;**41**:965–72.

125. Stroink H, Brouwer OF, Arts WF, et al. The first unprovoked, untreated seizure in childhood: a hospital based study of the accuracy of the diagnosis, rate of recurrence, and long term outcome after recurrence. Dutch study of epilepsy in childhood. *J Neurol Neurosurg Psychiatry* 1998;**64**:595–600.

126. Oguni H, Fukuyama Y, Tanaka T, et al. Myoclonic-astatic epilepsy of early childhood – clinical and EEG analysis of myoclonic–astatic seizures, and discussions on the nosology of the syndrome. *Brain Dev* 2001;**23**:757–64.

127. Zivin L, Marsan CA. Incidence and prognostic significance of 'epileptiform' activity in the EEG of non-epileptic subjects. *Brain* 1968;**91**:751–78.

128. Gilchrist JM. Arrhythmogenic seizures: diagnosis by simultaneous EEG/ECG recording. *Neurology* 1985;**35**:1503–6.

129. Nishino S, Ripley B, Overeem S, et al. Hypocretin (orexin) deficiency in human narcolepsy. *Lancet* 2000;**355**:39–40.

130. Mathias CJ, Polinsky RJ. Separating the primary autonomic failure syndromes, multiple system atrophy, and pure autonomic failure from Parkinson's disease. *Adv Neurol* 1999;**80**:353–61.

131. Maki BE, Holliday PJ, Topper AK. A prospective study of postural balance and risk of falling in an ambulatory and independent elderly population. *J Gerontol* 1994;**49**:M72–84.

132. Boers I, Gerschlager W, Stalenhoef PA, Bloem BR. Falls in the elderly. II. Strategies for prevention. *Wien Klin Wochenschr* 2001;**113**:398–407.

133. Lach HW, Reed AT, Arfken CL, et al. Falls in the elderly: reliability of a classification system. *J Am Geriatr Soc* 1991;**39**:197–202.

134. Martin TP, Hanusa BH, Kapoor WN. Risk stratification of patients with syncope. *Ann Emerg Med* 1997;**29**:459–66.

135. Kapoor WN, Hanusa BH. Is syncope a risk factor for poor outcomes? Comparison of patients with and without syncope. *Am J Med* 1996;**100**:646–55.

136. Silverstein MD, Singer DE, Mulley AG, et al. Patients with syncope admitted to medical intensive care units. *JAMA* 1982;**248**:1185–9.

137. Kapoor WN, Karpf M, Wieand S, et al. A prospective evaluation and follow-up of patients with syncope. *N Engl J Med* 1983;**309**:197–204.

138. Raviele A, Proclemer A, Gasparini G, et al. Long-term follow-up of patients with unexplained syncope and negative electrophysiologic study. *Eur Heart J* 1989;**10**:127–32.

17

Rehabilitation of balance disorders in the patient with vestibular pathology

MAROUSA PAVLOU, ANNE SHUMWAY-COOK, FAY B. HORAK, LUCY YARDLEY AND ADOLFO M. BRONSTEIN

INTRODUCTION

The often irreversible nature of lesions within the vestibular system makes rehabilitation an important therapeutic option. Vestibular disorders are a frequent cause of balance and related gait complaints in the general population.[1] In addition, lesions to peripheral and central vestibular structures frequently accompany central neural injury, affecting a patient's ability to recover from a traumatic brain injury.[2] Because of the scope and severity of the problem, interest in the development of rehabilitation programs directed at maximizing compensation for vestibular lesions has grown in recent years.[3]

This chapter describes a 'systems approach' to rehabilitation of balance disorders in patients with vestibular deficits. We begin by defining a 'systems approach', the physiological rationale upon which it is based, and the impairments associated with various vestibular pathologies. We then explain a variety of components required for a comprehensive assessment and identification of primary and secondary impairments constraining function. Finally, we describe the treatment of balance disorders in patients with vestibular deficits.

A systems approach to rehabilitation

A key aspect of a systems approach to rehabilitation of balance disorders is the understanding that control of posture and balance emerges from an interaction of many systems which are organized in accordance with the stability requirements inherent in the task being performed, and constrained by the environment (see Chapter 1). Since lesions of peripheral and central vestibular structures vary in their type and severity,

patients with vestibular disorders often show a wide range of functional limitations that must be assessed independently of one another.[4,5] Vestibular deficits affect stance, gait, eye–head coordination and provoke various vertiginous symptoms (see Chapters 6 and 9). The extent of these deficits are dependent on both the nature and extent of vestibular pathology and the individual's capacity to compensate for the pathology. Thus, a systems approach to balance rehabilitation begins with a comprehensive assessment to identify the signs and symptoms of vestibular pathology.

A thorough assessment involves a variety of tests, measurements and observations to: (1) document functional limitations (defined by the individual's capacity to perform everyday balance and gait activities without restriction,[6] and (2) determine specific impairments that constrain functional abilities.[7,8] Impairments are defined as psychological, physiological, or anatomical problems related to structure or function.[9] Impairments can be the direct result of vestibular pathology, as in the presence of vertigo or imbalance, or indirectly associated with pathology, such as the development of musculoskeletal problems in the neck region because of excessive splinting or guarding to minimize head movement-provoked dizziness, or cardiopulmonary deconditioning secondary to inactivity. Treatment involves an individualized program of exercises and activities aimed at (1) remediating direct and indirect impairments, (2) maximizing function, and (3) facilitating the natural compensatory process.

Physiological rationale

The purpose of a rehabilitation approach for vestibular problems is to facilitate the ability of the central nervous system (CNS) to compensate for vestibular deficits and to seek resolution of the underlying pathological mechanisms when possible. The best model for understanding CNS plasticity as the basis for recovery of function has been compensation for vestibular injury. Studies have shown that the neural basis for compensation is distributed throughout the nervous system such that lesions in or pharmacological depression of the cerebellum, cortex, spinal cord, brainstem or sensory systems can prevent or reduce the capacity for compensation. Inactivity, whether from bedrest, fear, anxiety or other factors, has also been demonstrated to delay and impair complete compensation.[10] Other factors, which can affect the capacity to compensate for a vestibular lesion, are listed in Table 17.1.

Several physiological mechanisms have been proposed to account for functional changes associated with CNS compensation, including (1) central sensory substitution, (2) rebalancing of tonic activity in central pathways (for review see Curthoys and Halmagyi)[11], and (3) physiological habituation:

1. Central sensory substitution mechanisms are the basis by which vision and somatosensory information can partly substitute for missing vestibular information for the purpose of dynamic and static orientation.[12,13] Studies have shown an increased reliance on visual information[14] or an increased responsiveness to somatosensory-triggered equilibrium responses following the absence of vestibular inputs.[15]
2. Rebalancing central tonic neural activity has been shown to accompany behavioral signs of recovery of function following vestibular injury. As recovery of

symmetric tonic activity in vestibular nuclei occurs, which is considered a direct measure of CNS compensation, abnormal eye movements and asymmetrical postures resolve following a unilateral vestibular lesion. Compensatory processes that re-establish symmetry of tonic vestibular nuclei activity include cerebellar disinhibition, increased sensitivity to visual and somatosensory input, and active sensorimotor activity.[10,11,16]

3. Physiological habituation is a decrease in response magnitude to repetitive sensory stimulation. Habituation of vertigo by systematically repeating the symptom provoking head movements or positions has been known for many years[17] and probably is the result of multiple physiologic mechanisms.

IMPAIRMENTS ASSOCIATED WITH VESTIBULAR PATHOLOGIES

Unilateral vestibular loss

Primary and secondary impairments in patients with unilateral vestibular loss (UVL) can involve all components listed in Table 17.2. Immediately after an acute

Table 17.1 *Factors interfering with clinical recovery following vestibular lesions*

Age	
CNS lesions	
Peripheral somatosensory disorders	
Visual disorders	Reduced visual acuity
	Modified optics (e.g. cataract operation)
	Strabismus
Visual dependence	
Cervical or other spine disorders	
Psychosocial factors	
Medical treatment	Inappropriate surgery
	Antivertiginous drugs
	Tranquilizers
	Anesthesia
Lack of mobility	Orthopedic
	Forced bedrest or patient advised not to move
	Psychological/fear

Table 17.2 *Balance impairments commonly associated with vestibular pathology*

I. Balance	
A. Musculoskeletal	1. Neck/back muscle tension
	2. Limited range of joint motion
	3. Pain (headache, neck/back pain, etc.)
B. Sensory	1. Visual dependence/visual vertigo
	2. Somatosensory dependence
	3. Poor use of vestibular information
	4. Inflexible sensory strategy
C. Motor	1. Poor alignment
	2. Excessive hip strategy
	3. Lack of hip strategy
	4. Lack of stepping strategy
	5. Inefficient, inflexible movement strategy
	6. Asymmetry
II. Eye–head coordination	
A. Poor gaze stabilization	1. External displacements
	2. Voluntary head movements
B. Poor head stabilization	
III. Abnormal perception of stability and motion	
A. Vertigo	1. Positional
	2. Movement related
B. Internal representation of posture	1. Poor sense of vertical
	2. Inaccurate sense of stability limits

UVL, patients have constant vertigo and lean their head and trunks and show spontaneous nystagmus to the side of the lesion. Although they are not able to stand in conditions requiring vestibular information for orientation for the first few weeks after UVL, this capacity often recovers when they are fully compensated.[18] Postural and locomotor ataxia is usually caused by left/right asymmetries and unsteadiness associated with head movements. Eye–head coordination during both voluntary and passive head movements is usually disturbed. Their internal perception of vertical and their stability limits may be skewed to one side, so they may actually throw themselves off balance by attempting a skewed equilibrium position.

Patients with unilateral loss of vestibular function often compensate with few long-term symptoms. In general, recovery of tonic impairments such as postural instability in quiet stance is faster and greater than that of dynamic impairments such as gait ataxia when patients move their heads. At the clinical level, well-compensated patients with complete UVL show either no spontaneous nystagmus or only some in the dark. The Romberg test is normal but some patients continue to report transient vertigo and oscillopsia during fast head movements as well as reduced postural balance during a demanding task. The way in which compensation for vestibular injuries occurs depends considerably on the time course of the disease process. Vestibular nerve lesions with slow rate of progression such as acoustic neuromas often cause little or no balance symptoms. Acute disruption of vestibular input, as in vestibular neuronitis, labyrinthitis, accidents or surgical trauma cause sudden, severe balance deficits. The intense initial symptoms resolve quickly over a few weeks but the presence of protracted, unresolved balance and dizziness symptoms is well known to clinicians.

Bilateral vestibular loss

Patients with bilaterally defective vestibular function are initially markedly unsteady but gradually recover. The degree of recovery depends on the cause and extent of bilateral vestibular loss (BVL).[19,20] When ototoxicity is the causative factor, improvement is often greater than when the cause of BVL is caused by a slowly progressive vestibular loss such as autoimmune or neurodegenerative disease.[20] If BVL is complete, patients will never recover the ability to balance when both vision and surface information is inadequate for an orientation reference, even with substantial improvements following rehabilitation. As a consequence, these patients need to be advised of dangerous environments and occupational situations such as swimming in the dark or underwater, walking on uneven surfaces in complex visual environments and working at heights. Perhaps because of an inability to optimally stabilize the head with reference to gravity, they may also be unable to generate appropriate hip/trunk movements to control equilibrium when a hip strategy is required (see below).[21,22] Individuals with BVL also experience falls to a greater extent than patients with UVL and should be informed about this increased risk and the use of assistive devices, especially for elderly patients.[23] If the loss of vestibular function occurs symmetrically and slowly these patients may never experience vertigo.

In the acute stages, these patients rely heavily on their visual system to control balance. Gradually, they become less unsteady in response to visual motion, suggesting that they progressively make better use of proprioceptive information from the lower limbs.[14,24] In patients with BVL, some postural response latencies are normal, even in the absence of vision.[25] Allum et al.[26] have suggested that abnormal magnitudes of muscular synergies are responsible for the unsteadiness in patients with BVL.

One consequence of sustaining BVL is oscillopsia, which is the unpleasant illusion of movement or blurring of images when travelling on vehicles, walking or performing head movements (see Chapter 7). The attenuation of this symptom with time may be partly due to the enhancement of the cervico-ocular reflex,[27,28] although a direct correlation between the magnitude of the cervico-ocular reflex and the intensity of the oscillopsia is not apparent.[29] Clinical evidence suggests that the cerebellum is necessary for the development of this neck afferent control of eye movements.[30] Other compensatory mechanisms that help to maintain gaze stability include reduced voluntary head movements (which is counterproductive for the rehabilitation of the patients),[29] substitution of slow phase compensatory eye movements by small, saccadic eye movements,[27,30,31] and an increased tolerance to retinal slip through a decreased sensitivity to visual motion.[32,33] Although most patients adapt to oscillopsia and some individuals experience a complete eradication of it,[34] others find that it remains a severe handicap, with a decrease in daily activities and the development of a more sedentary lifestyle.[29] It seems that a direct correlation exists between perceived disability due to oscillopsia and the degree of control patients feel they have over the situation: the less control an individual believes they have over their condition, the higher their perceived disability/handicap scores.[31] Thus, rehabilitation programs serve a dual purpose in the patient with vestibular pathology: they provide guidance with respect to exercises and activities that promote the compensatory process and provide patients with appropriate information about their condition and the expected outcome of treatment so they feel more in control of their symptoms (see Chapter 19).

Central vestibular disorders

Common central vestibular disorders associated with dizziness include cerebellar disease (multiple sclerosis, cerebellar degenerations, tumor and Chiari malformation), vascular disease (brainstem stroke and transient ischemic attack), migraine and head injuries (e.g. post-concussion syndrome). Patients complaining of dizziness following a head injury may have a combination of central and peripheral vestibular deficits as well as neck injury.[35] Although extensive evidence exists for the benefit of physical therapy intervention for peripheral vestibular disorders, only a few studies[36–39] have been done on the use of rehabilitation protocols in central vestibular disorders, and none of these studies included a control group. A recent study by Whitney et al.[40] looked at the effect of a customized vestibular physical therapy program for patients diagnosed with migraine-related vestibulopathy or vestibular dysfunction with a history of migraine headache. After treatment, both patient populations showed a significant decrease in risk of falls and perceived handicap from dizziness as well as an increase in balance confidence.[40] Furthermore, patients taking antimigraine medication in conjunction with physical therapy intervention showed greater improvement as opposed to the non-medicated group.[40] Studies including a heterogeneous population of peripheral, central and multiple deficits provide varying results, with some reporting poor outcome for the last two groups[3,41] and others reporting a similar degree of improvement as patients with stable peripheral vestibular disorders.[42,43] However, overall, patients with central vestibular disorders are expected to require a longer period for improvement and have worse outcomes of rehabilitation than patients with peripheral vestibular disorders.[3,41] These results may depend on the location and extent of the central deficit and the additional complications that result including cognitive and neuromuscular impairments. The degree of benefit that may be gained through physical therapy intervention will not truly be known until proper controlled clinical trials for central vestibular disorders are conducted.

Fluctuating vestibular deficits and benign paroxysmal positional vertigo

A minority of patients will have pure UVL or BVL. Many patients have incomplete damage, fluctuating function (Ménière's disease), benign paroxysmal positioning vertigo (BPPV) (see below and Chapter 9), and slowly progressive tumors and can show additional CNS, medical or psychological complications. It is much more difficult for the CNS to compensate for a fluctuating vestibular deficit (e.g. Ménière's disease) or for multiple deficits than for a steady loss of any kind. Although Black et al.[44] found that patients with fluctuating peripheral vestibular disorders show the same postural and symptomatic improvement as patients with a stable condition, Hahn et al.[45] using visuo-vestibular biofeedback found that postural control improvements in Ménière's disease

patients were transient in nature. In general, these patients are more difficult to treat with an exercise approach than those with a steady loss of function, except for specific exercises for BPPV (see below).

Balance impairments vary in patients with fluctuating, irritative vestibular lesions but often include postural instability under altered sensory environments such as in moving visual or surface environments. The patients often feel quite unsteady and over-respond to postural displacements. The dizziness is often associated with cognitive complaints such as inability to concentrate, poor memory, etc., especially during dynamic balancing tasks such as walking while moving their heads.

Visual vertigo

A subgroup of patients with balance disorders complain that their symptoms are precipitated or exacerbated by complex visual surroundings.[46,47] These include situations with repetitive or unstable visual patterns such as those encountered while walking down supermarket aisles, in crowds or viewing moving scenes.[46] Symptoms may also be precipitated by driving, particularly in certain conditions such as going over the brow of a hill or around bends in what is known as motorist disorientation syndrome.[48] Patients with vestibular disorders appear to rely more on visual cues for postural stability, showing greater postural sway in response to moving visual scenes than normal controls.[14,41,49,50] It has been suggested that visual vertigo (VV) results from an increased visual dependency for perception and postural control, which has a limiting effect on the process of compensation, especially in situations causing visual–vestibular conflict.[41,49] Visual vertigo has also been reported in patients with anxiety disorders[51–53] and motion sickness.[54] Patients diagnosed with VV are more destabilized by the visually disorienting stimuli than patients with labyrinthine deficiency[49] or vestibular patients without VV.[46] Visual vertigo leads to a significant degree of symptoms, perceived disability and lower activity levels that cannot be explained by a susceptibility to motion sickness and anxiety.[49] Rehabilitation with optokinetic stimulation provides a significant improvement in postural stability,[55,56] although comparable results are obtained with a customized vestibular exercise program.[57] In contrast, a rehabilitation program incorporating repeated progressive exposure to visual–vestibular stimulation during therapy provides substantially greater improvement in VV symptoms as opposed to therapy with vestibular exercises alone.[57]

Cervical vertigo

The existence of a vertigo disorder that is cervical in origin is a topic surrounded by controversy because of the inability of clinical studies to provide convincing evidence of a cervical mechanism and to confirm the diagnosis with a definitive diagnostic test.[58] Evidence suggests that cervical proprioception may influence vestibular function,[59,60] causing dizziness[61] and disequilibrium,[59,62,63] although oculomotor and vestibular testing is usually normal following cervical injury. Patients often present with symptoms of dizziness associated with neck pain, headache, decreased cervical motion, ataxia and/or gait unsteadiness, and increased postural sway with posturography testing.[62,63] Owing to the insufficient reliability of available tests and the similarity with symptoms common to vestibular disturbances, cervicogenic vertigo is a diagnosis contemplated only after extracervical causes (peripheral or central vestibular disorder) have been excluded, a history of prior neck injury or pathology exists, and there is a close association between neck pain and complaints of dizziness.[64,65] Cervical vertigo may be a result of cervical spine dysfunction, most often a whiplash injury[66] and, to a lesser extent, other types of cervical spine dysfunction (e.g. cervical spondylosis),[61] excessive lordosis of the cervical vertebral column[64] or muscle spasm in the neck region.[67] Treatment for cervicogenic dizziness includes interventions used for the relief of musculoskeletal pain (see below) in addition to postural re-education and balance exercises.[63–65,68,69] Controlled studies have shown that the majority of patients report a significant reduction in symptomology and neck pain following therapy[63,69] as well as an improvement in postural stability,[63] although postural stability remains below normal levels when a proprioceptive perturbation (vibration) is applied to the neck muscles.[63] These studies use traditional physical therapy interventions without the incorporation of vestibular rehabilitation (VR) as part of their treatment protocol. Wrisley et al.[65] and Clendaniel[68] advocate the additional use of vestibular exercises in order to reduce any motion sensitivity and to improve the use of vestibular and proprioceptive cues for balance. No randomized controlled studies have been conducted to determine whether a combination of manual therapy and VR can provide an even greater improvement of dizziness and postural stability compared with treatment using manual therapy alone. Nonetheless, despite the ambiguity surrounding the diagnosis of cervical vertigo and the limited controlled studies available, it seems logical to suggest that if a patient presents with cervical pain and imbalance, both conditions should be assessed by the therapist and treated accordingly. It would seem, therefore, that the current debate on the existence of cervicogenic dizziness, its relevance and mechanisms, is one of more theoretical interest rather than of practical significance.[58]

VESTIBULAR REHABILITATION

Vestibular rehabilitation is an exercise approach to treating primary and secondary symptoms associated with vestibular pathology. The purpose of VR is to stimulate central compensation and to provide a structured opportunity for the recovery of sensorimotor coordination over a wide range of orientations and movements. Vestibular rehabilitation was first employed as a method of speeding neurophysiological habituation following surgically induced UVL.[70] The treatment protocol used in this initial rehabilitation program came to be known as the Cawthorne–Cooksey exercises. The patient was asked to repeatedly perform a generic progressive sequence of eye, head and body movements in order to stimulate the vestibular system and enhance the natural

Table 17.3 *Range of movements typically included in vestibular rehabilitation (VR) programs*

Head exercises (performed with eyes open and eyes closed)	Bend head backwards and forwards
	Turn head from side to side
	Tilt head from one shoulder to the other
Fixation exercises	Move eyes up and down, side-to-side
	Perform head exercises while fixating stationary target
	Perform head exercises while fixating moving target
Positioning exercises (performed with eyes open and closed)	While seated, bend down to touch the floor
	While seated, turn to look over shoulder both to left and right
	Bend down with head twisted first to one side and then the other
	Lying down, roll from one side to the other
	Sit up from lying on the back and on each side
	Repeat with head turned to each side
Postural exercises (performed eyes open; eyes closed under supervision)	Practice static stance with feet as close together as possible
	Practice standing on one leg, and heel-to-toe
	Repeat head and fixation exercises while standing and then walking
	Practice walking in circles, pivot turns, up slopes, stairs, around obstacles
	Standing and walking in environments with altered surface and/or visual conditions with and without head and fixation exercises
	Aerobic exercises including alternative touching the fingers to the toes, trunk bends and twists, etc.

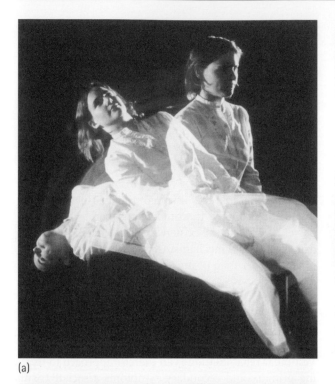

(a)

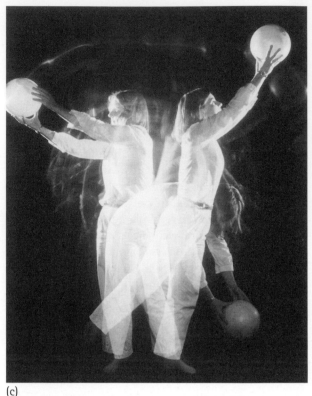

(c)

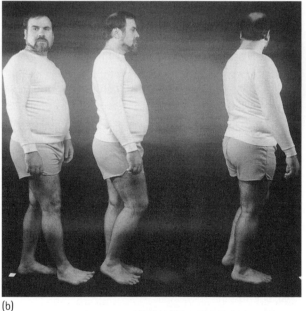

(b)

Figure 17.1 *Examples of exercises to habituate vertigo while improving balance with active head and center of body mass movements. (a) Repetition of the Hallpike position; (b) walking while turning the head to the left and right; and (c) large, circular motions of the head and trunk while maintaining visual fixation on a hand-held ball.*

process of central compensation for the asymmetry in the peripheral vestibular input. These exercises continue to remain popular today for many reasons. These include cost and time efficiency on behalf of the healthcare system since patients are educated in the exercises on a single visit, either in an individual or group setting, and then instructed to continue them in their home environment, often with no further supervision or follow-up. Table 17.3 and Fig. 17.1 include a sample of the type of symptom-provoking exercises that are usually included in VR programs and are based on the initial Cawthorne–Cooksey exercises.

Individualized therapy incorporating a combination of: (1) habituation, (2) adaptation exercises and (3) balance and mobility exercises are becoming more common, particularly in the light of recent studies showing that a customized therapy program results in greater improvement than a generic one.[71,72] In customized VR programs the exercises the patient is asked to perform are specific to those eye, head or body positions and movements that provoke vertigo. For example, if a patient complains of dizziness every time they reach up into a cupboard, that particular movement should be given as a specific exercise. In addition, VR includes exercises and activities customized to improve the particular balance and mobility problems associated with vestibular pathology.

Vestibular rehabilitation begins with a comprehensive rehabilitation assessment by a trained therapist. Results from this assessment are used to develop a customized treatment program.

Rehabilitation assessment

Assessment of the patient with vestibular pathology focuses on three main areas: balance and postural control underlying mobility skills, eye–head coordination and gaze stabilization, and vertigo.[4,5]

ASSESSING POSTURE AND BALANCE CONTROL

The assessment of posture and balance control in the patient with peripheral and or central nervous system deficit involves: (1) quantifying functional limitations and (2) identifying the underlying impairments that constrain the patient's ability to function independently. Since there is no single test that allows the clinician to quantify both functional limitations and underlying sensory, motor and cognitive impairments, a battery of tests and measurements must be assembled which enables clinicians to document problems at several levels of analysis.[7,8]

Quantifying functional abilities

A systems approach begins with assessment of functional abilities to determine how well a patient can perform a variety of skills that depend on balance.[73] A number of tests are available ranging from simple one-item screening tests to more comprehensive tests evaluating multiple aspects of balance.

The get up and go test

The get up and go test is a quick screening tool for detecting balance problems in the elderly.[74] This test requires the subject to stand up from a chair, walk 3 m, turn around, and return. Performance is judged subjectively and graded using the following scale: 1 = normal; 2 = very slightly abnormal; 3 = mildly abnormal; 4 = moderately abnormal; 5 = severely abnormal. The tool has been shown to be both reliable and consistent. It has been shown that older adults who scored 3 or higher on this test had an increased risk for falls.[74] The up and go test is a modification of the get up and go test, and adds a timing component to performance.[75] Neurologically intact adults that are independent in balance and mobility skills are able to perform the test in less than 10 s. This test correlates well with functional capacity. Adults that take longer than 30 s to complete the test are often dependent in activities of daily living and mobility skills.[75]

The functional reach test

The functional reach test[76] is a single-item test used to detect balance problems in older adults. In this test, the older adult is asked to stand with feet shoulder width apart, and with the arm raised to 90° to the front. Without moving the feet, the person is asked to reach as far forward as possible while still maintaining stability. The distance that can be reached is determined and compared with established norms. This test is also reliable and highly predictive of falls in the elderly.

The Tinetti balance and mobility scale

The Tinetti balance and mobility scale was also developed to screen for balance and mobility skills in older adults and determine the risk for falls.[77,78] The balance portion of Tinetti's scale rates performance on 11 different tasks and grades each item 0, 1 or 2. This scale is often used together with the Tinetti gait evaluation, and a total score is used to predict the risk for falls.

The dynamic gait index

The dynamic gait index[79] assesses an individual's ability to modify gait according to changing task demands, such as walking at varying gait speeds, while performing head movements or pivot turns. Performance is rated on a 4-point scale between 0 and 3. The test has shown to be a valid predictor of falls in both the elderly population[80] and patients with vestibular disorders.[81]

The functional balance scale

The functional balance scale developed by Berg[82] uses 14 different items, which are rated 0–4. The test is reported to have good test–retest and inter-rater reliability and has shown to be an effective predictor of falls in community-dwelling older adults.[80] However, there are no norms published for this test.

Fregly's ataxia test battery

Fregly's tests use a stopwatch to time the duration a patient can maintain a series of equilibrium positions such as one foot or heel/toe standing, eyes open and closed.[83] Normative values are published but need to be expanded at both ends of the age span and for women.

Evaluation of test results

Tests such as those presented above allow a clinician to determine the level of performance of functional tasks of balance in the patient with peripheral and or central neural lesions compared with standards established within normal subjects. Results can indicate the need for therapy, serve as a baseline level of performance and, when repeated at regular intervals, can provide both the therapist and patient with objective documentation about change in functional status. However, one must distinguish between static and dynamic balance tasks and consider these tests within the general context. Non-locomotor tests are often used to test for the risk of falls although the majority of falls occur during movement.[84] The functional reach test was developed to test dynamic balance, but Wernick-Robinson et al.[85] observed this test in healthy elderly individuals and patients with vestibular dysfunction, and found that both groups achieved the same functional reach distance without increasing the distance between the center of gravity and the center of pressure during or at the end of the movement. These results suggest that the functional reach test does not measure dynamic balance. In contrast, the get up and go test and the Berg balance scale are highly correlated with gait velocity, which has been described as a 'gold standard' for assessing balance in vestibular patients.[74,86] These findings suggest that a variety of static and dynamic balance measures are needed in order to gain a better understanding of the functional limitations resulting from different vestibular pathologies.[87,88] However, a variety of measurements are required in order to provide insight into the underlying sensory and motor impairments that constrain functional independence.

IDENTIFYING IMPAIRMENTS

Once functional limitations are quantified, assessment focuses on identifying the impairments in each of the systems essential to controlling posture and balance.

Musculoskeletal impairments

In patients with peripheral vestibular pathology, complaints of vertigo and oscillopsia often lead to compensatory strategies that restrict head and trunk movement.[5,29] This can lead to secondary musculoskeletal impairments including muscle tension, fatigue and pain in the cervical, and sometimes the thoracolumbar region.

Assessment of the musculoskeletal system includes evaluation of range of motion, flexibility and alignment, in as functional a situation as possible. Range of motion of joints should be evaluated both through slow, passive range and actively. For example, a patient may not be able to actively achieve full cervical range of motion owing to dizziness, pain, or co-contraction although passive range with the head supported against gravity is possible. Joint range can be measured quantitatively using equipment such as a goniometer, or can be described subjectively using an ordinal scale.[89,90] Lower limb muscle strength must also be examined. Many patients with vestibular deficits acquire a sedentary lifestyle that may lead to secondary muscle weakness and act as an additional contribution to the increased risk of falls.

Change in a patient's internal perception of vertical can lead to abnormal alignment of body parts with respect to each other and to the base of support. Abnormal alignment may place a patient close to their stability limits and alter the movement strategies necessary to move their center of mass.[91] The patient's alignment with respect to vertical and with respect to adjacent body segments needs to be observed in sitting and standing. A plumb line in conjunction with a grid can be used to quantify alignment at the head, shoulders, trunk, pelvis, hips, knees and ankle with photographs or videotapes. In standing, static force plates can be used to mea-

sure placement of the center of pressure or two standard scales can be used to determine if there is weight discrepancy between the two sides.[5,8] Body alignment provides the initial equilibrium position upon which motor and sensory strategies are related.

Neuromuscular impairments

Controlling the body's position in space for the purpose of balance and orientation requires motor coordination processes that organize muscles throughout the body into coordinated movement strategies. The three main postural response strategies used to recover stance balance in both the anterior/posterior and lateral directions are an ankle strategy, a hip strategy and a stepping strategy, which are illustrated in Fig. 17.2 (see Chapter 1).[92–95]

Although many CNS injuries such as stroke, head injury, and cerebral palsy result in improperly timed postural synergies, peripheral vestibular patients usually show normally coordinated muscle activation in the legs and trunk.[96–100] However, postural responses can be hypometric or hypermetric and the neck and trunk often exhibit abnormal co-contraction that stiffens joints. In addition, patients with vestibular pathology may show poorly coordinated head-in-space stability,[101,102] which further affects movement strategies for postural equilibrium.

Normal postural control requires the ability to adapt motor strategies to changing task and environmental demands. The inability to do this is a characteristic of many patients with neurological disorders. Pathology within the vestibular system can affect the selection of a movement strategy rather than the latency of onset or the temporal and spatial characteristics of the movement synergy itself.[4,5,100,103]

Assessment of neuromuscular impairments focuses on evaluating problems in the ability to generate and coordinate multijoint movements necessary for balance.[5,7,8] Postural movement strategies are examined under three different task conditions including: (1) self-initiated postural sway, (2) externally induced postural responses and (3) anticipatory postural adjustments accompanying a potentially destabilizing limb movement.[7]

A variety of clinical protocols are available for the evaluation of movement strategies.[8,104,105] For example, the clinician may hold the patient at the hips and displace them slightly forward, backward and side to side asking them to 'let me move you'. Externally induced postural responses are observed in response to pushes on the patient's shoulders, hips or sternum, in response to sudden tilts or translations of a patient's standing or sitting surface, or by suddenly releasing an isometric resistance against a standing patient's shoulders. Anticipatory postural adjustments are noted accompanying rapid elevation of the arms (with weighted hands if possible), rising to toes and holding, abducting one leg to the side or initiation of a step. Self-initiated postural movements include asking subjects to lean forward and backwards

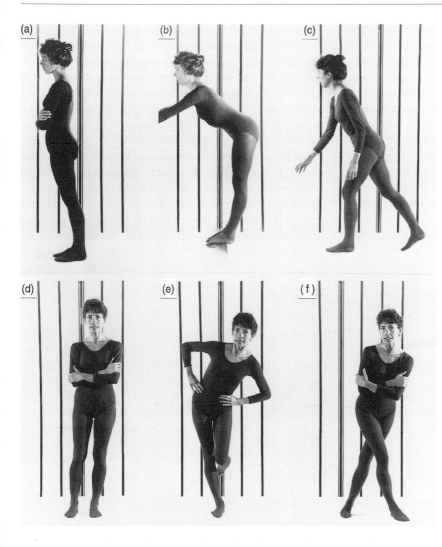

Figure 17.2 *Three movement strategies for recovery of balance; an ankle, hip and stepping strategy for the anterior/posterior direction (top) and for the lateral direction (bottom). In an ankle strategy, a vertical orientation of the trunk is preserved. In a hip strategy, vertical orientation of the trunk is compromised while the hips or lumbothoracic spine actively moves the center of mass. In a stepping strategy, the base of support moves under the falling center of body mass. (Reprinted with permission from ref. 4.)*

and laterally to their limits of stability and asking subjects to voluntarily sway sinusoidally at different speeds.

A coordinated adult responds to a small perturbation in the anterior/posterior direction by using sway principally about the ankles and in the lateral direction by using hip abduction/adduction. A therapist should carefully observe the ankle joints to determine if the tibialis anterior muscles are active in both legs in response to backward body sway. If knee and hip motion are minimal during these compensatory ankle sway movements this indicates that the appropriate proximal muscle synergists have been activated in addition to the ankle muscles. Larger displacements to stance posture with the feet planted on the surface cause greater amounts of hip and trunk responses – a hip strategy – as the subject attempts to maintain the center of mass within the base of support. Displacements that are large or fast may result in a stepping response. However, this hierarchy of responses does not manifest as a series of sequential responses (e.g. ankle, then hip, then step). Many individuals with normal balance function naturally respond to even small perturbations with a step, but when asked to maintain balance without initiating a step they are able to do this.[106] Runge et al.[107] report that all subjects with and without vestibular loss respond to large, forward sway displacements with a step at least once even though they have been instructed to try to avoid stepping.

Evaluating multijoint postural coordination requires careful observation and descriptive analysis. Many patients with CNS deficits will show uniquely uncoordinated movement strategies for postural control that cannot be classified as an ankle, hip or stepping strategy. For example, the clinician may note that during recovery of stance balance the patient demonstrates excessive knee flexion, asymmetric movements in the lower extremities, excessive flexion or rotation of the trunk, or excessive use of the arms.

Postural orientation impairments

Balance deficits can result from damage within individual sensory systems (vision, somatosensory and vestibular) which provide spatial orientation information, or from pathology affecting central sensory structures important in the interpretation and selection of sensory information for balance control. Disruption of sensory information processing may affect postural control in several ways: (1) a patient's ability to accurately determine the orientation of the body with respect to gravity and the environment may be disturbed; (2) a patient's ability to adapt sensory inputs to changes in task and environmental demands may be impaired; and (3) a patient's ability to anticipate instability based on prior experience may be affected.[5,7,108] Sensory adaptation problems can also manifest as an inflexible weighting of sensory information for orientation, and/or an inability to maintain balance in any environments where sensory information is inaccurately reporting self-motion.[30,46,109–112]

Assessment of the sensory components begins with an evaluation of the individual senses important to postural control. Particular attention is paid to evaluating somatosensation in the lower extremities. Commonly used tests are vibration or joint position sense. To test

joint position sense the examiner should lightly hold the sides of one of the patient's toes, then move it slightly up and down while asking the patient to report the direction of movement. Vibration sense may be tested by applying a tuning fork or neurothesiometer with constant pressure at the stimulating site until the individual reports that they can no longer perceive (tuning fork) or have just perceived (neurothesiometer) vibration.[113]

In order to determine how sensory information from visual, somatosensory and vestibular systems is utilized to maintain a vertical orientation, Shumway-Cook and Horak[73,112] designed the Clinical Test of Sensory Interaction and Balance, or CTSIB (Fig. 17.3), modeled after Nashner's[114,115] dynamic posturography, sensory

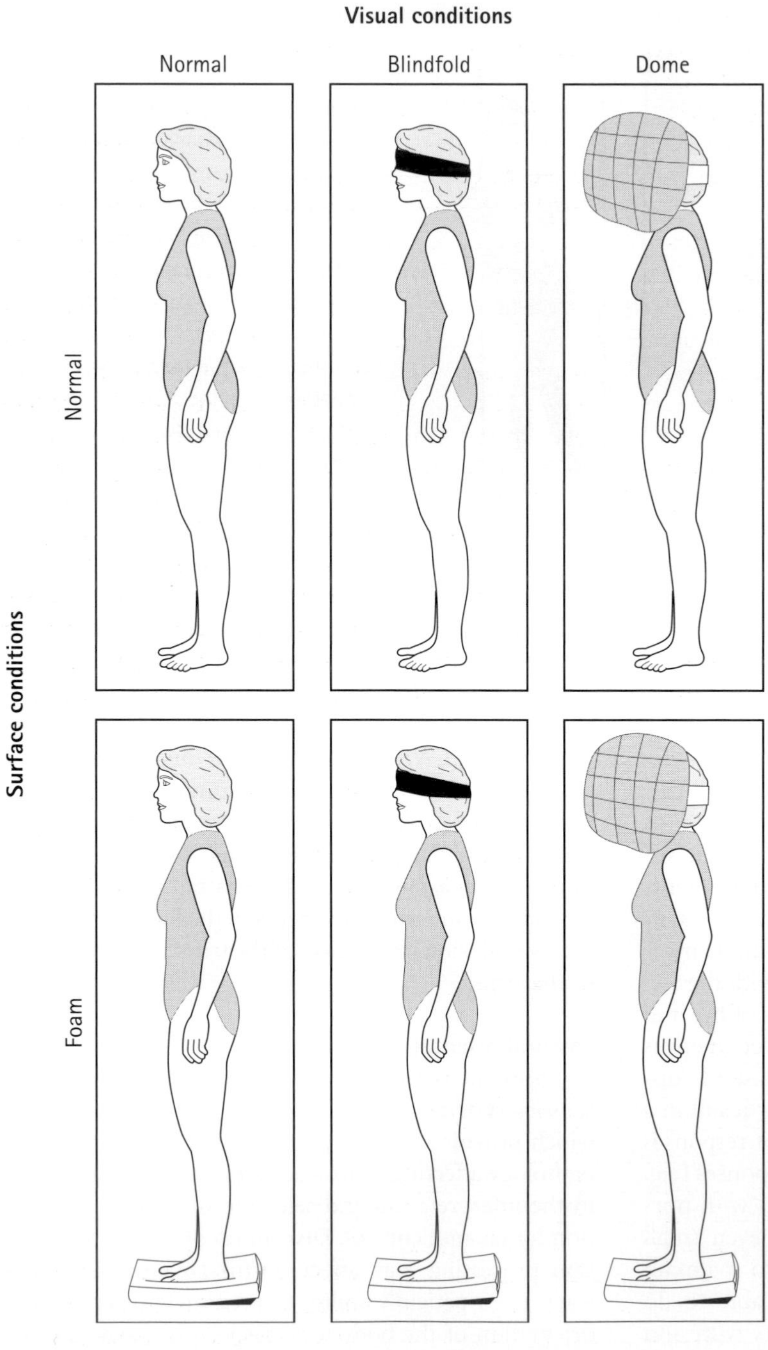

Visual conditions

Normal   Blindfold   Dome

Surface conditions

Normal

Foam

Figure 17.3 *A rehabilitation approach for testing the ability to maintain stance balance under altered sensory conditions, called the Clinical Test of Sensory Interaction and Balance (CTSIB). (Redrawn from Shumway-Cook A, Harak F. Assessing the influence of sensory interaction on balance.* Phys Ther *1986;* **66:** *1548–50 with permission of the American Physical Therapy Association.)*

organization protocol. Body sway is measured while the subject stands quietly for 20 s under six different conditions. Eye closure or blindfolds, a modified Japanese lantern (dome) and foam are used, respectively, to alter the availability and accuracy of visual and somatosensory inputs for postural orientation.

Patients are tested in an identical posture for all six conditions, for example, feet together with hands placed on hips. Using condition 1 as a baseline reference, the patient is observed for changes in the amount and direction of sway over the subsequent five conditions. If the patient is unable to stand for 20 s a second trial is given.[73] Differences in the amount of body sway in the various conditions are used to determine a subject's ability to organize and select appropriate sensory information for postural control. A single fall, regardless of the condition, is not considered abnormal.[97,110,116] However, two or more falls are indicative of difficulties adapting sensory information for postural control. Neurologically intact young adults are able to maintain balance for 20–30 s on all conditions, with minimal amounts of body sway.

A proposed model for interpreting results is summarized in Fig. 17.4. A visual or somatosensory dependency indicates an over-reliance on visual or somatosensory information from the feet, respectively, for postural control. A sensory selection problem is defined as an inability to effectively adapt sensory information for postural control whenever availability of sensory information is altered. Finally, falls in conditions 5 and 6 (Fig. 17.4) suggest an inability to utilize vestibular information for orientation.

Comparison of patients' performance in the CTSIB and dynamic posturography (Chapter 1) shows that they are not exactly equivalent (F. B. Horak, unpublished data).[41,117] More patients fall in the sway-referenced visual surround of dynamic posturography than in the dome during CTSIB. In the modified version of the CTSIB the dome is no longer used as it has not shown to be effective in identifying a visual dependency (A. Shumway-Cook, unpublished observations, 1997). In contrast, more patients tend to fall on the foam than on the sway-referenced platform. It must be kept in mind that standing on different surfaces changes the dynamics of force

production for control of equilibrium such that motor coordination deficits could affect performance in this condition. El-Kashlan et al.[117] found that the CTSIB shows a lower sensitivity towards the detection of postural control abnormalities and the definition of specific patterns of dysfunction in comparison to dynamic posturography. However, as Bronstein and Guerraz[118] commented, the results could just as easily indicate a false positive in dynamic posturography instead of a false negative in CTSIB.

In recent years much controversy has been generated over the usefulness of posturography tests. Dynamic posturography was developed to quantify the ability to balance in standing under altered surface and/or visual conditions. Some studies find a positive correlation between posturography scores and a patient's functional abilities, measured both objectively (gait velocity, tandem and single-leg stance, etc.) and subjectively (questionnaires)[117,119] but others find a poor to non-existent relationship between the various measurements.[86,87,120–123] Many VR studies use posturography as an outcome measure for functional performance.[20,41,42,44,117,124,125] The test has shown itself to be a reliable measurement for comparing pre- and post-therapy improvement in balance function as well as being able to distinguish malingerers[126,127] and individuals with secondary gain (e.g. worker's compensation, pending lawsuits)[128] from those with a real disability. Dynamic posturography produces perturbations in the pitch plane but real-life situations such as standing on an accelerating bus, provoke destabilizing forces in multiple directions. Furthermore, the postural responses required to stand on an uneven surface are different from those for walking or performing a reaching task on the same surface and cannot be assessed accurately by a single test. Therefore, posturography results should only be considered as an adjunctive contribution to the difficult and complex task of assessing a patient's functional disabilities and sensory deficits.[42,87]

In summary, a rehabilitation assessment of balance control focuses on evaluating functional abilities dependent on posture and balance control, and identifying the constellation of sensory and motor impairments which constrain independence in functional skills. Table 17.4

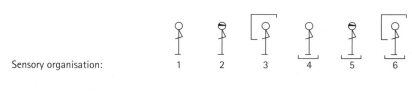

Sensory organisation: 1 2 3 4 5 6

Patterns of postural disorientation						
Visually dependent		?	*		?	*
Surface dependent				*	*	*
Vestibular loss					*	*
Sensory selection			*	*	*	*
* = Body sway excessive or falls						
? = May or may not show abnormal sway						

Figure 17.4 *Interpreting performance on tests examining the ability to stand under altered sensory conditions.*

Table 17.4 *Assessment of balance control*

Functional assessment	'Get Up and Go' Test
	Functional Reach Test
	Tinetti Balance and Mobility Scale
	Dynamic Gait Index
	Functional Balance Scale
	Fregly's Ataxia Test Battery
Systems assessment	Musculoskeletal system
	Range of motion, flexibility and alignment
	Neuromuscular system
	Strength and tone
	Coordination of movement strategies
	Timing, scaling and adaptation
	Sensory systems
	Orientation to somatosensory, vestibular and visual information

outlines the general categories of a balance assessment. A general problem in the management of vestibular patients is the lack of correspondence that often exists between vestibular-related eye movement assessment, balance tests and symptoms.[129] Therefore, eye–head coordination and complaints of dizziness in the patient with vestibular pathology must also be evaluated.

ASSESSING EYE–HEAD COORDINATION

Adequate head and gaze stability is required for complex tasks such as balancing on a beam or walking, although it may not be critical for postural stability in quiet stance.[22,31] During head movement, stability of the eyes in space depends on the vestibulo-ocular reflex, which rotates the eyes in the opposite direction to the head. Several aspects of eye–head coordination essential to the ability to stabilize gaze are evaluated to develop a customized VR programme (see also Chapter 7). Eye movements used to locate targets presented within both the central and peripheral visual fields are assessed first without any head movements. The patient is asked to keep the head still and move only the eyes. Saccadic eye movements to fixed targets, smooth pursuit eye movements used to track moving targets as well as the patient's ability to use the eyes to locate and maintain a stable gaze on a target are assessed (see Chapter 7). Eye movements are graded subjectively according to a three-point scale: intact, impaired, or unable and any subjective complaints related to blurred or unstable vision are recorded.

It is also important to evaluate the patient's ability to stabilize gaze either on an earth fixed target (e.g. stationary object in the room) and a target moving in phase with the head (e.g. walking and simultaneously reading a newspaper one is holding) during head movements. Task performance depends on the intactness of the vestibulo-ocular reflex and visual suppression of the vestibulo-ocular response respectively (see Chapter 7). Gaze stability is assessed in various directions, and at different amplitudes and speeds of head movement. Finally, the patient's ability to make eye/head/trunk movements necessary to locate targets oriented in the far periphery is tested.

Eye–head coordination is assessed in sitting, standing and walking (e.g. the patient is asked to look to the right or left, up or down while walking a straight path). The impact of head movements on stability is observed and reported. For example, head movements during gait often cause the patient to deviate from a straight path and in severe cases stagger and lose balance.

ASSESSING PERCEPTIONS OF STABILITY AND MOTION

Dizziness and vertigo

Central neural and vestibular lesions can also profoundly affect a patient's sense of self motion or environmental motion (see Chapters 7 and 9). Vertigo is the perception of motion, either self or environmental, in a stationary context. Dizziness can also be used to describe sensations such as rocking, tilting, lightheadedness and unsteadiness that can arise from either vestibular or central lesions or both.[130] The term rotational vertigo is reserved for a sensation of rotatory motion (spinning) of the environment and is often caused by semicircular canal pathology.

Dizziness and vertigo can be either spontaneous or provoked by a change in position or motion of the head. Sometimes, dizziness is provoked by an environmental change such as when visual or surface orientation cues are inaccurate for orientation. When dizziness is provoked while the patient is sitting, standing or walking unsupported, it is often a contributor to unsteadiness and loss of balance.[5] It is critical to evaluate systematically the particular environments, conditions, head movements and positions that provoke vertigo in order to design appropriate exercises and to counsel patients on how to control their symptoms. Assessment of dizziness begins with a careful history to determine the patient's perceptions of whether dizziness is constant or provoked, and the situations or conditions which stimulate dizziness. Questionnaires can be employed to provide a quantitative measure of the frequency and severity of symptoms and their effect on daily activities (see Chapter 19). Patients with psychiatric complications may experience a greater degree of handicap and prolonged recovery. Therefore, psychological and emotional status which affect treatment outcome must also be evaluated (see Chapter 19). The Situational Characteristics Questionnaire[51] may be used to identify symptoms provoked by disorienting environmental situations that can cause visual–vestibular conflict. The Vertigo Positions and Movement Test[131]

Table 17.5 *Vertigo positions and movement test*

	Intensity (0–10)	Duration (no. of seconds)	Imbalance (yes/no)
1. Baseline-seated (eyes open)			
2. Position provoked – look right			
3. Position provoked – look left			
4. Movement provoked – side to side			
5. Position provoked – look up			
6. Position provoked – look down			
7. Movement provoked – up and down			
8. Sit to supine			
9. Rolling to right			
10. Rolling to left			
11. Supine to sit			
12. Sit to stand			
13. Passive head/trunk rotation			
14. Passive trunk rotation – head still			
15. Bend to floor			
16. Standing – look over right shoulder			
17. Standing – look over left shoulder			
18. Walking – horizontal head turns			
19. Walking – vertical head turns			
20. Walking – change speed			
21. Walking – quick stop			
22. Walking – pivot turn			
23. Hallpike right			
24. Hallpike left			
Other:			

examines both the subjective intensity of dizziness on a scale of 0–10 (no dizziness to most severe possible) and its duration in response to movement and/or positional changes of the head and body (Table 17.5). The therapist records the presence of nystagmus, and notes autonomic nervous system signs such as sweating, pallor and nausea. A dizziness index can be calculated by multiplying the intensity by the duration and summing all the numbers.[132]

Internal representation of posture

A patient's subconscious internal representation of their stability limits and of their sensory and biomechanical capabilities may be distorted by a CNS lesion. When internal representation of stability limits is smaller than actual, patients minimize body sway and center of mass movements using excessive movement strategies for equilibrium; when it is larger than actual, patients easily exceed their limits of stability and fall without taking appropriate action.

The consistency between the patient's perceived versus actual stability limits is subjectively assessed for both the sitting and standing position using self-initiated postural movements. Alternatively, patients are asked to reach for an object held at the outer edge of their stability limits. The therapist observes the extent to which the patient is willing to move the center of mass, and makes a subjective judgement about whether the patient is moving to their full stability limits in all directions.

Internal sense of gravitational vertical can be affected by both vestibular and CNS lesions and is extremely disruptive to postural stability. If this sense of 'verticality' is tilted forward, backwards or to the side, patients will attempt to align their bodies in stance and sitting to this distorted sense of vertical. Therapists can assess a patient's internal sense of vertical by passively moving them off vertical in stance or sitting and asking them to voluntarily realign to vertical. Both surface orientation and visual information can be reduced in this assessment. The sense of left/right (roll) verticality can be quantified by asking patients to align a luminous line to the perceived vertical in the dark and then measuring the deviation from true vertical.[133,134] A visual dependency for perception of verticality may be assessed with the 'Rod and Frame' test. The patient is seated straight in front of the luminescent test apparatus in an otherwise dark room and is asked to set the rod to vertical independent of the tilted position of the frame.[49] Patients with a visual dependency show an increased tilt in the direction of the frame. When using visual vertical tests the examiner must remember that the subjective 'postural' vertical and 'visual' vertical are not necessarily correlated.[135,136]

In summary, a systems approach to rehabilitation assessment of balance control is directed at evaluating a patient's ability to perform functional balance tasks and to use and adapt strategies appropriately for changing task conditions. If functional performance is suboptimal, assessment aims to identify the sensory, motor and cognitive impairments responsible and to decide whether therapy will be able to improve functional task performance despite the existing impairments. If therapy is judged to be beneficial, the information gained through assessment is used to develop a comprehensive list of problems, establish short- and long-term goals, and formulate a plan of care for retraining posture control and decreasing symptoms.

Treatment

Vestibular rehabilitation uses exercises to: (1) facilitate neural compensation for vestibular pathology; (2) resolve or prevent impairments; (3) promote the development of effective strategies for recovery of functional skills in the face of potentially permanent impairments; (4) retrain functional goal-oriented tasks in a wide variety of environmental contexts; and (5) decrease the magnitude of symptoms experienced by the patient. During the course of treatment, therapists must constantly evaluate and monitor the changing constellation of impairments affecting each patient and adjust the treatment programme accordingly.

SPECIFIC COMPONENTS OF VR

Treating musculoskeletal impairments

Many musculoskeletal problems, including limited range of motion and decreased flexibility, can be completely remediated or prevented using traditional physical therapy techniques, including modalities such as heat, passive manipulation, massage, stretching exercises, casting and biofeedback. Muscle weakness owing to inactivity can be improved effectively with traditional strengthening exercises once full range of motion, if limited, has been achieved. Balance exercises often included in VR programs can further enhance muscle strength.

Musculoskeletal problems can also include problems in postural alignment. The goal when retraining alignment is to help the patient develop an initial position that: (1) is appropriate for the task, (2) is efficient with respect to gravity, that is, with minimal muscle activity requirements for maintaining the position, and (3) maximizes stability, that is, places the center of mass well within the patient's stability limits. A normal alignment allows the greatest range of movements for postural control.

There are a number of approaches that can be used to help patients develop a symmetrically vertical posture. Verbal and manual cues are often used to assist a patient in finding and maintaining an appropriate vertical posture. Patients practice with eyes open and closed, on firm or compliant surfaces, learning to maintain a vertical position in the absence of visual and/or somatosensory cues. Mirrors can also be used to provide patients with visual feedback about their position in space. Another approach to retraining vertical posture involves having patients stand (or sit) with their back against the wall, which provides enhanced somatosensory feedback about their position in space. This feedback can be further increased by placing a small protruding object vertically on the wall (e.g. yardstick or a rolled-up towel) and having the patient lean against it. Somatosensory feedback can be made intermittent by having the patient lean away from the wall, only occasionally leaning back to get knowledge of results.

Kinetic or force feedback devices are often used to provide patients with information about postural alignment and weight bearing status. Kinetic feedback can be provided with devices as simple as bathroom scales or alternatively, through limb load monitors,[137] or forceplate biofeedback systems.[138]

Retraining sensory and movement strategies

Retraining strategies for balance control involves helping a patient to recover, or develop, sensory and motor strategies that are effective in meeting the balance requirements of functional tasks. The nature of the underlying impairments determines whether the patient will be able to recover previously used strategies or will need to develop compensatory strategies, as in a BVL.

The goal when retraining movement strategies involves helping the patient develop coordinated movements effective in meeting the demands for posture and balance in sitting and in standing. Patients must develop movement strategies that are successful in controlling the center of mass relative to the base of support, including: (1) strategies which move the center of mass relative to a stationary base of support, in standing, for example, an ankle or hip strategy; and (2) strategies for changing the base of support, for example a stepping strategy in standing or a protective reach in sitting.

Developing a coordinated ankle strategy

When retraining the use of an ankle strategy during self-initiated sway, patients are asked to practice swaying back and forth, and side to side, within small ranges, keeping the body straight and not bending at the hips or knees. Knowledge of results regarding how far the center of mass is moving during self-initiated sway can be facilitated using static forceplate retraining systems,[138] which can effectively be used to retrain scaling problems.[7] Patients are asked to move the center of mass voluntarily to different targets displayed on a screen. Targets are made progressively smaller, and are placed closed together, requiring greater precision in force control. Knowledge of results is given with respect to movements which overshoot the target, indicating an error in amplitude scaling of postural synergies. Patients may also practice amplitude scaling by responding to perturbations of various amplitudes applied at the hips or shoulders. Small perturbations, such as a small pull or push at the hips or shoulders are used to practice the use of an ankle strategy to recover equilibrium. Feedback regarding the appropriateness of their response is provided by the clinician.

Finally, patients are asked to carry out a variety of manipulation tasks, such as reaching, lifting, and throwing, which help patients to develop strategies for anticipatory postural control. A hierarchy of tasks reflecting increasing anticipatory postural demands can be helpful when retraining patients in this important area. The magnitude of anticipatory postural activity is directly related to the potential for instability inherent in a task. Potential instability relates to speed, effort, degree of external support and task complexity. Thus, asking a patient who is externally supported by the therapist to lift a light load slowly requires minimal anticipatory postural activity. Conversely, an unsupported patient who must lift a heavy load quickly must use a substantial amount of anticipatory postural activity to remain stable.

Developing a coordinated hip strategy

A hip strategy can be facilitated by asking the patient to maintain balance without taking a step and using faster and larger displacements than those used for an ankle strategy. Use of a hip strategy can also be facilitated by restricting force control at the ankle joints by standing across a narrow beam, standing heel/toe or in single limb stance. Patients practice both voluntary sway and response to external perturbations on altered surfaces to relearn how to control a hip strategy. Attempts to stabilize the head and eyes in space by focusing on a visual target can also help to improve control of a hip strategy.

Developing a coordinated step strategy

Learning to step in response to a large perturbation is an essential part of balance retraining.[7,8] Both the preparatory postural adjustment toward the stance leg and the step itself can be practiced independently prior to putting them together. Stepping can be practiced by passively shifting the patient's weight to one side and then quickly bringing the center of mass back towards the unweighted leg, or in response to large backward or forward perturbations. If needed, manual assistance at the ankle can be used to facilitate a stepping response. In order to increase the size of a compensatory step, subjects can also practice stepping over a visual target or obstacle in response to the external perturbations.

When providing balance exercises, the environment must be modified to allow a patient to practice the exercises safely and without the continual supervision of a therapist. Patients that are very unsteady, or fearful of falling can practice movements while wearing a harness connected to the ceiling, in parallel bars, standing close to a wall or corner, with a chair or table in front of them.

Improving perception of orientation and movement

The goal when retraining perception of postural orientation in space is to help the patient learn to integrate sensory information effectively in a variety of altered environments. This necessitates correctly interpreting the body's position and movements in space. Treatment strategies generally require the patient to maintain balance during progressively more difficult static and dynamic movement tasks while the clinician systematically varies the availability and accuracy of sources of sensory information for orientation.

Patients that are surface dependent, that is, have difficulty balancing when surface characteristics are altered, are asked to perform tasks while sitting or standing on surfaces with disrupted somatosensory cues for orientation, such as carpets, compliant foam and moving surfaces (e.g. tilt board; Fig. 17.5).

Patients that are visually dependent are prescribed a variety of balance tasks when visual cues are absent (eyes closed or blindfolded) or reduced (blinders or diminished lighting). Alternatively, visual cues can be made inaccurate for orientation through the use of glasses smeared with petroleum jelly, prism glasses, vision-reversing plastic mirrors[139] or complex moving visual scenes (Fig. 17.6a–c). Decreasing a patient's sensitivity to visual motion cues in their environment can be done by asking the patient to maintain balance during exposure to optokinetic stimuli such as moving curtains with stripes, moving discs with multicolored and differently sized circles or even moving rooms.[4,5,56,57] Exposure to optokinetic stimuli in the home environment may be accomplished by having the patient watch videos with conflicting visual scenes, such as high-speed car chases either on a television screen or while wearing a head-mounted display (Fig 17.6c), 'busy' screen savers on a computer (multiple moving shapes or mazes), or moving large cardboard posters with vertical lines. Exposure to any complex visual stimulation should be gradual and involve maintaining visual fixation at varying distances (see below) from the visual scene while conducting exercises in sitting, standing and during walking, first alone and then in combination with voluntary head movements at progressively increasing frequencies.

Finally, in order to enhance the patient's ability to use remaining vestibular information for postural stability, exercises are given that ask the patient to balance while both visual and somatosensory are simultaneously reduced (Fig. 17.6d,e).

Learning to adapt strategies to changing contexts

Developing adaptive capacities in the patient is also a critical part of retraining balance. The ability to perform functional tasks in a natural environment requires that the patient modify strategies to changing task and environmental demands. Since the stability and orientation requirements vary with the task and the environment, a hierarchy of tasks can be used, beginning with tasks that have relatively few stability demands, and moving on to those that place heavy demands on the postural control system. For example, postural demands involved in maintaining an upright seated posture while in a semi-supported seated position are relatively few. In contrast,

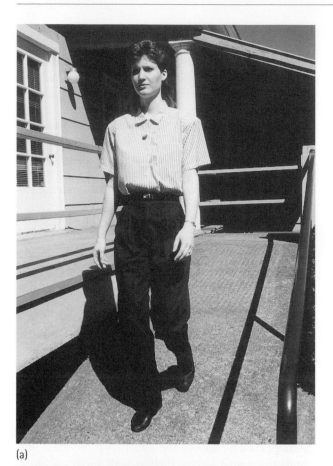

(a)

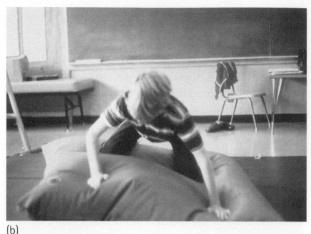

(b)

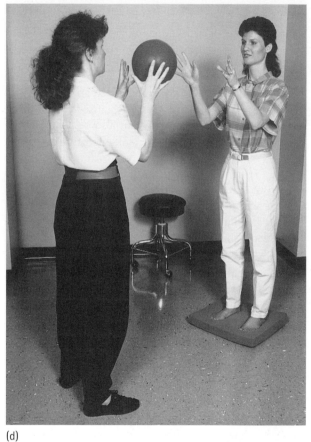

(d)

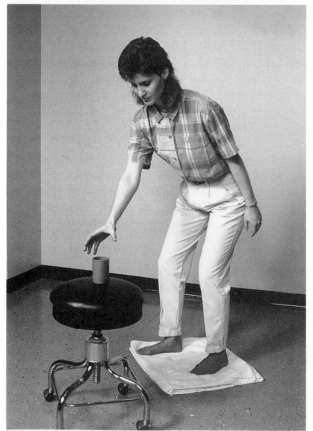

(c)

Figure 17.5 *Examples of exercises to reduce over-dependence on surface somatosensory cues for orientation: (a) patient walking on a tilted ramp; (b) child balancing on all fours on a large pillow; (c) patient reaching for a glass of water while balancing on compliant foam; (d) patient catching a ball while standing on compliant foam.*

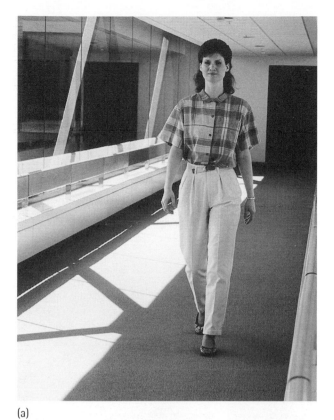

(a)

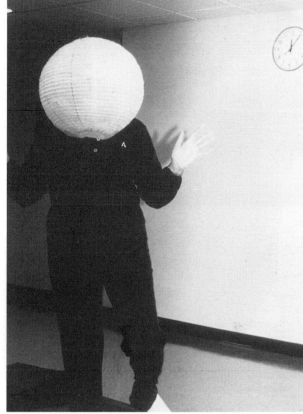

(b)

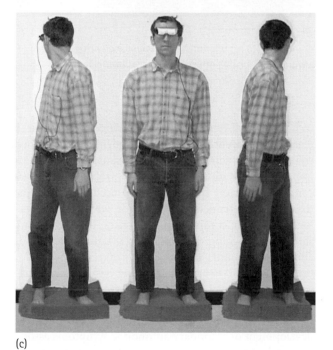

(c)

Figure 17.6 *Examples of exercises to reduce visual motion sensitivity: (a) walking across a windowed bridge with complex visual orientation information from shadow and traffic in the street below; (b) wearing a visual stabilization dome while balancing on one foot; (c) using a head-mounted display (Eye-Trek FMD-200, Olympus Optical Co. Ltd) for image projection. Patients may watch a video showing visually conflicting stimuli while performing head and body movements in sitting, standing, and walking. (Continued overleaf.)*

sitting on a moving tilt board while holding a cup of water has fairly rigorous stability requirements, reflecting the changing and unpredictable nature of the task. This requires constant adaptation of the postural system. Consequently, supported sitting would be a good task to begin with when working with a patient who has severe postural dyscontrol. Unilateral vestibular loss patients also require more time to complete a voluntary movement strategy[140] and gait tasks,[87] although they initiate their responses at the same time as normals.[140] Therefore, as the patient improves, more difficult and demanding tasks can be introduced using varying speeds of movement.

Thus, during balance retraining, patients practice a wide collection of functional tasks in a variety of contexts. This includes: (1) maintaining balance with a reduced base of support; (2) maintaining balance while

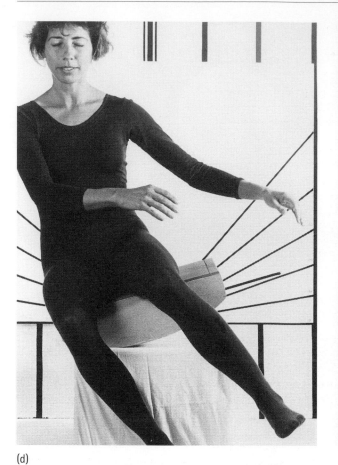

(d)

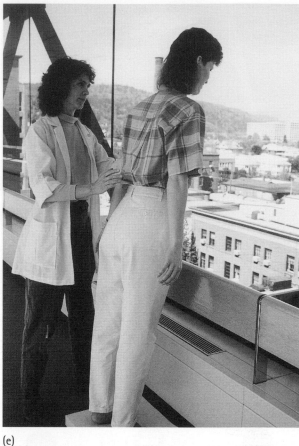

(e)

Figure 17.6 (continued) *Examples of therapy to force use of vestibular information for orientation: (d) balancing with eyes closed on a tilting board; (e) patient standing on compliant foam and swaying forward while looking down to the street traffic below.*

changing the orientation of the head and trunk; and (3) maintaining balance while performing a variety of upper extremity tasks.

Eye and head exercises

Adaptation exercises incorporating gaze fixation and head movements as well as eye movements and postural exercises are also prescribed to promote the recovery of normal vestibulo-ocular and vestibulospinal reflex function. Gaze fixation exercises are performed at varying distances from the target since vestibulo-ocular reflex (VOR) gain depends on target distance, with higher vestibulo-ocular reflex gains required the closer the target.[141,142] Fixation exercises are given to patients with oscillopsia and to patients with a decrease in vestibulo-ocular reflex gain, most often seen in peripheral vestibular disorders. When oscillopsia is a problem (e.g. BVL), voluntary head oscillation at progressively increasing frequency while maintaining visual fixation on textured objects or reading material can further promote habituation. (A. M. Bronstein and J. D. Hood, personal observation).

Relaxation exercises

There are a variety of reasons why particular patients with vertigo may benefit from being taught relaxation

techniques.[143,144] When dizziness is related to stress, neck tension, hyperventilation, or jaw-clenching or grinding, relaxation may directly remove a cause of vertigo or imbalance. For significant cervical problems a formal course of physical therapy may be needed, but simple techniques for reducing neck tension which can be performed before commencing exercises for vertigo are shoulder shrugging, shoulder/arm rotation (backwards and forwards), and gentle stretching exercises specific for the neck region. Relaxation training has also been suggested as a means of increasing tolerance of the symptoms provoked by exercise-based therapy.[145] In addition, relaxation techniques can help to reduce or prevent the development of secondary autonomic symptoms associated with anxiety arousal, which include nausea, breathing difficulties and feeling faint.

Therapies that have been used successfully to enable the patient to control arousal, hyperventilation and autonomic symptoms include various relaxation techniques, education in respiration control and biofeedback. One of the simplest and most widely used methods of relaxation is known as 'progressive relaxation'. This involves focusing on one set of muscles at a time, first deliberately clenching them, and then relaxing them. A

Table 17.6 *Stages of training in applied relaxation*

Stage	Target time	Relaxation method
1.	15 min	Clench, then relax: (a) feet, legs, hips, stomach, back, chest (b) hands, arms, shoulders, neck, face
2.	5 min	Directly relax these same muscle groups
3.	2 min	When relaxed, think 'relax' on each expiration, until relaxed state is associated with internal instruction to relax
4.	60–90 s	Practice maintaining/restoring relaxed state during/after making movements (for example vestibular rehabilitation exercises)
5.	20–30 s	Practice using internal instruction to relax in natural, non-stressful situations
6.		Apply relaxation in stressful situations (for example, during attack of vertigo)

training program known as 'applied relaxation'[146] can be used to teach the patient how to implement relaxation techniques in progressively more stressful situations (see Table 17.6).

Slow, diaphragmatic breathing is a vital component of relaxation. The aim is to establish a breathing pattern of 10–14 breaths a minute, by monitoring and then deliberately slowing the respiratory cycle. By placing one hand on the chest and the other on the stomach the patient can monitor whether their breathing is thoracic or diaphragmatic; if thoracic, they may need to be taught to draw in and expel air by deliberately inflating and compressing the stomach, while keeping the chest flat and motionless.

Biofeedback is a more elaborate technique for teaching relaxation, whereby the patient is attached to devices that monitor their physiological state (e.g. muscle tension, heart or respiratory rate) and provide a feedback signal, such as a light or tone, to inform the patient when they are progressing towards the relaxed state. Although biofeedback requires more resources than other relaxation training programs, in terms of equipment and therapist time, the technological aspect of the technique can help to motivate patients that are skeptical of the value of 'soft' therapies such as relaxation, and the objective feedback can be useful to individuals who have difficulty detecting their own internal anxiety state. Respiratory biofeedback with a handheld capnometry device has lately shown to be successful in decreasing panic and psychological symptoms associated with panic disorder.[147]

General aspects of VR

General characteristics of every exercise program include specificity, repetition, and progression. The patient is only given exercises that specifically provoke their symptoms. Norré and de Weerdt[148] found that the symptoms of patients that performed exercises not provoking symptoms resulted in unchanged vertigo, but after the same patients had practiced performing disorienting movements, their symptoms improved. The prescribed exercises are performed for at least 10–20 min, twice per day. Pacing of the exercises is crucial. Unless they are performed slowly at first, exercises may induce an unacceptable degree of vertigo and nausea. Since the aim is to stimulate the vestibular system, some clinicians prefer patients to cease taking vestibular sedatives before beginning treatment. As symptoms abate the patient gradually increases the pace and difficulty of the exercises. Patients may be advised to cease exercising and seek advice if during VR they experience severe pain in the neck, loss of consciousness or vision, or sensations of numbness, weakness or tingling in the face or limbs.

Performing specific head and body movements without dizziness means that those particular exercises have become easier, it does not guarantee that the patient will be able to go into visually conflicting surroundings without experiencing any adverse symptoms. Therefore, as patients become more accustomed to the exercises and their tolerance increases, they are advised to gradually expose themselves once again to everyday situations that they have come to avoid over time, such as supermarket aisles, crowds, and shopping malls. Once all the exercises can be performed without dizziness, it is important that patients maintain a high degree of physical activity (e.g. playing ball games, dancing, or other activities) in order to sustain compensation.

An essential part of VR involves educating the patient about the dynamic nature of vestibular compensation. This understanding is critical to forming positive but realistic expectations. For example, patients are warned that their symptoms may at first worsen, and that improvement may be uneven – they will probably experience good days and bad days. In addition, patients are cautioned that even after compensation is achieved, and symptoms have largely resolved, periods of stress, fatigue or illnesses may result in a temporary reoccurrence of symptoms.

Clinical studies on the efficacy of VR

Clinical trials of the efficacy of exercise programs typically report improvement in symptoms in over 80 per cent of those participating, but with complete elimination of vertigo in less than one-third.[148–150] Improvement refers to a reduction in movement-provoked vertigo or residual dizziness and unsteadiness, as exercise therapy is not expected to reduce the number or severity of spontaneous episodes of acute vertigo. Many trials now support the use of VR; however, outcomes of various trials must be reviewed carefully and not be taken at face value. For example, Blakely[151] reported a significant 66 per cent improvement in symptoms after 4 weeks of home exercises but no control group has been included to compare these results with. Inclusion of an appropriate control condition is important, since balance disorders are notoriously prone to fluctuations in symptomatology and placebo effects; indeed, the authors of a very carefully conducted trial of (drug) therapy for Ménière's disease[152] concluded that participation in any clinical trial appeared to be the best treatment. Placebo effects merit serious consideration, since they may actually reflect genuine improvement resulting from nonspecific features of therapy (see Chapter 19), including interest, information, or reassurance. The possibility of spontaneous remission must also be considered, especially when investigating vestibular disorders in the acute phase.

Some clinical trials have begun to remedy these methodological shortcomings. Horak et al.[124] have undertaken a comparison of vestibular exercises with either medication (valium or meclozine) or general conditioning exercises. Results from a small sample indicated that both objective assessments of postural stability and subjective ratings of symptom severity showed more improvement in the vestibular exercise group than in the other two. Shepard et al.[71] also found a higher rate of improvement among people recovering from vestibular neuritis who were given exercise therapy than among those that had an operation to section the vestibular nerve. More recently, Strupp et al.[153] assessed the effect of vestibular exercises on central compensation in patients with acute/subacute vestibular neuritis. Their results indicated that although function of the vestibulo-ocular system and perception returned to normal ranges within the same time frame in both groups (treatment and no treatment), postural stability or vestibulospinal compensation occurred to a significantly greater extent in patients that received VR. These findings advocate the initiation of treatment early after symptom onset.

Yardley et al.[154] conducted a large randomized controlled trial comparing the effect of an unsupervised home VR exercise program with a no-treatment group. They reported significantly greater improvements of the treatment population on practically all outcome measures of postural control, symptoms and emotional state, both at 6-week and 6-month follow-ups.[154] However, the authors note that the extent of the improvement was rather modest. They suggest this may be partly due to lack of patient motivation with a drop-out rate of one in four patients, which could potentially be reduced with closer monitoring and greater support.[154] More recently, Black et al.[44] were the first to include both normal and abnormal control/reference groups as well as to judge rehabilitation success by the return to normal ranges for scores on both objective and subjective measurements. Their findings support earlier observations that individualized VR treatment protocols notably improve symptoms, postural stability and the patients' ability to perform daily activities.

The success of vestibular exercises may also be influenced by their effect on patients' beliefs about the consequences of their dizziness. It has recently been shown that such beliefs predict handicap since the sedentary lifestyle many vestibular patients acquire is not only a result of the actual symptoms they experience but also of the anticipated consequences that patients believe these symptoms have during everyday activities (severe dizziness, falls, social embarrassment).[155] Following VR, negative beliefs are found to be significantly reduced and it is proposed the decrease in reported symptoms and handicap may be due to two factors: the physiological effects of treatment and the psychological component of therapy, which helps patients to obtain a sense of control over the situation and dispel their negative notions about the consequences of dizziness.[155]

There has been relatively little discussion of the issue of uptake, dropout and non-compliance rates, which pose a real problem not only in VR clinical trials but also in everyday clinical practice. Many people who are offered a therapy requiring them to deliberately induce dizziness for several weeks are initially dismayed; in one study only 54 per cent of patients accepted treatment by VR.[125] Yardley et al.[156] found that fewer than 2 per cent of dizzy people identified in a population survey were both suitable and willing to be assessed and treated in hospital. The majority of these eligible patients were not willing to attend for a hospital visit and, to a lesser extent, either failed to attend, declined treatment or were deemed unsuitable for the study for various reasons such as a non-vestibular diagnosis and taking psychoactive medication. The problem of acceptance and participation therefore deserves closer attention (see Chapter 19).

Owing to the varying and sometimes narrow selection criteria employed in VR clinical trials, it is difficult to estimate what percentage of a heterogeneous clinical population of dizzy patients could be expected to improve, although Yardley and colleagues[155] found that nearly four times as many treated as control patients improved in their controlled trial of treatment for an extremely heterogeneous sample of patients with dizziness in primary care. Ambivalent findings for more complex conditions involving patients with central vestibular deficits and fluctuating vertigo raise awareness that further studies are required to assess the true effectiveness of VR for varying diagnostic categories. Nonetheless, numerous studies have shown the substantial benefit of providing VR to patients of all ages[20,41,44] with vestibular dysfunction. Vestibular rehabilitation is now commonly used for a wide range of balance disorders and the only dizzy patients for whom VR is specifically contra-indicated are those in whom exercise and head movements might aggravate either the underlying cause of the dizziness (for example, patients with a suspected fistula) or other conditions (e.g. heart failure or severe cervical damage).

THERAPIES FOR BPPV

Benign paroxysmal positioning vertigo is one of the most common vestibular disorders. It is thought to arise as a result of the accumulation of debris (dislodged otoconia) in the posterior semicircular canal, although recent evidence shows that anterior and horizontal canal involvement may also occur, although to a much lesser extent.[157–159] The debris are thought to be adhered to the cupula or freely-moving in the canal (cupulo- or canal-lithiasis respectively), resulting in changes in the response of the cupula to reorientation with respect to gravity. Spontaneous remission of symptoms may occur, but for many the condition persists and requires treatment. The aim of the exercise therapies developed specifically for BPPV is to eliminate the root-cause of the vertigo by dispersing the debris.[160]

A single treatment technique known as the 'Liberatory Manoeuvre' has been suggested by Sémont et al.[161] (see Chapter 9 and Fig. 9.3). First, the Dix-Hallpike maneuver is used to identify the position provoking BPPV (Chapters 6 and 9). The therapist moves the patient quickly from the sitting position to the provoking position, which is maintained for 2 or 3 min. The patient's head is then rapidly rolled over to the opposite ear-down position, which is also maintained for several minutes. The recommendation that patients must try to keep their head vertical for 48 h, even at night, and avoid the provoking position for 1 week following treatment is now considered not to be necessary.

Epley[162] suggested an alternative repositioning maneuver to accomplish the same goal, displacement of debris from the posterior or anterior canal where it rests on the cupula to the utricular cavity where it becomes harmless. In the Epley maneuver, the patient is quickly tilted straight back with the symptomatic head-side tilted back and down, inducing an attack. Rotation of the head and trunk toward the unaffected ear then cause further movement of the debris downward toward the exit to the canal, resulting in more vertigo and nystagmus. Each position should be maintained for 2 min or at least

until the provoked vertigo and nystagmus subsides. The final uprighting of the patient causes the debris to enter the utricular cavity. The complete procedure should be repeated until no further symptoms are provoked, usually a maximum of two or three times in one session. During treatment, Epley[162] and Li[163] advocate the use of mastoid oscillation over the affected ear in order to facilitate the removal of the debris. However, more recent work comparing cure rates with and without the use of assistive devices concludes that mastoid vibration does not improve results and is therefore not necessary.[67,164]

Self-treatment techniques also exist for the treatment of BPPV. These exercises are usually prescribed for patients that have a recurrence of symptoms but are unable to visit their doctor or therapist[165] and for those patients with positive Hallpike signs remaining after attempting one of the following single treatment maneuvers. The first self-treatment approach was developed by Brandt and Daroff[166] who recommended positional exercises for BPPV based on the assumption that cupulothiasis was the underlying mechanism. The patient sits on the edge of a bed or couch, and moves rapidly from the sitting position to lie on the side provoking vertigo, with their head tilted downwards so that the lateral aspects of their occiput touch the bed. After 30 s the patient should resume the sitting position for 30 s, and then lie on the opposite side for 30 s. Brandt has recently modified this exercise to eliminate the stop in the sitting position (T. Brandt, personal communication). The whole sequence should be repeated 10 times, and the treatment is continued until it no longer provokes dizziness and nausea (normally between one and four weeks). Brandt notes that improvement tends to fluctuate and recovery is often abrupt, and reports that very few patients fail to respond to a prolonged course of this therapy. However, Radtke et al.[167] recently proposed a modified Epley maneuver for self-treatment at home, which they found to be more effective than the Brandt–Daroff exercises, with a significantly shorter remission time and higher success rate. The modifications to the original Epley maneuver include resting the head on the bed instead of the head-hanging position and the use of a pillow to support the patient's shoulder to achieve head reclination.[167,168]

The above procedures are not recommended for patients for whom restriction of violent movement is imposed by secondary conditions such as cervical or lumbar pain caused by injury or arthritis, unstable heart disease, anxiety, obesity, and an unwillingness of the individual to pursue a protracted program of exercises.[165,169,170] A canalith repositioning technique involving a 360° heels-over-head rotation of the posterior semicircular canal using a motion device[169,171] has shown to be an efficient method for treating BPPV and it has been suggested that it may be safely used with patients for whom traditional maneuvers are not advised.[169] However, it does not seem likely that this procedure will gain much popularity because of practical constraints such as the cost and space required for the equipment, and the proven efficacy of manual treatments.

Some clinicians describe very favorable results, with complete eradication of vertigo in over 90 per cent of suitable patients.[162,164,172,173] However, others have found it difficult to replicate this success rate.[170,174,175] Improvement percentages in these studies are still quite high and individual authors conclude that single treatment techniques are effective in the treatment of BPPV. Outcome variability may result from a number of factors such as correct technique when performing the maneuver, the repetition of the maneuver until symptoms resolve, number of treatment sessions, post-treatment instructions as well as a possibility that posterior canal BPPV may convert to horizontal or anterior canal BPPV after treatment.[158,176] If this occurs, separate procedures must be performed for alleviation of symptoms.

Two methods have been shown to be effective for the treatment of horizontal canal BPPV. A very simple method known as 'forced prolonged position' (FPP)[177] has the patient lie on their unaffected side for 12 consecutive hours. In the second procedure ('barbecue rotation') identified by Lempert and Tiel-Wilck,[178] the patient begins in a supine position and is rotated 270° around the longitudinal (yaw) axis toward the unaffected ear in three successive 90° steps at 30-s intervals. The patient is then brought to a sitting position with the head tilted slightly forwards. Both groups have reported treatment success.[177,178] A comparative study of the two procedures finds that FPP is slightly more successful but 'barbecue rotation' has the advantage of providing more immediate results.[179] Nuti et al.[179] suggest treating patients with both maneuvers in sequence – a barbecue rotation followed by FPP – even when no symptoms can be elicited after the initial procedure.

Postural instability is a common characteristic of BPPV that is well documented[109,180,181] but often neglected. Recent studies using dynamic posturography have shown that prior to treatment with a repositioning maneuver, patients display an inability to maintain balance when somatosensory cues are altered and postural control relies mainly on vestibular cues.[180,181] However, these findings do not extend to disorders of the horizontal semicircular canal where postural control remains unaffected both prior to and following therapy.[181] Following treatment using the Semont or Epley maneuver for individuals with posterior canal BPPV, authors in two independent studies[180,181] noted an overall improvement in postural stability, although many patients' scores remained below those for the control group. Therefore, patients should be assessed for any balance deficits that may remain after treatment for the BPPV and, if required, should be provided with the appropriate exercises to improve balance.

To summarize, a variety of simple and effective techniques are available for the treatment of BPPV. However, the selection of technique and the provision of any additional balance therapy should be based on a multifactorial assessment of the individual, rather than on theoretical predilections.[170,182]

CONCLUSIONS

There are a wide number of causes of balance disorders in patients with peripheral or CNS deficits, so no one set of exercises for retraining balance is appropriate. A balance rehabilitation program reflects the particular constellation of impairments and compensations specific for each patient and therefore, if possible, should be individually designed based on a systematic evaluation of each patient. In addition to the physiological reasons for developing individualized exercise programs, there may be more general benefits. Tailoring an exercise program entails working with the individual to discover their particular sensorimotor impairments, selecting exercises that directly address these, and discussing how the exercises may be expected to affect particular aspects of disorientation and disequilibrium. For example, the process of identifying those movements or perceptual conditions which provoke vertigo provides a concrete demonstration that the program is relevant to the person's problems, which may enhance adherence to the treatment by promoting confidence in the therapy and an understanding of the rationale for performing exercises.

REFERENCES

1. Herdman SJ. *Vestibular rehabilitation*. Philadelphia: FA Davis, 2000.
2. Shumway-Cook A. Vestibular rehabilitation in traumatic brain injury. In: Herdman SJ, ed. *Vestibular rehabilitation*. Philadelphia: FA Davis, 2000;476–93.
3. Konrad HR, Tomlinson D, Stockwell CW, et al. Rehabilitation therapy for patients with disequilibrium and balance disorders. *Otolarngol Head Neck Surg* 1992;**107**:105–8.
4. Shumway-Cook A, Horak FB. Vestibular rehabilitation: an exercise approach to managing symptoms of vestibular dysfunction. *Semin Hear* 1989;**10**:196–205.
5. Shumway-Cook A, Horak F. Rehabilitation strategies for patients with vestibular deficits. *Neurol Clin N Am* 1990;**8**:441–57.
6. Jette, AM. Physical disablement concepts for physical therapy research and practice. *Phys Ther* 1994;**74**:380–6.
7. Shumway-Cook A, Horak F. *Balance rehabilitation in the neurologic patient: course syllabus*. Seattle: NERA, 1992.
8. Shumway-Cook A, Woollacott M. *Motor Control: theory and practical applications*, 2nd edn. Philadelphia: Lippincott, Williams & Wilkins, 2001.
9. Nagi SZ. Some conceptual issues in disability and rehabilitation. In: Sussman MB, ed. *Sociology and rehabilitation*. Washington, DC: American Sociological Association, 1965;100–13.

10. Lacour M, Xerri C. Vestibular compensation: New perspective. In: Flohr H, Precht W, eds. *Lesion induced neuronal plasticity in sensorimotor systems.* New York: Springer Verlag, 1981;240–53.

11. Curthoys IS, Halmagyi GM. Vestibular compensation: a review of the oculomotor, neural and clinical consequences of unilateral vestibular loss. *J Vestib Res* 1995;**5**:67–107.

12. Marchand AR, Amblard B. Locomotion in adult cats with early vestibular deprivation: Visual cue substitution. *Exp Brain Res* 1984;**454**:395.

13. Pfaltz CR, Karnath R. Central compensation of vestibular dysfunction: peripheral lesions. *Adv Otorhinolarynogol* 1983;**30**:335.

14. Bles W, deJong JM, deWit G. Compensation for labyrinthine defects by use of a tilting room. *Acta Otolaryngol (Stockh)* 1983;**95**:576.

15. Horak FB, Shupert CL. Role of the vestibular system in postural control. In: Herdman SJ, ed. *Vestibular rehabilitation.* Philadelphia: FA Davis, 1994;22–46.

16. McCabe BF. Labyrinthine exercises in the treatment of disease characterized by vertigo: their physiologic basis and methodology. *Laryngoscope* 1970;**80**:1429.

17. Cawthorne T. Vestibular injuries. *Proc R Soc Med* 1945;**39**:270–3.

18. Black F, Peterka RJ, Shupert C, Nashner L. Effects of unilateral loss of vestibular function on the vestibulo-ocular reflex and postural control. *Ann Oto-Rhino-Laryngol* 1989;**98**:884–9.

19. Calder JH, Jacobson GP. Acquired bilateral peripheral vestibular system impairment: rehabilitative options and outcomes. *J Am Acad Audiol* 2000;**11**:514–21.

20. Gillespie MB, Minor LB. Prognosis in bilateral vestibular hypofunction. *Laryngoscope* 1999;**109**:35–41.

21. Horak FB, Shumway-Cook A, Crowe T, Black FO. Vestibular function and motor proficiency in children with hearing impairments and in learning disabled children with motor impairments. *Dev Med Child Neurol* 1988;**30**:64–79.

22. Schupert CL, Horak FB, Black FO. Hip sway associated with vestibulopathy. *J Vestib Res* 1994;**4**:231–44.

23. Herdman SJ, Blatt P, Schubert MC, Tusa RJ. Falls in patients with vestibular deficits. *Am J Otol* 2000;**21**:847–51.

24. Bronstein AM. Suppression of visually evoked postural responses. *Exp Brain Res* 1986;**63**:655–8.

25. Bisdorff AR, Bronstein AM, Gresty MA. Responses in neck and facial muscles to sudden free fall and a startling auditory stimulus. *Electro-encephalogr Clin Neurophysiol* 1994;**93**:409–16.

26. Allum JHJ, Honegger F, Pfaltz CR. The role of stretch and vestibulo-spinal reflexes in the generation of human equilibrating reactions. *Prog Brain Res* 1994b;**80**:399–409.

27. Kasai T, Zee D. Eye head coordination in labyrinthine defective human beings. *Brain Res* 1978;**81**:123.

28. Bronstein AM, Hood JD. The cervico-ocular reflex in normal subjects and patients with absent vestibular function. *Brain Res* 1986;**373**:399–408.

29. Bronstein AM, Hood JD. Oscillopsia of peripheral vestibular origin. *Acta Otolaryngol (Stockh)* 1987;**104**:307–14.

30. Bronstein AM, Mossman SS, Luxon LM. The neck-eye reflex in patients with reduced vestibular and optokinetic function. *Brain* 1991;**114**:1–11.

31. Berthoz A, Melvill Jones G. *Adaptive mechanisms in gaze control. Reviews in oculomotor research 1.* New York: Elsevier Science, 1985.

32. Grunfeld EA, Morland AB, Bronstein AM, Gresty MA. Adaptation to oscillopsia: a psychophysical and questionnaire investigation. *Brain* 2000;**123**:277–90.

33. Morland AB, Bronstein AM, Ruddock KH, Wooding DS. Oscillopsia: visual function during motion in the absence of vestibulo-ocular reflex. *J Neurol Neurosurg Psychiatry* 1998;**65**:828–35.

34. Hess K, Gresty MA, Leech J. Clinical and theoretical aspects of head movement dependent oscillopsia (HMDO). *J Neurol* 1978;**219**:151–7.

35. Furman JP, Whitney SL. Central causes of dizziness. *Phys Ther* 2000;**80**:179–87.

36. Gill-Body KM, Popat RA, Parker SW, Krebs DE. Rehabilitation of balance in two patients with cerebellar dysfunction. *Phys Ther* 1997;**77**:534–52.

37. Burton JM. Physical therapy management of a patient with central vestibular dysfunction: a case report. *Neurol Rep* 1996;**20**:61–2.

38. Fitzgerald DC. Persistent dizziness following head trauma and perilymphatic fistula. *Arch Phys Rehabil Med* 1995;**76**:1017–20.

39. Godbout A. Structured habituation training for movement provoked vertigo after severe traumatic brain injury: a single-case experiment. *Brain Inj* 1997;**11**:629–41.

40. Whitney SL, Wrisley DM, Brown KE, Furman JM. Physical therapy for migraine-related vestibulopathy and vestibular dysfunction with history of migraine. *Laryngoscope* 2000;**110**:1528–34.

41. Shepard NT, Smith-Wheelock M, Telian SA, Raj A. Vestibular and balance rehabilitation therapy. *Ann Oto-Rhino-Laryngol* 1993;**102**:198–205.

42. Cass SP, Borello-France D, Furman JM. Functional outcome of vestibular rehabilitation in patients with abnormal sensory-organization testing. *Am J Otol* 1996;**17**:581–94.

43. Cowand JL, Wrisley DM, Walker M, et al. Efficacy of vestibular rehabilitation. *Otolaryngol Head Neck Surg* 1998;**118**:49–54.

44. Black FO, Angel CR, Peszecker SC, Gianna C. Outcome analysis of individualised vestibular rehabilitation protocols. *Am J Otol* 2000;**21**:543–51.

45. Hahn A, Sejna I, Stolbova K, Cocek A. Visuo-vestibular biofeedback in patients with peripheral vestibular disorders. *Acta Otolaryngol (Stockh) Suppl* 2001;**545**:88–91.

46. Bronstein AM. The visual vertigo syndrome. *Acta Otolaryngol (Stockh) Suppl* 1995;**520**:45–8.

47. Jacob RG, Woody SR, Clark DB, et al. Discomfort with space and motion: a possible marker of vestibular dysfunction assessed by the Situational Characteristics Questionnaire. *J Psychopathol Behav Assess* 1993;**15**:299–324.

48. Page NGR, Gresty MA. Motorist's vestibular disorientation syndrome. *J Neurol Neurosurg Psychiatry* 1985;**48**:729–35.

49. Guerraz M, Yardley L, Bertholon P, et al. Visual vertigo: symptom assessment, spatial orientation and postural control. *Brain* 2001;**124**:1646–56.

50. Redfern MS, Furman JM. Postural sway of patients with vestibular disorders during optic flow. *J Vestib Res* 1994;**4**:221–30.

51. Jacob RF, Lilienfeld MA, Furman JMR, et al. Panic disorder with vestibular dysfunction: further clinical observations and

description of space and motion phobic stimuli. *J Anxiety Disord* 1989;**3**:117–30.

52. Jacob RG, Redfern MS, Furman JM. Optic flow-induced sway in anxiety disorders associated with space and motion discomfort. *J Anxiety Disord* 1994;**9**:411–25.

53. Yardley L, Luxon L, Lear S, et al. Vestibular and posturographic test results in people with symptoms of panic and agoraphobia. *J Audiol Med* 1994;**3**:48–65.

54. Yardley L. Motion sickness and perception: a reappraisal of the sensory conflict approach. *Br J Psychol* 1992;**83**:449–73.

55. Tsuzuku T, Vitte E, Sémont A, Berthoz A. Modification of parameters in vertical optokinetic nystagmus after repeated vertical optokinetic stimulation in patients with vestibular lesions. *Acta Otolaryngol (Stockh) Suppl* 1995;**520**:419–22.

56. Vitte E, Sémont A, Berthoz A. Repeated optokinetic stimulation in conditions of active standing facilitates recovery from vestibular deficits. *Exp Brain Res* 1994;**102**:141–8.

57. Pavlou M, Lingeswaran A, Davies RA, et al. Machine-based vs. customised rehabilitation for the treatment of chronic vestibular patients (Abstract). *Proceedings of the ISPG symposium, Maastricht, Netherlands.* Maastricht: ISPG, 2001.

58. Brandt T, Bronstein AM. Cervical vertigo. *J Neurol Neurosurg Psychiatry* 2001;**71**:8–12.

59. De Jong PTVM, de Jong JMBV, Cohen B, Jongkees, LBW. Ataxia and nystagmus induced by injection of local anaesthetics in the neck. *Ann Neurol* 1977;**1**:240–6.

60. Mergner T, Siebold C, Schweigart G, Becker W. Human perception of horizontal trunk and head rotation in space during vestibular and neck stimulation. *Exp Brain Res* 1991;**85**:389–404.

61. Ryan GMS, Cope S. Cervical vertigo. *Lancet* 1955;**ii**:1355–8.

62. Alund M, Ledin T, Odkvist L, Larsson SE. Dynamic posturography among patients with common neck disorders. A study of 15 cases with suspected cervical vertigo. *J Vestib Res* 1993;**3**:383–9.

63. Karlberg M, Magnusson M, Malmström E, et al. Postural and symptomatic improvement after physiotherapy in patients with dizziness of suspected cervical origin. *Arch Phys Rehabil Med* 1996;**77**:874–82.

64. Biesinger E. Vertigo caused by disorders of the cervical vertebral column: diagnosis and treatment. *Adv Oto-Rhino-Laryngol* 1988;**39**:44–51.

65. Wrisley DM, Sparto PJ, Whitney SL, Furman JM. Cervicogenic dizziness: a review of diagnosis and treatment. *J Orthopaed Sports Phys Ther* 2000;**30**:755–66.

66. Mallinson AI, Longridge NS. Dizziness form whiplash and head injury: differences between whiplash and head injury. *Am J Otol* 1998;**19**:814–18.

67. Hain TC, Helminski JO, Reis IL, Uddin MK. Vibration does not improve results of the canalith repositioning procedure. *Arch Otolaryngol Head Neck Surg* 2000;**126**:617–22.

68. Clendaniel RA. Cervical vertigo. In: Herdman SJ, ed. *Vestibular rehabilitation.* Philadelphia: FA Davis, 2000;494–509.

69. Galm R, Rittmeister M, Schmitt E. Vertigo in patients with cervical spine dysfunction. *Eur Spine J* 1998;**7**:55–8.

70. Cooksey FS. Rehabilitation in vestibular injuries. *Proc R Soc Med* 1945;**39**:273–8.

71. Shepard NT, Telian SA. Programmatic vestibular rehabilitation. *Otolaryngol Head Neck Surg* 1995;**112**:173–82.

72. Szturm T, Ireland DJ, Lessing-Turner M. Comparison of different exercise programs in the rehabilitation of patients with chronic peripheral vestibular dysfunction. *J Vestib Res* 1994;**4**:461–79.

73. Horak F. Clinical measurement of postural control in adults. *Phys Ther* 1987;**67**:1881–5.

74. Mathias, S, Nayak, U, Issacs, B. Balance in elderly patients: the 'Get-up and Go' test. *Arch Phys Rehabil Med* 1986;**67**:387–9.

75. Podsiadlo D, Richardson S. The timed 'Up &Go': a test of basic functional mobility for frail elderly persons. *J Am Geriatr Soc* 1991;**39**:142–8.

76. Duncan PW, Weiner DK, Chandler J, Studenski S. Functional reach: a new clinical measure of balance. *J Gerontol* 1990;**45**:192–5.

77. Tinetti ME. Performance oriented assessment of mobility problems in elderly patients. *J Am Geriatr Soc* 1986;**34**:119–26.

78. Tinetti ME, Ginter SF. Identifying mobility dysfunctions in elderly patients: standard neuromuscular examination or direct assessment? *JAMA* 1988;**259**:1190–3.

79. Shumway-Cook, A, Woollacott, M. *Motor control: theory and practical applications*, 1st edn. Philadelphia: Lippincott, Williams & Wilkins, 1995.

80. Shumway-Cook A, Baldwin M, Polissar NL, Gruber W. Predicting the probability for falls in community-dwelling older adults. *Phys Ther* 1997;**77**:812–19.

81. Whitney SL, Hudak MT, Marchetti GF. The dynamic gait index relates to self-reported fall history in individuals with vestibular dysfunction. *J Vestib Res* 2000;**10**:99–105.

82. Berg, K. Measuring balance in the elderly: validation of an instrument. Dissertation. Montreal: McGill University, 1993.

83. Fregly AR, Graybiel AR. An ataxia test battery not requiring rails. *Aerospace Med* 1968;**3**:277–82.

84. Tinetti ME, Douchette JT, Claus EB. The contribution of predisposing and situational risk factors to serious fall injuries. *J Am Geriatr Soc* 1995;**43**:1207–13.

85. Wernick-Robinson M, Krebs DE, Giorgetti MM. Functional reach: does it really measure dynamic balance? *Arch Phys Rehabil Med* 1999;**80**:262–9.

86. Evans MK, Krebs DE. Posturography does not test vestibulospinal function. *Otolaryngol Head Neck Sur* 1999;**120**:164–73.

87. Gill-Body KM, Beninato M, Krebs DE. Relationships among balance impairments, functional performance, and disability in people with peripheral vestibular dysfunction. *Phys Ther* 2000;**80**:748–58.

88. Allum JHJ, Adkin AL, Carpenter MG, et al. Trunk sway measures of postural stability during clinical balance tests: effects of a unilateral vestibular deficit. *Gait Posture* 2001;**14**:227–37.

89. Saunders D. Evaluation, treatment and prevention of musculoskeletal disorders. Minneapolis: Viking Press, 1991.

90. Magee DJ. *Orthopedic physical assessment.* Philadelphia: Saunders, 1987.

91. Horak FB, Moore SP. The effect of prior leaning on human postural responses. *Gait Posture* 1993;**1**:203–10.

92. Horak F, Nashner L. Central programming of postural movements: adaptation to altered support surface configurations. *J Neurophysiol* 1986;**55**:1369–81.

93. Nashner L, Woollacott M. The organization of rapid postural adjustments of standing humans: an experimental–conceptual model. In: Talbott RE, Humphrey DR, eds. *Posture and movement.* New York: Raven Press, 1979;243–57.

94. Nashner LM. Fixed patterns of rapid postural responses among leg muscles during stance. *Exp Brain Res* 1977;**30**:13–24.

95. Nashner L. Adapting reflexes controlling the human posture. *Exp Brain Res* 1976;**26**:59–72.

96. Nashner LM, Shumway-Cook A, Marin O. Stance posture control in select groups of children with cerebral palsy: deficits in sensory organization and muscular coordination. *Exp Brain Res* 1983;**49**:393–409.

97. DeFabio R, Badke MB.Relationship of sensory organization to balance function in patients with hemiplegia. *Phys Ther* 1990;**70**:543–52.

98. Horak FB, Shupert CL, Dietz V, Horstmann G. Vestibular and somatosensory contributions to responses to head and body displacements in stance. *Exp Brain Res* 1994;**100**:93–106.

99. Allum JHJ, Bloem BR, Carpenter MG, Honegger F. Differential diagnosis of proprioceptive and vestibular deficits using dynamic support-surface posturography. *Gait Posture* 2001;**14**:217–26.

100. Carpenter MG, Allum JH, Honegger F. Vestibular influences on human postural control in combinations of pitch and roll planes reveal differences in spatiotemporal processing. *Exp Brain Res* 2001;**140**:95–111.

101. Ito Y, Corna S, von Brevern M, et al. Neck muscle responses to abrupt free fall of the head: comparison of normal with labyrinthine-defective human subjects. *J Physiol* 1995;**489**:911–16.

102. Bronstein AM. Evidence for a vestibular input contributing to dynamic head stabilization in man. *Acta Otolaryngol (Stockh)* 1988;**105**:1–6.

103. Horak, FB, Diener, HC, Nashner, LM. Influence of central set on human postural responses. *J Neurophysiol* 1989;**62**:841–53.

104. Bobath B. *Adult hemiplegia: evaluation and treatment.* London: Heinemann Medical Books, 1978.

105. Carr JH, Shepherd RB. *Motor relearning program for stroke.* Rockville: Aspen Publications, 1983.

106. Maki BE, McIlroy WE. The role of limb movements in maintaining upright stance: The 'change-in-support' strategy. *Phys Ther* 1997;**77**:488–507.

107. Runge CF, Shupert CL, Horak FB, Zajac FE. Role of vestibular information in initiation of rapid postural responses. *Exp Brain Res* 1998;**122**:403 12.

108. Inglis JT, Horak FB, Shupert CL, Jones-Rycewicz C. The importance of somatosensory information in triggering and scaling automatic postural responses in humans. *Exp Brain Res* 1994;**101**:159–64.

109. Black FO, Shupert C, Horak FB, Nashner LM. Abnormal postural control associated with peripheral vestibular disorders. In: Pompeiano O, Allum J, eds. Vestibulo-spinal control of posture and movement. *Progress in brain research*, Vol. 76. Amsterdam: Elsevier Science Publishers, 1988;263–75.

110. Horak FB, Nashner LM, Diener HC. Postural strategies associated with somatosensory and vestibular loss. *Exp Brain Res* 1990;**82**:167–77.

111. Horak, F, Shupert, C, Mirka, A. Components of postural dyscontrol in the elderly: a review. *Neurobiol Ageing* 1989b;**10**:727–45.

112. Shumway-Cook A, Horak F. Assessing the influence of sensory interaction on balance. *Phys Ther* 1986;**66**:1548–50.

113. Bergin PS, Bronstein AM, Murray NMF, et al. Body sway and vibration perception thresholds in normal ageing and in patients with polyneuropathy. *J Neurol Neurosurg Psychiatry* 1995;**58**:335–40.

114. Nashner LM. 1982: Adaptation of human movement to altered environments. *Trends Neurosci* **5**:358–61.

115. Peterka RJ, Black FO. Age-related changes in human posture control: sensory organization tests. *J Vestib Res* 1990;**1**:73–85.

116. Cohen H, Blatchly C, Gombash L. A study of the clinical test of sensory interaction and balance. *Phys Ther* 1993;**73**:346–54.

117. El-Kashlan HK, Shepard NT, Asher AM. Evaluation of clinical measures of equilibrium. *Laryngoscope* 1998;**108**:311–19.

118. Bronstein AM, Guerraz M. Visual-vestibular control of posture and gait: physiological mechanisms and disorders. *Curr Opin Neurol* 1999;**12**:5–11.

119. Jacobson GP, Calder JH. A screening version of the Dizziness Handicap Inventory. *Am J Otol* 1998;**19**:804–8.

120. Cohen HS, Kimball KT, Adams AS. Application of the vestibular disorders activities of daily living scale. *Laryngoscope* 2000;**110**:1204–9.

121. Dobie RA. Does computerized dynamic posturography help us care for our patients? *Am J Otol* 1997;**18**:108–12.

122. O'Neill DE, Gill-Body DM, Krebs DE. Posturography changes do not predict functional performance changes. *Am J Otol* 1998;**19**:797–803.

123. Robertson DD, Ireland DJ. Dizziness handicap inventory correlates of computerized dynamic posturography. *J Otolaryngol* 1995;**24**:118–24.

124. Horak F, Jones-Rycewicz C, Black FO, Shumway-Cook A. Effects of vestibular rehabilitation on dizziness and imbalance. *Otolaryngol Head Neck Surg* 1992;**106**:175–80.

125. Keim RJ, Cook M, Martini D. Balance rehabilitation therapy. *Laryngoscope* 1992;**102**:1302–7.

126. Goebel JA, Sataloff RT, Hanson JM, et al. Posturographic evidence of nonorganic sway patterns in normal subjects, patients, and suspected malingerers. *Otolaryngol Head Neck Surg* 1997;**117**:293–302.

127. Krempl GA, Dobie RA. Evaluation of posturography in the detection of malingering subjects. *Am J Otol* 1998;**19**:619–27.

128. Gianoli G, McWilliams S, Soileau J, Belafsky P. Posturographic performance in patients with the potential for secondary gain. *Otolaryngol Head Neck Surg* 2000;**122**:11–8.

129. Stephens SDG, Hogan S, Meredith R. The desynchrony between complaints and signs of vestibular disorders. *Acta Otolaryngol (Stockh)* 1991;**11**:188–92.

130. Gresty MA, Bronstein AM, Brandt T, Dieterich M. Neurology of otolith function: peripheral and central disorders. *Brain* 1992;**115**:647–73.

131. Norré ME. Treatment of unilateral vestibular hypofunction. In: Osterveld WJ, ed. *Otoneurology.* New York: John Wiley and Sons, 1984;23–29.

132. Norré M. Rationale of rehabilitation treatment for vertigo. *Am J Otolaryngol* 1987;**8**:31.

133. Friedmann G. The judgement of the visual vertical and

horizontal in peripheral and central vestibular lesions. *Brain* 1970;**93**:313–28.

134. Brandt T. *Vertigo: its multisensory syndromes.* London: Springer-Verlag, 1991.

135. Anastasopoulos D, Bronstein A, Haslwanter T, et al. The role of somatosensory input for the perception of verticality. *Ann N Y Acad Sci* 1999;**871**:379–83.

136. Mittelstaedt H. The information processing structure of the subjective vertical. A cybernetic bridge between its psychophysics and its neurobiology. In: Marko H, Hauske G, Struppler A, eds. *Processing structures for perception and action.* Wenheim: VCH Verlagsgesellschaft, 1988;217–63.

137. Herman R. Augmented sensory feedback in control of limb movement. In: Fields WS, ed. *Neural organization and its relevance to prosthetics.* New York: Intercontinental Medical Book Corp, 1973.

138. Shumway-Cook A, Anson D, Haller S. Postural sway biofeedback, its effect on reestablishing stance stability in hemiplegic patients. *Arch Phys Rehabil Med* 1988;**69**:395–41.

139. Yardley L, Lerwill H, Hall M, Gresty M. Visual destabilisation of posture. *Acta Otolaryngol (Stockh)* 1992;**112**:14–21.

140. Borello-France DF, Gallagher JD, Redfurn M. Voluntary movement strategies of individuals with unilateral peripheral vestibular hypofunction. *J Vestib Res* 1999;**9**:265–75.

141. Crane BT, Demer JL. Gaze stabilization during dynamic posturography in normal and vestibulopathic humans. *Exp Brain Res* 1998;**122**:235–46.

142. Herdman SJ. Advances in the treatment of vestibular disorders. *Phys Ther* 1997;**77**:602–18.

143. Beyts JP. Vestibular rehabilitation. In: Stephens D, ed. *Adult audiology, Scott-Brown's Otolaryngology,* 5th edn. London: Butterworths, 1987.

144. Ödkvist I, Ödkvist LM. Physiotherapy in vertigo. *Acta Otolaryngol (Stockh) Suppl* 1988;**455**:74–6.

145. Leduc A, Decloedt V. La kinesitherapie en ORL. *Acta Otorhinolaryngol Belg* 1989;**43**:381–90.

146. Ost, L-G. Applied relaxation: description of a coping technique and review of controlled studies. *Behav Res Ther* 1987;**25**:397–409.

147. Meuret AE, Wilhelm FH, Roth WT. Respiratory biofeedback-assisted therapy in panic disorder. *Behav Modif* 2001;**25**:584–605.

148. Norré ME, de Weerdt W. Treatment of vertigo based on habituation. 2. Technique and results of habituation training. *J Laryngol Otol* 1980;**94**:971–7.

149. Cohen H. Vestibular rehabilitation reduces functional disability. *Otolaryngol Head Neck Surg* 1992;**107**:638–43.

150. Shepard NT, Telian SA, Smith-Wheelock M. Habituation and balance training therapy. *Neurol Clin N Am* 1990;**8**:459–75.

151. Blakeley, BW. Vestibular rehabilitation on a budget. *J Otolaryngol* 1999;**28**:205–9.

152. Schmidt JTH, Huizing EH. The clinical drug trial in Ménière's disease with emphasis on the effect of betahistine SR. *Acta Otolaryngol (Stockh) Suppl* 1992;**497**:1–189.

153. Strupp M, Arbusow V, Maag KP, et al. Vestibular exercises improve central vestibulospinal compensation after vestibular neuritis. *Neurology* 1998;**3**:838–44.

154. Yardley L, Beech S, Evans T, Weinman J. A randomized controlled trial of exercise therapy for dizziness and vertigo in primary care. *Br J Gen Pract* 1998;**48**:1136–40.

155. Yardley L, Beech S, Weinman J. Influence of beliefs about the consequences of dizziness on handicap in people with dizziness, and the effects of therapy on beliefs. *J Psychosomat Res* 2001;**50**:1–6.

156. Yardley L, Burgneay J, Anderson G, et al. Feasibility and effectiveness of providing vestibular rehabilitation for dizzy patients in the community. *Clin Otolaryngol* 1998b;**23**:442–8.

157. Fife TD. Recognition and management of horizontal canal benign positional vertigo. *Am J Otol* 1998;**19**:345–51.

158. Herdman SJ, Tusa RJ. Complications of the canalith repositioning procedure. *Arch Otolaryngol Head Neck Surg* 1996;**122**:281–6.

159. McClure JA. Horizontal canal BPV. *J Otolaryngol* 1985;**14**:30–35.

160. Troost BT, Patton JM. Exercise therapy for positional vertigo. *Neurology* 1992;**42**:1441–4.

161. Sémont A, Freyss G. Vitte E. Curing the BPPV with a Liberatory manoeuvre. *Adv Otorhinolaryngol* 1988;**42**:290–3.

162. Epley EM. The canalith repositioning procedure for treatment of benign paroxysmal positional vertigo. *Otolaryngol Head Neck Surg* 1992;**107**:399–404.

163. Li JC. Mastoid oscillation: a critical factor for success in the canalith repositioning procedure. *Otolaryngol Head Neck Surg* 1995;**112**:670–5.

164. Nunez RA, Cass SP, Furman JM. Short- and long-term outcomes of canalith repositioning for benign paroxysmal positional vertigo. *Otolaryngol Head Neck Surg* 2000;**122**:647–53.

165. Furman JP, Cass SP. Benign paroxysmal positional vertigo. *N Engl J Med* 1999;**341**:1590–6.

166. Brandt T, Daroff RB. Physical therapy for benign paroxysmal positional vertigo. *Arch Otolaryngol* 1980;**106**:484–5.

167. Radtke A, Neuhauser H, von Brevern M, Lempert T. A modified Epley's procedure for self-treatment of benign paroxysmal positional vertigo. *Neurology* 1999;**53**:1358–60.

168. Radtke A, Neuhauser H, von Brevern M, Lempert T. Self-treatment of benign positional vertigo [Online]. Berlin, Germany: Neurologische Klinik, Charité, 2002; http://www.charite.de/ch/neuro[2002:Jan 15]

169. Furman JP, Cass SP, Briggs BC. Treatment of benign positional vertigo using heels-over-head rotation. *Ann Otol Rhinol Laryngol* 1998;**107**:1046–53.

170. Herdman S, Tusa RJ, Zee DS, et al. Single treatment approaches to benign paroxysmal positional vertigo. *Arch Otolaryngol Head Neck Surg* 1993;**119**:450–4.

171. Lempert T, Wolsley C, Davies R. et al. Three-hundred and sixty-degree rotation of the posterior semicircular canal for treatment of benign positional vertigo: a placebo-controlled trial. *Neurology* 1997;**49**:729–33.

172. Aranda-Moreno C, Jauregui-Renaud K. Epley and Semont maneuvers in the treatment of benign paroxysmal postural vertigo. *Gaceta medica de Mexico* 2000;**136**:433–9.

173. Wolf JS, Boyev KP, Manokey BJ, Mattox DE. Success of the modified Epley maneuver in treating benign paroxysmal positional vertigo. *Laryngoscope* 1999;**109**:900–3.

174. Froehling DA, Bowen JM, Mohr DN, et al. The canalith repositioning procedure for the treatment of benign paroxysmal positional vertigo: a randomized controlled trial. *Mayo Clin Proc* 2000;**75**:695–700.

175. Wolf M, Hertanu T, Novikov I, Kronenberg J. Epley's

manoeuvre for benign paroxysmal positional vertigo: a prospective study. *Clin Otolaryngol* 1999;**24**:43–6.

176. Macias JD, Lambert KM, Massingale S. et al. *Laryngoscope* 2000;**110**:1921–4.

177. Vannucchi P, Giannoni B, Pagnini P. Treatment of horizontal semicircular canal benign paroxysmal positional vertigo. *J Vestib Res* 1997;**7**:1–6.

178. Lempert T, Tiel-Wilck K. A positional maneuver for treatment of horizontal-canal benign positional vertigo. *Laryngoscope* 1996;**106**:476–8.

179. Nuti D, Agus G, Barbieri MT, Passali D. The management of horizontal-canal paroxysmal positional vertigo. *Acta Otolaryngol (Stockh)* 1998;**118**:455–60.

180. Blatt PJ, Georgakakis GA, Herdman SJ, et al. The effect of the canalith repositioning maneuver on resolving postural instability in patients with benign paroxysmal positional vertigo. *Am J Otol* 2000;**21**:356–63.

181. Di Girolamo S, Ottaviani F, Scarano E, et al. Postural control in horizontal benign paroxysmal vertigo. *Eur Arch Otorhinolaryngol* 2000;**257**:372–5.

182. Herdman SJ, Tusa RJ. Assessment and treatment of patients with benign paroxysmal positional vertigo. In: Herdman SJ, ed. *Vestibular rehabilitation*. Philadelphia: FA Davis, 2000;451–75.

18

Neurological rehabilitation of gait and balance disorders

KARL-HEINZ MAURITZ, STEFAN HESSE AND CORDULA WERNER

INTRODUCTION

Restoration of mobility is a major goal in neurological rehabilitation, preventing long-term disability and handicap. Mobility includes walking, standing up, sitting down, weight shifting from one leg to the other, turning around, initiating and stopping locomotion, as well as climbing stairs. Therapeutic methods to retrain gait functions in the most common syndromes will be presented (i.e. in hemiplegia caused by stroke or traumatic brain injury, paraplegia caused by spinal cord injuries and in Parkinson's disease). Goals of therapy include security and safety, speed and endurance, accuracy and low variability, flexibility and adaptability to the surroundings.

The achievement of these goals depends on a complex interaction between the neurological deficit, other physical and cognitive deficits, training procedures, compensation strategies, psychological factors and the social environment. An effective rehabilitation program has to take into account the personal needs and goals of the individual patient. Mobility training also includes the use of technical aids such as walkers, canes or the application of orthoses, and has to consider the prevention of falls. A wide variety of therapeutic procedures is available and has to be adapted to the individual situation: different concepts of physiotherapy stressing different features, such as force exercise, reduction of spasticity, gait symmetry, utilization of equilibrium reflexes, stepping automation, endurance training, repetition of rhythmic movements, etc. The spectrum of available therapies was recently widened by treadmill training with partial body-weight support, gait machines, by functional electrical stimulation (FES), locomotor pharmacotherapy,

selective reduction of spasticity by botulinum toxin injections, by acoustic and visual cuing and biofeedback. Those methods pertaining to gait improvement will also be described.

Before starting with therapy, a comprehensive assessment is necessary to evaluate the deficits and the remaining functions. These assessment methods are also crucial in monitoring the progress and selecting the most appropriate strategies. Since neurological and orthopedic evaluation methods are described elsewhere in this book, only the specific assessment methods of rehabilitation will be mentioned.

GENERAL PRINCIPLES OF GAIT REHABILITATION

Gait impairment very often results in long-term disability and handicap. One-third of patients with acute stroke are not ambulatory at least 3 months after admission to a general hospital.[1] In patients that have partly recovered (above 60 points in the Barthel Index) major problems are unsafe walking and difficulties in stair climbing.[2] Therefore, restoration of mobility is crucial for independent living and gait training is an essential part of neurological rehabilitation. The efforts by intensive rehabilitation programs pay off because many patients with lesions of the nervous system improve considerably in their mobility.

'Quality of movement' vs. task–specific repetitive approach

There are two different approaches in regaining mobility. One aims at restoration of physiological gait functions and stresses 'quality of movement', avoiding substitute mechanisms and technical assists as far as possible, whereas the main goal of the other approach is to get the patient to move and walk even with compensatory and substitute movements and technical aids. These two different approaches result in quite different rehabilitation programs. Proponents of the first 'school', for example, may even immobilize some patients in case they acquired a 'pathological gait pattern', in order to make them unlearn these unwanted walking strategies. The second strategy follows a task-specific repetitive approach in line with modern principles of motor rehabilitation. Intensity of therapy correlated with the motor outcome and a transfer from one motor task to another was questioned by studies of Winstein et al.[3] and by Dean and Shepherd.[4] These workers elegantly showed that the practice of balance while standing or sitting improved these specific tasks, while gait symmetry remained unchanged.

Physiotherapy and gait training

Several schools of physical therapy have often polarized opinions concerning the techniques used in gait training. There are functionally oriented traditional approaches and other techniques based on neurophysiological models. A frequently used concept is the neurodevelopmental technique (NDT) according to Bobath.[5,6] The NDT stresses the reduction of spasticity and the symmetry of gait, whereas force development, speed and endurance are considered to be of secondary importance.[5,6] Other treatment designs are the Brunnstroem method, the PNF concept or the Rood method.[7-9]

Despite theoretical and practical differences a superiority of a particular procedure has not been proven in terms of 'activities of daily living' (ADL), including general mobility.[10] A further development of physical therapy based on rational guidelines therefore seems necessary for the future. Specifically for gait functions it could be shown that newer approaches are very efficient at regaining mobility in non-ambulatory stroke patients[11-13] and in spinal cord injured patients.[14-16]

Energy considerations and fatigue

Patients with gait disturbances are less able to use gravity and inertia in ambulation and therefore must resort to actual muscle work, which means that they have to spend more energy covering a certain distance. It was shown that handicapped ambulators as well as able-bodied walkers[14] usually need four to five multiples of the basal metabolic rate for walking. This means that handicapped walkers have to settle for lower speed in order not to exceed these energy expenditures. At comparable speeds, hemiparetic patients expend 65 per cent more energy than normal subjects, which can be reduced to 52

per cent by the use of an ankle–foot orthosis. With more severe deficits, gait velocities are progressively lower to a point when wheelchair ambulation becomes a faster and less strenuous alternative. Wheelchair ambulation requires no more energy than normal walking at the same speed.[18]

In physical therapy the interdependence of speed, stride length and energy expenditure has to be taken more into account for a correct interpretation of therapeutic effects. Speed is a very important variable in unstable movements such as walking, standing up and sitting down. Gravity, inertia and momentum define many aspects of gait. Therefore, training at low velocities, which is requested in some physiotherapeutic concepts, makes the performance often more difficult.[19] Accordingly one study revealed that hemiparetic subjects consumed less energy per distance covered when they were walking faster.[20]

Technical aids for mobility

Early ambulation has many advantages for the musculoskeletal, cardiovascular, pulmonary and renal systems, and in many neurological gait disorders crutches, canes or orthoses may be the only possible way to regain ambulation. These technical aids should be used early in the rehabilitation program. Gait analysis studies could not confirm often-expressed fears that the use of canes or orthoses resulted in an unphysiological gait pattern: it has been found that hemiparetic patients wearing ankle–foot orthoses walked more safely, more symmetrically and less spastically.[21,22] With respect to costs, a prospective study of 466 stroke patients (from 1 year in a German rehabilitation hospital)[23] found that the per capita costs for technical aids were not even 10 per cent of the costs for inpatient treatment. Considering the positive effects for mobility and independence, these figures could alleviate fears of overstretching health budgets since an early prescription can result in a reduction of the length of stay. Prescription of technical aids requires specialized knowledge. It is deplorable that in many countries the technical aids for a considerable percentage of patients are not adequately selected for their requirements.[24]

Canes, crutches and walkers

Canes and crutches can only be used by patients with normal upper limb function who have the cognitive abilities to learn skillful handling. Canes should be carried on the side opposite the weak limb. There are several models of canes and crutches, which should be carefully selected for the individual patient. The use of canes resulted in an unloading of approximately 15 per cent irrespective of the height of the aid; gait symmetry and trunk kinematics were not negatively affected.[21]

Most standard walkers provide a high stability, but the patient has to learn to maneuver it. Before prescribing a particular model the patient should train with it. Cognitive functions, proper balance, vision and upper limb functions have to be taken into consideration in addition to the size of the patient's apartment and personal needs. (For a more detailed description of technical aids see ref. 25.)

Wheelchairs

A standard wheelchair has a sling back and sling seat, and folds easily. Depending on the age, deficits and individual needs, a hand-propelled model or an electrical wheelchair will be selected. There are several thousand models currently on the market and each physician prescribing wheelchairs should be familiar with sizes, models, mechanical parts and seating systems. (For a short review see ref. 26.)

Clinical assessment of gait functions

For assessment of the functional deficit, for adapting therapy to the individual needs and for monitoring progress, measurement of walking ability and gait endurance are important. Both measures offer simple and reliable quantification for clinical purposes in rehabilitation units.

Temporal–distance measurement is a clinically feasible and quantitative approach for kinematic gait analysis. Parameters are velocity, cadence, step length, stride length, stride length/lower extremity length, step time, step time differential. Timed walking tests (5 m, 10 m, 20 m) and the Rivermead Mobility Index[27] are standardized and recommended for routine quantification of mobility. The Functional Ambulation Categories (FAC; see Table 18.1) are designed to give detailed information about the physical support needed by patients who are walking.[28] The 6-min walking test (measuring the maximum uninterrupted walking distance covered within 6 min) is most suitable to assess gait endurance.[29]

Table 18.1 *Functional ambulation classification (FAC)*

0	Patient cannot walk, or requires help of two or more people
1	Patient requires firm continuous support from one person who helps carrying weight and with balance
2	Patient needs continuous or intermittent support of one person to help with balance or coordination
3	Patient requires verbal supervision or stand-by help from one person without physical contact
4	Patient can walk independently on level ground, but requires help on stairs, slopes or uneven surfaces
5	Patient can walk independently anywhere

Falls

Rehabilitation of gait disturbances must also include the prevention of falls, which are very common in elderly patients after stroke or in parkinsonism. Therefore, safety evaluation of the home, installation of handrails, changes in the bathroom, repair of uneven floors and elimination of rugs should be planned by experienced therapists.

However, gait training always poses some risks of falling and unnecessary restrictions should be avoided. One may even assume that the incorporation of gait perturbations in gait practice may be beneficial to minimize the risk of falls.

MAJOR NEUROLOGICAL SYNDROMES RESULTING IN BALANCE AND GAIT DISABILITY

Hemiparesis

One of the most common gait disturbances is caused by hemiparesis due to stroke, and gait training is an essential part of physiotherapy in stroke rehabilitation. One-third of patients with acute stroke are not ambulatory at least 3 months after admission to a general hospital.[1]

SITTING/SIT–TO–STAND TRANSFER

Activities controlling the trunk in a sitting position are practiced in the beginning. Once these tasks are accomplished, activities preparing the patient to stand up from sitting should follow.

Hemiparetic patients rise slowly; they are insecure and tend to put more weight on the unaffected limb.[30,31] During standing-up, patients are normally encouraged by physiotherapists to put weight on both lower limbs, to incline forward and to avoid mediolateral displacement of the head-arm-trunk segment.[5,6] A dynamic analysis of standing-up by right and left sided hemiparetics found that patients with right-hemispheric lesions put more weight on the unaffected leg compared with patients that had lesions in the left hemisphere.[32] The method applied also included visualization of the dynamics of weight distribution and lateral body shift in the rising hemiparetic patient particularly during the unstable two-base support after seat-off. Since the dynamics of standing-up are much slower in patients, energy consumption is higher and symmetry as well as balance is more precarious. If the patients were encouraged to rise faster, their energy consumption was lower and the displacement of the center of pressure became more symmetric.

GAIT TRAINING

The main physical therapy approaches that are used today for hemiparetic patients were developed by Bobath, Brunnstroem, Rood and Knott; most of these concepts were developed for patients with stroke.[7-9]

One of the main goals is the restoration of physiological gait patterns, in particular gait symmetry. For normal subjects symmetry of kinematic, kinetic and to some degree electromyograph (EMG) data can be documented. Asymmetry of the hemiparetic gait is well established for kinematic and kinetic data. The NDT requires reflex inhibitory movement patterns to be invoked in order to normalize tone. During gait training, symmetric weight acceptance and push-off are strictly controlled and a 'non-use' of the paretic limb is avoided.

More recently, these concepts have been questioned by newer data on motor learning, skill acquisition and results of modern neuroscience.

Hesse et al.[33,34] found that, after a 4-week intensive inpatient training program, there was no significant improvement in the gait symmetry parameters. An explanation for the lack of improvement of gait symmetry might lie in the therapy itself. During a typical physiotherapy session, tone-inhibiting maneuvers and advanced postural reactions are applied during sitting and standing in order to normalize muscle tone. Practicing gait is only a minor part and the patient is strictly encouraged to walk in a slow, controlled way. Forssberg and Hirschfield[35] looked at gait training in cerebral palsy children and noted that, although they can be taught a normal gait during the therapy sessions, the old pathological pattern returns as soon as the child is no longer concentrating on walking. The same seems to hold true for gait training after stroke. Therefore it seems inefficient to spend too much time and energy on normalizing gait. Instead the therapist should focus on the functional level of locomotion, improving gait speed and endurance.

TREADMILL TRAINING

Animal experiments on adult spinal cats had shown that an interactive locomotor training using a treadmill and body-weight support improved locomotor performance. A motor-driven treadmill and suspension system[36] also proved to be effective in the treatment of spinal cord injured patients with various degrees of spastic paresis.[37]

In the rehabilitation of non-ambulatory hemiparetic subjects, treadmill training with partial body-weight support (BWS) combined with enforced stepping movements has gained greater acceptance since its first description in 1994.[6] As a task-specific training it allows practice of complete gait cycles with many repetitions instead of single elements or preparatory maneuvers at an early stage of gait rehabilitation. The harness substitutes for deficient equilibrium reflexes, the body weight is reduced according to the degree of paresis and the

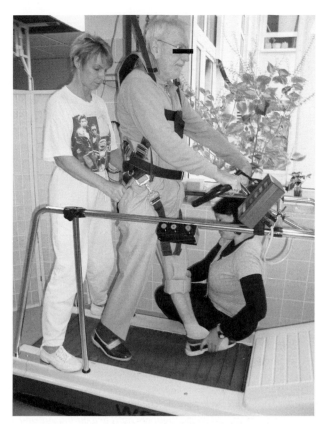

Figure 18.1 *Treadmill training with partial body-weight support. The patient stands on a motor-driven treadmill with variable speed control (range 0.01–2.25 m/s) and is supported by a modified parachute harness suspended by a set of pulleys.*

motor-driven treadmill enforces locomotion (Fig. 18.1). The finding that balance training while standing could improve balance symmetry without improving gait symmetry in hemiparetic patients[3] further supports the specificity of the task-specific training concept, which can be translated into the slogan: 'who wants to regain walking ability, has to walk'.

Two therapists provide manual help in the beginning to correct gait deviations. One therapist, sitting by the paretic side, facilitates the swing of the paretic limb, pays attention that its initial contact is made with the heel, prevents knee hyperextension during mid-stance and encourages symmetry of step length and stance duration. The second therapist stands on the treadmill behind the patient and facilitates weight-shift onto the stance limb, hip extension, pelvic rotation and trunk erection. Hip extension can be increased passively by the treadmill and manual prolongation of the stance phase. Treadmill speed should be adjusted to a comfortable cadence and stride length of each patient and the mean BWS should be between 25 per cent and 40 per cent at the beginning. The support must be reduced as soon as possible to enable full load of the lower limbs. Gait analysis studies showed that hemiparetic patients walked more symmetrically and less spastically on the treadmill

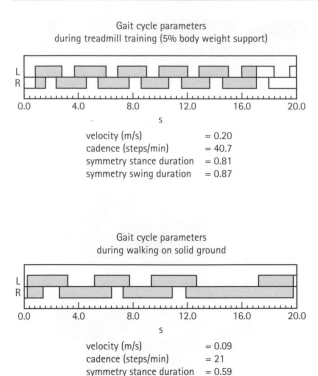

Gait cycle parameters
during treadmill training (5% body weight support)

velocity (m/s)   = 0.20
cadence (steps/min)   = 40.7
symmetry stance duration = 0.81
symmetry swing duration   = 0.87

Gait cycle parameters
during walking on solid ground

velocity (m/s)   = 0.09
cadence (steps/min)   = 21
symmetry stance duration = 0.59
symmetry swing duration   = 2.65

Figure 18.2 *Gait cycle parameters during treadmill training (5 per cent body-weight support) (upper half) and during walking on solid ground (lower half) in a patient with left-sided hemiparesis. The symmetric stepping conditions in the treadmill training can be observed.*

compared with floor walking, thus allaying often-expressed fears of an unphysiological gait pattern on the belt (Fig. 18.2).[38]

The first clinical studies – a baseline-treatment study (n = 9) and two single case design studies (n = 14) – dealt with chronic non-ambulatory hemiparetic subjects (Fig. 18.3). They revealed that the therapy was extremely promising with regard to restoration of gait ability and the improvement of ground walking velocity.[39,40] The single-case design studies followed an A–B–A design. During the A-phases, treadmill therapy was applied alone (n = 7) or in combination with functional electrical stimulation (FES) on the belt (n = 7), the patients did not receive any additional single physiotherapy (Fig. 18.4). During the B-phases, the patients received physiotherapy following a conservative Bobath concept of the same time extent. Each phase lasted 3 weeks. The FES helped to facilitate the movement on the belt, for example the stimulation of the nervus peroneus during the swing phase assisted the dorsiflexion of the foot. The results showed that the patients improved their gait ability and ground level walking velocity considerably during the first 3-week A-phase (A1) of exclusive daily treadmill training alone or in combination with FES. During the subsequent period of 3 weeks of conventional physiotherapy (B) gait ability did not change,

whereas the second A-phase further enhanced walking ability. All subjects that had been wheelchair-bound before therapy became ambulatory at least with verbal support at the end of the study. During one 30-min session of treadmill training with BWS, the patients could practice up to 1000 gait cycles compared with a median of less than 50 gait cycles during one regular physiotherapy session. Other motor functions improved steadily, whereas the muscle tone remained unchanged. With a minimum stroke interval of 3 months before study admission, spontaneous recovery alone could not have explained the observed beneficial effects. Another study in 30 chronic non-ambulatory subjects showed that the combination of treadmill therapy and focused gait rehabilitation on the floor resulted in better gait improvement compared with treadmill therapy alone. The result favors a more intense approach on the one side and the combination of interactive locomotor therapy and conventional gait training on the other.[41]

In acute stroke patients, several randomized controlled studies have investigated the potential of the locomotor therapy. A large Canadian study in 100 acute stroke patients compared treadmill therapy with and without BWS.[42] Following randomization, 50 patients were trained to walk with up to 40 per cent of their body weight supported (BWS group), and the other 50 subjects were trained to walk bearing full on their lower limbs (no-BWS group). After a 6-week training period, the BWS group scored significantly higher than the no-BWS group for functional balance (P = 0.001), motor recovery (P = 0.001), over-ground walking speed (P = 0.029) and over-ground walking endurance (P = 0.018). The follow-up evaluation 3 months later revealed that the BWS group continued to have significantly higher scores for overground walking speed (P = 0.006) and motor recovery (P = 0.039).

Kosak and Reding[43] published the first controlled study comparing treadmill therapy with BWS vs. physiotherapy in 56 acute stroke patients.[39] Physiotherapy included aggressive early therapy-assisted ambulation using knee–ankle combination bracing and hemi-bar if needed (i.e. the approach was definitely different from a classic NDT one with tone-inhibiting and gait preparatory maneuvers dominating). Treatment sessions in both groups lasted up to 45 min per day, 5 days a week until patients could walk over ground unassisted. Although the outcome of the two groups as a whole did not differ, a subgroup with major hemispheric stroke, defined by the presence of hemiparesis, hemianopic visual deficit and hemihypesthesia, who received more than 12 treatment sessions, showed significantly better over-ground endurance (90 ± 34 m vs. 44 ± 10 m) and speed scores (12 ± 4 m/min vs. 8 ± 2 m/min) for the treadmill vs. the physiotherapy group.

Nielsson and co-workers[44] conducted the first multicenter trial. Seventy-three acute stroke patients participated. The patients were either allocated to the treadmill

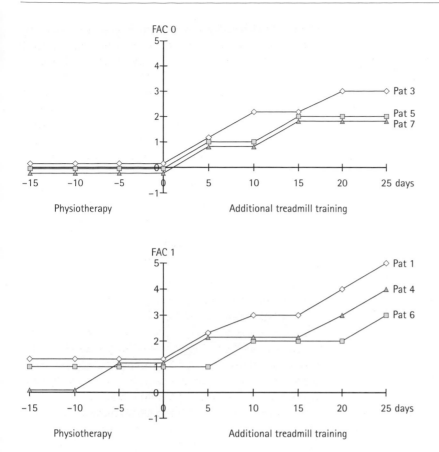

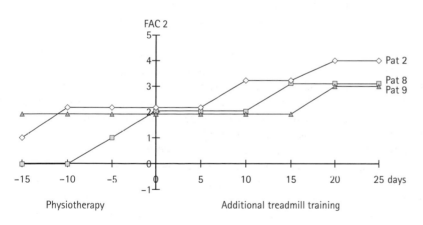

Figure 18.3 *Functional ambulation categories (FAC) levels before and during treadmill training of hemiparetic patients (Pat 1–9) with FAC levels of 0, 1 and 2 on day 1. A FAC level of 0 describes a patient that cannot walk or requires help of two or more people. At level 1, a patient needs continuous support from one person. At level 2, a patient needs continuous or intermittent support of one person to help with balance or coordination. The results show a marked improvement in the FAC levels during treadmill training, but not during conventional physical therapy.*

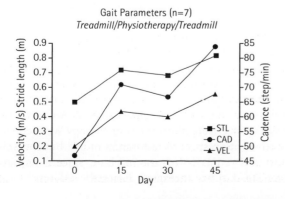

Figure 18.4 *Gait parameters (stride length, velocity, cadence) for seven hemiparetic patients in an A–B–A study showing the positive effects of treadmill training. In the first 15 days (treadmill training) a large improvement can be observed, then during conventional physiotherapy (days 16–30) stagnation, followed by another significant improvement in the second treadmill phase (days 31–45).*

or to the physiotherapy group; treadmill training and physiotherapy were both 30 min every workday for 2 months. Physiotherapy followed the Motor Relearning Program stressing the repetitive practice of gait on the floor and on the stairs. Treadmill training following the above-mentioned principles were continued at least until the patients were able to walk unsupported on the belt; gait therapy then continued on the ground. Dependent variables were the FAC, the walking velocity and the Fugl-Meyer Motor Scale. At the end of the study and at follow-up both groups had improved considerably but did not differ with respect to any of the chosen variables.

Most recently, Pohl and co-workers[45] investigated treadmill training in ambulatory hemiparetic subjects as a tool to increase speed and endurance. The experimental group ($n = 20$) underwent stepwise speed training on the treadmill. At the end of the study they not only walked faster but had also reached a significantly higher mobility level compared with the control group ($n = 20$).[45] Furthermore, open studies showed that hemiparetic subjects could improve their cardiovascular fitness following a several months' aerobic training on the treadmill.[46]

GAIT MACHINES

In considering all the advantages of this approach, some disadvantages could also be observed. One of the major disadvantages of treadmill training is the effort required by two or three therapists to assist the gait of severely affected subjects, when setting the paretic limbs and controlling trunk movements. Therefore, our group designed and constructed an electromechanical gait trainer (Gait Trainer GT I; Reha-Stim company, Berlin, Germany) (Fig. 18.5).[47] The harness-secured subject was positioned on two footplates whose movements simulated stance and swing in a symmetric manner with a ratio of 60 per cent to 40 per cent between stance and swing. The cadence and stride length can be set in a stepless manner within a speed range of 0.1–2.8 km/h according to individual needs. A servo-controlled drive mechanism assisted the gait-like movement according to abilities and the vertical and horizontal movements of the trunk were controlled in a phase-dependent manner. Phase-dependent electrical stimulation of the quadriceps muscle during the stance phase can help to stabilize the knee; alternatively the therapist sits in front and controls the knee movement.

The sagittal joint kinematics and the dynamic electromyogram of selected lower limb muscles in control subjects have been shown to closely mimic normal gait. Severely affected hemiparetic subject needed less help on the gait trainer compared with assisted treadmill walking, while the movement was more symmetric and the single-stance phase of the paretic limb lasted longer on the gait trainer entraining the weight-bearing muscles effectively.

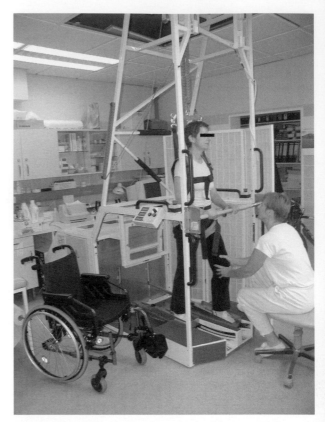

Figure 18.5 *A left-hemiparetic patient walks on the gait trainer GT I with the help of one therapist controlling the movement of the paretic knee.*

The dynamic electromyogram of the lower limbs revealed a comparable activation of the trunk and thigh muscles. The plantarflexor spasticity was less on the gait trainer. The activity of the tibialis anterior muscle was diminished on the gait trainer as the patients could put some weight on the footplate during the 'swing phase' despite the controlled horizontal trunk movement.

Subsequent clinical results have shown marked improvements in gait ability of severely affected hemiparetic subjects. A first baseline treatment study (3 weeks of conventional therapy followed by 4 weeks of additional therapy on the gait trainer) with 14 non-ambulatory hemiparetic patients (mean stroke interval 11.2 weeks) could confirm the potential of this novel approach.[48] The 4 weeks of physiotherapy and gait training resulted in a significant improvement in gait ability in all subjects. Velocity, cadence and stride length improved significantly. The kinesiological electromyogram of selected lower limb muscles revealed a more physiological pattern of the thigh and shank muscles. A recent study compared gait trainer therapy (A) and treadmill training (B) in 30 non-ambulatory subacute stroke survivors with the help of an A–B–A and B–A–B design respectively. Both types of therapy were equally effective with respect to restoration of gait but therapist effort was reduced with the machine, since it required one instead of two therapists during the sessions.[45]

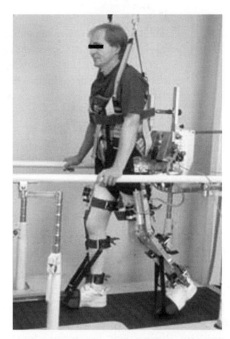

Figure 18.6 *Paraparetic subject practicing on the Lokomat, an exoskeleton with powered drives to bend the hip and knee during the swing phase.*

Colombo and co-workers[50] suggested another solution to the problem of reducing intensive efforts from the therapists (Fig. 18.6). They used a hybrid system consisting of a motor-driven treadmill (to promote the stance phase) and a powered exoskeleton with drives flexing the hip and knee during the swing phase. So far, the system is purely passive; a force-control sensing the patient's effort will be a next step for clinical testing. Another potential solution is a robot arm which places the limbs during their swing phases, as has been shown successfully in spinalized rats (at the laboratory of Dr V. Edgerton, UCLA, Los Angeles, CA, USA).

FUNCTIONAL ELECTRICAL STIMULATION IN HEMIPLEGIC PATIENTS

Functional electrical stimulation (FES) was developed more than 30 years ago[51] as an electronic orthotic device preventing the foot drop in hemiparetic stroke patients. Present gait stimulation programs have been research oriented, either using the surface or indwelling electrodes.[52–54] The stimulators were complicated and bulky,[55] and large numbers of electrodes at predetermined stimulation sites often did not allow simple positioning. Despite favorable effects of functional stimulation, its clinical application was restricted to a limited number of well-trained persons.[56,57] In a new attempt it was therefore decided to thoroughly

adjust the stimulation parameters to the individual needs of the patient and to reduce the number of stimulation channels with regard to optimum efficiency. Simple lightweight dual-channel stimulators, which can be fully programmed and adapted to the patient's cadence,[58] were connected together, thus rendering a viable solution for clinical use.

Restoration of standing and weight-shift was achieved by stimulation of gluteus maximus, quadriceps and hamstring muscles.[59] The stimulation stabilized the pelvis and knee, enabling better standing symmetry and faster weight-shift. A carry-over effect was observed after the stimulation procedure.

It has also been shown that five- to six-channel electrical stimulation of the main lower extremity muscle groups, synchronized with the phases of stride, could successfully initiate the gait pattern and antigravity support in hemiparetic patients after stroke and other brain injuries. When applied in kinesiologically correct sequences it could restore their gait faster and further than conventional physiotherapeutic techniques within a few weeks. Eventually, it could provide an independent ambulation with or even without a cane or crutch in severely affected hemiparetic patients that would otherwise have remained wheelchair-bound.[52,53,55]

In addition to the functional gait improvement documented by the increase in stride parameters, the gait pattern was also restored (Fig. 18.7). This was documented by the clinical analysis[60] and the symmetry ratios, as the key elements of healthy gait.[61,62] However, the ratio of the self-adopted and the maximum speed did not change considerably after the treatment. The restoration of motor functions was shown by the hierarchical Rivermead test for hemiparetic patients.[27] Scores on the Ashworth Scale[63] documented that spasticity decreased in the hip and knee joints during treatment. These effects could be ascribed to the therapy as the post-stroke interval exceeded 12 weeks, during which 80 per cent of spontaneous recovery should have occurred.[1]

The combined shoulder–arm stimulation, with one large electrode on the supraspinatus and the other on the deltoideus and triceps brachii muscles, in addition to the leg stimulation, alleviated the problem of the depressed shoulder and induced the reciprocal arm swing during gait.[59] It also helped the elbow extension. In addition, a sustained trunk erection was observed during the stimulation, providing a stable trunk and pelvic alignment as an integral part of the physiological gait. As a consequence, a pelvic rotation could be initiated in some patients.

It has been shown that standing and weight-shift can be improved by FES in hemiparetic patients. It can be administered in addition to physical therapy, in particular for severely affected patients that require considerable physical effort from the therapists.

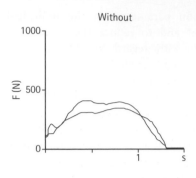

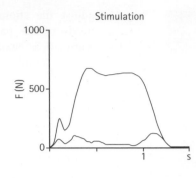

Figure 18.7 *Mean vertical ground reaction forces and their standard deviations during gait in a hemiparetic patient without and with four-channel functional electrical stimulation (FES). Note an increase of 140 N in the midstance of the affected leg and a much smaller standard deviation. Better gait dynamics are reflected in the loading and push-off peaks during stimulation.*

ORTHOSES

A common problem is spastic inversion of the foot. The objective is to achieve primary heel strike with the foot in a plantigrade position. Figure 18.8 shows the beneficial effect of a metal ankle–foot orthosis (AFO). Further, gait analysis with and without an AFO showed that their use rendered the gait more efficient and safer, facilitated muscle activation of the quadriceps muscle, reduced ankle spasticity and increased walking velocity considerably.[22] If spasticity is not severe, an AFO is the appropriate technical aid. There are different models of AFOs. The metal AFO is connected to the shoe with a riveted 'stirrup' that articulates to an ankle joint. This metal AFO has many advantages. It is adjustable in the ankle joint and it offers the highest rigidity and therefore is preferable in patients with severe spastic inversion of the foot. Since this orthosis is adjustable, it should be preferred when the condition may change. Thermoplastic orthoses have less weight and are preferred by patients because of their better cosmetic appearance.

BOTULINUM TOXIN AND OTHER CHEMICAL AGENTS

Botulinum toxin A injection has been used successfully in the treatment of focal dystonias. First studies on the treatment of spasticity reported a significant tone reduction of leg adductors; upper limb flexor spasticity and spastic drop-foot.[12,64–67] Problems associated with plantar flexor spasticity during gait are a fore-foot contact, reduced loading and stance duration on the affected limb, a stance equinus, poor progression of the body with reduced stride length, lack of push-off and dragging of the toes.[60]

For the spastic drop-foot, several open studies showed that the intramuscular injection of botulinum toxin into the plantarflexors reduced muscle tone, diminished ankle clonus and painful toe clawing, improved the mode of initial contact and improved ankle range of motion, with better advancement of the body, gait symmetry and walking velocity for up to 4 months (Fig. 18.9). Dynamic EMG recordings revealed a preferential diminution of the so-called premature activity of the plantarflexors originating in the terminal swing.[68]

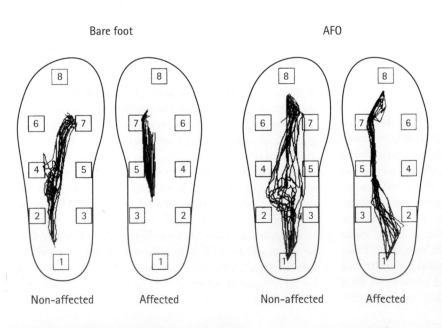

Figure 18.8 *Effect of an ankle–foot orthosis (AFO) on the gait pattern of a right-sided hemiparetic patient. Trajectories of the center of pressure under both feet during consecutive strides, bare-footed and with AFO. The recordings demonstrate that the patient regains initial heel contact. The length and pattern of the trajectory also improved on the non-affected side.*

Before injection   After injection

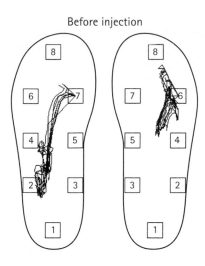
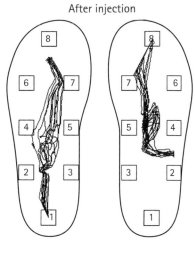

Figure 18.9 *Effect of botulinum toxin injection on the gait pattern of a right-sided hemiparetic patient. Trajectories of the center of pressure under both feet during consecutive strides, before and 2 weeks after botulinum toxin injection into the calf muscles. The recordings demonstrate that the length and pattern of the trajectory improved on both sides.*

Burbaud and co-workers[69] conducted a double blind, placebo-controlled study in 24 individuals suffering from a spastic drop-foot. The authors injected EMG-guided placebo or a total dosage of 1000 units Dysport into the musculus soleus, gastrocnemius, tibialis posterior and flexor digitorum longus. Patients reported a clear subjective improvement in foot spasticity after botulinum toxin but not after placebo administration. Significant changes were noted in Ashworth scale values for ankle extensors and invertors, and for active ankle dorsiflexion up to 3 months after injection. Gait velocity was slightly but not significantly improved after the injection of botulinum toxin.

To increase the effectiveness of the costly toxin, patients should walk vigorously after injection, referring to the positive correlation between terminal nerve end activity and toxin uptake. When the patients are unable to walk, an electrical stimulation of the injected muscles (trains of 3 s, 25 Hz, 0.2 ms, above motor threshold) has also been recommended five times for 30 min each day for 3 days after injection.[70] Further, the exclusive injection of the gastrocnemius muscle bellies is not sufficient in most cases, the soleus, tibialis posterior, long toe flexor and, for severe ankle inversion, the tibialis anterior muscle should be also treated. To address the accompanying mechanical changes of spastic muscles, Reiter and co-workers[71] studied the effects of a tonic stretch of the injected muscles. The authors compared two groups of hemiparetic patients with a spastic drop-foot. One group received the injection of a high dose of botulinum toxin into the plantarflexors while the second group received a smaller dose of 50 per cent plus a tonic stretch with the help of a tape. Both groups showed similar effects on muscle tone and gait function. In summary, functional activity, electrical stimulation, a proper muscle selection and a tonic stretch should help to promote the effectiveness of the treatment. (Note, one should not shake the vials after dilution, otherwise the toxin may stick to the walls of the vial.)

ANESTHETICS

Topical applied anesthetics on the skin of lower limbs of chronic stroke and head trauma patients can result in a considerable improvement of limb mobility and gait.[72] The effect arises from reduced muscle rigidity and augmentation of joint mobility. Physical therapy exercises performed during the effective period of the anesthetic rendered long-lasting improvement in the patients' ability to ambulate.

SERIAL CASTING

In traumatic brain injuries the development of contractures often prevent the patient from regaining mobility. It is painful and time consuming to overcome these contractures and to restore functional movement. Serial casting, whereby the limb is held in a progressively corrected position by a plaster cast is now the method of choice to correct severe contractures in the lower limbs (Fig. 18.10). Serial plastering with circular casts can be successfully used to overcome contractures in the knee flexion or plantarflexion of the ankle.[73] Common protocols recommend that the cast is changed each week with an increased angle; about 6 weeks are usually required to overcome a contracture. Recently, Pohl and co-workers[74] investigated shorter intervals of 2–3 days and found deformity corrections of a similar extent while side-effects such as scars occurred less.

AUDITORY CUING AND BIOFEEDBACK

Auditory (musical) rhythm as a peripheral pacing signal for hemiparetic stroke patients resulted in a significant increase in weight-bearing stance time on the paretic side, improved stride symmetry with rhythmic cuing, an increase in the muscle activation during midstance/push-off on the affected side, a decreased EMG variability during midstance/push-off phase on the hemiparetic side and other normalizations of the gait pattern.[75]

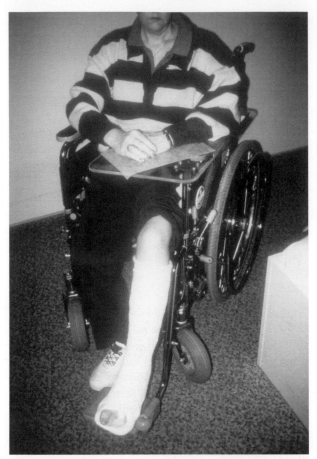

Figure 18.10 *Serial casting of the lower extremity to overcome severe contractures of the ankle joint. The plaster cast is changed every 3 days and the ankle angle is gradually improved to a normal position over a treatment period of 6 weeks.*

Visual and auditory feedback of knee angle during different phases of gait relative to the desired target was given to hemiparetic stroke patients in order to increase knee flexion during the push-off and pull-off. After 4 weeks the patients' gait velocity, stride length and transfers between kinetic and potential energy were significantly improved. The total energy cost was lower.[76]

Paraplegia

For most patients with spinal cord injuries recovery of locomotor function has the highest priority. The likelihood of achieving this goal depends on several factors, such as on the level of the injury, the completeness of the lesion, the muscle tone, the associated complications (heterotopic ossification, contractures, etc.), age and weight of a patient, and on their determination and motivation in the therapy. Patients with spinal cord injuries above T2 will not regain locomotor functions because trunk stability is missing. Patients with lesions at midthoracic or lower thoracic levels are often able to ambulate with long leg-braces. However walking with knee–ankle–foot orthoses (KAFOs) is in most cases done

only as an exercise since it is very strenuous. Therefore it is more economic to use an appropriate wheelchair.

Burke et al.[77] reported in a large sample of spinal cord injured patients that 37 per cent could not walk at discharge from a rehabilitation center, 24 per cent could walk but used a wheelchair for daily locomotion and 39 per cent were functional walkers.

Intensive rehabilitation programs for spinal cord injured patients include passive rage of motion (PROM) exercises, strength and endurance training of partly paralyzed muscles and also of the upper extremities, antispastic medication, corrective surgery, if necessary, tilt table standing, use of orthotic devices and of crutches and learning of compensatory strategies.

The KAFO and the reciprocating gait orthosis are the most commonly used orthotic aids. The latter have recently gained popularity because of the more normal gait pattern and lower energy costs.

New advances have been made for locomotor rehabilitation of spinal cord injured patients.[11] They include treadmill training with partial body-weight support, pharmacotherapy of locomotion and FES.

Treadmill training

In patients with incomplete and even complete paraplegia, coordinated stepping movements can be induced by weight support and standing on a motor-driven treadmill. Body-weight support is provided by a modified parachute harness suspended by a set of pulleys. The harness allows the free movement of the lower limbs and of the arms (method is similar to that shown in Fig. 18.1). The pattern of leg muscle EMG was comparable to that seen in healthy subjects. Patients with incomplete paraplegia profited from the training program in that their walking on a stationary surface improved even when unsupported.[17,37] By this new training method, gait could be effectively restored in spinal cord injury patients with various degrees of spastic paresis within 1.5 to several months.[37] The method implies that gait retraining may be initiated early in the rehabilitation period,[14] and peripheral stimulation may facilitate muscle activation during the stance and swing phase. A large randomized trial is being conducted in the USA; to date, only open studies have shown the potential of the locomotor therapy in paraparetic subjects.[78] For paraplegic subjects, Dietz and co-workers[79] showed that a several-month-long treadmill training elicited rhythmic activation patterns of lower limb muscles similar to those seen in healthy subjects, the functional gait ability, however, did not change.

PHARMACOTHERAPY OF LOCOMOTION

In a small sample of patients with incomplete spinal cord injury it was shown that clonidine was associated with the initiation of locomotion.[80] Similar results for a

Canadian multicenter trial with cyproheptadine, a serotonergic antagonist, suggest that, as in the cat noradrenergic and serotonergic drugs have a powerful effect on the modulation of locomotor patterns.[81] The combined effect of new medications together with a locomotor training using body-weight support and treadmill walking showed an improvement in gait with full weight bearing and in walking speed.[82] It therefore seems that the interactive locomotor training using body-weight support in combination with certain drugs could be a powerful approach for neurological rehabilitation.[14]

FUNCTIONAL ELECTRICAL STIMULATION

Kantrowitz reported in a short publication for the first time that stimulation of the quadriceps and the glutei enabled a T-3 paraplegic patient to stand.[83] Clinically complete spinal cord injury patients can regain their standing and walking ability by FES of their lower limbs.[11] However FES has not yet become a widely accepted therapeutic technique in neurological rehabilitation, although recent results show beneficial effects on speed, energy consumption, and postural stability.[12,84,85] Many different stimulation systems were described, with surface stimulation, with transcutaneous electrodes and fully implantable systems.[86,87] For clinical purposes, a four-channel surface electrical stimulation method including both quadriceps muscles can provide standing, while stepping is induced by the stimulation of combined ankle dorsal flexion and flexion withdrawal response at the peroneal nerve. Alternating stimulation between the quadriceps muscle and peroneal nerve on both lower limbs is controlled with manual switches by patients themselves (Fig. 18.11).[48,56] Currently used stimulation protocols include an initial strengthening program of the antigravity muscles. The patients are treated by cyclic stimulation of the quadriceps muscle while lying or sitting before the electrically induced standing. The strengthening might last weeks or even months before initiation of the stimulated gait.[86]

In contrast, it was demonstrated in chronic non-ambulatory hemiparetic patients that immediate walking with FES without previous strengthening of the muscles could restore gait functions within 2–3 weeks, so that patients could walk without assistance.[52,56] Immediate standing assisted by FES without prior conditioning of the muscles was recently also shown for paraplegic patients.[13] After about 2 weeks they started to walk with electrical stimulation. Diminished limb flexion during the swing phase due to habituation of the flexor reflex after prolonged use was overcome by stimulation frequencies above 20 Hz. Individual patients were described to cover long distances and walk for hours. Most patients, however, perform FES standing and gait for exercise purposes with the effect of a reduced spasticity, strengthened muscles and improved self-esteem. Better mineralization of the bones, enhanced bowel and

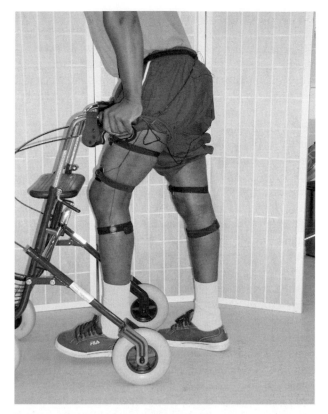

Figure 18.11 *Functional electrical stimulation for restoration of standing and gait in a paraplegic patient. Two commercially available ALT-2 dual channel stimulators are fastened to a belt and used for the alternating surface stimulation of quadriceps muscle and peroneal nerve on both sides, which can be triggered by the patient via switches in both crutches.*

bladder functions, better thermoregulation and reduced urinary infections are other beneficial effects. Following a 6-week inpatient training program, 16 paraplegic patients had a mean standing duration of 22.6 min. The gait velocity of 12 patients ranged from 2.9 to 24.2 m/min, the maximum walking distance ranged from 4 to 335 m. Further positive effects of FES-assisted standing and walking were strengthening of lower limb muscles, prophylaxis of thrombosis, osteoporosis and joint contracture, improvement of skin and muscle blood perfusion and improved thermoregulation. Nevertheless, because of flexor spasm and unrealistic expectations, eight of the 16 patients stopped the program completely and only seven patients practiced FES-assisted standing after 1 year. One patient continued FES walking. In incomplete paraparetic and tetraparetic patients, FES could help to restore voluntary motor function of the lower limbs. Four patients with an incomplete cervical lesion, who had been able to walk a short distance before treatment, improved their gait velocity/walking distance without FES with a mean of 33.3 per cent/163.8 per cent after 6 weeks of FES treatment.[88]

Basal ganglia disorders

The characteristics of parkinsonian gait and the pharmacotherapy of the disorder have been described elsewhere. Therefore, only physiotherapeutic exercises will be discussed here. The goals include increased movement and range of motion, improved equilibrium and better gait functions. Only a few studies have examined the efficacy of physical therapy in Parkinson's disease and there are contradictory results.[89] Nonetheless, physical therapy is an integral part of neurological rehabilitation and most patients benefit because (at least) musculoskeletal complications are prevented and the incidence of falling is reduced. Palmer et al.[90] studied patients with Parkinson's disease treated with two different training procedures. One group was treated according to a program designed by the Parkinson Foundation of the USA and the other group received karate training. Both groups showed increases in gait velocity and in general well-being. Outpatient physical therapy improved flexibility, posture and gait. The self-care skills were also increased.[91] In contrast, Pedersen et al.[92] examined the effects of a physical therapy regimen with gait exercises, foot extension tasks and walking tasks and found no change in maximum gait velocity and stride length; patients even worsened after training. Recently, it was shown in a randomized, single blind and crossover study[93] that patients receiving 4-weeks' intensive physical therapy showed significant improvement in the Unified Parkinson's Disease Rating Scale (UPDRS), ADL and motor scores, but no change in mentation score. During the following 6 weeks, when patients did not regularly exercise, these scores returned to baseline. Therefore, patients improved by physical therapy, but this improvement is not sustained when normal activity is resumed.

The focus of the gait training should be on active arm swings, increasing stride length, turning, starting and stopping. The use of assistive devices such as a walker or a cane has to be learned. Auditory and visual cuing are also very effective means to improve gait performance. A study by Richards et al.[94] demonstrated that auditory cues could dramatically modify gait movements and muscle activation in parkinsonian patients.

Falling is a serious problem in parkinsonism and therefore risks have to be minimized by installation of handrails. Some specialists encourage parkinsonian patients to learn karate, tai chi or judo techniques for safe falling.

Miyai and co-workers conducted a prospective crossover trial in 10 Morbus Parkinson patients, moderately affected with a Hoehn and Yahr stage 2.5 or 3 and that were not demented.[95] Patients were randomized to receive either a 4-week program of treadmill therapy with body-weight support followed by 4 weeks of conventional physiotherapy, or the same treatments in opposite order. Irrespective of the order of the treatment blocks, treadmill therapy produced a significantly larger effect on ambulation and the mean motor score of the UPRDS. The authors concluded that treadmill therapy produced greater improvements in activities of daily living, motor performance and ambulation compared with conventional physical therapy. All patients felt most comfortable when walking with 20 per cent body-weight support and were most uncomfortable with 30 per cent body-weight support.[96]

CONCLUSION

Neurological rehabilitation of gait disturbances has to consider the etiology, severity of the functional deficit, cognitive abilities, age and several other factors. Therefore, a functional assessment of postural capabilities and gait functions has to be done at the beginning in order to select an individual mobility program. Only a thorough biomechanical understanding of the gait cycle will allow prescription of the best mobility aid for the patient and to adapt it to their requirements. The skills of the doctor are needed to combine the suitable therapies and the best technical aids for the individual patient. In recent years new ideas have emerged. Training procedures in physical therapy should stress active exercises to increase force in the paretic limb, as well as the repetition of gait cycles. Technical aids should be prescribed earlier, since their costs are usually almost negligible compared with the costs of a prolonged inpatient treatment. Treadmill training with partial body-weight support in a parachute harness allows early training of postural reactions and of stepping. The gait pattern can be considerably improved by FES. A new approach is mechanical- and computer-controlled training machines and robots to enable the repetitive training of complex gait cycles without overstressing therapists. First results demonstrate positive effects beyond the classical retraining procedures. Specific drugs with local, intrathecal or systemic application can further increase locomotor abilities and reduce spasticity. The new methods described in this chapter increase the therapeutic spectrum considerably. However, rehabilitation of gait functions has to become more creative in finding the best combination of these effective therapies.

REFERENCES

1. Wade DT, Wood VA, Heller A, et al. Walking after stroke. Measurement and recovery over the first 3 months. *Scand J Rehabil Med* 1987;**19**:25–30.
2. Granger CV, Hamilton BB, Gresham GE. The stroke rehabilitation outcome study. Part I: general description. *Arch Phys Med Rehabil* 1988;**69**:506–9.
3. Winstein CJ, Gardner ER, McNeal DR, et al. Standing balance training: effect on balance and locomotion in hemiparetic adults. *Arch Phys Med Rehabil* 1989;**70**:755–62.

4. Dean C, Shepherd R. Task-related training improves the performance of seated reaching tasks following stroke: a randomised controlled trial. *Stroke* 1997;**28**:722–8.

5. Davies PM. *Steps to follow. A guide to the treatment of adult hemiplegia.* Berlin: Springer-Verlag, 1985.

6. Davies PM. *Right in the middle; selective trunk activity in the treatment of adult hemiplegia.* Berlin: Springer-Verlag, 1990.

7. Bobath B. *Adult hemiplegia: evaluation and treatment,* 2nd edn. London: William Heineman Medical Books, 1978.

8. Brunstrom S. *Movement therapy in hemiplegia: a neurophysiological approach.* New York: Harper and Row, 1970.

9. Voss DE, Ionta MK, Meyers BJ. *Proprioceptive neuromuscular facilitation,* 3rd edn. Philadelphia: Harper and Row, 1985.

10. Mauritz KH. General rehabilitation. *Curr Opin Neurol Neurosurg* 1990;**3**:714–18.

11. Hesse S, Bertelt C, Schaffrin A, et al. Restoration of gait in nonambulatory hemiparetic patients by treadmill training with partial body weight support. *Arch Phys Med Rehabil* 1994;**75**:1087–93.

12. Hesse S, Lücke D, Malezic M, et al. Botulinum toxin treatment for lower limb spasticity in chronic hemiparetic patients. *J Neurol Neurosurg Psychiatry* 1994;**57**:1321–4.

13. Malezic M, Hesse S, Schewe H, Mauritz KH. Restoration of standing, weight-shift and gait by multichannel electrical stimulation in hemiparetic patients. *Int J Rehabil Res* 1994;**17**:169–79.

14. Barbeau H, Rossignol S. Enhancement of locomotor recovery following spinal cord injury. *Curr Opin Neurol* 1994;**7**:517–24.

15. Malezic M, Hesse S. Restoration of gait by functional electrical stimulation in paraplegic patients – modified program of treatment. *Paraplegia* 1995;**33**:126–31.

16. Dietz V, Colombo G, Jensen L. Locomotor activity in spinal man. *Lancet* 1994;**344**:1260–3.

17. Corcoran PJ, Brengelmann GL. Oxygen uptake in normal and handicapped subjects, in relation to speed of walking beside velocity-controlled cart. *Arch Phys Med Rehabil* 1970;**51**:78–87.

18. Fisher SV, Gullickson G. Energy cost of ambulation in health and disability: a literature review. *Arch Phys Med Rehabil* 1978;**59**:124–33.

19. Pai YC, Rogers MW. Control of body mass transfer as a function of speed of ascent in sit-to-stand. *Med Sci Sports Exerc* 1990;**22**:378–84.

20. Hesse S, Werner C, Paul T, et al. Influence of lower limb muscle activity and energy consumption during treadmill walking of hemiparetic patients. *Arch Phys Med Rehabil* 2001;**82**:1547–50.

21. Tyson S. The influence of different walking aids on hemiplegic gait. *Clin Rehabil* 1998;**12**:395–401.

22. Hesse S, Werner C, Konrad M, et al. Non-velocity related effects of a rigid double-stopped ankle-foot orthosis on gait and lower limb muscle activity of hemiparetic patients with an equinovarus deformity. *Stroke* 1999;**30**:1855–1861.

23. Hesse S, Gahein-Sama AL, Mauritz KH. Technical aids in hemiparetic patients: prescription, expenses and usage. *Clin Rehabil* 1996;**10**:328–333.

24. Perks BA, Macintosh R, Steward CPU, Bardsley GI. A survey of marginal wheelchair users. *J Rehabil Res Dev* 1994;**31**:297–302.

25. Basmajian JV, Wolf SL. *Therapeutic exercise,* 5th edn. Baltimore: Williams and Wilkins, 1990.

26. Laven L. Adaptive equipment. In: Good DC, Couch JR, eds. *Handbook of neurorehabilitation.* New York: Marcel Dekker, 1994;317–41.

27. Collen FM, Wade DT, Bradshaw CM. Mobility after stroke: reliability of measures of impairment and disability. *Int Disabil Stud* 1990;**12**:6–9.

28. Wade DT. *Measurement in neurological rehabilitation.* Oxford, New York, Tokyo: Oxford University Press, 1992.

29. Lipkin PD, Scriven AJ, Crake T, Poole-Wilson PA. Six minute walking test for assessing capacity in chronic heart failure. *BMJ* 1986;**292**:653–5.

30. Engardt M, Olsson E. Body weight-bearing while rising and sitting down in patients with stroke. *Scand J Rehabil Med* 1992;**24**:67–74.

31. Yoshida K, Iwakura H, Inoue F. Motion analysis in the movements of standing up from and sitting down on a chair. *Scand J Rehabil Med* 1983;**15**:133–40.

32. Hesse S, Schauer M, Malezic M, et al. Quantitative analysis of rising from a chair in healthy and hemiparetic subjects. *Scand J Rehabil Med* 1994;**26**:161–6.

33. Hesse S, Jahnke M, Schreiner C, Mauritz KH. Gait symmetry and functional walking performance in hemiparetic patients prior to and after a 4-week rehabilitation program. *Gait Posture* 1993;**1**:166–71.

34. Hesse S, Jahnke M, Bertelt CM, et al. Gait outcome in ambulatory hemiparetic patients after a 4-week comprehensive rehabilitation program and prognostic factors. *Stroke* 1994;**25**:1999–2004.

35. Forssberg H, Hirschfeld H. *Movement disorders in children.* Basle: Karger Verlag, 1990.

36. Barbeau H, Wainberg W, Finch L. Description and application of a system for locomotor rehabilitation. *Med J Biol Engineer Computer Sci* 1987;**25**:341–4.

37. Wernig A, Müller S. Laufband locomotion with body weight support improved walking in persons with severe spinal cord injuries. *Paraplegia* 1992;**30**:229–38.

38. Hesse S, Konrad M, Uhlenbrock D. Treadmill walking with partial body weight support versus floor walking in hemiparetic subjects. *Arch Phys Med Rehabil* 1999;**80**:421–7.

39. Hesse S, Malezic M, Schaffrin A, Mauritz KH. Restoration of gait by a combined treadmill training and multichannel electrical stimulation in non-ambulatory hemiparetic patients. *Scand J Rehabil Med* 1995;**27**:199–205.

40. Hesse S, Bertelt C, Jahnke MT, et al. Treadmill training with partial body weight support as compared to physiotherapy in non-ambulatory hemiparetic patients. *Stroke* 1995;**26**, 976–81.

41. Werner C, von Frankenberg S, Treig T, et al. Treadmill training with partial body weight support and an electromechanical gait trainer for restoration of gait in subacute stroke patients. A randomized crossover study. *Stroke* 2002;**33**:867–973.

42. Visintin M, Barbeau H, Korner-Bitensky N, Mayo NE. A new approach to retrain gait in stroke patients through body weight support and treadmill stimulation. *Stroke* 1998;**29**:1122–8.

43. Kosak MC, Reding MJ. Comparison of partial body weight-supported treadmill gait training versus aggressive bracing assisted walking post stroke. *Neurorehabil Neural Repair* 2000;**14**:13–19.

44. Nilsson L, Carlsson J, Danielsson A, et al. Walking training of patients with hemiparesis at an early stage after stroke: a comparison of walking training on a treadmill with body

weight support and walking training on the ground. *Clin Rehabil* 2001;**15**:515–27.

45. Pohl M, Mehrholz J, Ritschel C, Rückriem S. Speed-dependent treadmill training in ambulatory stroke patients: a randomized controlled trial. *Stroke* 2002;**33**:553–8.

46. Macko RF, DeSouza CA, Tretter LD. Treadmill aerobic exercise training reduces the energy expenditure and cardiovascular demands of hemiparetic gait in chronic patients: a preliminary report. *Stroke* 1997;**28**:326–30.

47. Hesse S, Uhlenbrock D, Werner C, Bardeleben A. A mechanized gait trainer for restoring gait in non-ambulatory subjects. *Arch Phys Med Rehabil* 2000;**81**:1158–61.

48. Hesse S, Werner C, Uhlenbrock D, et al. An electromechanical gait trainer for restoration of gait in hemiparetic stroke patients: preliminary results. *Neurorehabil Neural Repair* 2001;**15**:37–48.

49. Werner C, von Frankenberg S, Treig T, et al. Treadmill training with partial body weight support and an electromechanical gait trainer for restoration of gait in subacute stroke patients. A randomized crossover study. *Stroke* 2002;**33**:867–973.

50. Colombo G, Wirz M, Dietz V. Driven gait orthosis for improvement of locomotor training in paraplegic patients. *Spinal Cord* 2001;**39**:252–5.

51. Liberson WT, Holmquest HJ, Scott D, Dow M. Functional electrotherapy, stimulation of peroneal nerve synchronized with the swing phase of the gait of hemiplegic patients. *Arch Phys Med Rehabil* 1961;**42**:101–5.

52. Bogataj U, Gros N, Malezic M, et al. Restoration of gait during two to three weeks of therapy with multichannel electrical stimulation. *Phys Ther* 1989;**69**:319–27.

53. Malezic M, Kljajic M, Acimovic-Janezic R, et al. Therapeutic effects of multisite electric stimulation of gait in motor-disabled patients. *Arch Phys Med Rehabil* 1987;**68**:553–60.

54. Marsolais EB, Kobetic R, Barnicle K, Jacobs J. FNS application for restoring function in stroke and head-injury patients. *J Clin Eng* 1990;**15**:489–96.

55. Trnkoczy A, Stanic U, Malezic M. Present state and prospects in design of multichannel FES stimulators for gait correction in paretic patients. *TIT J Life Sci* 1978;**8**:17–27.

56. Malezic M, Bogataj U, Gros N, et al. Evaluation of gait with multichannel electrical stimulation. *Orthopedics* 1987;**10**:769–72.

57. Malezic M, Stanic U, Kljajic M, et al. Multichannel electrical stimulation of gait in motor disabled patients. *Orthopedics* 1984;**7**:1187–95.

58. Malezic M, Bogataj U, Gros N, et al. Application of a programmable dual-channel adaptive electrical system for the control and analysis of gait. *J Rehabil Res Dev* 1992;**29**:41–53.

59. Hesse S, Malezic M, Mauritz KH. Multichannel electric stimulation in hemiparetic patients. In: Edwards J, ed. *Muscular components in functional electrical stimulation.* Brussels: Commission of the European Communities concerted Action, 1994;87–92.

60. Perry J. *Gait analysis; normal and pathological function.* Thorofare: Slack Inc, 1992.

61. Hannah RE, Morrison JB, Chapman AE. Kinematic Symmetry of the lower limbs. *Arch Phys Med Rehabil* 1984;**65**:155–58.

62. Murray MP, Drought AB, Kory RC. Walking patterns of normal men. *J Bone Joint Surg* 1964;**46**:335–60.

63. Bohannon RW, Smith MB. Interrater reliability of a modified Ashworth spastic scale of muscle spasticity. *Phys Ther* 1987;**67**:206–7.

64. Das TK, Park DM. Botulinum toxin in treating spasticity. *Br J Clin Pract* 1989;**43**:401–2.

65. Snow BJ, Tsui JL, Bhatt MH, et al. Treatment of spasticity with botulinum toxin:a double blind study. *Ann Neurol* 1990;**28**:512–15.

66. Dengler R, Neyer U, Wohlfarth K, et al. Local botulinum toxin in the treatment of spastic drop foot. *J Neurol* 1992;**239**:375–8.

67. Hesse S, Friedrich H, Domasch C, Mauritz KH. Botulinum toxin therapy for upper limb flexor spasticity: preliminary results. *J Rehabil Sci* 1992;**5**:98–101.

68. Hesse S, Krajnik J, Luecke D, et al. Ankle muscle activity before and after botulinum toxin therapy for lower limb extensor spasticity in chronic hemiparetic patients. *Stroke* 1996;**27**:455–60.

69. Burbaud P, Wiart L, Dubos JL, et al. A randomised, double blind, placebo controlled trial of botulinum toxin in the treatment of spastic foot in hemiparetic patients. *J Neurol Neurosurg Psychiatry* 1996;**61**:265–9.

70. Hesse S, Jahnke MT, Lücke D, Mauritz KH. Short-term electrical stimulation enhances the effectiveness of Botulinum toxin in the treatment of lower limb spasticity. *Neurosci Lett* 1995;**201**:37–40

71. Reiter F, Danni M, Lagalla G, et al. Low-dose botulinum toxin with ankle taping for the treatment of spastic equinovarus foot after stroke. *Arch Phys Med Rehabil* 1998;**79**:532–5.

72. Sabbahi MA, DeLuca CJ. Topical anesthetic-induced improvement in the mobility of patients with muscular hypertonicity: preliminary results. *J Electromyogr Kinesiol* 1991;**1**:41–48.

73. Davies PM. *Starting again.* Berlin: Springer Verlag, 1994; 299–381.

74. Pohl M, Ruckriem S, Mehrholz J, et al. Effectiveness of serial casting in patients with severe cerebral spasticity: a comparison study. *Arch Phys Med Rehabil* 2002;**83**:784–90.

75. Thaut MH, McIntosh GC, Prassas SG, Rice RR. Effect of rhythmic auditory cueing on temporal stride parameters and EMG patterns in hemiparetic gait of stroke patients. *J Neurol Rehabil* 1993;**7**:9–16.

76. Olney SJ, Colborne GR, Martin CS. Joint angle feedback and biomechanical gait analysis in stroke patients: a case report. *Phys Ther* 1989;**69**:863–70.

77. Burke DC, Burley HT, Ungar GH. Data on spinal injuries: Part II. Outcome of the treatment of 352 consecutive admissions. *Austr N Z J Surg* 1985;**55**:377–82.

78. Wernig A, Nanassy A, Müller S. Maintenance of locomotor abilities following Laufband (treadmill) therapy in para- and tetraplegic persons:follow- up studies. *Spinal Cord* 1998;**36**:744–9.

79. Dietz V, Colombo G, Jensen L, Baumgartner L. Locomotor capacity of spinal cord in paraplegic patients. *Ann Neurol* 1995;**37**:574–82.

80. Steward JE, Barbeau H, Gauthier S. Modulation of locomotor patterns and spasticity in spinal cord injured patients. *Can J Neurol Sci* 1991;**18**:321–32.

81. Norman KE, Barbeau H. Comparison of cyproheptadine, clonidine and baclofen on the modulation of gait pattern in subjects with spinal cord injury. In: Thilmann AE, Burke DJ, Rymer WZ, eds. *Spasticity: mechanisms and management.* Berlin; Springer-Verlag, 1993;410–25.

82. Fung J, Steward JE, Barbeau H. The combined effect of clonidine and cyproheptatine with interactive training on the

modulation of locomotion in spinal cord injured subjects. *J Neurol Sci* 1990,**100**:85–93.

83. Kantrowitz A. *Electronic physiologic aids. Report of the Maimonides Hospital. Brooklyn.* New York: Maimonides Hospital 1960;4–5.

84. Stein RB, Bélanger M, Wheeler G, et al. Electrical systems for improving locomotion after incomplete spinal cord injury: an assessment. *Arch Phys Med Rehabil* 1993;**74**:954–9.

85. Granat MH, Ferguson ACB, Andrews BJ, Delargy M. The role of functional electrical stimulation in the rehabilitation of patients with incomplete spinal cord injury – observed benefits during gait studies. *Paraplegia* 1993;**31**:207–15.

86. Kralj A, Bajd T. *Functional electrical stimulation: standing and walking after spinal cord injury.* Boca Raton: CRC Press, 1989.

87. Mauritz KH. Restoration of posture and gait by functional neuromuscular stimulation (FNS). In: Bles W, Brandt T, eds. *Disorders of posture and gait.* Amsterdam: Elsevier Science, 1986;367–85.

88. Hesse S, Malezic M, Lücke D, Mauritz KH. Value of functional electrostimulation in paraplegic patients. *Nervenarzt* 1998;**69**:300–5.

89. Hömberg V. Motor training in the therapy of Parkinson's disease. *Neurology* 1993;**43**(Suppl 6):S45–6.

90. Palmer SS, Mortimer JA, Webster DD, Bistevins R, Dickinson GL. Exercise therapy for Parkinson's disease. *Arch Phys Med Rehabil* 1986;**67**:741–5.

91. Barnes W, Seiz J, Kiel D, Elble RJ, Manyam BV. Outpatient Parkinson disease rehabilitation program. *Arch Phys Med Rehabil* 1991;**72**:796.

92. Pedersen SE, Öberg B, Isulander A, Vretman M. Group training in parkinsonism: quantitative measurements of treatment. *Scand J Rehabil Med* 1990;**22**:207–11.

93. Comella CL, Stebbins GT, Brown-Toms N, Goetz CG. Physical therapy and Parkinson's disease:a controlled clinical trial. *Neurology* 1994;**44**:376–78.

94. Richards CL, Malouin F, Bedard PJ, Cioni M. Changes induced by L-Dopa and sensory cues on the gait of Parkinsonian patients. In: Woollacott M, Horak F, eds. *Posture and gait: control mechanisms.* Eugene: University of Oregon Books, 1992.

95. Hoehn MM, Yahr MD. Parkinsonism: onset, progression, and mortality. *Neurology* 1967;**17**:427–42.

96. Miyai I, Fujimoto Y, Yamamoto H, et al. Long-term effect of body weight-supported treadmill training in Parkinson's disease: a randomized controlled trial. *Arch Phys Med Rehabil* 2000;**83**:1370–3.

19

Psychosocial aspects of disorders affecting balance and gait

LUCY YARDLEY, MARJAN JAHANSHAHI AND RICHARD S. HALLAM

19
Introduction	360
Psychosocial problems associated with vestibular disorder	361
Psychosocial aspects of vestibular rehabilitation	365
The psychosocial impact of neurological disorders of balance and gait	370
Summary	378
References	378

INTRODUCTION

This chapter reviews the psychosocial factors and psychological therapies which are relevant to two groups of people with balance disorders. The first consists of people with dizziness and imbalance caused by vestibular dysfunction. In this clinical population psychosocial factors often play a key role in handicap and recovery. Whereas Chapter 15 addresses psychosomatic processes in this population (i.e. the way in which psychological factors contribute to complaints of dizziness or imbalance), this chapter discusses somatopsychic processes – the way in which psychological factors can aggravate or alleviate the course of an organic disorder. The second group comprises people whose balance and gait problems are caused by central neurological disorders. Balance and gait impairment can be associated with hemiparesis following stroke and are features of the middle to late stages of disorders such as Parkinson's disease, Huntington's disease, cerebellar disease, multiple sclerosis and motor neuron disease. Postural instability and falls occur early in the course of progressive supranuclear palsy and can help to differentiate this disorder from other parkinsonian syndromes where these symptoms occur somewhat later such as multiple system atrophy and cortico-basal-degeneration and from idiopathic Parkinson's disease where recurrent falls appear much later.[1–3] In these patients psychosocial problems are typically less central to the symptomatology and progression of the disorder, but can still have an important impact on quality of life.

There are some parallels between the problems encountered by people with vestibular dysfunction and those with neurological disorders causing postural instability and gait impairment. Both groups may become uncertain of their own capabilities, concerned about the likely reactions of others to their infirmity and anxious about the significance of their symptoms. In both cases, these fears may result in secondary psychological disturbance and excessive restriction of activity. Therefore, some of the psychological techniques used to reduce anxiety, promote confidence and encourage activity are suitable for both populations.

Nevertheless, there are also a number of distinctive features of the experience of vertigo caused by vestibular disorder which demand a specialized therapeutic approach rather different from that adopted for neurological balance disorders. For example, acute vertigo attacks are generally infrequent but also unpredictable and violent, which causes difficulties entirely dissimilar to the often chronic disability that results from many neurological balance and gait disorders. Despite the frightening and unpleasant nature of the symptoms of vestibular dysfunction, the prognosis is generally self-limiting and benign, whereas the reverse may be true in the case of those with balance and gait problems caused by more serious and progressive neurological disorders. The goal of rehabilitation in the two populations may also be quite different. There is often a realistic possibility of restoring normal function in the case of those with vestibular disorders, whereas the goal of therapy for progressive neurological disorders is to minimize and cope with an unavoidable degree of disability.

In order to do justice to the important differences between these two patient groups, this chapter will first outline the particular psychosocial factors that contribute to the problems of people with vestibular disorder, and some specific therapeutic techniques which can be used to relieve or eliminate their difficulties, and will then consider the somewhat different problems and therapeutic approaches relevant to patients with neurological disorders.

PSYCHOSOCIAL PROBLEMS ASSOCIATED WITH VESTIBULAR DISORDER

The experience of vertigo

The impact of psychosocial factors on the patient's experience of balance disorder fundamentally influences the meaning and consequences of an episode of disorientation or imbalance. Three key components of the psychosocial experience of balance disorder can be distinguished (see Fig. 19.1). The first is subjective complaints, which are the product not only of the biological processes amply covered elsewhere in this book, but also the perceptual and emotional factors detailed below. Second, the term psychological distress is employed here to designate the affective aspect of the experience, and beliefs, inferences and expectations which contribute to negative emotional reactions. The third component comprises the functional, behavioral and social sequelae of balance disorder commonly referred to as disability and handicap.

Pre-existing and coexisting psychosocial characteristics or circumstances will partly determine the vulnerability of an individual to each aspect of the experience. For example, occupational demands will moderate the degree of handicap, while concurrent stress may undermine the capacity to cope with symptoms. The physical environment is also relevant, since exposure to perceptually complex or challenging situations can provoke latent symptoms and disability. In addition, the three main elements of the psychosocial experience of balance disorder can have bidirectional interactive effects (illustrated by the arrows linking the elements in Fig. 19.1); for example, persistent attacks of dizziness and imbalance can undoubtedly result in anxiety, but at the same time the apprehensive introspection which frequently accompanies anxiety may contribute to an exaggerated awareness of illness. The reciprocal causal links between the emotional, behavioral, and social consequences of disequilibrium can thus readily create or maintain an escalating cycle of symptoms, handicap and distress. In the following sections the specific factors and processes contributing to each aspect of this potential vicious cycle are considered in more detail.

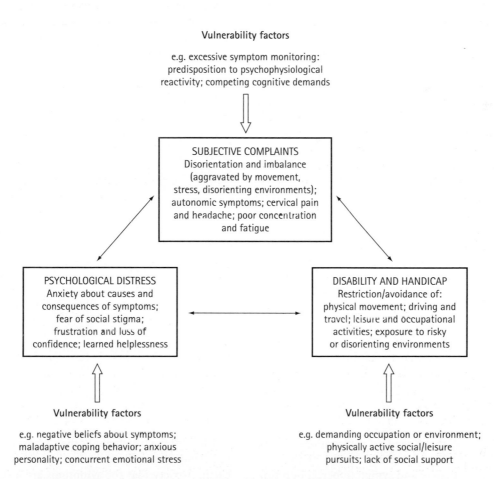

Figure 19.1 *Three key interrelated components of the psychosocial experience of balance disorder and contributory vulnerability factors.*

Subjective complaints

In addition to the core symptoms of disorientation and disequilibrium, people with balance disorders (in particular, vestibular dysfunction) frequently complain of a range of ancillary symptoms such as nausea, vomiting, diarrhea, sweating, trembling, palpitations, difficulty breathing, loss of concentration, and general lightheadedness and malaise.[4] The autonomic symptoms can be triggered directly in response to disorientation, but they are also characteristic of the physiological arousal associated with anxiety and have been shown to correlate with complaints of anxiety in patients with balance disorder.[5] Even when symptoms are ancillary to a primary diagnosis of vestibular disorder, a high level of reported somatic anxiety (i.e. numerous physical manifestations of anxiety) has proved to be a relatively powerful predictor of future patient well-being, predicting change in self-rated vertigo severity and handicap better than either initial vertigo severity or anxiety-provoking thoughts.[6,7]

Three complementary psychological mechanisms can help to explain why subjective reports of anxiety-related symptoms are associated with disequilibrium and handicap. First, high scores on self-report measures of somatic anxiety might indicate an excessive awareness and fear of physical symptoms. It has been suggested that the tendency to focus upon oneself is inevitably associated with distress and handicap, either because anxious self-monitoring of one's physical status is itself a sign of underlying psychological difficulties, or because constant self-evaluation draws attention to internal states which could be interpreted negatively.[8] Sensitivity to disequilibrium could therefore be enhanced by an internal focus of attention, or by a predisposition to evaluate sensations and events as potentially threatening, or to detect and monitor perceived sources of threat.[9,10]

Alternatively, or additionally, the high somatic anxiety symptom scores might reflect actual psychophysiological arousal. Arousal may directly enhance disorientation via the numerous reciprocal connections between the vestibular system, cerebellum and autonomic brainstem structures,[11] perhaps by inhibiting central habituation and suppression of disorienting vestibular signals, or by disrupting central integration of information for orientation.[12,13] Moreover, somatic symptoms of arousal in vestibular patients have been shown to be associated with an increased respiration rate,[14] and this may result in hyperventilation (overbreathing leading to alkalosis). This may itself cause disorientation and unsteadiness, and disinhibition of central suppression of peripheral vestibular imbalance.[15,16]

Finally, both of the foregoing explanations can be incorporated within an interactive model of the relationship between anxiety and symptom perception similar to that proposed by Clark[17] to account for the development of panic attacks. Clark suggests that negative perceptions of the physiological signs of arousal can themselves give rise to heightened anxiety, leading to an escalating cycle of symptoms and fear of what they might signify. In the case of patients with vestibular disorder, autonomic symptoms might originally form part of the syndrome of spontaneous acute vertigo, but might thereafter become part of a panic reaction to the milder disorientation provoked by movement, disorienting situations, or perhaps fatigue and stress (see below).

The psychophysiological processes described above provide a possible explanation for the covariation of stress and disorientation frequently reported by patients. However, subjective descriptions of an association between stress and attacks of dizziness and disequilibrium often confound emotional arousal with mental (cognitive) exertion or fatigue. Recent research suggests that orientation may require some cognitive effort.[18] It is therefore possible that it is actually the cognitive load imposed by distressing events that is most relevant to the difficulties experienced during stress, since emotionally challenging events generally involve urgent requirements for information-processing. The possibility that overcoming disorientation requires mental effort is consistent with patients' accounts of a bidirectional association between cognitive effort and disorientation; not only can demanding tasks provoke disorientation, but people with chronic balance disorders often complain of inability to concentrate and mental fatigue.[19]

Psychological distress

The form of psychological distress most commonly associated with balance disorders is anxiety, whether manifested in the form of somatic complaints, panic attacks, phobia, or generalized anxiety disorder. Studies of the psychological status of people referred to specialist balance clinics have consistently identified clinically significant levels of anxiety, panic disorder or other psychological disturbance in from one- to two-thirds of the patients.[20,21] Anxiety is typically associated with an actual or anticipated threat, where there is some perceived possibility of attaining safety or relief. The appraisal of threat is commonly supposed to comprise two stages; first, assessment of the degree of threat posed by the potential stressor, and second an appraisal of the capacity to cope effectively with this threat.[22] Hence, psychological distress in people with balance disorders is related to beliefs about the dangers and difficulties posed by disequilibrium, and evaluations of personal and situational resources for averting or coping with these threats.

Many of the beliefs about the dangers of dizziness and imbalance naturally center around the fear of physical harm. Anxiety that the symptoms are a sign of sinister disease is very common, and is frequently resistant to routine reassurance.[23] Patients are also often concerned that they might fall and hurt themselves, or are apprehensive that an unexpected attack might occur while they are involved in some potentially hazardous activity such as driving, scaling heights or operating dangerous machinery. However, the beliefs that are most closely linked to handicap in people with balance disorders relate to fear of losing control when in public,[24,25] concern about the social embarrassment and shame that might ensue, and a dread of being perceived as abnormal, neurotic, drunk or otherwise incompetent. These beliefs not only lead to distress, but may be associated with increases in psychophysiological arousal (discussed above) and can motivate restriction of activity (see the following section).

Further anxiety may arise as a result of uncertainty regarding the meaning and future course of the illness.[26] Authentication of the physical origin of illness is prerequisite for psychosocial adjustment, as it provides an acceptable explanation for deviations from normality and a well-established model for future conduct and social relations. However, in many cases of balance disorder it can be very difficult for the physician confidently to identify the etiology, predict the prognosis or the success of treatment, or even to confirm the impairment. The ambiguous status of their illness denies many patients with balance disorders the clearly defined sick role which would normally absolve them of personal responsibility for their symptoms; in the absence of a firm diagnosis, the suspicion that emotional weakness is the imputed or actual cause of their symptoms becomes an additional source of distress. Moreover, the unpredictability of attacks and uncertainty about the future course of the illness can make it difficult to plan for either the near or the distant future. Research has shown that an unexplained, unpredictable experience attributed to internal origin (whether a physical or a mental defect) is much more likely to cause anxiety than is a circumscribed, well-understood and ultimately controllable external set of circumstances.[27,28] Hence, the uncertainty surrounding the probable cause and course of the illness can make it more difficult to adjust and adapt to balance disorder than to equally disabling but more inexorable, and therefore predictable, chronic medical conditions.

Naturally, personality factors are likely to play a part in the development of fears relating to balance disorder; apprehension about the significance and possible consequences of symptoms will be more pronounced in people whose genetic make-up or learning experiences have predisposed them to anxiety or phobia. This is one possible explanation for the relatively high incidence of previous psychiatric problems observed among vestibular patients referred to specialist neuro-otological clinics;[20,21] the people who eventually require referral to a specialist on account of balance disorder may be predominantly those that are prone to become anxious or that have poor coping skills (see also Chapter 15).

In cases of chronic balance disorder, depression may also ensue. Depression can be a reaction to loss (including loss of physical health), or a sign of what has been called 'learned helplessness' – a condition of passive despair which occurs in circumstances that seem to offer no opportunity for active coping.[29] Hence, if the individual considers that their balance disorder has adverse consequences over which they have absolutely no control, and if these consequences are perceived as having an extensive and long-lasting negative impact on their lifestyle, then depression is likely to ensue. The following section examines the way in which common beliefs about the causes and consequences of disorientation promote a passive coping style which fosters handicap and depression.

Disability and handicap

The World Health Organization (WHO)[30] defines 'disability' as the impact of 'impairment' (i.e. the immediate effects of symptoms) on daily activities, while 'handicap' reflects effects on broad spheres of life, such as social roles and relationships and economic self-sufficiency.[30] However, the level of disability and handicap associated with vestibular disorder has been shown to be more closely related to fear of symptoms and their possible consequences than to the actual severity of the symptoms themselves,[25] since acute, disabling attacks of vertigo are seldom very frequent or prolonged.[7] The problem is that the strategies which most patients employ to cope with the threat of disequilibrium actually tend to promote the excessive avoidance of activities and places often referred to, respectively, as 'anticipatory disability' and 'agoraphobia'. In their attempts to avoid disclosure or exposure of their condition, people with balance disorders may relinquish a wide range of social engagements, from parties to evening classes. Concern about the possibility of a sudden attack dissuades them from undertaking activities perceived as responsible or potentially dangerous, such as driving, climbing, operating machinery or caring for children. A further motive for retiring from a variety of valued social and occupational activities originates from the desire to avoid provoking disorientation, whether by exertion, travel, stress or exposure to disorienting environments.

The restrictions on lifestyle following from these coping strategies can be understood as the consequence of a set of self-generated rules governing behavior, based on beliefs concerning the available courses of action and their potential consequences.[31] Unfortunately, those that experience unexpected attacks of disorientation or imbalance tend to apply these rules over a wider range of situations and longer time-scale than may be strictly necessary in order to avoid dizziness and social exposure. Such blanket prohibition of activity is a logical strategy for coping with symptoms that are perceived to be unpredictable, but the avoidance behavior limits opportunities for testing or extending the boundaries of possible action, and may thus perpetuate a vicious circle of diminished self-confidence.[32] For example, the residual symptoms provoked by vigorous movement or disorienting environments are often mistaken for warnings of an imminent attack. Since the rational response is to withdraw from the provocative situation (just as any sensible person with back pain desists from lifting heavy objects) the individual never has an opportunity to learn that they could cope with and overcome the mild disorientation that would result, but instead gains the impression that a severe attack has been averted by prudent self-handicapping behavior.

The application of self-generated rules for coping with dizziness or imbalance in a rigid and unnecessary fashion can lead to frustration and depression, as these rules may lead to excessive constraints upon behavior that are often far more extensive than the direct effects of the balance disorder warrant. The result may be an apparently insoluble dilemma in which people are torn between the fear of provoking disorientation or being socially discredited by an attack of dizziness in public, and the desire to escape a depressingly constrictive lifestyle. The consequent behavioral impasse may ultimately result in the condition of 'learned helplessness' described in the previous section. Alternatively, one response to the psychosocial conflict posed by this dilemma is to adopt the role of an invalid. This solution provides the individual with a new identity and a less ambitious set of goals, and thereby minimizes the risk of failure. Such behavior can have agreeable consequences such as receiving attention and sympathy or being absolved from unpleasant or stressful duties, but the costs include relinquishing the prospect of fulfilling many normal roles, accepting the stigma attached to this departure from normal behavior, and putting strain on social or family relationships. External circumstances and support can crucially affect the ability of an individual to reconcile social and practical demands with the limitations imposed by illness. For example, a person living alone in a tenth floor apartment or an individual whose occupation involves long hours and extensive travel is likely to encounter more difficulty adjusting to a balance disorder than someone with a flexible employer, supportive family and sedentary job.

Disability and handicap maintain or fuel the cycle of psychosocial distress associated with balance disorder not only by perpetuating the anxiety and depression caused by symptoms, but also by exacerbating the symptomatology itself. Restriction of head movement and avoidance of exertion can result in a variety of secondary symptoms, ranging from simple loss of fitness to neck tension and headache. Moreover, limitation of physical activity and avoidance of disorienting environments prolongs the duration of residual disorientation due to balance system dysfunction by retarding compensation and preventing the development of adapted, skilled perceptual–motor coordination. Hence, as long as the individual continues to avoid particular movements and situations, these will continue to provoke dizziness and imbalance.

A multidisciplinary approach to management

The guiding principle of the biopsychosocial approach is the assumption that every patient complaining of dizziness or imbalance is likely to have both a genuine orientation problem and related psychosocial difficulties; both of these elements of patients' problems merit investigation and some form of assistance. An immediate benefit of this approach is that it generally proves much more welcome to patients than either medical or psychological treatment alone. People with authenticated balance disorders are eager to receive advice on how to cope with their symptoms and disability, while anxious patients with less well-defined balance problems are relieved to have their complaints taken seriously. When there is a lack of evidence of physical dysfunction to account for symptoms, simple reassurance that there is no organic basis for sensations which the patient regards as signs of physical disorder may be interpreted as a failure of diagnosis on the part of the doctor and/or an implicit accusation of emotional weakness or malingering. Acknowledging the validity of the patient's perception of their illness is therefore an essential first step towards gaining their trust and confidence in the recommended therapy.

This approach to rehabilitation is particularly well suited to the treatment of balance disorders, since therapies designed to promote neurophysiological adaptation and enhance sensorimotor capabilities and skills are likely also to exert a variety of valuable psychosocial effects. These covert benefits of physiotherapy may include increasing tolerance of physical symptoms, reducing anxiety about their significance, promoting confidence in balance, and minimizing restriction of physical and social activity. Of course, the wide-ranging benefits of rehabilitation for balance disorders already constitute part of the rationale for recommending balance exercises for patients that are not expected to achieve complete functional compensation, such as those with bilateral hypofunction. However, it is advantageous to explore the range and nature of the latent psychological effects of physiotherapy in a more explicit and systematic manner in order to be able to fully exploit the psychosocial aspects of rehabilitation and supplement the physiotherapy with appropriate, targeted psychotherapeutic techniques.

Recognition of the importance of psychosocial factors in rehabilitation does not necessarily demand the direct participation of a psychiatrist or psychologist in the management of patients. Indeed, referral to a psychiatrist or clinical psychologist can actually be unhelpful if the patient perceives the implication of emotional disorder as erroneous and stigmatizing. Conversely, guidance offered sensitively by the doctor, occupational or behavioral therapist, physiotherapist, or audiologist may be more readily accepted and less damaging to the patient's self-esteem. Group sessions and self-help organizations may also help to build confidence at the same time as enabling sufferers to share their experiences and offer mutual advice and support. To identify and address the psychosocial aspects of balance disorders it is therefore simply necessary to ensure that: (1) adequate time, attention and resources are specifically allotted to the assessment and treatment of psychosocial problems; (2) liaison with psychiatric and psychological personnel is sufficiently close to permit communication and advice concerning circumscribed psychosocial problems and appropriate referral of more difficult cases; and (3) all medical and ancillary staff involved in rehabilitation receive education on the common links between physical and psychological factors in dizziness and imbalance and basic training in their identification and management. The purpose of the remainder of this chapter is to provide an elementary guide to some of the techniques which can be employed to assess and alleviate handicap and distress.

PSYCHOSOCIAL ASPECTS OF VESTIBULAR REHABILITATION

While the core physiotherapeutic element of vestibular habituation usually takes the form of a series of daily exercises (see Chapter 17), when conceived broadly vestibular rehabilitation (VR) encompasses an attempt to deal with all the psychosocial consequences of a balance disorder, including family and work-related problems associated with disability. The primary goals of VR are to improve balance in the specific contexts in which deficits are observed and render balance and postural control an automatic unconscious activity rather than a deliberate achievement, to reduce motion provoked symptoms and/or help the patient to cope with them better, to educate the patient about the causes of symptoms and, in general, to improve functional capacity and promote resumption of normal activities without undue emotional distress. These are all aims in which psychological factors should be considered.

Educating the patient and maximizing motivation

One psychological characteristic of the equilibrial sense is that it is normally taken for granted – it is spatial disorientation and loss of equilibrium that is signaled to the organism. Moreover, given that the senses can compensate for each other (and that compensation may be acquired gradually if systemic deterioration is gradual) symptoms of dizziness or imbalance may be revealed only in conditions of sensory conflict, sensory impoverishment, or in cognitively or physically demanding conditions. For this reason, the patient may be at a loss to explain the nature of their experiences and difficulties. Educating the patient about the nature of their disability therefore assumes great importance.

Explanation of the distinction between spontaneous and provoked vertigo and imbalance can be particularly helpful. Without knowledge of balance system function, the natural assumption is that any dizziness or unsteadiness may be the early sign of a spontaneous attack. Many patients therefore desist from activities which provoke even mild symptoms, hence preventing or retarding compensation. Simply informing patients that mild, provoked dizziness is a natural and necessary part of the process of compensation can break this cycle of restriction of activity and persisting residual symptoms. In addition, an understanding of how movement and environmental factors can provoke vertigo and imbalance often greatly reduces anxiety, as it enables the patient to anticipate and account for symptoms that previously appeared unpredictable and inexplicable. If the therapist is able to help the patient to identify the triggers for their dizziness, this reassures them that the therapist does indeed have an expert understanding of the causes of their problem, which is no longer viewed as a mysterious and potentially sinister disorder. The more the patient comes to understand what may influence their symptoms, the greater their sense of control over the situation.

Patient education also plays an important part in shaping the positive but realistic expectations needed to ensure adherence to any program of treatment.[33] Patients who remain partly unconvinced of the efficacy of VR, or who encounter unexpected and unpleasant side-effects, are unlikely to carry out the exercises as prescribed. Since patients are usually wary of revealing their non-compliance,[34] the result can be an apparent failure of treatment which may lead the clinician to question the efficacy of rehabilitation. It is therefore vital before commencing VR to convince the patient that it is the appropriate form of treatment, to warn them that an initial increase in symptoms may occur at first, and to teach them how to pace the exercises so that the dizziness provoked is not intolerably severe.

The response to VR will vary according to the patient's home environment, level of social support, daily activity level, cognitive abilities and motivation for recovery. Although compensation for equilibrial dysfunction can be fairly rapid (e.g. after labyrinthectomy) it will be slowed by pathology or degenerative changes in the central nervous system. Recurrent malfunction will impede the development of compensation and will also reduce motivation to engage in the necessary rehabilitation exercises. Educating the patient in the underlying causes and environmental triggers of their symptoms, and in the rationale of VR, is therefore vital to ensure that motivation is maintained. Chronically high levels of autonomic nervous system arousal and/or tendency to hyperventilate are also thought by some authors to retard the process of compensation.[12,13] In addition, maladaptive adjustments to dizziness and imbalance such as avoidance of rapid movement, a rigid head posture, and over-reliance on visual guidance of movement are likely to impede recovery of function. Older patients may have multisensory deficits, cognitive impairment and other physical conditions that have additional destabilizing influences and hamper recovery.[35] To avoid disillusionment and premature rejection of VR it is necessary to advise patients of the factors that may affect the speed of recovery, and forewarn them if improvement is likely to be slow and partial.

Alleviating symptoms and anxiety

Given that balance performance in everyday activities is strongly correlated with expressed confidence in balance and generalized anxiety,[36] it seems possible that the efficacy of the exercises may be attributable in some measure to psychological factors. Behavioral psychologists have theorized that an automatic emotional and physiological response can be learned through repeated experience of an association between somatic sensations and an aversive experience. The possibility that this form of learning (known as 'classical conditioning') may contribute to the experience of vertigo can be inferred from occasional reports by patients that they have developed an aversion to tastes or smells that happened to precede the onset of their first vertiginous episode. Jacob[13] has proposed that some patients with balance disorders may develop a learned panic response to attacks of vertigo, and that this panic reaction may later become a generalized response to any form of dizziness or unsteadiness, such as the slight sensations of disorientation which may be experienced in environments characterized by complex orientation and motion cues (e.g. escalators or motorways).

If panic becomes a learned response to dizziness, a psychological barrier of caution and fear may have to be broken before the neurophysiological processes of compensation for a balance disorder can begin to take effect. The therapeutic principle that forms the basis for this procedure is 'extinction' – that is, repeated presentation of the somatic sensation of dizziness and imbalance (the 'conditioned stimulus') in the absence of the aversive experience that has previously followed it (the 'unconditioned stimulus'), which in this case is fear and panic. According to behavioral theory, exposure to the relevant somatic sensation (vertigo) without accompanying fear is therefore the crucial element of VR, rather than any objective improvement in balance performance. However, it is most probable that during VR the psycho-

logical and physical effects of exposure have reciprocal benefits. The gradual lessening in fear resulting from repeated, controlled experience of dizziness in a safe environment will be accompanied by a reduction in anxiety-related symptomatology, while the decrease in both apprehension and symptoms encourages the patient to persist with the physiotherapeutic exercises, hence achieving organic compensation.

Any movement-based rehabilitation technique guarantees exposure to the relevant disorienting stimulus, although careful control of duration of exposure is desirable. In order to ensure that the sensation of vertigo is not accompanied by fear, it may be necessary to teach the patient a method of 'applied relaxation' (see Chapter 17). At first, the relaxation is practiced in isolation, but once mastered it is then applied in the situations that provoke anxiety, such as when dizzy. In addition, research indicates that this 'extinction' or 'desensitization' approach may be enhanced by cognitively preparing the patient in a way that dispels unrealistic fears, corrects unfounded beliefs and inspires confidence in the ability to cope with emotional distress and disorienting sensations.[37,38]

It is useful for the clinician and therapist to be able to identify patients that have particularly high levels of anxiety. A number of short psychological scales are available for assessing psychological distress, and many of these provide validated 'cut-off points' for detecting clinically significant anxiety and depression requiring treatment.[39,40] In the case of symptoms such as nausea, sweating, palpitations, or malaise, which are of equivocal etiology, it may be possible to attribute them to psychological or physical causes, or at least to identify triggering events. A more accurate attribution makes it easier for the patient to tackle excessive fears or adapt to symptoms that may have to be accepted rather than controlled. Detection of anxiety-related symptoms also alerts the clinician to the need for VR to be supplemented by therapies such as relaxation or cognitive–behavioral therapy (see below). The absence of conscious 'psychological' antecedents for such symptoms (over and above those of a sensory, perceptual or postural kind) need not imply the absence of a psychological aspect to their etiology, since anxiety can be experienced and expressed entirely as physical symptomatology.[41] The tendency to complain of somatic symptoms that have no identifiable organic basis can be detected using established 'somatization' scales,[42,43] and there are also scales that assess physical signs of anxiety,[44] as well as specific psychological problems such as panic disorder and agoraphobia.[45,46]

A disadvantage of most psychological measures of somatic anxiety is that they class 'dizziness' and 'nausea' as signs of anxiety, whereas in balance disorder patients these symptoms may actually have an organic etiology. The 'Vertigo Symptom Scale' (VSS) solves this problem by providing two subscales that are specifically designed to discriminate between symptoms of balance system dysfunction and of anxiety, and to give a measure of the severity of each (see Appendix 19.1). The 'Anxiety' subscale has been shown to be highly correlated with other psychological measures of anxiety, while the 'Vertigo' subscale is related to objective measures of vestibular function and clinical classifications of vertigo.[5,6,47] The 'Anxiety' subscale assesses both excessive complaints of diverse somatic symptoms (from backache to chest pain) and the presence of psychophysiological symptoms of anxiety, such as a pounding heart. A further advantage of the VSS is that it appears to the patient to be simply assessing the severity of symptoms typical of balance disorder. In contrast, it is fairly obvious in the case of most psychological questionnaires that they are measuring anxiety, panic or hypochondria; consequently, patients that are already worried that people do not believe their symptoms are organic may become resentful and suspicious when given such a questionnaire, and may deny any anxiety.

Hyperventilation can be a contributory factor to symptoms experienced during episodes, which may be exacerbated by changes in the pattern of breathing associated with the emotional response to the episode. The signs of chronic hyperventilation are extremely variable but typically include tingling sensations in the extremities, numbness of the skin, lightheadedness, breathing difficulties and tightness in the throat or chest. The possibility that hyperventilation contributes to the symptom pattern can be tested by asking the patient to over-breathe at a rate of 30 breaths per minute for 3 min (or until the patient feels unable to continue). The reliability, sensitivity and specificity of this 'hyperventilation provocation test' has been called into question, and remains a topic for heated debate.[48] However, by careful questioning it should be possible to determine the extent to which the effects of hyperventilation mimic typical episodes of dizziness or disorientation. Similarly, the role of hyperventilation in producing vestibular-type symptoms is still uncertain, but it may nevertheless be useful to demonstrate to the patient that their apparently sinister and mysterious symptoms can be caused – and more importantly controlled – by something as simple and innocuous as a change in breathing pattern.

Where hyperventilation is suspected, relaxation and slow diaphragmatic breathing should be taught. The effectiveness of slowing breathing down (or rebreathing exhaled air in a paper bag) in removing these sensations quickly may help to convince the patient of this new interpretation of the cause of their symptoms. With regard to teaching relaxation and a slower, less effortful, diaphragmatic style of breathing, this can usually be achieved within a few sessions of demonstration and reinforced by practice at home with audio-recorded instructions. However, a minority of patients find this extremely difficult and require extensive training.

Alleviating handicap and encouraging activity

Although the psychosocial consequences of balance disorders are quite variable, the following considerations may help to guide management of the individual case. First, the patient may benefit from a clarification and objective assessment of the actual degree of handicap and how it might be overcome. A detailed functional analysis of the triggers and consequences of episodes of dizziness and imbalance can also reveal the patient's coping resources and how they might be improved. Patients can be asked about recent, typical or initial episodes, or instances that have been significant in shaping their psychological response. There are a number of questionnaires suitable for assessing disability and handicap,[23,48,49] and they are a quick and economical method of assessment of patients problems. As reliable and quantifiable measures of patient well-being, properly developed and validated questionnaires are also a useful means of monitoring long-term changes in patient status and improvements following treatment. However, the administration of questionnaires should be followed up by a clinical interview with the patient for clarification and discussion of the problems they identify.

The patient might be unaware of strategies for managing these problems that others have found useful or they might be overactively applying preferred techniques. The problem of travel-induced symptoms is a common one, as is a fear of loss of control while driving a car. In the latter case, the assessment of danger may be magnified by the patient especially if a warning of an impending episode is always received, giving adequate time to pull over and stop. The desire to appear normal and a fear of embarrassment may mean that patients fail to share their difficulties with family, friends, or employer who, in reality, may be more charitably disposed and willing to make adjustments than the patient expects. The patient may report experiences of having been perceived as incompetent, neurotic, drunk or drugged. Sensitive exploration of these memories may reveal that the 'persecutor's' perceptions arose out of ignorance of their condition which, it is well recognized, is not commonly understood. A joint interview with a partner or confidante can assist in the process of objective assessment of handicap and facilitate self-disclosure. The potential benefits here are the alleviation of fears others may have about the patient's potential dependence on them, a better understanding of the condition and its implications for the future, and the identification of more effective means of coping with symptoms or social embarrassment.

A considerable proportion of patients feel obliged to give up their job or change the nature of their employment. This may be due to the stress and fatigue of ill-health or due to travel restrictions, repeated absences from work or interference with work efficiency itself. In this area too, objective assessment of the handicap and counseling to examine the possibility of compromise arrangements or flexible working should be explored. Letters to employers from medical or other specialists (with explicit guidance from the patient) can sometimes relieve these and other seemingly intractable situations.

It can be helpful to supplement the specific physiotherapeutic exercises of VR with a program of physical activity outside the home. The activities used to extend and generalize restoration of physical confidence may be as simple as walking, or as demanding as ball games or ballroom dancing, in which rhythm and touch may assist the patient to maintain good balance while practising both novel and well-rehearsed movements. Patients are likely to benefit most when exercises build on existing habits and interests and exploit whatever resources are available for maintaining motivation. Spouses, partners or friends may play an important role in prompting and encouraging activities and in providing a bridge of reassurance until confidence is regained. For example, a partner may prompt a patient to follow a prearranged program of activities designed to develop confidence in negotiating environmental challenges (steps, slopes, uneven ground, etc.) or in extending the patient's territorial boundaries. Most patients feel more confident when tackling these in the company of trusted others; eventually, sufficient confidence is gained for them to be tackled alone.

A group of patients has been identified who respond with disorientation and fear to stimuli normally involved in the perception of space and motion, and movement through space.[50,51] These patients seem to experience excessive disorientation and dizziness when exposed to incongruity between cues in different sensory modalities, to the absence of strong visuospatial cues (such as in open spaces), or to the vestibular stimulation resulting from rapid change of speed and direction, as experienced in vehicular transportation. Other patients are sensitive to minor 'obstacles' such as curbs that have to be negotiated while walking. The patient sometimes seeks out cues that strongly signal horizontal and vertical planes, and also a means of support when loss of balance is feared. The patient may cling tenaciously to walls or hand rails, although a walking stick, shopping basket or close presence of another person may suffice to restore confidence in balance.

The etiology of this fear of space and motion cues is unclear; it might arise as a secondary consequence of previous falls, vertiginous episodes or panic attacks or may reflect a primary impairment of the processing of space and motion cues. Dependence on visual cues or oversensitivity to moving visual stimuli can be addressed at the level of perceptual–motor functioning by balance retraining (see Chapter 17). However, fear of space and motion cues bears many similarities to the psychological condition known as 'panic disorder with agoraphobia'.[52,53] People with such phobias may therefore also benefit from a number of well-validated psychological therapies for agoraphobia.[54,55] For example, a program of 'graded exposure' to the feared environments may be agreed with the patient. The therapist and patient jointly construct a hierarchy of progressively more anxiety-provoking tasks for the patient to accomplish; for a patient whose target goal was to travel by bus to a nearby town, the hierarchy might start with simply walking to the bus-stop, which once successfully completed would then be followed by getting on the bus, travelling to the next bus-stop, and so on. This can be undertaken under the supervision of a psychologist or behavioral therapist, and it is often advisable to enlist the support of family members.

Cognitive–behavioral therapy

Although VR addresses many of the anxieties and avoidance habits of patients, a more comprehensive and individually tailored approach that follows established cognitive–behavioral principles[36,56] may be required if the patient has deeply entrenched unrealistic fears about potential dangers or personal embarrassment. These interventions are usually short-term in nature, although longer-term support is occasionally helpful. They are probably best performed by a professional working alongside the medical team so that information from each source can contribute to an effective management approach. However, the subject of psychological therapy must be broached with great sensitivity, since patients that attribute their psychological difficulties to somatic causes are likely to resist non-medical referral if they feel that their somatic concerns are not being seriously investigated. It is usual in the psychological management of these patients to take the somatic complaints seriously and to confront rationally the medical evidence and fears of illness. At the same time, it is important to avoid confirming suspicions of serious illness by over-investigation of physical complaints, which can be interpreted by the patient as evidence that their symptoms must be sinister.[57] For patients that are antagonistic to the idea of psychological treatment, vestibular rehabilitation may be particularly useful since it can address some psychological aspects of balance disorder yet has a clear somatic rationale.[34] However, the problem of switching the patient's focus from somatic to psychological concerns can be achieved in most cases.

The cognitive–behavioral approach involves three principal components. The first element of therapy is a gradual confrontation of patients' idiosyncratic fear-provoking and disorienting cues while 'safety cues' are gradually withdrawn. A 'safety-cue' in this context can be defined as any aspect of the situation which reduces the magnitude or probability of threat; for example, the presence of a trusted companion, the close proximity of an exit point, or a physical support such as wall or walking stick. The second component of cognitive–behavioral therapy consists of rational challenges to unrealistic fears and a cognitive 'restructuring' of mistaken causal attributions. In addition to threats already mentioned, these commonly include a fear of life-threatening illness, death, loss of control or madness and public humiliation or embarrassment. Therapy entails a systematic gathering and disputing of evidence for the patient's beliefs through open-ended Socratic questioning. Alternative interpretations of the evidence are entertained, disputed and tested out. 'Behavioral experiments' may be used to test the validity of beliefs the patient holds. For example, a dizzy patient may have developed a fear of crossing busy roads, and this fear may persist despite considerable improvement in objective balance function following VR. In this case, the belief that a sudden and dangerously disabling attack of dizziness might still occur when crossing a road would first be confronted verbally by discussing the true likelihood and probable consequences of such an eventuality. The patient might then be asked to empirically test their belief that they cannot cross a road safely; a few successful crossings made on quiet roads or with a companion can provide the necessary evidence that this belief was erroneous.

Third, the patient may benefit from training in techniques for coping with distress itself, such as applied relaxation or distraction. Distraction techniques might include switching attention to neutral aspects of the situation rather than the self (e.g. talking to someone, looking in shop windows or listening to a portable stereo). A different mental attitude to the distressing experience is encouraged which can be summed up as 'detached acceptance', backed up by previously rehearsed verbal statements. These are either mentally repeated or read from a cue-card. Examples here might include 'This is unpleasant but it will pass', 'I know this is another dizzy attack but it won't physically hurt me'.

Psychosocial case studies

CASE 1

Mr S is a man in his late twenties with a history of vertigo associated with middle ear disease since childhood, for which he had been hospitalized on a number of occasions for treatment by antibiotics and surgery. Previously, he recovered well with no residual symptoms or disability, but following the last inpatient treatment he complained of persistent marked giddiness, headaches, and pain and fullness in the ear, and felt unable to return to work. On referral to a specialist balance clinic he was visibly agitated, flushed and trembling, and when told that no physical cause had been found for his symptoms burst into tears.

He was referred for vestibular rehabilitation, and because of his conviction that further medication and surgery was needed was at first hostile and suspicious that his symptoms were being dismissed as psychological. The somatic rationale for postoperative VR was therefore explained at length. At first the exercises caused a worsening in his aural pain and headaches and renewed anxiety, and the patient angrily rejected the suggestion that headache was a secondary tension-related symptom rather than a sign of internal damage (although the headache could be relieved by neck massage). However, after 6 weeks of VR his symptoms started to improve, with a resulting increase in his motivation and confidence. After 8 weeks he was experiencing much reduced symptoms, the most severe being headaches following exercising at the gym. At this point the patient spontaneously asked whether he might benefit from psychological therapies, and was taught relaxation and breath control. Daily practice with the aid of tape-recorded instructions resulted in further improvement, and in lieu of returning to his previous occupation the patient started training as a counselor.

CASE 2

Mrs B is a 70-year-old widow who was until recently a physically active woman. At the time of referral she was having increasing difficulty in walking downstairs, stepping off curbs, getting off buses, and walking on sloping terrain. Despite a previous stapedectomy and the possibility of a perilymph leak a major psychological contribution to her imbalance was suspected. Faced with obstacles she experienced nausea, dizziness and a fear of falling, which was intensified by three actual previous falls. Concerned about hurting herself and creating a humiliating public spectacle she therefore avoided obstacles and stayed at home, if possible, venturing out only when accompanied. She stated that she had lost confidence in herself, and that even imagining an obstacle caused emotional distress.

Her abilities were assessed on steps and slopes around the hospital, and on a single step of 2, 4, 6, 8 and 10 cm in height. Ratings of her anxiety were taken on a simple scale, and the time taken for task completion was recorded in order to establish a baseline against which to measure improvement. She was unable to walk downstairs without holding the banister and tended to shuffle and lean forward.

A program of graded exposure in ascending steps at a normal pace and with normal posture was arranged, beginning with the 2-cm step and proceeding to the higher steps. Feedback was given on progress and praise was given for her efforts. She made rapid progress over six sessions. This was evident also in her home environment where she no longer spent time planning routes and was able to take buses alone. She reported that the nausea disappeared and she 'felt taller'.

THE PSYCHOSOCIAL IMPACT OF NEUROLOGICAL DISORDERS OF BALANCE AND GAIT

From the text above it is evident that there is a sizeable body of research on the psychosocial impact of vestibular disorders. The core aspect of this work relates to how symptoms such as dizziness, vertigo and balance problems affect the daily activities, social functioning and emotional well-being of the person with vestibular dysfunction. While the psychosocial impact of neurological disorders affecting balance and gait has also been extensively investigated in a number of illnesses such as Parkinson's disease, the focus of this work has not been specifically on the effects of the balance and gait problems on daily life. Instead, the net effect of all the symptoms of the disorder on the daily living of the individual has been studied. For example, in idiopathic Parkinson's disease, measures of disability[58] have examined the total impact of symptoms such as rigidity, tremor, bradykinesia, dysphonia, micrographia and the emphasis has not been solely on the balance and walking problems of these patients. Nevertheless, given the primacy of mobility for independent living, balance and gait problems have undoubtedly been key contributors to the disability associated with these disorders. Bearing in mind this difference in emphasis, in the remainder of this chapter we first review the psychosocial sequelae of neurological disorders of gait and balance and then consider various approaches to their management.

Neurological disorders affecting gait and balance are diverse in their etiology. They also differ in terms of when in their course, balance and gait problems first appear. These differences in the precise nature, extent, and time of onset of balance and gait problems are likely to have implications for the way in which the disorder affects the individual's psychosocial functioning and quality of life. Ideally, the psychosocial features of each of these neurological disorders of balance and gait should be considered separately, since there are likely to be major similarities as well as notable differences in the way in which motor neuron disease, Parkinson's disease, post-cerebrovascular accident (CVA), hemipareis, multiple sclerosis, and progressive supranuclear palsy, to take a few examples, affect the daily activities, emotional well-being and quality of life of the patients. For instance, the often short and aggressively progressive course of motor neuron disease may lead one to expect that the disability associated with symptoms such as speech impairment, reduced mobility and respiratory distress may cause greater emotional upset and poorer quality of life than in other neurological disorders affecting balance and gait. In the case of Huntington's disease, the genetic basis of the disorder and its implications for the rest of the family can be a key feature of the psychological burden. Even within a single neurological disorder affecting balance and gait, such as multiple sclerosis, the course of the illness and hence the psychosocial consequences can vary enormously from one person to another, ranging from mild and remitting symptoms for 30 years to a rapidly progressive and disabling disease within 5 years. However, consideration of the psychosocial consequences of each of the neurological disorders of balance and balance is beyond the scope of the present chapter. In the following sections we will mainly consider the psychosocial features of Parkinson's disease for several reasons. First, Parkinson's disease is one of the most prevalent of the neurological disorders affecting balance and gait.[59,60] Second, while impairment of balance, falls and inability to walk occur in the middle to late stages of Parkinson's disease and can help differentiate the disorder from other parkinsonian syndromes such as progressive supranuclear palsy in which falls occur early,[1-3] other gait-related symptoms such as slowness of walking, lack of arm swing, a shuffling gait, and start hesitation can be present from the earlier stages of the illness.[61-64] Third, the psychosocial impact of Parkinson's disease on the sufferers has been studied more extensively than the other disorders. Fourth, the focus of our own work has primarily been on the impact of Parkinson's disease on psychosocial functioning and quality of life. However, before reviewing the specific psychosocial features of Parkinson's disease, particularly the implications of the gait and balance problems, we will review the general framework within which the effects of disorders of balance and gait on daily life can be evaluated which is applicable across all these neurological disorders.

The stress of chronic, progressive neurological illness and factors determining its effects on daily life

When some major change occurs in our lives, regardless of whether it is pleasant or unpleasant, we have to make some effort to adjust to the new circumstances. During this process of adjustment, we draw on personal resources, physical, mental or social. Such a 'change' becomes a stress when there is a marked imbalance between the effort required to adjust, and the personal resources available for doing so. The most stressful life events are those that are unexpected and over which we have less control.[65,66] This is why the onset of a chronic neurological illness is experienced as stressful, because it is usually unexpected and we have little control over it.

Acute and chronic illness differ in fundamental ways. An acute illness such as appendicitis results in intense pain that comes on suddenly and is quickly resolved by medical intervention and treatment. The person is ill only for a short period, and once the illness is treated and cured, they resume their previous roles and return to normal function. In contrast, with chronic illness, since the symptoms usually develop gradually, there is no clear event that marks the transition of the individual from being well to being ill, other than the diagnosis by a doctor. Also, when chronic illness is progressive, the symptoms will become worse over time. This means that daily activities, social and occupational functioning will not return to a familiar version of normality, but instead will also show gradual decline, as it becomes necessary to give up familiar roles at work, at home and socially.

The rate of progression of the illness is a major determinant of the psychosocial effects of the illness.[67-69] Disorders that progress rapidly give the person little time to adjust emotionally to the loss of normal function and ensuing disability and for this reason are, in many cases, more likely to be associated with emotional distress. The demands and challenges posed by chronic illness change with the 'phase of illness'. For example, in the early phase shortly after diagnosis, when the symptoms are relatively mild, people have to alter their future plans and expectations to adjust to the knowledge that they are no longer healthy. Practical arrangements may have to be made to prepare for the prospect of future unemployment and loss of earnings and increasing disability and loss of mobility. The middle phase, which is usually the longest, is associated with moderately severe symptoms and disability, as a result of which key social and occupational roles may have to be given up. A sudden or severe worsening of symptoms during this phase may result in depression. By the late phase, the illness progresses to produce severe symptoms that are no longer controlled by medical treatment. Loss of autonomy and increasing dependence may characterize the later phases of chronic illness. Emotionally, this phase may be associated with feelings of helplessness as the disease, in a sense, 'takes over' and the degree of physical dependence increases. Therefore, coping with a chronic neurological illness is not a 'one-off' challenge, but a continuous and on-going process of adjustment with many emotional ups and downs in its course.[69]

The symptoms of chronic illness result in loss of normal function and disability in daily activities. Familiar ways of living and well-established habits may have to be abandoned and new adjustments made. Over time, familiar personal, occupational and social roles may have to be given up. Future expectations and aspirations require fundamental revision after the onset of a chronic illness. All of these changes can create a sense of emotional loss in the person who has a chronic illness. People's reactions to loss, whether the death of a loved one or loss of normal function and roles through chronic illness, are similar. Loss is associated with grieving which has four phases: (1) shock, disbelief and denial; (2) anger; (3) mourning and depression; and (4) acceptance and adjustment. The pace of psychological transition through these phases varies from person to person and may be as brief as a few months and as long as many years. Also, as the nature and severity of problems posed by a chronic illness such as Parkinson's disease change over time, people may find that they occasionally revert temporarily to an earlier phase of emotional reaction, for example, when new or more severe symptoms develop.[69]

The ways in which different people cope with the stress of chronic illness are very individual and in some way unique. But research in a range of chronic disorders has established that a number of factors influence how well people adjust to and cope with chronic illness.[70-76] Personal characteristics of individuals such as their sense of self-esteem, their beliefs about how much personal control they have over life situations, their appraisal or personal perception/interpretation of the stressful event, and their habitual patterns of emotional and practical coping are important in this respect.[70,71,74] The environment in which the person lives (for example the suitability of housing for mobility problems), their extent of financial security, and access to appropriate social support – that is, availability of family/friends on whom the person can rely for sympathy, understanding, emotional and practical support – are other features that will determine the degree of adjustment to the stress of chronic illness.[71,74,76] The characteristics of the chronic illness, particularly the rate of progression and the controllability of symptoms are also important variables.[67,68] Therefore, given these plethora of factors that can influence adjustment to chronic illness, the impact of chronic illness on people's well-being is not straightforward but can be modified by many complex routes.

The World Health Organization model of chronic illness – impairment, disability and handicap

The majority of the neurological disorders affecting balance and gait are progressive and often chronic. The WHO has suggested a useful way of thinking about the consequences of chronic illness by focusing on the distinction between impairment, disability and handicap.[30] (More recently, the terms 'activity' and 'participation' were proposed instead of disability and handicap.) While impairment is the combined effects of the symptoms of the illness, disability refers to the way in which impairment affects daily activities. Handicap reflects the impact of the disease in its widest personal and social sense and the restrictions experienced by the individual. The handicap associated with a chronic illness and its impact on quality of life (Qol) are considered in relation to broad spheres of life and social roles such as mobility, work, social and leisure activities, relationship with others, physical independence, and economic self-sufficiency. While impairment and disability are measured against some general reference of normality, handicap can only be adequately judged in relation to each individual's life circumstances, immediate social context and future expectations. That is, in terms of how that person functioned, worked and played before the onset of the illness or the life they would be expected to be leading if the illness had not occurred. Impairment, disability and handicap do not have a direct relationship to each other. Only some impairments result in disability and the disabling effects of some impairments may be greater than others. For example, impairments of balance and gait, which often lead to restriction of mobility and so have implications for independent living, are more disabling than impairments associated with other symptoms such as 'masked facies'. The association between impairment, disability and handicap varies from one person to another. For example, some people with multiple sclerosis may be greatly disabled and restrict their lives although the impairment is mild, whereas others may not be handicapped despite severe impairment and disability. This is where the personal characteristics and resources of the individual play a key role in determining the impact of chronic illness.

As noted above, the personal characteristics (age, self-esteem, beliefs, goals, motives, appraisal of illness, etc.) and life circumstances of the individual (marital status, nature of job and financial security), the physical and social setting in which they live (house/flat, lift or facilities for wheelchair, living alone or not and social support network), all play a part in preventing or producing handicap. The important contribution of these other factors means that although the degree of impairment and disability are undoubtedly important, but they do not inevitably lead to handicap. Instead, individuals have the opportunity to make use of their personal and social resources to prevent impairment and disability from producing handicap because the psychological make-up of the individual, their appraisal of their situation and the coping strategies they use are important in determining handicap. Figure 19.2 shows the factors that contribute to the development of depression in Parkinson's disease. Of course, when balance and gait problems become severe enough to make the use of walking aids such as a cane, Zimmer frame or a wheelchair necessary, other factors, such as social prejudice, and environmental obstacles, such as inadequate transport facilities and access to buildings, all contribute to the creation of handicap.

Disability in Parkinson's disease

The symptoms of Parkinson's disease result in significant disability in a range of self-care (washing, dressing and feeding) and daily activities (getting out of a chair, mobility inside and outside the house and engagement in social activities).[58,78,79] There is evidence that such disability, as measured by the Schwab and England[80] scale, is greater in people with Parkinson's disease that had experienced falls than in those that had not,[61] perhaps partly because of the longer duration and severity of illness in the fallers.

A number of studies have focused on describing the social impact of PD on patients' daily lives.[81,82] Singer[82] reported that patients with Parkinson's disease were less likely to work, to have a circle of friends, and do household duties, and more likely to engage in stationary and

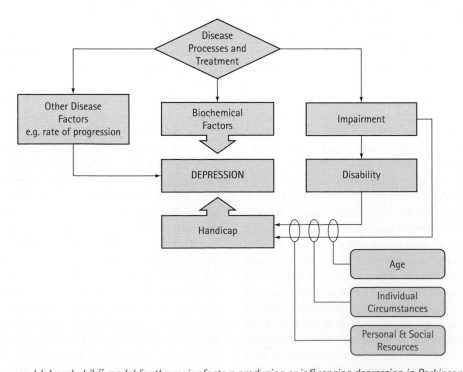

Figure 19.2 *Brown and Jahanshahi's[77] model for the major factors producing or influencing depression in Parkinson's disease.*

solitary activities, such as watching television and reading, a pattern considered to reflect 'premature social ageing' in their sample of younger patients. The level of disability in daily activities associated with Parkinson's disease is similar to that found in other chronic illnesses such as arthritis.[78] As would be expected from a progressive disorder, a 2-year longitudinal study of 132 patients with Parkinson's disease showed that disability increased over the follow-up period.[79] Increasing imbalance and gait problems characterize progression of Parkinson's disease[83] and it is likely that these symptoms form a core component of the increased disability experienced by patients over time. In a prospective assessment of falls, Bloem et al.[64] found fear of falling in the future to be common among patients with Parkinson's disease (reported by 46 per cent of the 59 patients studied) and to lead to restriction of activities and in some cases to social isolation.

Depression and factors related to adjustment to illness in Parkinson's disease

Depression is common in Parkinson's disease, although there is no agreement about its rate or its etiology. Estimates of prevalence of depression in Parkinson's disease vary considerably, ranging from 20 per cent[84] to 90 per cent.[85] Similarly, there is an ongoing debate about whether depression is a sequela of the biochemical deficiency giving rise to the motor symptoms of Parkinson's disease or a reaction to the onset of and experience of living with the chronic and disabling illness.[77]

As noted above, there are major individual differences in adjustment to chronic illness. This is also the case in Parkinson's disease and Dakof and Mandelshon[86] described four patterns of adjustment to the illness: sanguine and engaged, depressed and apprehensive, depressed and misunderstood, passive and resigned. The four groups were distinguished in terms of presence/absence and severity of depression as well as disease severity but not demographic and health variables. The 'sanguine and engaged' subgroup appeared well-adjusted and had the least severe Parkinson's disease. An unsuccessful struggle to cope with the illness and anxiety about the future was characteristic of the 'depressed and apprehensive' subgroup. The 'depressed and misunderstood' group was the most severely disabled, depressed and socially isolated, showing a marked withdrawal from participation in previous personal, family and social roles. In contrast, the 'passive and resigned' subgroup had accepted and resigned themselves to their dependence on others for self-care and daily activities. Other studies assessing a range of psychiatric symptoms have also shown that depression is the most frequently encountered psychiatric problem among patients with Parkinson's disease. Brown and MacCarthy[87] used a standardized psychiatric interview, the 'Present State Examination' with 40 patients with Parkinson's disease and found depression and anxiety to be the most common. Using the Neuropsychiatric Inventory, Aarsland et al.[88] assessed 139 patients with Parkinson's disease and reported at least one psychiatric symptom in 61 per cent of the sample, with depression (38 per cent) being the most common.

The qualitative characteristics of the depression experienced by patients with Parkinson's disease has been described by Gotham et al.[78] Pessimism and hopelessness, decreased motivation and drive, and increased concern with health were the main features of depression in Parkinson's disease, while negative feelings of guilt, self-blame and worthlessness were absent. This pattern was confirmed by Huber et al.[89] who also found that sadness and hopelessness and somatic symptoms such as fatigue and concern about health were the most common aspects of the experience of depression in Parkinson's disease, while self-reproach and vegetative symptoms such as sleep disturbance or weight loss were least common. Gotham et al.'s[78] sample of patients with Parkinson's disease was also significantly more anxious than age-matched normals. Other studies have also found anxiety to be a common experience in patients with Parkinson's disease.[90] Although, to our knowledge, no study has examined the influence of stage of illness or the symptoms or psychosocial factors that influence the development of anxiety in Parkinson's disease, as will be discussed below, disturbance of posture and balance and difficulty with walking are among the symptoms likely to contribute to anxiety through 'fear of falling'. These symptoms are perceived as making mobility around the house and outside prone to falls and hence risky and to be avoided.

Given that Parkinson's disease is a chronic and progressive disorder, the impact of the illness on daily activities and psychosocial functioning is likely to change over time. Consequently, a number of studies have examined how disability and depression change over time with progression of the illness. In a longitudinal follow-up study of 132 patients over a 2-year period, Brown et al.[79] found that both baseline and follow-up levels of depression were significantly related to levels of disability in activities of daily living. The results also showed that the relative level and rate of increase in disability across time may be a better predictor of depression than its absolute level. Huber et al.[89] also examined how the qualitative experience of depression changes with progression of the illness. While negative mood and self-reproach were present in the early phases of the illness, vegetative symptoms of depression appeared in the later stages of Parkinson's disease and only somatic symptoms of depression showed increase with progression of the neurological disorder. In their longitudinal follow-up of a sample of 92 patients with Parkinson's disease for a period of 12 months, Starkstein et al.[91] found that those with major depression at the time of initial assessment

374 Psychosocial aspects of disorders affecting balance and gait

showed a significantly greater deterioration in activities of daily living, further progression of illness, as indexed by the Hoehn and Yahr scale,[83] and greater cognitive decline than patients with minor depression or no depression.

As previously discussed, a complex web of inter-related social and personal factors operate to determine coping and adjustment to chronic illnesses such as Parkinson's disease. To date, the most comprehensive study of the psychosocial determinants of depression and adjustment of illness in Parkinson's disease has been the report by MacCarthy and Brown.[71] They examined the association between disability, self-esteem, attributions and perceived control, social support, coping strategies and depression and adjustment to illness in 136 patients with Parkinson's disease. Disability in activities of daily living, self-esteem and use of maladaptive coping strategies such as wishful thinking or denial accounted for 44 per cent of the variance of depression in Parkinson's disease. Disability and maladaptive coping were also major predictors of adjustment of illness and practical social support contributed to positive well-being in this sample. Age of onset of Parkinson's disease is another factor that has been shown to influence the extent of depression and its correlates. Starkstein et al.[92] found that patients with early-onset Parkinson's disease (onset before age 55 years) were significantly more depressed than patients with late-onset Parkinson's disease, even after controlling for differences in duration of illness. Furthermore, while in the late-onset group of patients, depression significantly correlated with impairments in activities of daily living, in the early-onset group, cognitive impairment and duration of illness were the main correlates of depression. In a population-based study, Schrag et al.[93] examined prevalence of depression in 97 patients with Parkinson's disease. Moderate to severe depression was reported by about 20 per cent of the sample. Greater depression was experienced with advancing disease severity, recent disease deterioration, presence of cognitive impairment and higher akinesia. The most important finding in relation to the influence of balance and walking problems on depression was that the incidence of depression was higher among patients that had experienced falls than among those that had not fallen, and was higher for the subgroup of patients with postural instability than those without. Furthermore, the mobility subscore of a disease-specific measure of quality of life was significantly worse for the depressed patients than those patients who were not depressed, suggesting that poorer mobility differentiated the depressed and non-depressed patients. Schrag et al.[93] further established that indices of quality of life explained a greater proportion of the variance in depression (53 per cent) than measures of disability (34 per cent) or impairment (28 per cent) respectively quantified using the Schwab and England[80] and the Hoehn and Yahr scales.[83] This suggests, that as proposed by the

Brown and Jahanshahi[77] model of depression shown in Fig. 19.2, the experience of depression in Parkinson's disease is more closely related to the individual's perception of the implications of the illness for their quality of life and less directly associated with impairment and disability. This conclusion is a opportune point for turning to the discussion of the concept of quality of life in chronic illness and more specifically in Parkinson's disease, which we will consider next.

Quality of life in Parkinson's disease

Traditionally, the medical model of disease has been concerned with acute illness. Within this model, the person falls ill, undergoes drug therapy or surgery, recovers quickly and their contact with the medical profession ends when the episode of acute illness is over. This traditional medical model does not fit the course of events in chronic illness, and the WHO considers it to be inappropriate for managing chronic illness. According to the WHO, in chronic disease, in addition to medical treatment of the symptoms, the primary concern of management should be promoting a good 'quality of life' for the ill person, their principal carer and their family. Quality of life does not have a simple definition or single meaning. Under normal circumstances, the person's quality of life is related to how they function and feel, and it encompasses their physical and mental health, social activities and relationships, work, financial and living circumstances. When a person becomes ill, the term health-related 'quality of life' captures the sum total effect of the illness and its subsequent treatment on the individual's physical, psychological, social and occupational functioning, as perceived by the person. For the chronically ill, 'quality of life' also incorporates the personal and emotional reactions of an individual to the differences they perceive between their actual and their desired activities. Like handicap, quality of life is extremely individual. For this reason, many of the factors outlined above are likely to also influence the impact of chronic illness on a person's quality of life.

In recent years, with the realization that quality of life measures are better indices of the impact of chronic illness than measures of impairment or disability, the focus has shifted to the assessment of quality of life. Using the SF-36 (Medical Outcomes Study 36-item Short Form),[94] a generic measure of quality of life, Karlsen et al.[95] found that all dimensions of quality of life were impaired in 233 Parkinson's disease patients relative to 100 healthy elderly people, with physical mobility being the most significantly affected, with 80 per cent of the patients compared with 41 per cent of the healthy elderly subjects reporting mobility problems. Schrag et al.[93,96,97] used Parkinson's disease quality of life – 39 items (PDQ-39)[98] a disease-specific quality of life measure and two generic measures of quality of life, the SF-36[94] and the EURO-Qol[99] in a population-based study of Parkinson's disease to identify the demographic and disease-related determinants of quality of life in Parkinson's disease. Their results demonstrated that Parkinson's disease patients have a poorer quality of life compared with the general population of the same age, particularly in the areas of physical mobility and social functioning.[93] Physical mobility was reported to be impaired by 100 per cent of the Parkinson's disease patients compared with 57 per cent of the general population, while the respective figures for impairment of social functioning were 85 per cent and 44 per cent. Relative to the general population, poorer quality of life was evident for all age groups and was similar for male and female patients, but the differences from the general population were particularly marked for the younger patients.[93]

Using the SF-36, Chriscilles et al.[100] have shown that stage of illness, as measured by the Hoehn and Yahr scale,[83] had a significant effect on quality of life as well as on direct (e.g. emergency room visits, use of community services, modification of home/car, use of aids and equipment) and indirect (e.g. days bedridden, retirement/ unemployment) economic measures for people with Parkinson's disease. Schrag et al.[93] also confirmed that quality of life deteriorated with increasing disease severity. Emergence of postural imbalance and increasing mobility problems are some of the characteristics of progressive stages of illness in Parkinson's disease, as defined by the Hoehn and Yahr scale,[83] and the influence of stage of illness on quality of life, probably partly reflects the contribution of the increasingly compromised balance and mobility. More direct evidence for this is provided by Schrag et al.'s.[96] finding that postural instability and experience of falls were two factors that had a significant impact on quality of life of the Parkinson's disease patients; with on–off fluctuations, cognitive impairment, recent deterioration or symptoms and experience of hallucinations being the other pertinent factors influencing quality of life in Parkinson's disease. Schrag et al.[97] found that postural instability was one of the predictors of quality of life in PD, which, together with depression, disability and cognitive impairment, accounted for 72 per cent of the variance of quality of life scores. These results clearly demonstrate that postural instability and the experience of falls are crucial determinants of quality of life in people with Parkinson's disease.

Bloem et al.[63] have proposed that fear of falling, which is common in patients with Parkinson's disease operates in a vicious circle to contribute to greater postural instability and risk of fractures after a fall. The restriction of activity associated with the fear of falling is proposed to lead to the development of muscle weakness and osteoporosis which, respectively, contribute to postural instability and increase the risk of fractures, and together with the resultant social isolation reduce the quality of life of the patients (Fig. 19.3). There is some evidence from our own work in support of this hypothesis. As noted above, Schrag et al.[96] found that postural instability and falls

were two of the factors that resulted in significantly poorer quality of life in Parkinson's disease.

Management of the psychosocial sequelae of neurological disorders of balance and gait

Medical treatment to improve the symptoms of Parkinson's disease and to reduce their impact on daily activities is likely to be of value in the management of the psychosocial sequelae of the illness. Nevertheless, as the sole course of action, such a medical approach is unlikely to be completely effective for preventing disability and depression and promoting good quality of life in Parkinson's disease for several reasons. First, the key symptoms of the disorder, such as postural instability and gait problems, which contribute to disability and poor quality of life, are the least responsive to levodopa[61–64] and surgical intervention.[101] Second, the relationship between the impairment associated with the symptoms, the resulting disability and depression is not necessarily direct. This was shown in a longitudinal follow-up study of 132 patients with Parkinson's disease by Brown et al.[79] They established that over a period of 2 years, disability had significantly increased whereas overall levels of depression remained relatively constant. They found that change in depression was not linearly dependent on change in disability and that in terms of development of depression the absolute change in disability may be less important than the relative change

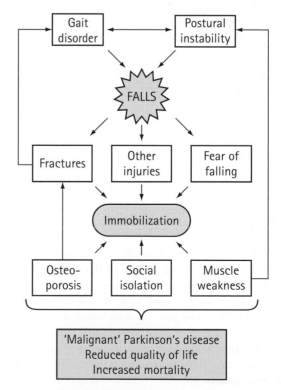

Figure 19.3 *The vicious cycle of postural instability and falls in Parkinson's disease.*[63]

and the rate of change. Third, as noted above, in addition to the severity and rate of progression of the symptoms, a multitude of other person-related, social and environmental factors operate to influence and determine an individual's adjustment to Parkinson's disease. Fourth, more specifically in relation to balance and gait problems, it is possible for anticipatory fear of falling to operate to promote avoidance and restriction of activity, which, as noted above, in the long-term would further exacerbate balance and mobility problems and increase the risk of fractures through the development of muscle weakness and osteoporosis.[63,64] For these reasons, direct management of the psychosocial sequelae of the illness is crucially important as it cannot be assumed that the interference with daily activities, the anxiety and the depression that patients may be experiencing would simply disappear with medical treatment of the core symptoms of Parkinson's disease. In this respect, various approaches are important: informing and educating the patient; ensuring access to adjunct therapy; and use of cognitive–behavioral therapy. As these partly overlap with the approaches appropriate for the rehabilitation of vestibular disorders which were outlined above in some detail, they will only be briefly considered below with respect to the management of Parkinson's disease and other neurological disorders associated with balance and gait problems.

Informing and educating the patient

Providing the patient with information about the symptoms and the likely course and progression of the illness may be helpful in several ways. First, it may prepare the patient, their carer and family for what to expect in the coming years. Second, it may allow them to recruit the personal, social, environmental and financial resources that may be essential for coping with the impact of the illness on their daily activities, work and social relationships. This would in turn promote a greater sense of personal control and overcome feelings of helplessness. In relation to balance and gait problems, teaching the patient the following general principles outlined by Morris et al.[102] is likely to be of value:

- Breaking down complex actions into a number of steps and then performing one step at a time.
- Ensuring that they do not do two things at once. For example, if walking and buttoning up a shirt at the same time, either the buttoning will become slower or the walking will become more clumsy. When mobile, the patient should just focus on walking.
- Paying attention to each movement as they perform them. Talking through movements is a good way of making sure that the patient pays attention to their performance.
- Consciously rehearsing difficult movements before performing them.

In addition, a number of specific strategies exist that the patient with Parkinson's disease can apply to their mobility problems.[69] Some of these strategies are:

- Imagining lines on the floor and high stepping over them to transform the shuffling gait into a more normal stride.
- To overcome start hesitation, rocking gently forward and backward before taking the first step, or starting to walk in time with a tune or stepping over a real object.
- Thinking 'heel first' while walking and consciously trying to walk with a long stride.
- To turn safely and reduce the risk of falls, walking in a large circle and avoiding sudden changes in direction.
- Avoiding carrying things while walking and using a small rucksack for this purpose. In this way, the patient's arms and hands are free for steadying themselves if they lose their balance and for holding on to rails on public transport or when climbing up or down steps.
- Keeping feet about 8 inches (c. 20 cm) apart to produce a more stable base.
- Standing to one side when opening doors, so that it is not necessary to take a backward step.

While some control over the layout of the home environment is possible, this is not the case when walking outside. However, when walking outside and/or using public transport, a number of general guidelines may prove valuable and reduce the risk of falls:

- Timing journeys outside the home to coincide with the patient's periods of maximum mobility.
- Allowing plenty of time for travelling so that there is no rush since this haste can make walking stressful and more prone to falls.
- Paying attention to obstacles and overcompensating movements accordingly, for example, to step over a curb, deliberately lifting the feet extra high, which would probably make them just about right given that movements in Parkinson's disease are ordinarily hypometric.

Since anticipatory fear of falling plays such a key role in exacerbating problems through restriction and avoidance of activity, educating the patient about the part it plays in their problems would be a first step in any cognitive–behavioral intervention program (see below). Evidence suggests that while psychiatric morbidity is high among patients with various neurological disorders, in the majority of cases it remains unrecognized by neurologists.[103] Patients need to be made aware that communication with doctors is a two-way process, in which they can play a major role. It is therefore, important for them to communicate explicitly any anxiety or depression they may be feeling to their general practitioner or neurologist so that this can be directly treated.

Ensuring access to adjunct therapy

There is some evidence of the value of physical therapy in reducing falls and improving mobility. Compared with a control group, 153 elderly people living in the community who received a 'risk factor reduction' intervention program of physical therapy had significantly fewer falls over a period of 12 months.[104] For patients with multiple sclerosis, facilitation (impairment-based) and task-oriented (disability-focused) physiotherapy treatment approaches have been compared and shown to be equally effective in improving walking.[105] More recent evidence from a randomized crossover trial has established that compared with no therapy, an 8-week course of physiotherapy at home or in the hospital is associated with improved mobility and mood in patients with multiple sclerosis, with the former being more costly because of staff travelling time.[106] While the evidence for the value of such adjunct forms of therapy in Parkinson's disease is less systematic,[107–110] these therapies may be of some value to patients. Bone density in the hip is reduced in Parkinson's disease,[111] which increases the risk of fractures with falls. Physiotherapy in the earlier stages of the illness may be helpful in preventing such bone loss. Physiotherapy exercises can also reduce joint stiffness, increase range of joint movements and prevent muscle weakness. To improve walking, physiotherapists teach PD patients to counteract the forward-leaning and stooped posture that results in the displacement of the center of gravity and to strike their heel down while walking and to think 'heel first' with each step. The physiotherapist can also demonstrate appropriate protective responses in case of a fall to the patient and teach them the best ways of getting up if falls occur. Such training may help alleviate some of the patient's anxieties about the consequences of falling and reduce fear of falling, which can lead to restriction of activities and social isolation.

Evidence suggests that in Parkinson's disease falls are related to postural instability and that hypotension and external factors are not major contributors.[61] Nevertheless, consultation with an occupational therapist may prove of value. Ankle pumps and hand-clenching exercises may prove of some value in alleviating hypotension when present. The occupational therapist can also advise the patient and carer about modifications to their living environment to minimize the risk of falls, for example by securing loose cables or introducing night lights, and selecting appropriate shoes to minimize 'stickiness' of the feet, which may contribute to 'freezing'. In the later stages of the illness, when postural instability and gait problems appear, the occupational therapist can also help the patient select appropriate walking aids such as wheeled walkers or a wheelchair. As the use of walking aids are perceived as indicators of disability by some patients, there may be initial unwillingness to use them.

The timing of their first use is of vital importance: if introduced too early they may result in premature loss of residual abilities, if left too late, the patient may be at risk of falling and fractures.

Cognitive–behavioral therapy

Fear of falling is common among patients with Parkinson's disease who have experienced falls in the past, with many patients confining themselves to their homes and becoming socially isolated.[61] Fear of falling is not fully explained by falling history and emotional and psychological variables contribute to it to a great extent. In common with other forms of fear and anxiety, fear of falling has cognitive, physiological and behavioral elements. A detailed analysis of the core cognitive components of fear of falling has been undertaken in an elderly population.[112] This revealed fear of 'damage to identity' (e.g. feeling foolish, feeling embarrassed and losing confidence) and 'functional incapacity' (e.g. helplessness, loss of independence and becoming disabled) as the two major factors contributing to fear of falling. These two factors, together with age, gender and falling history explained a good proportion of the variance of restriction of activity in the elderly population. Over time, the physiological response of heightened arousal and hyperventilation associated with fear of falling may operate to encourage the behavioral sequelae of escape and avoidance. In this way, a vicious cycle of escalating fear and avoidance will be set up with substantial restriction of activity, which will in turn affect mobility because of the risk of loss of bone density, muscle weakness and incoordination due to inactivity.[63]

The approach for management of fear of falling would be similar to the therapy used for other forms of anxiety. First, the person needs to be made aware of the relationship between their anxious cognitions, bodily symptoms signaling heightened arousal, and escape and avoidance behaviors. Cognitive re-structuring, with a focus on 'damage to identity' and 'functional incapacity' as two of the cognitive components of fear of falling, would be useful. Perceived self-efficacy, indicating the individual's confidence in their ability to perform specific activities, has been shown to be closely associated with fear of falling.[113–115] Therefore, increasing the person's perceived self-efficacy with regard their ability to control their balance and mobility could be another focus of therapy. Since the perception of the consequences of falling is an important element of fear of falling, discussing the immediate aftermaths of falling, for example how to summon help and how to get up, with the patient may help alleviate some of the anxiety associated with this. Patients need to learn to identify anxious cognitions and to use positive self-talk to contest and replace such negative thoughts. Relaxation training for counteracting any symptoms of arousal which can act to heighten fear would also be of value. Where severe avoidance and restriction of activity have developed, systematic desensitization or 'graded exposure' to the feared situations may be called for.

Depression, which is a relatively common psychosocial sequela of neurological disorders affecting balance and gait, would also benefit from cognitive–behavioral intervention. As a first step, the patient needs to come to terms with the reality of the illness and accept the limitations imposed by it and find ways of working around these. For example, people with Parkinson's disease can adjust their daily routine to accommodate slowness and increased fatigue. Acceptance of the illness also ensures that people set themselves realistic goals and standards which will prevent disappointment and self-blame if previous standards are not achieved. With the appreciation that thoughts, feelings and actions are closely related, patients can start to monitor their thoughts to establish how what they think affects the way they feel and behave. The negative thinking style characteristic of depression means that the depressed individuals perceive themselves, the world and the future in negative terms.[116,117] With training, depressed patients can learn to identify and challenge negative thoughts and the errors of thinking that result in biased interpretations of reality. To protect their sense of self-esteem, patients need to realize that despite the physical changes produced by the illness, their past achievements have not been altered and that there are no obstacles to reaching new and realistic goals. In light of the other factors that contribute to the development of depression (Fig. 19.2), patients should also be encouraged to remain active and not to give up professional or social roles prematurely. New activities and hobbies can be pleasurable in the short-term and also help promote a sense of control and achievement. Given the importance of practical and emotional social support in 'buffering' the stress of chronic illness, patients should maintain their social ties with friends and family. In light of the progressive and chronic nature of the majority of disorders affecting balance and gait, the process of adjustment has to be ongoing. The different phases of the illness are likely to make different demands on the patients' personal and emotional resources and patients have to be prepared for a continuous and ongoing process of adjustment.

A program of training in coping skills incorporating stress inoculation, positive thinking, social skills training, modeling and role play, and muscle relaxation was used by Ellgring et al.[90] to teach 25 patients with Parkinson's disease to accept the reality of their illness, cope with being in public places, and deal with difficult situations. Although the value of the program delivered as five 2-h seminars in the course of 2 months was not systematically assessed, it was rated as very helpful by the patients.

SUMMARY

Management of the psychosocial aspects of vertigo and imbalance can be summarized as three core elements. First, education about balance system function can help to reduce the anxiety caused by symptoms that are poorly understood and to motivate the patient to resume activity (normally as part of a supervised programme of vestibular rehabilitation). Second, the simultaneous reduction of symptoms of dizziness and anxiety can be achieved by combining repeated provocation of dizziness by movement with techniques for reducing fear and inducing relaxation. Finally, psychosocial problems at home and work can be directly addressed by discussing strategies for coping with practical problems and by enlisting the assistance of relatives and employers. Patients that restrict their activities unduly because of an excessive fear of vertigo may benefit from well-established psychological treatments such as graded exposure and cognitive–behavioral therapy.

It is evident that the psychosocial impact of neurological disorders affecting balance and gait is multifactorially determined and for this reason susceptible to large individual differences. Nevertheless, a management approach focused on informing and educating the patient, ensuring access to adjunct therapy, and cognitive–behavioral therapy for fear of falling and depression is likely to be of benefit in the majority of cases. What is required is more systematic evidence for the efficacy of such management programs in these disorders.

REFERENCES

1. Litvan I, Campbell G, Mangone CA, et al. Which clinical features differentiate progressive supranuclear palsy (Steele–Richardson–Olszewski syndrome) from related disorders? A clinicopathological study. *Brain* 1997;**120**;65–74.

2. Wenning GK, Ebersbach G, Verny M, et al. Progression of falls in postmortem-confirmed parkinsonian disorders. *Mov Disord* 1999;**14**(6):947–50.

3. Wenning GK, Ben Shlomo Y, Hughes A, et al. What clinical features are most useful to distinguish definite multiple system atrophy from Parkinson's disease? *J Neurol Neurosurg Psychiatry* 2000;**68**(4):434–40.

4. O'Connor KP, Hallam R, Beyts J, Hinchcliffe R. Dizziness: behavioural, subjective and organic aspects. *J Psychosom Res* 1988;**32**:291–302.

5. Yardley L, Masson E, Verschuur C, et al. Symptoms, anxiety and handicap in dizzy patients: development of the Vertigo Symptom Scale. *J Psychosom Res* 1992;**36**:731–41.

6. Brookes GB, Faldon M, Kanayama R, et al. Recovery from unilateral vestibular nerve section in human subjects evaluated by physiological, psychological and questionnaire assessments. *Acta Otolaryngol* 1994;**513**(Suppl):40–8.

7. Yardley L, Luxon L, Haacke NP. A longitudinal study of symptoms, anxiety and subjective well-being in patients with vertigo. *Clin Otolaryngol* 1994;**19**:109–16.

8. Bass, C. *Somatization*. Oxford: Blackwell Scientific Publications, 1990.

9. Cioffi, D. Beyond attentional strategies: a cognitive–perceptual model of somatic interpretation. *Psychol Bull* 1991;**109**:25–41.

10. Ingram RE. Self-focused attention in clinical disorders: review and a conceptual model. *Psychol Bull* 1990;**107**;156–76.

11. Jacob RG, Furman JMR, Clark DB, et al. Psychogenic dizziness. In: Sharpe JA, Barber HO, eds. *The vestibulo-ocular reflex and vertigo*. New York: Raven Press, 1993.

12. Beyts JP. Vestibular rehabilitation. In . Stephens D, ed. *Scott-Brown's otolaryngology: adult audiology*, 5th edn. London: Butterworths, 1987.

13. Jacob RG. Panic disorder and the vestibular system. *Psychiatr Clin N Am* 1988;**11**:361–74.

14. Yardley L, Gresty M, Bronstein A, et al. Changes in heart rate and respiration rate in patients with vestibular dysfunction following head movements which provoke dizziness. *Biol Psychol* 1998;**49**:95–108.

15. Sakellari V, Bronstein AM, Corna S, et al. The effects of hyperventilation on postural control mechanisms. *Brain* 1997;**120**;1659–73.

16. Evans, RW. Neurologic aspects of hyperventilation syndrome. *Semin Neurol* 1995;**15**:115–25.

17. Clark DM. A cognitive approach to panic. *Behav Res Ther* 1986;**24**:461–70.

18. Yardley L, Gardner M, Lavie N, Gresty M. Attentional demands of passive self-motion in darkness. *Neuropsychologia* 1999;**37**:1293–301.

19. Yardley L, Burgneay J, Nazareth, I, Luxon, L. Neuro-otological and psychiatric abnormalities in a community sample of people with dizziness: a blind, controlled investigation. *J Neurol Neurosurg Psychiatry* 1998;**65**:679–84.

20. McKenna L, Hallam RS, Hinchcliffe R. The prevalence of psychological disturbance in neuro-otology outpatients. *Clin Otolaryngol* 1991;**16**:452–6.

21. Asmundson GJG, Larsen DK, Stein MB. Panic disorder and vestibular disturbance: an overview of empirical findings and clinical implications. *J Psychosom Res* 1998;**44**:107–20.

22. Lazarus RS. *Emotion and adaptation*. Oxford: Oxford University Press, 1991.

23. Yardley L, Putman J. Quantitative analysis of factors contributing to handicap and distress in vertiginous patients: a questionnaire study. *Clin Otolaryngol* 1992;**17**:231–6.

24. Yardley L. Contribution of symptoms and beliefs to handicap in people with vertigo: a longitudinal study. *Br J Clin Psychol* 1994;**33**:101–13.

25. Yardley L, Beech S, Weinman J. Influence of beliefs about the consequences of dizziness on handicap in people with dizziness, and the effect of therapy on beliefs. *J Psychosom Res* 2001;**50**,1–6.

26. Leventhal H, Nerenz DR. The assessment of illness cognition. In Karoly P, ed. *Measurement strategies in health psychology*. New York: Wiley, 1985.

27. Miller SM. Controllability and human stress: method, evidence and theory. *Behav Res Ther* 1979;**17**:287–304.

28. Steptoe A, Appels, A, eds. *Stress, personal control and health*. Chichester: Wiley, 1989.

29. Abramson LY, Seligman MEP, Teasdale JD. Learned helplessness in humans: critique and reformulation. *J Abnorm Psychol* 1978;**87**:49–74.

30. World Health Organization. *International classification of impairments, disabilities and handicaps. A manual of classification relating to the consequences of disease*. Geneva: World Health Organization, 1980.

31. Zettle RD, Hayes SC. Rule-governed behaviour: a potential theoretical framework for cognitive–behavioral therapy. In: Kendall PC, ed. *Advances in cognitive–behavioral research and therapy*, Vol 1. New York: Academic Press, 1982.

32. Bandura A. Self-efficacy mechanism in human agency. *Am Psychol* 1982;**37**:122–47.

33. Ley, P. *Communicating with patients*. London: Croom Helm, 1988.

34. Yardley L, Luxon LM. Rehabilitation for dizziness. *BMJ* 1994;**308**:1252–3.

35. Woolacott MH, Shumway-Cook A. *Development of posture and gait across the life span*. South Carolina: University of South Carolina Press, 1989.

36. Hallam RS. *Counselling for anxiety problems*. London: Sage, 1992.

37. Dobie TG, May JG, Fischer WD, et al. A comparison of two methods of training resistance to visually-induced motion sickness. *Aviat Space Environ Med* 1987;**58**(Suppl.); A34–41.

38. Dobie TG, May JG, Fisher WD, Bologna NB. An evaluation of cognitive–behavioral therapy for training resistance to visually-induced motion sickness. *Aviat Space Environ Med* 1989;**60**:307–14.

39. Goldberg DP, Huxley, P. *A user's guide to the General Health Questionnaire*. Windsor: NFER–Nelson, 1988.

40. Zigmond AS, Snaith RP. The Hospital Anxiety and Depression Scale. *Acta Psychiatr Scand* 1983;**67**:361–70.

41. Russell JL, Kushner MG, Beitman BD, Bartels KM. Non-fearful panic disorder in neurology patients validated by lactate challenge. *Am J Psychiatry* 1991;**148**:361–4.

42. Derogatis LR, Lipman RS, Rickels K, et al. The Hopkins symptom checklist (HSCL): a self-report symptom inventory. *Behav Sci* 1974;**19**:1–15.

43. Kirmayer LJ, Robbins JM, Dworkind M, Yaffer MJ . Somatization and the recognition of depression and anxiety in primary care. *Am J Psychiatry* 1993;**150**:734–41.

44. Schwartz GE, Davidson RJ, Coleman DJ. Patterning of cognitive and somatic processes in the self-regulation of anxiety: effects of mediation versus exercise. *Psychosom Med* 1978;**40**, 321–8.

45. Chambless DL, Caputo GC, Jasin SE, et al. The Mobility Inventory for Agoraphobia. *Behav Res Ther* 1985;**23**:35–44.

46. Norton GR, Dorward J, Cox BJ. Factors associated with panic attacks in nonclinical subjects. *Behav Ther* 1986;**17**:239–52.

47. Yardley L, Burgneay J, Andersson G, et al. Feasibility and effectiveness of providing vestibular rehabilitation for dizzy patients in the community. *Clin Otolaryngol* 1998;**23**:442–48.

48. Jacobson GP, Newman CW. The development of the Dizziness Handicap Inventory. *Arch Otolaryngol Head Neck Surg* 1990;**116**:424–7.

48. Hornsveld H, Garssen B, Dop MF, van Spiegel P. Symptom reporting during voluntary hyperventilation and mental load: implications for diagnosing hyperventilation syndrome. *J Psychosom Res* 1990;**34**:687–97.

49. Cohen, H. 1992. Vestibular rehabilitation reduces functional disability. *Otolaryngol Head Neck Sur* 1992;**107**:638–43.

50. Jacob RG, Lilienfeld SO, Furman JMR, et al. Panic disorder with vestibular dysfunction: further clinical observations and description of space and motion phobic stimuli. *J Anxiety Disord* 1989;**3**:117–30.

51. Redfern M, Yardley L, Bronstein A. Visual influences on balance. *J Anxiety Disord* 2002;**42**:17–23.

52. Yardley L, Luxon L, Lear S. et al. Vestibular and posturographic test results in people with symptoms of panic and agoraphobia. *J Audiol Med* 1994;**3**;48–65.

53. Yardley L, Britton J, Lear S. et al. Relationship between balance system function and agoraphobic avoidance. *Behav Res Ther* 1995;**33**:435–9.

54. Andersson G, Yardley L. Combined cognitive–behavioural and physiotherapy treatment of dizziness: a case–report. *Behav Cogn Ther* 1998;**26**:365–9.

55. Jeans V, Orrell MW. Behavioural treatment of space phobia: a case report. *Behav Psychother* 1991;**19**;285–8.

56. Beck AT, Emery G, Greenberg RL. *Anxiety disorders and phobias: a cognitive perspective*. New York: Basic Books, 1985.

57. Warwick HMC, Salkovskis PM. Reassurance. *BMJ* 1985;**290**:1028.

58. Brown RG MacCarthy B Jahanshahi M Marsden CD. The accuracy of self-reported disability in patients with Parkinson's disease. *Arch Neurol* 1989;**46**:955–9.

59. MacDonald BK, Cockerell OC, Sander JW, Shorvon SD. The incidence and lifetime prevalence of neurological disorders in a prospective community-based study in the UK. *Brain* 2000;**123**:665–76.

60. Errea JM, Ara JR, Aibar C, de Pedro Cuesta J. Prevalence of Parkinson's disease in lower Aragon, Spain. *Mov Disord* 1999;**14**:596–604

61. Koller WC, Glatt S, Vetere-Overfield B, Hassanein R. Falls and Parkinson's disease. *Clin Neuropharmacol* 1989;**12**(2): 98–105

62. Rogers MW. Disorders of posture, balance, and gait in Parkinson's disease. *Clin Geriatr Med* 1996;**12**(4): 825–45.

63. Bloem BR, van Vugt JPP, Becklley DJ. Postural instability and falls in Parkinson's disease. *Adv Neurol* 2001.

64. Bloem BR Grimbergen YAM, Cramer MC, et al. Prospective assessment of falls in Parkinson's disease. *J Neurol* 2001; **248**(11):950–8.

65. Paykel ES. The Interview for Recent Life Events. *Psychol Med* 1997;**27**(2):301–10.

66. Paykel ES, Cooper Z, Ramana R, Hayhurst H. Life events, social support and marital relationships in the outcome of severe depression. *Psychol Med* 1996;**26**(1):121–33.

67. Mindham RH, Bagshaw A, James SA, Swannell AJ. Factors associated with the appearance of psychiatric symptoms in rheumatoid arthritis. *J Psychosom Res* 1981;**25**:429–35.

68. Moos RH, Solomon GF. Personality correlates of the degree of functional incapacity of patients with physical disease. *J Chronic Dis* 1965;**18**:1019–38.

69. Jahanshahi M, Marsden CD. *Living and coping with Parkinson's disease: a self-help guide for patients and their carers. Human horizon series.* Souvenir Press, 1998.

70. Felton BJ, Revenson TA. Coping with chronic illness: a study of illness controllability and the influence of coping strategies on psychological adjustment. *J Consult Clin Psychol* 1984;**52**:343–53

71. MacCarthy B, Brown R. Psychosocial factors in Parkinson's disease. *Br J Clin Psychol* 1989;**28**:41–52.

72. Jahanshahi M, Marsden CD. Body concept, disability and depression in torticollis. *Behav Neurol* 1990;**3**;117–31.

73. Jahanshahi M, Marsden CD. A longitudinal follow-up study of depression, disability and body concept in torticollis. *Behav Neurol* 1990;**3**;233–46.

74. Jahanshahi M. Psychosocial correlates of depression in torticollis. *J Psychosom Res* 1991;**35**:1–15.

75. Folkman S, Lazarus RS. If it changes it must be a process: study of emotion and coping during three stages of a college examination. *J Pers Soc Psychol* 1985;**48**:150–70.

76. McIvor GP, Riklan M, Reznikoff M. Depression in multiple sclerosis as a function of length and severity of illness, age, remissions, and perceived social support. *J Clin Psychol* 1984;**40**:1028–33.

77. Brown RG, Jahanshahi M. Depression in Parkinson's disease: a psychosocial viewpoint. In: Weiner WJ, Lang AE, eds. *Behavioural neurology of movement disorders. Advances in neurology*, Vol 65. New York: Raven Press, 1995.

78. Gotham AM, Brown RG, Marsden CD. Depression in Parkinson's disease: a quantitative and qualitative analysis. *J Neurol Neurosurg Psychiatry* 1986;**49**(4):381–9.

79. Brown RG, MacCarthy B, Gotham AM, et al. Depression and disability in Parkinson's disease: a follow-up of 132 cases. *Psychol Med* 1988;**18**(1):49–55.

80. Schwab RS, England AC. Projection technique for evaluating surgery in Parkinson's disease. In: Gillingham FJ, Donaldson IML, eds. *Third Symposium on Parkinson's disease.* Edinburgh: Churchill Livingstone, 1969, 152–7.

81. Oxtoby M. *Parkinson's disease patients and their social needs.* Town?: Parkinson's Disease Society, 1982.

82. Singer E. Social costs of Parkinson's disease. *J Chron Dis* 1973;**26**:243–54.

83. Hoehn MM, Yahr MD. Parkinsonism: onset, progression and mortality. *Neurology* 1967;**17**:427–42.

84. Patrick HT, Levy DM. Parkinson's disease: a clinical study of 146 cases. *Arch Neurol Psychiatry* 1922;**7**:711–20.

85. Mindham RH. Psychiatric syndromes in Parkinsonism. *J Neurol Neurosurg Psychiatry* 1970;**30**:188–91.

86. Dakof GA, Mendelsohn GA. Patterns of adaptation to Parkinson's disease. *Health Psychol* 1989;**8**:355–72.

87. Brown RG, MacCarthy B. Psychiatric morbidity in patients with Parkinson's disease. *Psychol Med* 1990;**20**(1):77–87.

88. Aarsland D, Larsen JP, Lim NG, et al Range of neuropsychiatric disturbances in patients with Parkinson's disease. *J Neurol Neurosurg Psychiatry* 1999;**67**:492–96.

89. Huber SJ, Friedenberg DL, Paulson GW, et al. The pattern of depressive symptoms varies with progression of Parkinson's disease. *J Neurol Neurosurg Psychiatry* 1990;**53**;275–8

90. Ellgring H, Seiler S, Nagel U, et al. Psychosocial problems of Parkinson patients: Approaches to assessment and treatment. In: Streifler MH, Korczyn AD, Melamed E, Youdim MHH, eds. *Parkinson's disease: anatomy, pathology and therapy. Advances in neurology*, Vol 53. New York: Raven Press,1998.

91. Starkstein SE, Mayberg HS, Leiguarda R, et al. A prospective longitudinal study of depression, cognitive decline, and physical impairments in patients with Parkinson's disease. *J Neurol Neurosurg Psychiatry* 1992;**55**:377–82.

92. Starkstein SE, Berthier ML, Bolduc PL, et al. Depression in patients with early versus late onset of Parkinson's disease. *Neurology* 1989;**39**;144–5.

93. Schrag A Jahanshahi M Quinn N. How does Parkinson's disease affect quality of life? A comparison with quality of life in the general population. *Mov Disord* 2000;**15**:1112–18.

94. Jenkinson C, Coulter A, Wright L. Short Form 36 (SF36) health survey questionnaire: normative data for adults of working age. *BMJ* 1993;**306**:1437–44.

95. Karlsen KH, Larsen JP, Tandberg E, Maeland JG. Influence of clinical and demographic variables on quality of life in patients with Parkinson's disease. *J Neurol Neurosurg Psychiatry* 1999;**66**:431–5.

96. Schrag A, Selai C, Jahanshahi M, Quinn NP. The EQ-5D – a generic quality of life measure – is a useful instrument to measure quality of life in patients with Parkinson's disease. *J Neurol Neurosurg Psychiatry* 2000;**69**:67–73.

97. Schrag A Jahanshahi M Quinn NP. What contributes to quality of life in patients with Parkinson's disease? *J Neurol Neurosurg Psychiatry* 2000;**69**:308–12.

98. Peto V, Jenkinson C, Fitzpatrick R, Greenhall R. The development and validation of a short measure of functioning and well being for individuals with Parkinson's disease. *Qual Life Res* 1995;**4**:241–8.

99. EuroQoL Group. EuroQoL: a new facility for the measurement of health-related quality of life. *Health Policy* 1990:**16**:199–208

100. Chriscilles EA, Rubenstein LM, Voelker MD, et al. The health burdens of Parkinson' disease. *Mov Disord* 1998;**13**:406–13.

101. Melnick ME, Dowling GA, Aminoff MJ, Barbaro NM. Effect of pallidotomy on postural control and motor function in Parkinson disease. *Arch Neurol.* 1999;**56**(11):1361–5.

102. Morris M, Iansek R, Kirkwood B. *Moving ahead with Parkinson's disease.* Kingston Centre, 1995.

103. Bridges KW, Goldberg DP. Psychiatric illness in inpatients with neurological disorders: patients' views on discussion of emotional problems with neurologists. *BMJ* 1984;**289**:656–8.

104. Tinetti ME, Baker DI, McAvay G, et al. Multifactorial intervention to reduce the risk of falling among elderly people living in the community. *N Engl J Med* 1994;**331**:821–7.

105. Lord SE, Wade DT, Halligan PW. A comparison of two physiotherapy treatment approaches to improve walking in multiple sclerosis: a pilot randomized controlled study. *Clin Rehabil* 1998;**12**(6):477–86.

106. Wiles CM, Newcombe RG, Fuller KJ, et al. Controlled randomised crossover trial of the effects of physiotherapy on mobility in chronic multiple sclerosis. *J Neurol Neurosurg Psychiatry* 2001;**70**:174–9.

107. Gibberd FB, Page NGR, Spencer KM, et al. Controlled trial of physiotherapy and occupational therapy for Parkinson's disease. *BMJ* 1981;**282**:1196.

108. Szelesky BC, Kosanovish NN, Shepherd W. Adjunctive treatment in Parkinson's disease: physical therapy and comprehensive group therapy. *Rehabil Lit* 1982;**43**:72–76.

109. Palmer SS, Mortimer JA, Webster DD, et al. Exercise therapy for Parkinson's disease. *Arch Phys Med Rehabil* 1986;**67**;741–5.

110. Banks X, Caird FI. Physiotherapy benefits patients with Parkinson's disease. *Clin Rehabil* 1989;**3**:11–6.

111. Taggart H, Crawford V. Reduced bone density of the hip in elderly patients with Parkinson's disease. *Age Ageing* 1995;**24**(4):326–8.

112. Yardley L, Smith H. A prospective study of the relationship between feared consequences of falling and avoidance of activity in community-living older people. 2002;17–23.

113. Tinetti ME, Mendes de Leon CF, Doucetter JT, Baker DI. Fear of falling and fall-related efficacy in relationship to functioning among community living elders. *J Gerontol* 1994;**49**;140–7.

114. Myers AM, Powell LE, Maki BE, et al. Psychological indicators of balance confidence: relationship to actual and perceived abilities. *J Gerontol* 1996;**51A**:M37–43.

115. Mendes de Leon CF, Seeman TE, Baker DI, et al. Self-efficacy, physical decline and change in functioning in community-living elders: a prospective study. *J Gerontol* 1996;**51B**:5183–90.

116. Beck AT. *Depression: causes and treatment.* Philadelphia: University of Pennsylvania Press, 1972.

117. Beck AT *Cognitive therapy and the emotional disorders.* New York: International Universities Press, 1976.

118. Yardley L, Medina SMG, Jurado CS, et al. Relationship between physical and psychosocial dysfunction in Mexican patients with vertigo: a cross-cultural validation of the Vertigo Symptom Scale. *J Psychosom Res* 1999;**46**:63–74.

119. Yardley L, Beech S, Zander L. et al. A randomised controlled trial of exercise therapy for dizziness and vertigo in primary care. *Br J Gen Pract* 1998;**48**:1136–40.

Appendix 19.1

The Vertigo Symptom Scale (VSS) is given on the page opposite. The discriminant, concurrent and predictive validity of the VSS have been confirmed cross-culturally. Both scales distinguish between patients complaining of disorientation and healthy controls.[14,52,53,118] The vertigo scale is unrelated to standard measures of anxiety and depression, but is correlated with handicap and with objective measures of perceptual disorientation following vestibular surgery.[5,6] The autonomic/anxiety scale is correlated with measures of anxiety and depression and with objective measures of psychophysiological arousal.[52,53] The short form (VSS-S) is suitable for use to assess benefits of therapy.[119]

Scoring and administration

To obtain a measure of vertigo severity, simply sum the patient's responses to the following items: 1a–1e, 4, 5, 7a–7e, 11, 15, 18a–18e. A measure of somatic anxiety can be obtained by summing items 2, 3, 6, 8 to 10, 12 to 14, 16, 17, 19 to 22. Sum all items on the VSS-S.

Statistical properties and normative values (based on a sample of 120 outpatients referred for investigation of balance disorder)[5]

The VSS subscales have very good statistical reliability (Cronbach's alpha was 0.88 for the vertigo scale, 0.85 for the anxiety scale) and the two scales were only modestly correlated (0.33). The mean normalized scores (i.e. scale scores divided by the number of scale items) were 1.12 on the vertigo scale (standard deviation = 0.75) and 1.33 on the anxiety scale (standard deviation = 0.79). The short form is also reliable (Cronbach's alpha is 0.88) and sensitive to therapy effects.[47,119]

VERTIGO SYMPTOM SCALE

Please circle the appropriate number to indicate about how many times you have experienced each of the symptoms listed below **during the past 12 months** (or since the vertigo started, if you have had vertigo for less than 1 year).

The range of responses are:

	0 Never (1–3 times a year)	1 A few times (4–12 times a year)	2 Several times (on average, more than once a month)	3 Quite often (on average, more than once a week)	4 Very often
How often in the past 12 months have you had the following symptoms:					
1. A feeling that things are spinning or moving around, lasting: (PLEASE ANSWER ALL THE CATEGORIES)					
(a) less than 2 minutes	0	1	2	3	4
(b) up to 20 minutes	0	1	2	3	4
(c) 20 minutes to 1 hour	0	1	2	3	4
(d) several hours	0	1	2	3	4
(e) more than 12 hours	0	1	2	3	4
2. Pains in the heart or chest region	0	1	2	3	4
3. Hot or cold spells	0	1	2	3	4
4. Unsteadiness so severe that you actually fall	0	1	2	3	4
5. Nausea (feeling sick), stomach churning	0	1	2	3	4
6. Tension/soreness in your muscles	0	1	2	3	4
7. A feeling of being light-headed, 'swimmy' or giddy, lasting: (PLEASE ANSWER ALL THE CATEGORIES)					
(a) less than 2 minutes	0	1	2	3	4
(b) up to 20 minutes	0	1	2	3	4
(c) 20 minutes to 1 hour	0	1	2	3	4
(d) several hours	0	1	2	3	4
(e) more than 12 hours	0	1	2	3	4
8. Trembling, shivering	0	1	2	3	4
9. Feeling of pressure in the ear(s)	0	1	2	3	4
10. Heart pounding or fluttering	0	1	2	3	4
11. Vomiting	0	1	2	3	4
12. Heavy feeling in arms or legs	0	1	2	3	4
13. Visual disturbances (e.g. blurring, flickering, spots before the eyes)	0	1	2	3	4
14. Headache or feeling of pressure in the head	0	1	2	3	4
15. Unable to stand or walk properly without support	0	1	2	3	4
16. Difficulty breathing, short of breath	0	1	2	3	4
17. Loss of concentration or memory	0	1	2	3	4
18. Feeling unsteady, about to lose balance, lasting: (PLEASE ANSWER ALL THE CATEGORIES)					
(a) less than 2 minutes	0	1	2	3	4
(b) up to 20 minutes	0	1	2	3	4
(c) 20 minutes to 1 hour	0	1	2	3	4
(d) several hours	0	1	2	3	4
(e) more than 12 hours	0	1	2	3	4
19. Tingling, prickling or numbness in parts of the body	0	1	2	3	4
20. Pains in the lower part of your back	0	1	2	3	4
21. Excessive sweating	0	1	2	3	4
22. Feeling faint, about to black out	0	1	2	3	4

VERTIGO SYMPTOM SCALE (SHORT FORM)

We would like to know what dizziness-related symptoms you have had just recently. Please circle the appropriate number to indicate about how many times you have experienced each of the symptoms listed below **during the past month.**

The range of responses are:

	0 Never	1 A few times	2 Several times (every week)	3 Quite often (most days)	4 Very often
How often **in the past month** have you had the following symptoms:					
1. A feeling that either you, or things around you, are spinning or moving, lasting **less** than 20 minutes	0	1	2	3	4
2. Hot or cold spells	0	1	2	3	4
3. Nausea (feeling sick), vomiting	0	1	2	3	4
4. A feeling that either you, or things around you, are spinning or moving, lasting **more** than 20 minutes	0	1	2	3	4
5. Heart pounding or fluttering	0	1	2	3	4
6. A feeling of being dizzy, disorientated or 'swimmy', lasting **all day**	0	1	2	3	4
7. Headache, or feeling of pressure in the head	0	1	2	3	4
8. Unable to stand or walk properly without support, veering or staggering to one side	0	1	2	3	4
9. Difficulty breathing, short of breath	0	1	2	3	4
10. Feeling unsteady, about to lose balance, lasting **more** than 20 minutes	0	1	2	3	4
11. Excessive sweating	0	1	2	3	4
12. Feeling faint, about to black out	0	1	2	3	4
13. Feeling unsteady, about to lose balance, lasting *less* than 20 minutes	0	1	2	3	4
14. Pains in the heart or chest region	0	1	2	3	4
15. A feeling of being dizzy, disorientated or swimmy, lasting **less** than 20 minutes	0	1	2	3	4

20

Balance control in older adults

PEI-FANG TANG AND MARJORIE H. WOOLLACOTT

INTRODUCTION

Incidence and impact of falls in older adults

Approximately 30 per cent of community-dwelling people over the age of 65 years fall at least once a year.[1–5] The incidence of falling increases to approximately 40 per cent or greater in community-dwelling people 80 years and older or in institutionalized older adults.[1,5–11] Falling accidents in the older population not only cause injuries, decreased mobility, reduced independence, changes in self-efficacy and lifestyles, and even deaths in older individuals, but also increase the needs and costs of geriatric health care in society.[5,7,12] The profound medical and social impact of accidental falls in older adults has brought to the attention of researchers and clinicians the need to develop effective methods to identify fall predisposing factors in this population.

Relationship between balance control abilities and falls in older adults

To date, numerous research studies have strongly suggested that poor balance control ability and impaired functional mobility in the elderly are among the most common precipitating factors for their recurrent falls.[1,5,13–17] Age-related changes in balance control abilities and functional mobility significantly compromise the abilities of older adults to perform safely everyday activities or interact with various types of environments in daily living. Thus, understanding the relevant issues and mechanisms related to balance and mobility control in older adults is the first important step in solving fall-related problems in order adults.

Purposes

The purposes of this chapter are twofold. First, we will discuss important conceptual issues in research on aging and balance control. Second, we will explore the mechanisms and functions of the aging balance control systems to facilitate the understanding of the causes of age-related changes in balance control abilities. Evidence of age-related changes in balance control systems will be discussed from the systems theory perspective. It is expected that with both the theoretical background and knowledge from empirical evidence, clinicians will be able to design clinical assessment tools and intervention regimens to effectively predict and prevent falls in older adults.

CURRENT RESEARCH ISSUES ON AGING AND BALANCE CONTROL

Before we discuss the nature of aging-related changes within the balance control systems, it is important to understand that the concepts of 'aging' and 'balance control' are rather complex and multifaceted. Therefore, in this chapter, we will discuss the definitions of 'aging' and 'balance control' first.

Issues on aging

Most researchers studying human aging agree that when examining the effects of the aging process on human functions, one should separate the aging effects from those due to pathological influences associated with diseases, even though many chronic diseases are commonly observed in older adults. However, researchers have also questioned whether older subjects selected based only on a disease-free criterion are truly representative of the majority of the healthy older population, whose physiological and psychological functions are considered merely affected by the intrinsic aging process.[18]

To solve this issue, two human aging models should be understood first. The first (genetic or program) model proposes that the function of human body systems are genetically programmed to decline linearly or curvilinearly with advancing age (see Fig. 20.1). Not until such natural decline reaches a certain threshold, do we see evident impairment in a person's function. Researchers advocating this model argue that the normal aging process involves an inevitable and irreversible subclinical decline in body functions. According to this model, the criteria for recruiting representative older subjects – those with normal aging processes – would be based on age-adjusted norms of disease-free older individuals.[19,20] Some researchers also define these older adults as undergoing 'usual aging.'[18]

The second (error or catastrophe) model of aging hypothesizes that human body systems continue to function at a level as high as young adults until death, unless an individual encounters disease(s) and/or environmental catastrophe(s), after which a rapid decline in behavioral function results.[21] Researchers supporting this model argue that not all of the body systems show a decline in function with aging. With proper diet, exercise, lifestyle and psychosocial support, it is possible that the physical and cognitive functions of older adults are comparable to those of young adults. Thus, the normal aging process is not completely inevitable and irreversible. In contrast, this process is modifiable. According to this model, the selection of representative older adults would be based on stringent criteria and

only disease-free, healthy older subjects whose functional levels are as high as young adults would be considered.[22,23] Rowe and Kahn[18] defined these older adults as undergoing 'successful aging.'

Conceivably, research findings on the effects of aging obtained from experiments using these aging models could be very different, even though both approaches exclude older adults that have overt diseases. Results of the large-scale 'MacArthur Studies of Successful Aging' have provided evidence for the distinction in physical and cognitive functions between older adults with 'usual' and 'successful' aging.[24–27] These issues regarding aging remind us that when studying literature on age-related changes in balance control abilities, one should be cautious about the selection criteria of older subjects and factors, such as exercises and lifestyle, which might affect balance control in the selected older adults. The interpretation and comparison of studies and extrapolation from a single study to the general aging population should also be made with caution. In this chapter, we mainly discuss balance control in older adults without pathology and those that belong to the usual aging group.

Definition of balance

Similar to the concept of aging, human 'balance control' is also a complex process that requires the integration of multiple body systems (cognitive, sensorimotor, and musculoskeletal systems). Traditionally, 'balance' has often been defined as a task of maintaining a person's center of gravity (COG) over the base of support (BOS) in an upright posture so that a fall would not happen.[28] However, this definition does not apply to all types of upright activities or sports skills of human beings. For example, during walking, the COG of the whole body moves forward along or close to the medial border of the supporting foot rather than passing through the base of the supporting foot as shown in Fig. 20.2. In such a dynamic task, the integration of posture and voluntary movement and maintaining a dynamic relationship between the body COG and base of support appear to be much more important than maintaining the COG within the base of support.

The contemporary research concept of 'balance (or postural equilibrium)' is different from the traditional one. It is now considered that balance consists of both static and dynamic components.[30] Static balance is defined as the status of the body in which all forces acting on the body are balanced, where the body remains static in an intended position or orientation; dynamic balance is referred to as the status in which the summed forces on the body allow the body to move in a controlled manner.[30] According to this definition, balance control abilities are fundamental to a wide range of daily activities ranging from static to dynamic ones. Good balance control abilities would indicate that successful pos-

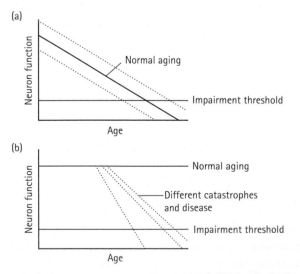

Figure 20.1 *Two models for human aging: (a) genetic model, in which the function of the nervous system declines linearly with age; (b) catastrophe model, in which nervous function continues at a high level until death, unless one encounters environmental catastrophe(s) or disease(s).*

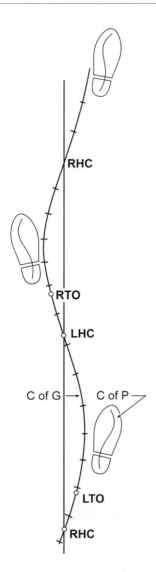

Figure 20.2 *A plot showing the relationship between center of gravity (C of G) path and foot placement during walking. During the double support phase, the C of G path moves between two feet contact, while during the single support phase, the C of G path never passes through the base of the support foot. RHC, right heel contact; RTO, right toe-off; LHC, left heel contact; LTO, left toe-off; C of P, center of pressure. (Reproduced from ref. 29, with permission.)*

ture–voluntary movement integration is achieved so that a person is able to fulfill the goal of a voluntary task in a safe manner. This definition also implies that the nature of balance control mechanisms is task-specific. People that have better static balance control do not necessarily show better dynamic balance control, and vice versa.[31]

Scope of balance control studies

To understand the entire range of balance function in older individuals, performance in a variety of tasks or tests ranging from those requiring static balance to those

requiring functional and dynamic balance adjustments should be considered. Patla and associates[32] classified the wide range of balance tests/tasks into the following categories: static–unperturbed balance tests; static–perturbed balance tests; balance control during unperturbed voluntary movements; and balance control during perturbed voluntary movement. The static–unperturbed balance tests are those in which a person's COG and BOS are not disturbed and their goal is to maintain the COG and BOS as steady for as long as possible. Many of the currently available clinical assessment tools of balance, such as two-legged stance, one-legged stance and tandem stance tests are examples of static-unperturbed balance tests. The length of time and steadiness that a person can maintain the testing position are often recorded in these tests. While these balance tests can be easily implemented in the clinic to detect changes or improvement in balance function of older adults, they have several limitations.[33] First, results of these tests do not explain the mechanisms that contribute to the observed age-related changes in balance function. Second, the relationship between performance on these tests and the behavioral outcome (fall versus no fall) remains controversial.[8,34–37] Older adults whose performance is worse than normal (showing greater sway or maintain the position for shorter period of time) on these static balance tests are not necessarily more prone to falls. Thus, clinicians who simply use this type of balance test would have difficulty in either identifying older adults that are in need of balance training or in identifying the body systems that should be targeted in balance training for the older adult.

The static-perturbed tests are those in which a person's COG or BOS is expectedly or unexpectedly perturbed while not performing any voluntary task except for maintaining an upright posture. Empirical research paradigms, such as the platform perturbation paradigm (perturbing BOS) and postural stress test (perturbing COG), belong to this category.[38,39] Intensive research has been done to investigate age-related changes in balance control abilities in these static-perturbed tests.[40–44] Results from these studies shed light on the mechanisms, the motor coordination mechanisms in particular, that older adults use to maintain balance under these perturbed stance conditions. Some researchers have also modified the perturbation paradigms by incorporating different combinations of sensory conditions to examine the abilities of older adults to make use of available senses to maintain balance.[42,44–47] Therefore, using these research paradigms, the mechanisms underlying balance control in older adults have become better understood.

The next category of balance test that requires dynamic balance control assesses balance control while performing voluntary movements without external perturbations. It is well perceived that the execution of a voluntary movement *per se* is already a perturbation to a person's balance. Past research has shown ample evidence for anticipatory postural adjustments that human beings adopt to overcome the disturbance accompanied with the upcoming voluntary movements in a feed-forward manner.[48] The existence of anticipatory postural adjustments reflects the ability of one's nervous system to integrate effectively postural and voluntary movement control so that voluntary movements can be achieved in a safe manner. Research studying age-related changes in anticipatory postural adjustments allows the examination of such integrative abilities in older adults.[49,50] Most of these studies have asked subjects to make simple arm movements while standing. In recent years, researchers also have noted the importance of investigating balance control during even more dynamic tasks such as reaching forward, turning, standing up, sitting down, and walking.[51–62] The ability to integrate balance control with these daily, functional, and dynamic tasks is also termed 'functional mobility' by many researchers.[51,52,59] Results from these studies have revealed a close relationship between the functional mobility of older adults and their likelihood of experiencing falls.[5,63–66] Thus, this functional mobility approach not only allows clinicians to accurately identify older fallers but also the types of dynamic balance and mobility tasks in which older adults have the greatest difficulty in maintaining balance.

Finally, the most challenging balance tests are those that require balance control during perturbed voluntary movements. One common example of balance tests in this category is balance control required in recovering from a slip or trip during walking. In such tasks, a person would use anticipatory postural adjustments to ensure the proper execution of the intended voluntary movements and at the same time use reactive postural adjustments to correct for postural disturbance caused by the external perturbations. Balance tests of this category may simulate the situations in which a fall most frequently occurs. Failure to control balance in such situations is very likely to result in a fall. Recently, researchers have just begun to examine balance control abilities of older adults in slip- or trip-like balance tests.[67–73] Significant age-related differences were evident in balance adjustments required in these most challenging balance tests.

The aforementioned four categories of balance tests encompass a wide scope of balance control mechanisms, ranging from the most static control mechanisms to the most dynamic ones. To comprehensively understand age-related changes in static and dynamic balance control mechanisms, older adults' performance in a wide range of static and dynamic balance tests should all be considered. However, although these categories provide a battery/hierarchy of balance tests that clinicians may use for testing older adults' balance control systems, some theoretical framework is still needed to systematically examine changes in their balance control systems. For this purpose, we will discuss this theoretical issue from the systems theory perspective.

SYSTEMS APPROACH TO STUDYING BALANCE CONTROL IN OLDER ADULTS

The systems perspective

The systems theory of motor control was first proposed by Bernstein.[74] According to this theory, human movements are not only the result of physiological processes, but are also constrained by biomechanical factors, such as internal (moment of inertia and mass) and external forces (ground reaction forces, friction, etc.).[75] Coordinated movements are organized around the functional goal of the movement as a result of the interactions among the multiple physiological subsystems and biomechanical factors. When this theory is applied to the study of balance control, it is suggested that multiple physiological subsystems and environmental factors interact to achieve the task goal of maintaining balance.[76,77] The primary physiological subsystems that have been identified to be involved in balance control are sensory organization and perception of orientation, motor coordination, predictive central set, musculoskeletal subsystems and environmental adaptation as shown in Fig. 20.3.[78] Since older adults may show deterioration in the function of these physiological subsystems related to balance control, the systems perspective is helpful in understanding subsystems that primarily contribute to the decreased balance control in this population. Age-related changes in balance control subsystems and the subsequent influences on balance control in older adults are discussed in the following text.

Age-related changes in sensory systems for balance control

The somatosensory, visual, and vestibular systems are the three main balance senses. The somatosensory system provides information on the position or motion of the

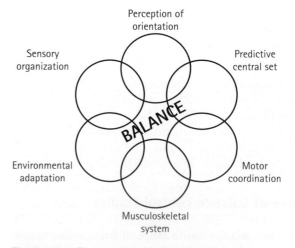

Figure 20.3 Six interrelated balance control systems. (Reproduced from ref. 79 with permission of the APTA.)

body with respect to the supporting surface and the position or motion of body segments with respect to each other. The visual system provides information on the orientation and motion of the body with respect to global space. The vestibular system senses the linear and angular acceleration of the head as well as the head position relative to gravity. Normally, these three senses work together to detect relevant peripheral sensory information from the environment, to develop an internal representation of the body in global space, and to trigger proactive or reactive balance adjustments, in an attempt to maintain static and dynamic balance under certain task and environmental contexts.[40,80,81]

With the existence of multiple sensory systems for balance control, redundant or conflicting sensory information may be provided by these three senses concurrently. With redundant sensory information, reduction of sensory input from one of the senses may be compensated for by the remaining senses and thus does not necessarily cause discernible changes in a person's balance. When there are conflicts between information provided by the different senses, a higher-level sensory organization or integration system is used to adjust the weighting on different sensory inputs. For example, when a person is standing in a stationary train and at the same time watching another train passing by, the visual and somatosensory inputs are in conflict. While somatosensory input informs the person that they are not moving, the visual input causes the illusion of self-motion. In this case, normally the higher-level sensory organization would increase weighting on the somatosensory system and decrease weighting on the visual system to prevent the person from increasing body sway in response to the illusive visual information.

There is ample evidence for age-related changes in the three balance-related sensory systems. The effects of these changes on balance control during various static and dynamic tasks in older adults are discussed below.

In the somatosensory system, decreased vibration sense (especially in the lower extremities), proprioception, and tactile sensation have been documented for older adults free from neurological diseases.[82–88] Reduced vibration sense was found to be correlated with increased postural sway while older adults were standing with the eyes open or closed on a firm or compliant surface.[89–91] Age-related decrease in vibration sense was also related to impaired mobility, such as walking, and falls in older adults.[92,93] Researchers have suggested that proprioception is the primary sense responsible for maintaining static standing balance or for triggering automatic postural responses when a standing adult experiences a sudden horizontal support surface displacement.[45,94–96] Joint position sense was also commonly found to decline with age.[84,91] This is exemplified in a significant increase in body sway when older adults stand with eyes closed compared with eyes open. In a retrospective study, Lord and colleagues[97] reported that older fallers appeared to

have poorer joint position sense than older non-fallers. In addition, lower extremity proprioception was also found to be one of the independent predictors of lateral stability when older adults were standing in a near-tandem stance.

Multiple parallel processing exists in the visual system. Within this processing of visual inputs the focal (foveal) vs. ambient (peripheral) modes of processing appear to be most related to balance control. Paulus and colleagues[98] examined the effect of focal vision on postural steadiness in normal stance by systematically reducing visual acuity using semitransparent plastic foils. The foils were placed close to the eyes of the subjects to reduce the general visual acuity without influencing the visual field. Reduced visual acuity appeared to be accompanied by increased postural sway, particularly in the antero-posterior direction. Age-related decreases in visual acuity, visual field, depth perception and contrast sensitivity at the intermediate and high spatial frequencies are commonly reported in older adults.[99–101] In a retrospective study, Lord et al.[97] reported that older fallers appeared to have poorer visual acuity than older non-fallers. Poor visual acuity was also found to have significant influence on the stair-descending performance of older adults.[102] It is thus hypothesized that a decline in balance control abilities in older adults may be partly attributable to the functional decrements in focal vision.

Ambient vision is primarily responsible for the perception of motion and spatial orientation and thus, is also important for control of balance.[103–105] Researchers have found that older adults show diminished sensitivity to a moving object with low spatial frequencies, especially when this object moves at a high speed.[106] Another type of visual perception, the perception of verticality and horizontality, has also been found to be impaired in older fallers compared with older non-fallers.[107] In addition, older adults also have difficulty in perceiving self-motion with reference to external space. Warren et al.[108] found age-related increases in the threshold to perceive the direction of self-motion resulting from optical flow information created by computer-simulated translational and curvilinear movement images. In contrast to these findings, other researchers using a moving visual room paradigm (the walls and ceiling moved, but the floor was stationary) found that older adults, with or without a history of imbalance, were more sensitive than young adults to a moving visual scene during standing, especially when the somatosensory input from the support surface was unreliable or the support surface was unstable.[109,110] Thus, older adults tend to over-rely on visual input, even though the visual information is illusive, especially when the somatosensation system does not provide an adequate reference frame for balance.[92,94,109,111] Although controversy exists over the threshold of older adults in detecting self-motion from ambient vision, the above-mentioned findings suggest that age-related decrements in the accuracy of visual perception of motion and spatial orientation may have a significant impact on balance control in older adults.

The vestibular system senses the position and motion of the head relative to external space, and the vestibulospinal reflex is important for triggering automatic postural responses when the head position is suddenly disturbed.[95,112–114] Because the gravitational reference that the vestibular system is based upon remains largely unaltered on earth, the vestibular system is also believed to play an important role in resolving sensory conflicts resulting from altered or distorted visual and/or somatosensory information.[115] In other words, the vestibular system is considered to play an important role in higher-level sensory integration.

For example, Lord and Ward[92] showed that level of vestibular function predicted the balance performance of older adults while standing on a foam surface with eyes closed. In addition, research has shown that patients with peripheral vestibular deficits have difficulty in suppressing unreliable visual and proprioceptive inputs.[116] However, Bronstein[117] showed that when the angular and linear acceleration of the head was smaller than the threshold for the vestibular system, it was the somatosensory system, not the vestibular system, that was involved in solving sensory conflict conditions. For example, when a healthy subject stands in a 'moving' room which is moving at a very slow speed (peak velocity 2–3 cm/s), the subject first incorrectly perceives body sway, and then corrects for it. A patient with vestibular dysfunction was found also to be able to correct the perceived sway; however, a patient deprived of proprioception from the lower legs failed to do so. Apparently, in this case, the somatosensory system, rather than the vestibular system, modulates the postural responses induced by illusive visual information.

Rosenhall[118] reported that the number of vestibular hair cells is reduced 20–40 per cent in healthy adults 70 years and older when compared with young adults.

The number of vestibular nerve fibers has also been found to decrease with age.[119] Neuronal loss of the medial, lateral, and inferior vestibular nuclei in advanced human aging has also been reported recently.[120] Thus, age-related declines in the ability to correctly detect head position and motion in space, to elicit vestibular spinal reflexes, or to solve sensory conflicts are not uncommon.

Researchers have used the Sensory Organization Test (SOT) to further investigate the age-related changes in the function of the vestibular system for solving sensory conflicting conditions in various balance tasks.[28,44,115] The SOT includes six sensory conditions, each involving different combinations of available balance senses. Therefore, the SOT permits a systematic examination of the contribution and interactions of individual senses in balance function. In the SOT, subjects stand on a movable platform surrounded by a visual enclosure. Both the platform and the visual enclosure can move in direct correlation with antero-posterior sway of the body, and thus induce inaccurate somatosensory or visual information for spatial orientation. The six sensory conditions of the SOT are: (1) normal vision, normal support surface (VnSn); (2) eyes closed, normal support surface (VcSn); (3) visual enclosure 'servoed' (rotating to follow the subject's postural sway), normal support surface (VsSn); (4) normal vision, support surface servoed (rotating to follow the subject's postural sway) (VnSs); (5) eyes closed, support surface servoed (VcSs); and (6) visual enclosure and support surface both servoed (VsSs). In the first three conditions, the visual input is manipulated, while in the last three conditions, the somatosensory input is manipulated in conjunction with a normal or altered visual input. In particular, because accurate visual and somatosensory inputs are unavailable in conditions 5 and 6, subjects have to shift their reliance (weighting) on these senses to a reliance on the vestibular system for maintaining an upright posture while standing on the platform. Figure 20.4 shows the six sensory conditions of the SOT.

| 1. Normal vision. Fixed support. | 2. Absent vision. | 3. Sway referenced vision. Fixed support. | 4. Normal vision. Sway-referenced support. | 5. Absent vision. Sway-referenced support. | 6. Sway-referenced vision and support. |

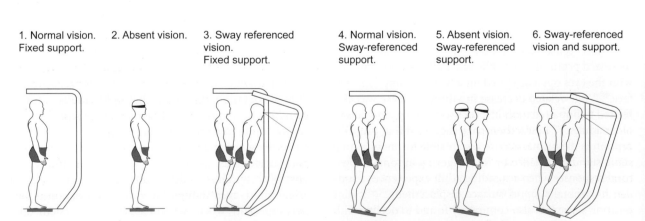

Figure 20.4 *Six conditions of the Sensory Organization Test (Reproduced from Nashner LM. Sensory, neuromuscular, and biomechanical contributions to human balance. In: Duncan PW, ed. Balance. Alexandria: American Physical Therapy Association, 1989: 5–12.*

Several researchers have found that in the SOT, healthy older adults showed only a slight increase in the amount of sway in the first four sensory conditions compared with young adults. However, older adults demonstrated a significantly much greater increase in the amount of sway in conditions 5 and 6 of the SOT compared with young adults (see Fig. 20.5). Some older subjects even lost their balance when they first experienced these conditions.[44,46,47] This is especially true for older adults with a history of falls.[45] These findings suggest that when the vestibular sense is available along with accurate vision or somatosensory information, older adults can maintain their upright balance. When both visual and somatosensory inputs are eliminated or inaccurate, leaving the vestibular system as the sole available and reliable sense, older adults start to show great difficulty in maintaining upright posture. Therefore, the higher-level sensory reweighting function of the vestibular system in healthy older adults appears to be depressed to a certain degree. Peterka and Black[121] found that some of the older adults that fell under sensory conditions 5 and 6 also presented with impaired vestibulo-ocular and optokinetic reflexes. More systematic analyses on the correlation between performance of older adults in the SOT test and clinical vestibular tests are needed to elucidate the contribution of the vestibular system or the interaction between the vestibular and visual systems to balance deterioration in older adults.

In summary, similar to young adults, for older adults, the somatosensory system remains as the most predominant sensory system among the three sensory systems used for maintaining static balance. When older adults are moving in the environment or are perturbed during standing, however, researchers have found that older adults tend to use a so-called 'head stabilization strategy' to stabilize their gaze and geographic orientation to enhance the accuracy and reliability of the visual and vestibular inputs.[122,123] For older adults, the role of vision becomes more prominent when the somatosensory system is unreliable or the support surface is unstable; in such cases, over-reliance on vision is often found. Finally, given the multisensory nature of balance control, when the environment can provide many different sensory cues, the impact of reduction in a single balance sensory system with age may be less discernible because of the redundant or compensatory sensory mechanisms. When more than one sensory system is altered, however, age-related changes in balance control become evident immediately.[42,47] This is particularly true when both visual and somatosensory inputs are altered or reduced, leaving the vestibular system the primary and solely sense for balance control.

Age-related changes in motor organization for balance control

From the systems perspective, the activation of a set of associated muscles or joints, called a 'synergy', to achieve the goal of a functional task under certain environmental contexts is essential to successful motor performance.[74] The use of synergies for various postural and voluntary movement tasks helps to solve the problem of controlling a multitude of degrees of freedom in postural and movement tasks. Researchers have devised various 'postural perturbation paradigms' to investigate how humans integrate sensory–motor information and coordinate muscular and joint actions in balance tasks. In many of the perturbation paradigms, mechanical perturbations are applied to either a body part, such as the head or trunk, to disturb the body's center of mass, or to the support surface to disturb the base of support.[38,39,43,80,124–128] Such mechanical perturbations are delivered in various forms, such as a push, a pull, a release of a pull or a displacement of the supporting surface, etc.

Using the support surface (or platform) perturbation paradigm and instructing subjects not to move the legs during the experiment, Nashner[125] and Horak and Nashner[126] observed two relatively stereotyped and dis-

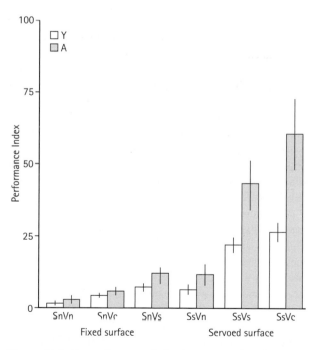

Figure 20.5 *The performance index (as measured by the area under the rectified and integrated sway curve) of the young (Y) and older (A) adult groups in six sensory organization conditions. In the first three conditions, the support surface remains fixed (Sn), and the visual conditions are changed from normal (Vn), to eyes closed (Vc), and to Vs (visual surround servoed). In the next three conditions, the support surface is servoed (Ss), and the same three visual conditions are used. Older adults show a significant increase in the amount of sway in the SsVs and SsVc conditions as compared with young adults. (Reproduced from ref. 44, with permission.)*

tinct muscle activation and joint movement patterns in the balance control repertoire of standing humans. A movable platform, which permitted anterior–posterior translation and upward–downward rotation, was used to test standing subjects' postural responses to a sudden movement of the platform. In response to a small forward platform translation, which induced backward body sway, young subjects were found to first activate the ankle dorsiflexor, tibialis anterior (TA) muscle, at a latency of 90–120 ms, followed by the activation of the quadriceps (Q) by a time lag of 20 ms or so. A similar distal-to-proximal muscle activation pattern (gastrocnemius (G) to hamstring, (H)) was observed in the backward platform translation trials. The distal-to-proximal muscle activation pattern is primarily accompanied by joint movement around the ankle joints, and termed the ankle strategy.[129] Further, because of the long onset latency of the first muscle response, these automatic postural responses are not simple spinal reflexes, but rather involve supraspinal or transcortical control.

When the platform perturbation became larger and faster or if the subject was standing on a relatively short beam compared with the foot length, muscles around the trunk and hip were activated first at similar latencies, followed by the distal leg muscles. Postural movement about the hip joint, called the hip strategy, often accompanies such a proximal-to-distal activation sequence.[126] It was also predicted that as the perturbation becomes very large or fast and the ankle and hip strategies are no longer sufficient for one to maintain balance, the stepping strategy would be used.[41]

Over the past two decades, the concepts of postural muscle synergies and movement strategies have been continually revisited and are still evolving. Rather than considering the ankle, hip, and stepping synergies and strategies as distinct and inflexible postural control strategies, researchers now believe that it may be more accurate to treat these postural control strategies as parts of the continuum of the balance control repertoire of human beings. The selection of one strategy over others in certain circumstances is determined by multiple factors, such as the subject's intention, experience, physical conditions or the received instructions, in addition to the characteristics of perturbations.[38] For example, it has been found that the stepping strategy is more frequently used than ankle or hip strategies when a perturbation is novel and when the subjects have not received any instruction to constrain their use of stepping strategy. This is true even when the perturbation is small.[130,131]

The perturbation paradigms allow researchers to examine age-related changes in motor organization for reactive balance control. In particular, studies in this area have focused on the ability of older adults to select an appropriate postural strategy and muscle synergy and to generate rapid and effective postural responses in response to a particular perturbation, and to adapt to changes in perturbation parameters or contexts.[41,44,72,73,132]

Several significant alterations have been reported in the movement strategies and muscular response characteristics of older adults in reaction to sudden platform perturbations during stance or walking.

With regard to movement strategies, it has been found that when no particular constraints or instructions are given, both older and young adults are most likely to use the stepping strategy for balance recovery in response to anterior and posterior platform translations of moderate magnitude and velocity.[133] However, while the majority of young adults are often able to fully regain balance with a single compensatory stepping after the perturbations, older adults are twice as likely to take multiple steps to regain stability. These additional steps are often directed laterally, indicating poorer control of lateral stability in older adults while using the stepping strategy.[130,131] In response to large backward pulls at the waist level, older adults are also found to be more likely to take multiple small steps to regain balance than young adults.[127] Similarly, when older adults are experiencing lateral platform perturbations during stance, they are also more likely to take multiple lateral steps or use arm reactions to regain balance.[134] Furthermore, collisions between the two feet while taking these laterally directed compensatory steps are much more prevalent in older adults than in young adults, suggesting significant motor deficits of older adults in generating safe and efficient lateral stepping.[135]

Together, results of these studies suggest that stepping is an important and common balance recovery strategy used by older adults in natural and unconstrained environments. To date, it remains unclear why older adults select a stepping strategy over other balance recovery strategies even when the perturbation does not cause the body COG to exceed the boundary of the BOS and a stepping strategy appears to be less safe and more attention-demanding for older adults.[133–136] Studies investigating this issue have now been undertaken by several researchers.[43,137–139]

Another way to investigate age-related changes in the motor organization of balance control is to examine the ability of older adults to use appropriate muscle synergies and to generate rapid and effective postural responses in reaction to perturbations. It has commonly been found that when experiencing platform translations during stance or walking, older adults show slower onset latencies of the distal postural muscles, compared with young adults.[44,72,121] The delayed onset latency of postural muscles may be caused by decreased somatosensory sensitivity to detect perturbation onset, delayed central processing time or delayed motor neuron recruitment time.

However, researchers generally agree that the slightly increased onset latency in muscle postural responses alone may not be the key factor that causes imbalance in older adults after experiencing external perturbations. Rather, it may be the decreased magnitude of postural responses and breakdown in the timing and sequencing of muscle synergies that place a significant impact on the ability of older adults to efficiently regain balance.[42,72,140] Older adults were found to more likely demonstrate a temporal reversal (i.e. a proximal to distal sequence) of muscle activation and a longer time of co-activation between agonist and antagonist postural muscles in their postural responses to platform translations.[42,44,72,140] The use of a proximal to distal muscle activation sequence may indicate that older adults are more likely to use the hip strategy to maintain balance.[42] The hip strategy is hypothesized to generate a large compensatory horizontal shear force against the support surface and thus may be a biomechanically inefficient or unstable strategy to be used in response to a relatively small perturbation.[41] Co-activation of agonist and antagonist postural muscles will increase joint stiffness, slow down the process of restoring joint positions during normal standing or walking, and thus increase the energy expenditure to regain balance. The presence of these temporal and spatial alterations in the organization of older adults' postural responses suggests changes in their central mechanisms in coordinating different muscles.

In addition, Tang and Woollacott[72] also found that the bursts of postural muscle responses of older adults were typically of smaller magnitude and longer duration, compared with those of young adults, in response to platform perturbation during walking (see Fig. 20.6). It is possible that older adults attempt to use a longer duration of muscle contractions to compensate for the smaller rate of muscle response generation. The difficulty with generating fast and powerful reactive postural responses in older adults could originate from peripheral mechanisms such as a loss of fast twitch muscle fibers[141]

or central mechanisms such as a decreased descending drive to recruit motor neurons. As a whole, the combination of longer-onset latency, smaller burst magnitude, and co-activation of agonist and antagonist muscles in the postural synergies of older adults is likely to result in inefficient postural responses.

In addition to the analysis of muscle synergies and movement strategies, researchers have recently started to examine joint torques generated in response to platform perturbations during stance. Interestingly, Hall and associates[142] found no age-related difference in the rate and magnitude of active ankle torque generation in response to platform translations, when comparisons were made between balance trials in which the same balance strategy (stepping or non-stepping strategy) was used by older and young adults. This result appears to be quite different from the above-mentioned findings in postural muscle responses and previous reports on the decreased ability of older adults to voluntarily generate rapid ankle torque.[143] More research is needed to clarify such seemingly contradictory findings among the different levels of analyses on motor organization in aging balance control. Table 20.1 summarizes the results of these studies.

Age-related changes in the musculoskeletal system for balance control

The musculoskeletal system is another important subsystem contributing to balance control. A number of studies have shown age-related changes in joint flexibility, muscle strength, and speed of muscle contrac-

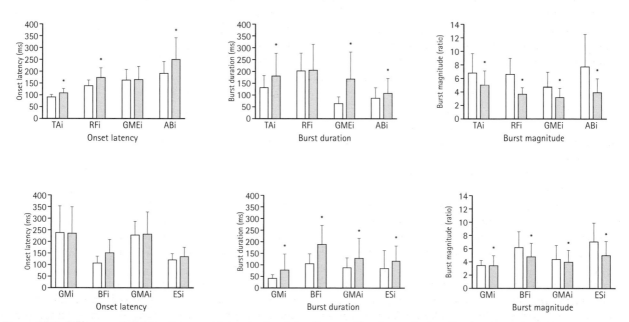

Figure 20.6 *Differences in contraction onset latencies, burst durations and burst magnitudes of postural muscles between young (open bars) and older (shaded bars) adults when reacting to a forward slip at heel-strike during gait. AB, abdominis muscles; BF, biceps femoris; ES, erectus spinae; GM, gastrocnemius medialis; GMA, gluteus maximus; GME, gluteus medius; i, ipsilateral; RF, rectus femoris; TA, tibialis anterior.*

Table 20.1 *Summary of research data on age-related changes in the subsystems contributing to balance control*

	Subsystem	Age-related changes	References
Sensory	Vision	Decreased visual acuity, visual field, depth perception, and contrast sensitivity at the intermediate and high spatial frequencies, in addition to diminished sensitivity to visual flow. Poor visual acuity correlated with falls, poor stair climbing performance	98,99,100,101,102,106,107
	Vestibular	Reduced vestibular hair cells, reduced neurons in vestibular nuclei. Loss correlated with increased sway on compliant (foam) surface with eyes closed	118,119
	Somatosensory	Decreased vibration, proprioception and tactile sensibility, joint position sense. Correlated with increased postural sway, falls and impaired mobility	89,91,93,97
Motor	Motor coordination	Increased COP movement and sway during quiet stance; Slowing and reduced amplitude of reactive postural responses during quiet stance and walking (with increased burst duration to compensate), with more steps taken during recovery from moderate amplitude balance threats; slowing and disorganization of proactive postural responses	44,49,72,73,133,134,144
Cognitive	Higher level sensory adaptation	Decreased ability to shift from the use of one sensory input to another for postural control; impairment associated with disturbed vestibulo-ocular and optokinetic reflexes	44,46,47,47,121
	Attention	Increased attention required for postural control, reflected in poorer performance in dual task situations for cognitive task, postural task or both. Cognitive task performance deteriorates further as complexity of postural task increases	136,145,146,147,148
Musculoskeletal	Muscle strength	Reduced muscle strength, and speed of muscle contraction; decreased ability to generate rapid ankle torque; Reduced muscle strength correlated with balance loss	11,47,92,143,149
	Range of motion	Reduced joint flexibility	148

tion.[150–153] Decreased joint flexibility, selective type II (fast-twitch) muscle fiber atrophy, and reduced muscle strength with concentric, eccentric and isokinetic contractions were found in subjects with advancing age.

To further investigate whether and how these decrements in the musculoskeletal system relate to balance control in aging, researchers have compared these musculoskeletal changes in older fallers and non-fallers.[149,154] Among these changes, the relationship between muscle strength and muscle power with balance control abilities is most often investigated. Muscle strength has been found to be an important predictor for losses of balance of older adults while being tested in the SOT conditions.[47] Lord and Ward[92] discovered that muscle strength contributes to balance performance of older adults while standing on foam with the eyes open. These findings suggest that muscle strength appears to be an important factor in balance tasks in which normal sensory conditions are altered.

Using an isokinetic muscle testing procedure, Whipple and associates[154] reported a reduced peak torque and power generated by the ankle and knee muscles of older fallers as compared with non-fallers. This difference was greater during faster (120°/s) joint movements than during slower (60°/s) movements. Similarly, studies by Thelen and associates[143] also demonstrated decreased ability of older adults to generate rapid ankle torque in voluntary mode. These results suggest that muscle power, which measures the rate of force generation, may be a more important factor than muscle strength in predicting balance abilities of older adults.[155] Clearly, as mentioned earlier, rapid generation of large muscle responses (i.e. high muscle power) is crucial for balance recovery from a postural perturbation.

As to which muscle(s) are most important for balance control, researchers have suggested that it depends upon the balance task being performed.[156] For example, in a retrospective study, Lord et al.[97] reported that older fallers appeared to have poorer quadriceps strength than older non-fallers. They also found that quadriceps strength was one of the independent predictors for lateral stability in near-tandem stance of older adults. In contrast, Whipple and colleagues[154] found that the strength of the ankle dorsiflexor appeared to be reduced the most among all muscles in the lower extremity of older fallers. In addition, the distal leg muscles, ankle dorsiflexors and plantarflexors, have been found to be important predictors of performance in dynamic functional mobility tests, namely the Berg Balance Scale and the Get Up and Go test, respectively.[156] Thus, although it is generally agreed that the lower extremity muscle strength was important for balance control in older adults,[5] it appears that different balance tasks place specific stress on strength of different muscles. Table 20.1 summarizes the results of these studies.

Age–related changes in environmental adaptation for balance control

Given the deterioration in balance control abilities of older adults, an important clinical question is whether these changes can be altered or improved by repeatedly exposing these older subjects to certain balance tasks. To answer this question, the rotational mode of the platform perturbation paradigm has been used to specifically test the adaptation abilities of one's motor organization of postural responses.[157] When young adults standing on the platform experienced an upward (ankle dorsiflexing) platform rotation, some of them exhibited muscle activation of the gastrocnemius. This gastrocnemius muscle activity was not desirable since it further increased the backward body sway originally induced by the platform movement and therefore destabilized the body to a greater extent. After repeated exposures to this rotational platform perturbation, the activity of the gastrocnemius muscle became progressively attenuated in young adults.[157] Older adults were found to be more likely to fall than the young adults when they first encountered the same rotational platform perturbation. However, with repeated exposures, they were also able to attenuate the undesirable activity of the gastrocnemius muscle (Fig. 20.7).[44]

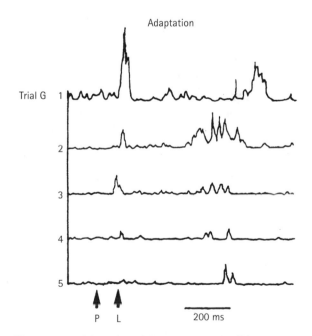

Figure 20.7 *Adaptation of the gastrocnemius (G) muscle activity to repeated ankle dorsiflexion perturbations of normal stance in an older subject. Since the activity of the G muscle further augments postural instability caused by the platform upward rotation, this activity is not desirable. Older adults are able to adapt to the stability needs and show attenuation of the G cavity across five consecutive trials. P indicates the onset of the platform movement and L indicates the onset of the long latency response of the G muscle. (Reproduced from ref. 44, with permission.)*

When investigating the adaptability of the motor organization of postural responses, researchers have also studied how young and older adults may change the desirable postural responses after repeated exposures to the same platform perturbations. Using a perturbed walking paradigm to simulate a forward slip, Tang and associates[71] discovered that young adults were able to reduce the activation duration and magnitude of the primary postural muscle responses of the tibialis anterior, rectus femoris and rectus abdominis across four repeated, yet non-consecutive, trials of the anterior perturbation occurring at heel-strike. Older adults decreased the duration and magnitude of only the tibialis anterior and/or rectus femoris responses and only when the perturbation was given in consecutive trials. These results suggest that while young adults are able to adopt the most parsimonious postural response strategies over only a few repeated (although non-consecutive) exposures to the same postural threats, older adults appear to have reduced adaptability when the same environmental experience is not given immediately following the previous experience. This difficulty with adapting to balance threats might account for their increased risk of falling when walking in a hazardous environment. Age-related decreases in learning and memory ability might contribute to such a decline in motor organization adaptability.

With regard to older adults' adaptability in sensory integration, Woollacott et al.[44] found that older adults who initially lost their balance in the sensory conditions where only the vestibular system could give accurate balance information were able to maintain their balance during subsequent consecutive exposures to the same sensory conflicting conditions. However, it remains unknown whether older adults would show similar adaptability if the same sensory conditions were not given consecutively.

Together, the above-mentioned findings indicate that although there is a decline in the adaptability in motor organization and sensory integration of the older adults, such adaptability is not completely lost in older adults. Thus, balance training to improve such adaptability may be possible. Moreover, it is important for balance training protocols designed for older adults to take into consideration the particular learning and memory characteristics of these older adults.

Age-related changes in predictive central set for balance control

Central set has been referred to as the higher level predictive processing of the central nervous system that sends out descending commands to the peripheral sensory and motor systems to prepare for an anticipated stimulus or voluntary task. Using the platform perturbation paradigm, Horak et al.[144] studied the effect of changes in central set on automatic postural responses of young adults 22–41 years of age. Significant differences in the magnitude of automatic postural responses imposed randomly versus serially, or imposed expectedly versus unexpectedly, were found. The influence of central set on automatic postural responses in older adults has not yet been systematically investigated.

An alternative method to examine the effect of central set on balance control in aging is to examine anticipatory postural responses in this population. It has been well documented that anticipatory postural responses precede the upcoming voluntary muscle activity and are task-specific.[48,158]. This task-specific property of anticipatory postural responses allows the body to anticipate and overcome the disequilibrium induced by the voluntary movement *per se*. While executing voluntary movements, the existence of central set helps to facilitate the development of anticipatory postural adjustments, which in turn, improve the coordination between voluntary movement and balance control.

Inglin and Woollacott[49] adopted the reaction-time paradigm, in which a specific reaction is expected to occur in response to a designated stimulus, to assess the effect of central set on anticipatory postural responses. Four reaction-time conditions (simple arm pull, simple arm push, choice arm pull and choice arm push) were tested on 15 young and 15 older subjects. In the simple reaction-time conditions, subjects were informed of the movement direction in advance, and all of the push or pull trials were performed consecutively. In the choice reaction-time conditions, no such information was provided and the push and pull trials were tested at random. Thus, central set was expected to be set at a lower level in the choice conditions than in the simple conditions. The results revealed that for the choice conditions, older adults showed a significantly greater increase in onset latencies of the postural and focal (primary mover) muscles than young adults in both the arm pull and push conditions (see Fig. 20.8). However, for the simple conditions, significant age differences were only found for arm push trials. Thus, the age differences in postural and voluntary performance were greater under the unpredictable, low-level central set choice reaction-time conditions than under the predictable, high-level central set simple reaction-time conditions.

Using the SOT paradigm, Teasdale and colleagues[159] evaluated the ability of young and older adults to quickly reconfigure the postural set when experiencing successively reduced or augmented visual sensory conditions. They found that both young and elderly adults increased the sway dispersion when the sensory condition was suddenly changed from the with-vision to no-vision condition. When the sensory condition was suddenly changed from the no-vision to with-vision condition, young adults were able to adapt rapidly and reduced their sway dispersion whereas older adults demonstrated an increased sway dispersion. The inabil-

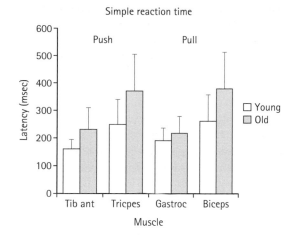

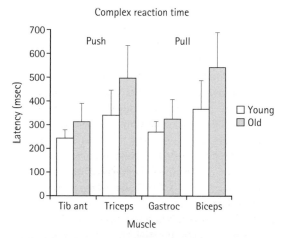

Figure 20.8 *Mean onset latencies (ms) and standard deviations of postural and focal (prime mover) muscles in young and older adults for simple vs. choice (complex) reaction time movements in which they pushed or pulled on a handle while standing. Tib ant, tibialis anterior; Gastroc, gastrocnemius.*

ity of older adults to adapt to an augmented sensory condition suggests that they may have a deficit related to changing their sensorimotor set when the environment is suddenly altered.

As a whole, these findings imply that older adults may be more sensitive to the level of central set or have greater difficulty in reconfiguring central set according to environmental and task demands than young adults. When the environmental and task conditions are more predictable (i.e. with a high level of central set) older adults were able to successfully and efficiently integrate postural and voluntary movement control. However, when the conditions become unpredictable, such integration suffers to a great extent. These age-related differences in the influence of central set on postural control may also account for the decreased environmental adaptability of older adults as mentioned above. Table 20.1 summarizes the results of these studies.

Age-related changes in cognitive demands for balance control

Scientists used to believe that balance control in healthy adults, because of its being practiced daily, required minimum cognitive processing. Over the past decade, however, studies using the dual-task paradigm revealed that the processing involved in balance control requires attention. Attentional demands have been found to increase with an increase in balance requirements of a task. That is, the more complex and dynamic balance tasks are more attention-demanding than the simple and static balance tasks.[145,160] For example, it has been found that attentional demands are greatest when a person is in the single support phase of walking, followed by the double support phase of walking, then by standing with a wide base of support and then by standing with feet together; they are least when the person is sitting.[145,160]

With advanced aging, attentional demands for a given balance task are, in general, increased.[146,147] It has been hypothesized that the need for greater amounts of attention with advanced aging is due to the poorer balance control of older adults. This hypothesis is supported by the following two studies. Using a dual-task paradigm, Shumway-Cook and colleagues[148] compared standing balance performance among healthy young adults, older non-fallers and older fallers. The results showed that the introduction of a secondary cognitive task, such as a sentence completion or a visual spatial orientation task, significantly affected both groups of older adults, especially those older adults with a history of falls. Although the center of pressure (COP) path increased significantly from performing the postural task alone to performing dual-tasks for both the balance groups of older adults, this increase was significantly much greater for impaired older adults. Similarly, Lundin-Olsson and associates[161] found that older adults that were more easily affected by the addition of a secondary motor task (carrying a tumbler of water, during the Timed Up-and-Go mobility test) were more likely to fall in a 6-month follow-up period.

In addition, the sensitivity of attentional demands to the complexity of a balance task is often more obvious for older adults than for young adults. For example, Lajoie et al.[147] found that, in the dual-task research paradigm, older adults showed greater reduction in the performance of the secondary verbal cognitive task than young adults as the primary balance task changed from standing with wide base of support to standing with narrow base of support. The reduction of the performance in the secondary task is considered a reflection of the need for greater demands of attentional allocation to the primary balance task when standing with a narrow support base. Similarly, Teasdale et al.[145,146] found a significantly greater reduction of performance on the secondary verbal task in older adults, compared with young adults, when they were changing from standing with normal vision and surface conditions to standing with no vision or altered surface conditions.

Shumway-Cook and Woollacott[162] tested the ability of young adults, healthy older adults and older adults with a history of falls to simultaneously perform a standing balance task in six sensory conditions and a verbal cognitive task. The six sensory conditions used were: (1) firm surface with the eyes open; (2) firm surface with the eyes closed; (3) firm surface with optokinetic stimulation; (4) sway-referenced surface with the eyes open; (5) sway-referenced surface with the eyes closed; and (6) sway-referenced surface with optokinetic stimulation. It was found that while postural performance of the young adults was not affected by the introduction of the secondary task in any of the six sensory conditions, the effects of the introduction of the secondary task on postural stability of older adults depended greatly on the sensory conditions. Postural stability of healthy older adults was affected by the secondary verbal task only when both the visual and somatosensory information was altered. For older fallers, however, the introduction of the secondary task significantly impaired their balance performance in all six sensory conditions, indicating that the attentional demands for balance tasks in older fallers are highly susceptible to any changes in sensory information.

Recently, another line of research has investigated whether age-related increases in attentional demand for postural tasks place significant impacts on the ability of older adults to recover their balance after experiencing a postural threat. Brown and colleagues[136] compared the attentional demands required for using the ankle, hip and stepping strategy between healthy older and young adults when regaining balance after a translational platform perturbation. A backward-counting mathematical task was used as the secondary cognitive task. While it was found that the attentional demands for regaining balance were not different among the types of balance-recovery strategies being used for young adults, using the stepping strategy to regain balance appeared to require a greater amount of attention than using other strategies for older adults. In addition, the use of the stepping strategy was significantly more attentionally demanding for the older adults than for the young adults. Given the known preference for using the stepping strategy for balance recovery in older adults, it was suggested that older adults may become more prone to falling if adequate attentional resources cannot be allocated in time for the preparation and execution of the stepping strategy.[136] A recent study investigating the neuromuscular postural responses of young and older adults in the same dual-task condition as that in the study by Brown and associates[136] showed that older adults did present significant difficulty in allocating more attentional demands to postural tasks when a secondary cognitive task was added.[163] When the backward

counting task was added to the balance recovery task, it was found that older adults showed a significantly greater reduction in the primary postural responses than young adults. Table 20.1 summarizes the results of these studies.

Clinical implications

The systems approach provides a useful guideline to investigate the complex nature of the age-related changes in balance control subsystems as well as the interaction mechanisms among these changes. It has to be kept in mind that a dramatic decline in balance control abilities may not be evident in older adults with a deficit in a single balance-related subsystem. It is often the age-related decline in multiple balance-associated systems that lead to a significant balance and functional decline in older adults.[164] Thus, clinicians may apply this approach to examining the function of the various balance-related subsystems in older adults. With this approach, clinicians will be able to identify the specific underlying causes of different balance problems and develop task- and individual-specific balance-training protocols.

A comprehensive assessment of balance function from the systems perspective would include examining the older adult performing a range of balance tasks under a variety of contexts. By varying the contexts the clinician can examine musculoskeletal, sensory, motor and cognitive components of balance control. Of course, safety is a primary concern when examining older adults with balance disorders, since they are at high risk for falls. Thus, they must be protected at all times, wearing an ambulation belt, with the clinician staying close to them during assessment, but not touching them, in order to accurately measure their balance abilities. Balance tasks to be assessed would include steady state (quiet stance), reactive and proactive balance control. The underlying components of balance control to be assessed include the musculoskeletal, sensory, motor and cognitive systems.[77]

There are a variety of functional tests of balance that can be used to assess balance performance. Self report measures include the Activities-specific Balance Confidence (ABC) Scale,[165] which tests the confidence of an older adult in their ability to carry out activities such as walking around the house (steady state and proactive balance), going up and down stairs (steady state and proactive balance), bending to pick up a slipper (proactive balance), getting in and out of a car (proactive balance), walking in a crowd and being bumped (reactive balance) and walking on an icy surface (reactive balance).

Performance measures include the Berg Balance Scale,[51] which evaluates balance by examining performance on 14 different tasks which are scored from 0 to 4. These include such tasks as standing unsupported (steady state), reaching forward with the outstretched arm (proactive), picking up an object off the floor (proactive) and standing on one leg (steady state and proactive). Note that this scale does not have any tasks that test reactive balance. The Performance-Oriented Mobility Assessment[59] does, however, include a reactive measure, in which the clinician nudges the sternum of the patient to give them a balance perturbation and determines the extent to which they recover balance in an efficient manner (steady, staggers, or begins to fall).[77] In addition to these tests, a very quick test, the Timed Up and Go Test[58] is a quick screening tool for detecting balance problems in elderly patients. The clinician simply times the patient as they stand up from a chair, walk 3 m, turn around and return. Healthy adults are able to perform the test in less than 10 s. Adults taking more than 30 s to complete the test are considered dependent in most activities of daily living.

It is also important to assess underlying sensory (visual, somatosensory and vestibular), neuromuscular (coordination of balance responses and the ability to use an ankle, hip or step strategy in response to a nudge to the sternum) and musculoskeletal components (strength, ROM and alignment) contributing to balance function, in order to determine the underlying factors contributing to decreases in balance performance, as measured by the above performance tests.[77]

CONCLUSIONS

In this chapter, we have reviewed the important issues and findings pertaining to aging and balance control in older adults. Both aging and balance control are multifactorial processes. Although it is common to discover age-related changes in balance control subsystems, recent studies have shown that older age is not uniformly associated with reductions in the ability to perform functional activities.[26,27] It is important to keep in mind that not all of the age-related changes in balance subsystems are inevitable or irreversible. With sufficient intensity of exercise and changes in lifestyle such as diet and activity level, it is possible to improve balance and mobility performance in older adults and decrease the incidence of falls in this population.[27] Balance control mechanisms are task-specific. Balance tasks range from being dynamic and complex to simple and static. Using the systems approach, researchers are able to identify a variety of balance control subsystems and age-related changes in these subsystems for the wide variety of balance tasks. By systematically examining each balance control subsystem, clinicians are able to make a more thorough assessment of balance control mechanisms. Task- and individual-specific interventions can thus be developed. Thus, it is recommended that a battery of balance assessments, ranging from simple static tasks to complex dynamic tasks, be used in clinics.

ACKNOWLEDGEMENTS

This work was supported by NIH grant AG05317 to Dr M. Woollacott.

REFERENCES

1. Campbell AJ, Reinken J, Alan BC, Martinez GS. Falls in old age: a study of frequency and related clinical factors. *Age Ageing* 1981;**10**:264–70.
2. Gryfe CI, Amies A, Ashley MJ. 1977. A longitudinal study of falls in an elderly population: I. Incidence and morbidity. *Age Ageing* **6**:201–10.
3. Lord SR, Ward JA, Williams P, Anstey KJ. An epidemiological study of falls in older community-dwelling women: the Randwick falls and fractures study. *Aust J Public Health* 1993;**17**(3):240–5.
4. Prudham D, Evans JG. Factors associated with falls in the elderly: a community study. *Age Ageing* 1981;**10**:141–6.
5. Tinetti ME, Speechley M, Ginter SF. Risk factors for falls among elderly persons living in the community. *N Engl J Med* 1988;**319**(26):1701–7.
6. Aronow WS, Abn C. Association of postprandial hypotension with incidence of fall, syncope, coronary events, stroke, and total mortality at 29-month follow-up in 499 older nursing home residents. *J Am Geriatr Soc* 1997;**45**:1051–3.
7. Baker SP, Harvey AH. Fall injuries in the elderly. *Clin Geriatr Med* 1985;**1**(3):501–11.
8. Fernie GR, Gryfe CI, Holliday PJ, Llewwllyn A. The relationship of postural sway in standing to the incidence of falls in geriatrics subjects. *Age Ageing* 1982;**11**:11–16.
9. Nevitt MC, Cummings SR, The study of osteoporotics fractures research group. Falls and fratures in older women. In: Vellas B, Toupet M, Rubenstein L, et al., eds. *Falls, balance and gait disorders in the elderly*. Paris: Elsevier, 1992;69–80.
10. Nyberg L, Gustafson Y, Janson A, Sandman PO, Eriksson S. Incidence of falls in three different types of geriatric care. A Swedish prospective study. *Scand J Soc Med* 1997;**25**(1):8–13
11. Wickham C, Cooper C, Magretts BM, Barker DJP. Muscle strength, activity, housing and risk of falls in elderly people. *Age Ageing* 1989;**18**:47–51.
12. Sattin RW, Huber DAL, DeVito CA, et al. The incidence of fall injury events among the elderly in a defined population. *Am J Epidemiol* 1990;**131**(6):1028–37.
13. Lipsitz LA, Jonsson PV, Kelley MM, Koestner JS. Causes and correlates of recurrent falls in ambulatory frail elderly. *J Gerontol* 1991;**46**(4):M114–22.
14. Rubenstein LZ, Josephson KR, Robbins A. Falls in the nursing home. *Ann Intern Med* 1994;**121**:442–51.
15. Rubenstein LZ, Josephson KR, Osterweil D. Falls and fall prevention in the nursing home. *Clin Geriatr Med* 1996;**12**(4):881–902.

16. Sheldon JH. On the natural history of falls in old age. *BMJ* 1960;December:1685–90.

17. Wolfson LI, Whipple R, Amerman P, et al. Gait and balance in the elderly. *Clin Geriatr Med* 1985;1(3):649–59.

18. Rowe JW, Kahn RL. Human aging: Usual and successful aging. *Science* 1987;237:143–9.

19. Calne DB, Calne JS. Normality and disease. *Can J Neurol Sci* 1988; 15: 3–4.

20. Calne DB, Eisen A, Meneilly G. Normal aging of the nervous system. *Ann Neurol* 1991; 30: 206–7.

21. Woollacott MH. Aging, posture control, and movement preparation. In: Woollacott MH, Shumway-Cook A, eds. *Development of posture and gait across the life span.* Columbia: University of South Carolina Press, 1989;155–75.

22. Sawle GV, Brooks DJ. Normal aging of the nervous system. *Ann Neurol* 1992;31(5):575–7.

23. Sawle GV, Colebatch JG, Shah A, et al. Striatal function in normal aging: implications for Parkinson's disease. *Ann Neurol* 1990;28:799–804.

24. Berkman LF, Seeman TE, Albert M, et al. High, usual and impaired functioning in community-dwelling older men and women: findings from the Macarthur Foundation research network on successful aging. *J Clin Epidemiol* 1993;46(10):1129–40.

25. Schoenfeld DE, Malmrose LC, Blazer DG, et al. Self-rated health and mortality in the high-functioning elderly-a closer look at healthy individuals: MacArthur Field study of successful aging. *J Gerontol Med Sci* 1994;49(3):M109–15.

26. Seeman TE, Charpentier PA, Berkman LF, et al. Predicting changes in physical performance in a high-functioning elderly cohort: MacArthur studies of successful aging. *J Gerontol Med Sci* 1994;49(3):M97–108.

27. Seeman TE, Berkman LF, Charpentier PA, et al. Behavioral and psychosocial predictors of physical performance: MacArthur studies of successful aging. *J Gerontol Med Sci* 1995;50A(4):M177–83.

28. Nashner LM. Practical biomechanics and physiology of balance. In: Jacobson GP, Newman CW, Kartush JM, eds. *Handbook of balance function testing.* St Louis: Mosby Year Book, 1993;261–79.

29. Winter DA, MacFayden BJ, Dickey JP. Adaptability of the CNS in human walking. In: Patla AE, ed. *Adaptability of human gait.* Amsterdam: Elsevier, 1991;127–44.

30. Horak FB, Macpherson JM. Postural orientation and equilibrium. In: Rowell LB, Shepard JT, eds. *Handbook of physiology. Volume Section 12: exercise: regulation and integration of multiple systems.* New York: Oxford University Press, 1996;255–92.

31. Patla AE, Winter DA, Frank JS, et al. Identification of age-related changes in the balance-control system. In: Duncan PW, ed. *Balance.* Alexandria: American Physical Therapy Association, 1989;43–55.

32. Patla AE, Frank J, Winter DA. Assessment of balance control in the elderly: major issues. *Physiother Can* 1990;42(2):89–97.

33. Tang P-F, Woollacott MH. Balance control in the elderly. In: Bronstein AM, Brandt T, Woollacott MH, eds. *Clinical disorders of balance, posture and gait.* London: Arnold, 1996;268–86.

34. Briggs RC, Gossman MR, Birch R, Drews JE, Shaddeau SA. Balance performance among noninstitutionalized elderly women. *Phys Ther* 1989;69(9):748–56.

35. Heitmann DK, Gossman MR, Shaddeau SA, Jackson JR. Balance performance and step width in noninstitutionalized, elderly, female fallers and nonfallers. *Phys Ther* 1989;69(11):923–31.

36. Maki BE, Holliday PJ, Fernie GR. Aging and postural control. *J Am Geriatr Soc* 1990;38:1–9.

37. Overstall PW, Exton-Smith AN, Imms FJ, Johnson AL. Falls in the elderly related to postural imbalance. *BMJ* 1977;January:261–4.

38. Horak FB, Henry SM, Shumway-Cook A. Postural perturbations: New insights for treatment of balance disorders. *Phys Ther* 1997;77(5):517–33.

39. Wolfson LI, Whipple R, Amerman P, Kleinberg A. Stressing the postural response: a quantitative method for testing balance. *J Am Geriatr Soc* 1986;34:845–50.

40. Gu MJ, Schultz AB, Shepard NT, Alexander NB. Postural control in young and elderly adults when stance is perturbed: Dynamics. *J Biomech* 1996;29(3):319–29.

41. Horak FB, Shupert CL, Mirka A. Components of postural dyscontrol in the elderly: A review. *Neurobiol Aging* 1989;10:727–38.

42. Manchester D, Woollacott MH, Zederbauer-Hylton N, Marin O. Visual, vestibular and somatosensory contributions to balance control in the older adults. *J Gerontol Med Sci* 1989;44(4):M118–27.

43. Pai YC, Rogers MW, Patton J, et al. Static versus dynamic predictions of protective stepping following waist-pull perturbations in young and older adults. *J Biomech* 1998;31:1111–8.

44. Woollacott MH, Shumway-Cook A, Nashner LM. Aging and posture control: changes in sensory organization and muscular coordination. *Int J Aging Hum Dev* 1986;23(2):97–114.

45. Anacker SL, Di Fabio RP. Influence of sensory inputs on standing balance in community-dwelling elders with a recent history of falling. *Phys Ther* 1992;72(8):575–84.

46. Camicioli R, Panzer VP, Kaye J. Balance in the healthy elderly: posturography and clinical assessment. *Arch Neurol* 1997;54(8):976–81.

47. Judge JO, King MB, Whipple R, et al. Dynamic balance in older persons: effects of reduced visual and proprioceptive input. *J Gerontol* 1995;50A(5):M263–70.

48. Massion J. Movement, posture and equilibrium: Interaction and coordination. *Prog Neurobiol* 1992;38:35–56.

49. Inglin B, Woollacott MH. Age-related changes in anticipatory postural adjustments associated with arm movements. *J Gerontol* 1988;41(4):M105–13.

50. Rogers MW, Kukulka CG, Soderberg GL. Age-related changes in postural responses preceding rapid self-paced and reaction time arm movements. *J Gerontol* 1992;47(5):M159–65.

51. Berg K, Wood-Dauphinee SL, Williams JI. Measuring balance in the elderly: validation of an instrument. *Can J Public Health* 1992;83(Suppl 2):S7–11.

52. Duncan PW, Weiner DK, Chandler J, Studenski S. Functional reach: a new clinical measure of balance. *J Gerontol* 1990;45(6):M192–7.

53. Ikeda E, Schenkman M, Riley PO, Hodge WA. Influence of age on dynamics of rising from a chair. *Phys Ther* 1991;71(6):473–81.

54. Mathias S, Nayak USL, Issacs B. Balance in elderly patients: the 'Get-up and Go' test. *Arch Phys Med Rehabil* 1986;67:387–9.

55. Millington PJ, Myklebust BM, Shambes GM. Biomechanical analysis of the sit-to-stand motion in elderly persons. *Arch Phys Med Rehabil* 1992;**73**:609–17.

56. Pai YC, Naughton BJ, Chang RW, Rogers MW. Control of body centre of mass momentum during sit-to-stand among young and elderly adults. *Gait Posture* 1994;**2**:109–16.

57. Papa E, Cappozzo A. Sit-to-stand motor strategies investigated in able-bodied young and elderly subjects. *J Biomech* 2000;**33**:1113–22.

58. Podsiadlo D, Richardson S. The timed 'Up & Go': A test of basic functional mobility for frail elderly persons. *J Am Geriatr Soc* 1991;**39**:142–8.

59. Tinetti ME. Performance-oriented assessment of mobility problems in elderly patients. *J Am Geriatr Soc* 1986;**34**:119–26.

60. Vander Linden DW, Brunt D, McCulluoch MU. Variant and invariant characteristics of the sit-to-stand task in healthy elderly adults. *Arch Phys Med Rehabil* 1994;**75**:653–60.

61. VanSwearingen JM, Paschal KA, Bonino P, Yang J-F. The modified gait abnormality rating scale for recognizing the risk of recurrent falls in community-dwelling elderly adults. *Phys Ther* 1996;**76**(9):995–1002.

62. Wolfson LI, Whipple R, Amerman P, Tobin JN. Gait assessment in the elderly: a gait abnormality rating scale and its relation to falls. *J Gerontol Med Sci* 1990;**45**(1):M12–19.

63. Duncan PW, Studenski S, Chandler J, Prescott B. Functional reach: predictive validity in a sample of elderly male veterans. *J Gerontol* 1992;**47**(3):M93–8.

64. Shumway-Cook A, Baldwin M, Polissar NL, Gruber W. Predicting the probability for falls in community-dwelling older adults. *Phys Ther* 1997;**77**(8):812–19.

65. Shumway-Cook A, Brauer S, Woollacott M. Predicting the probability of falls in community-dwelling older adults using the Timed Up and Go test. *Phys Ther* 2000;**80**(9):896–903.

66. Studenski S, Duncan PW, Chandler J, et al. Predicting falls: The role of mobility and nonphysical factors. *J Am Geriatr Assoc* 1994;**42**:297–302.

67. Chen HC, Ashton-Miller JA, Alexander NB, Schultz AB. Stepping over obstacles: gait patters of healthy young and old adults. *J Gerontol* 1991;**46**:M196–203.

68. Chen H-C, Ashton-Miller JA, Alexander NB, Schultz AB. Age effects on strategies used to avoid obstacles. *Gait Posture* 1994a;**2**:139–46.

69. Chen HC, Ashton-Miller JA, Alexander NB, Schultz AB. Effects of age and available response time on ability to step over an obstacle. *J Gerontol* 1994;**49**(5):M227–33.

70. Chen HC, Schultz AB, Ashton-Miller JA, et al. Stepping over obstacles: dividing attention impairs performance of old more than young adults. *J Gerontol Med Sci* 1996;**51A**(3):M116–22.

71. Tang P-F, Woollacott MH, Chong RKY. Decreased adaptation to repeated surface perturbations during walking in older adults. In: *Society for Neuroscience Abstracts. New Orleans, Louisiana, October 25–30, 1997*;1562. New Orleans: Society for Neuroscience.

72. Tang P-F, Woollacott MH. Inefficient postural responses to unexpected slips during walking in older adults. *J Gerontol Med Sci* 1998;**53A**(6):M471–80.

73. Tang P-F, Woollacott MH. Phase-dependent modulation of proximal and distal postural responses to slips in young and older adults. *J Gerontol Med Sci* 1999;**54A**(2):M89–102.

74. Bernstein N. *The co-ordination and regulation of movements*, 1st edn. Oxford: Pergamon Press, 1967.

75. Kugler PN, Kelso JAS, Turvey MT. On the control and co-ordination of naturally developing systems. In: Kelso JAS, Clark JE, eds. *The development of movement control and co-ordination*. Chichester: John Wiley and Sons, 1982;5–78.

76. Woollacott MH, Shumway-Cook A. Changes in posture control across the life span – a systems approach. *Phys Ther* 1990;**70**(12):799–53–807/61.

77. Shumway-Cook A, Woollacott MH. *Motor control: theory and practical application*. Philadelphia: Lippincott, Williams and Wilkins, 2001.

78. Harak F. Clinical assessment of balance disorders. *Gait Posture* 1997;**6**:76–84.

79. Horak FB. Assumptions underlying motor control for neurologic rehabilitation. In: Lister MJ, ed. *Contemporary management of motor control problems: proceedings of the II STEP conference*. Alexandria: Foundation of Physical Therapy, 1991;11–27.

80. Nashner LM. *Analysis of movement control in man using the movable platform*. New York: Raven Press, 1983.

81. Patla AE. Age-related changes in visually guided locomotion over different terrains: major issues. In: Stelmach GE, Homberg V, eds. *Sensorimotor impairment in the elderly*. Dordrecht: Kluwer Academic Publishers, 1993;231–52.

82. Birren JE. Vibratory sensibility in the aged. *J Gerontol* 1974;**2**:267–8.

83. De Michele G, Filla A, Coppola N, et al. Influence of age, gender, height and education on vibration sense. A study by tuning fork in 192 normal subjects. *J Neurol Sci* 1991;**105**(2):155–8.

84. Kokmen E, Bossemeyer RW, Williams WIJ. Quantitative evaluation of joint motion sensation in an aging population. *J Gerontol* 1978;**33**(1):62–7.

85. MacLennan MJ, Timothy JI, Hall MRP. Vibration sense, proprioception and ankle reflexes in old age. *J Clin Exp Gerontol* 1980;**2**:159–71.

86. Potvin AR, Syndulko K, Tourtellotte WW, et al. Human neurologic function and the aging process. *J Am Geriatr Soc.* 1980;**28**(1):1–9.

87. Skinner HB, Barrack RL, Cook SD. Age-related decline in proprioception. *Clin Orthop* 1984;**184**:208–11.

88. Waite LM, Broe GA, Creasey H, et al. Neurological signs, aging, and the neurodegenerative syndromes. *Arch Neurol* 1996;**53**(6):498–502.

89. Bergin PS, Bronstein AM, Murray NM, et al. Body sway and vibration perception thresholds in normal aging and in patients with polyneuropathy. *J Neurol Neurosurg Psychiatry.* 1995;**58**(3):335–40.

90. Brocklehurst JC, Robertson D, James-Groom P. Clinical correlates of sway in old age-sensory modalities. *Age Ageing* 1982;**11**:1–10.

91. Lord SR, Clark RD, Webster IW. Postural stability and associated physiological factors in a population of aged persons. *J Gerontol Med Sci* 1991;**46**(3):M69–76.

92. Lord SR, Ward JA. Age-associated differences in sensori-motor function and balance in community dwelling women. *Age Ageing* 1994;**23**:452–60.

93. Lord SR, Lloyd DG, Li SK. Sensori-motor function, gait patters and falls in community-dwelling women. *Age Ageing* 1996;25:292–9.

94. Colledge NR, Cantley P, Peaston I, et al. Ageing and balance: the measurement of spontaneous sway by posturography. *Gerontology* 1994;40(5):273–8.

95. Horak FB, Shupert CL, Dietz V, Horstmann G. Vestibular and somatosensory contributions to responses to head and body displacements in stance. *Exp Brain Res* 1994;100:93–106.

96. Inglis JT, Horak FB, Shupert CL, Jones-Rycewicz C. The importance of somatosensory information in triggering and scaling automatic postural responses in humans. *Exp Brain Res* 1994;101:159–64.

97. Lord SR, Rogers MW, Howland A, Fitzpatrick R. Lateral stability, sensorimotor function and falls in older people. *J Am Geriatr Soc* 1999;47:1077–81.

98. Paulus WM, Straube A, Brandt Th. Visual stabilization of posture: physiological stimulus characteristics and clinical aspects. *Brain* 1984;107:1143–63.

99. Gittings NS, Fozard JL. Age related changes in visual acuity. *J Gerontol* 1986;21:423–33.

100. Owsley C, Sekuler R, Siemsen D. Contrast sensitivity throughout adulthood. *Vis Res* 1983; 23: 689–99.

101. Pitts DG. Visual acuity as a function of age. *J Am Optom Assoc* 1982;53:117–24.

102. Simoneau GG, Cavanagh PR, Ulbrecht JS, et al. The influence of visual factors on fall-related kinematic variables during stair descent by older women. *J Gerontol* 1991;46(6):M188–95.

103. Leibowitz HW, Shupert CL. Spatial orientation mechanisms and their implications for falls. *Clin Geriatr Med* 1985;1(3):571–80.

104. Amblard B, Carblanc A. Role of foveal and peripheral visual information in maintenance of postural equilibrium in man. *Percept Mot Skills* 1980;51:903–12.

105. Stoffregen TA. Flow structure versus retinal location in the optical control of stance. *J Exp Psychol Hum Percept Perform* 1985;11(5):554–65.

106. Sekuler R, Hutman LP, Owsley CJ. Human aging and spatial vision. *Science* 1980;209(12):1255–6.

107. Brownlee MG, Banks MA, Crosbie WJ, et al. Consideration of spatial orientation mechanism as related to elderly fallers. *Gerontology* 1989;35:323–31.

108. Warren JWH, Blackwell AW, Morris MW. Age differences in perceiving the direction of self-motion from optical flow. *J Gerontol Psychol Sci* 1989;44(5):147–53.

109. Borger LL, Whitney SL, Redfern MS, Furman JM. The influence of dynamic visual environments on postural sway in the elderly. *J Vestib Res* 1999;9(3):197–205.

110. Sundermier L, Woollacott MH, Jensen JL, Moore S. Postural sensitivity to visual flow in aging adults with and without balance problems. *J Gerontol* 1996;51A(2):M45–52.

111. Ring C. Visual push: a sensitive measure of dynamic balance in man. *Arch Phys Med Rehabil* 1988;69:256–60.

112. Horstmann GA, Dietz V. The contribution of vestibular input to the stabilization of human posture: A new experimental approach. *Neurosci Lett* 1988;95:179–84.

113. Allum JHJ, Pfaltz CR. Visual and vestibular contributions to pitch sway stabilization in the ankle muscle of normals and patients with bilateral peripheral vestibular deficits. *Exp Brain Res* 1985;58:82–94.

114. Allum JHJ, Honegger F, Pfaltz CR. The role of stretch and vestibulo-spinal reflexes in the generation of human equilibriating reactions. *Prog Brain Res* 1989;80:399–409.

115. Nashner LM. Computerized dynamic posturography. In: Jacobson GP, Newman CW, Kartush JM, eds. *Handbook of balance function testing*. St Louis, MO: Mosby Year Book, 1993:280–307.

116. Black FO, Peterka RJ, Shupert CL, Nashner LM. Effects of unilateral loss of vestibular function on the vestibulo-ocular reflex and postural control. *Ann Otol Rhinol Laryngol* 1989;98:884–9.

117. Bronstein AM. Suppression of visually evoked postural responses. *Exp Brain Res* 1986;63:655–8.

118. Rosenhall U. Degenerative patterns in the aging humanvestibular neuro-epithelia. *Acta Otolaryngol* 1973;76:208–20.

119. Bergstrom B. Morphology of the vestibular nerve II: The number of myelinated vestibular nerve fibers in man at various ages. *Acta Otolaryngol* 1973;76(2):173–9.

120. Alvarez JC, Diaz C, Suarez C, et al. Aging and the human vestibular nuclei: morphometric analysis. *Mech Ageing Dev* 2000;114(3):149–72.

121. Peterka RJ, Black FO. Age-related changes in human posture control: Sensory Organization Test. *J Vestib Res* 1990;1:73–85.

122. Di Fabio RP, Emasithi A. Aging and the mechanisms underlying head and postural control during voluntary motion. *Phys Ther* 1997;77(5):458–75.

123. Nardone A, Grasso M, Tarantola J, et al. Postural coordination in elderly subjects standing on a periodically moving platform. *Arch Phys Med Rehabil* 2000;81:1217–23.

124. Do MC, Breniere Y, Brenguier P. A biomechanical study of balance recovery during the forward fall. *J Biomech* 1982;15(13):933–9.

125. Nashner LM. Fixed patterns of rapid postural responses among leg muscles during stance. *Exp Brain Res* 1977;30:13–24.

126. Horak FB, Nashner LM. Central programming of postural movements; Adaptation to altered support-surface configuration. *J Neurophysiol* 1986;55(6):1369–81.

127. Luchies CW, Alexander NB, Schultz AB, Ashton-Miller JA. Stepping responses of young and old adults to postural disturbances: Kinematics. *J Am Geriatr Soc* 1994;42:506–12.

128. Thelen DG, Wojcik LA, Schultz AB, et al. Age differences in using a rapid step to regain balance during a forward fall. *J Gerontol Med Sci* 1997;52A(1):M8–13.

129. Nashner LM, McCollum G. The organization of human postural movements: a formal basis and experimental synthesis. *Behav Brain Sci* 1985;8:135–72.

130. McIlroy WE, Maki BE. Task constraints on foot movement and the incidence of compensatory stepping following perturbation of upright stance. *Brain Res* 1993;616:30–8.

131. McIlroy WE, Maki BE. Adaptive changes to compensatory stepping responses. *Gait Posture* 1995;3:43–50.

132. Tang P-F, Woollacott MH, Chong RKY. Control of reactive balance adjustments in perturbed human walking: roles of proximal and distal postural muscle activity. *Exp Brain Res* 1998;119(2):114–52.

133. McIlroy WE, Maki BE. Age-related changes in compensatory stepping in response to unpredictable perturbations. *J Gerontol* 1996;51A(6):M289–96.

134. Maki BE, McIlroy WE. The role of limb movements in

maintaining upright stance: The 'change-in-support' strategy. *Phys Ther* 1997;**77**(5):488–507.

135. Maki BE, Edmondstone MA, McIlroy WE. Age-related differences in laterally directed compensatory stepping behavior. *J Gerontol Med Sci* 2000;**55A**(5):M270–7.

136. Brown LA, Shumway-Cook A, Woollacott MH. Attentional demands and postural recovery: the effects of aging. *J Gerontol : Med Sci* 1999;**54A**(4):M165–71.

137. McIlroy WE, Maki BE. The control of lateral stability during rapid stepping reactions evoked by antero-posterior perturbation: does anticipation play a role? *Gait Posture* 1999;**9**:190–8.

138. Pai YC, Maki BE, Iqbal K, et al. Thresholds for step initiation induced by support-surface translation: a dynamic center-of-mass model provides much better prediction than a static model. *J Biomech* 2000;**33**:387–92.

139. Rogers MW, Hain TC, Hanke TA, Janssen I. Stimulus parameters and inertial load: effects on the incidence of protective stepping responses in healthy human subjects. *Arch Phys Med Rehabil* 1996;**77**:363–8.

140. Stelmach GE, Phillips J, Di Fabio RP, Teasdale N. Age, functional postural reflexes, and voluntary sway. *J Gerontol Biol Sci* 1989;**44**(4):B100–6.

141. Lexell J. Human aging, muscle mass, and fiber type composition. *J Gerontol Ser A* 1995;**50A**(Spec Iss):11–6.

142. Hall CD, Woollacott MH, Jensen JL. Age-related changes in rate and magnitude of ankle torque development: implications for balance control. *J Gerontol Med Sci* 1999;**54A**(10):M507–13.

143. Thelen DG, Schultz AB, Alexander NB, Ashton-Miller JA. Effects of age on rapid ankle torque development. *J Gerontol Med Sci* 1996;**51A**(5):M226–32.

144. Horak FB, Diener HC, Nashner LM. Influence of central set on human postural responses. *J Neurophysiol* 1989;**62**(4):841–53.

145. Teasdale N, Lajoie Y, Bard C, et al. Cognitive processes involved for maintaining postural stability while standing and walking. In: Stelmach GE, Homberg V, eds. *Sensorimotor impairment in the elderly*. Dordrecht: Kluwer Academic Publishers, 1993;157–68.

146. Teasdale N, Larue J, Bard C, Fluery M. On the cognitive penetrability of posture control. *Exp Aging Res* 1993;**19**:1–13.

147. Lajoie Y, Teasdale N, Bard C, Fleury M. Attentional demands for walking: age-related changes. In: Ferrandez AM, Teasdale N, eds. *Changes in sensory motor behavior in aging*. Amsterdam: Elsevier Science, 1996;235–56.

148. Shumway-Cook A, Woollacott M, Kerns KA, Baldwin M. The effects of two types of cognitive tasks on postural stability in older adults with and without a history of falls. *J Gerontol Med Sci* 1997;**52A**(4):M232–40.

149. Gehlsen GM, Whaley MH. Falls in the elderly: Part II, balance, strength, and flexibility. *Arch Phys Med Rehabil* 1990;**71**:739–41.

150. Larsson L, Grimby G, Karlsson J. Muscle strength and speed of movement in relation to age and muscle morphology. *J Appl Physiol* 1979;**46**(3):451–6.

151. Vandervoort AA, McComas AJ. Contractile changes in opposing muscles of the human ankle joint with aging. *J Appl Physiol* 1986;**61**:361–7.

152. Vandervoort AA, Hill K, Sandrin M, Vyse VM. Mobility impairment and falling in the elderly. *Physiother Can* 1990;**42**(2):99–107.

153. Walker JM, Sue D, Miles-Elkousy N, et al. Active mobility of the extremities in older subjects. *Phys Ther* 1984;**64**(6):919–23.

154. Whipple RH, Wolfson LI, Amerman PM. The relationship of knee and ankle weakness to falls in nursing home residents: an isokinetic study. *J Am Geriatr Soc* 1987;**35**:13–20.

155. Foldvari M, Clark M, Laviolette L, et al. Association of muscle power with functional status in community-dwelling elderly women. *J Gerontol Med Sci* 2000;**55A**(4):M192–9.

156. Daubney ME, Culham EG. Lower-extremity muscle force and balance performance in adults aged 65 years and older. *Phys Ther* 1999;**79**(12):1177–85.

157. Nashner LM. Adapting reflexes controlling the human posture. *Exp Brain Res* 1976;**26**:59–72.

158. Cordo PJ, Nashner LM. Properties of postural adjustments associated with rapid arm movements. *J Neurophysiol* 1982;**47**(2):287–302.

159. Teasdale N, Stelmach GE, Breunig A, Meeuwsen HJ. Age differences in visual sensory integration. *Exp Brain Res* 1991;**85**:691–6.

160. Lajoie Y, Teasdale N, Fleury CBM. Attentional demands for static and dynamic equilibrium. *Exp Brain Res* 1993;**97**:139–44.

161. Lundin-Olsson L, Nyberg L, Gustafson Y. Attention, frailty, and falls: the effect of a manual task on basic mobility. *J Am Geriatr Soc* 1998;**46**:758–61.

162. Shumway-Cook A, Woollacott M. Attentional demands and postural control: the effect of sensory context. *J Gerontol Med Sci* 2000;**55A**(1):M10–16.

163. Rankin JK, Woollacott MH, Shumway-Cook A, Brown LA. Cognitive influence on postural stability: a neuromuscular analysis in young and older adults. *J Gerontol Med Sci* 2000;**55A**(3):M112–19.

164. Duncan PW, Chandler J, Studenski S, et al. How do physiological components of balance affect mobility in elderly men? *Arch Phys Med Rehabil* 1993;**74**:1343–9.

165. Powell LE, Myers AM. The Activities-specific Balance Confidence (ABC) Scale. *J Gerontol* 1995;**50A**:M28–34.

21

Falls and gait disorders in the elderly – principles of rehabilitation

PETER OVERSTALL

INTRODUCTION

The last 10 years have seen a major change in our attitude to falls. Geriatricians have long known them to be an important problem for older people and have recognized the effectiveness of the multidisciplinary approach but the development of a coherent evidence-based falls prevention strategy is something new. There is now a substantial laboratory and health service literature and this has resulted in evidence-based guidelines for the prevention of falls jointly published by the American and British Geriatrics Societies and the American Academy of Orthopedic Surgeons.[1] Preventing falls and providing effective treatment and rehabilitation is one of the key requirements in the UK National Service Framework for Older People.[2] The frequency of the problem, the high burden of morbidity and the evidence of preventability justify a widespread preventive strategy.

Disability can be thought of as the ecological gap between what an environment demands of a person and what the person is capable of doing,[3] and in this sense the individual with recurrent falls is truly disabled. Disability or frailty is the result usually of impairment in multiple systems, aggravated by the lack of adaptability typical of aging processes. Thus, we find disability in the elderly characterized by cognitive impairment,[4] falls, incontinence and functional dependence.[5] Our recognition that falls cannot be seen in isolation and that the elderly faller needs to be viewed comprehensively marks an important turning point. A history of recurrent falls is simply a convenient marker for the presence of widespread health defects.

FALLS AND THEIR CONSEQUENCES

About one-third of all people over the age of 65 fall each year and about half of these have recurrent falls.[6–8] Many studies[6,9,10] but not all[11] report a higher rate in women and a rising incidence with increasing age. In a prospective community study, the incidence rate of falls among home-dwelling men was 368/1000 person-years (py) and in women was 611/1000 py. The incidence rates in institutions were much higher, with the men experiencing 2021 falls/1000 py and women 1423/1000 py. There is a decline in fall rate in institutions in the very elderly suggesting that these residents are very frail and probably chair- or bed-bound, thus reducing the opportunities for falling.[10] Falls among people living at home most commonly occur in the day during periods of maximal activity.[8,10] Most falls occur when the person is walking and are caused by trips and slips.[11] In institutions night-time falls have been linked to visits to the toilet,[12] but urgency associated with an overactive bladder is not confined to institutions and weekly or more frequent urge incontinence is an independent risk factor for falling among community-dwelling women.[13]

Injury

Serious injury following a fall is comparatively rare with fractures occurring in about 5 per cent of falls among older persons living at home.[7,10] Serious injury following a fall is more likely to occur in people living in institutions, although the risk is mainly confined to residents that are frail, but still ambulatory. Risk factors for serious injury in the community include female sex, low body mass and cognitive impairment.[14] In a prospective community study, men living at home experienced 42 major soft tissue injuries/1000 py and 12 fractures/1000 py. Institutionalized men had 122 major soft tissue injuries/1000 py and 41 fractures/1000 py. Women living at home had 65 major soft tissue injuries/1000 py and 33 fractures/1000 py. Institutionalized women had 131 major soft tissue injuries/1000 py and 58 fractures/1000 py.[15] The risk of severe head injury is greatest in people living in institutions and increases with age with an overall incidence for both sexes of 29/1000 py for those aged 70–79 years and 72/1000 py for those aged 80 years or older.[16]

Mortality following a fall is low, but nonetheless the complications caused by falls are the leading cause of death from injury in men and women over the age of 65 in the US. In the UK falls are the third highest cause of injury/death (after motor vehicle traffic crashes and suicide) in the over 65s for both sexes (greater than 2.5 per 100 000 for males; greater than 1.6 per 100 000 for females). Falls are, however, the leading cause of injury hospitalizations in those aged 65 and over for both sexes (greater than 2.1 per 1000 for males; greater than 4.2 per 1000 for females).[17] A prospective primary care study found that the risk of death in recurrent fallers was increased at 1 year by up to 2.6-fold and increased by 1.9-fold at 3 years. Those that reported more than one fall in the previous 3 months had an average mortality of 16.4 per cent in the next year compared with 8.5 per cent for non-fallers. There was no relationship between a single fall and mortality.[18] Multiple falls or a single fall causing a serious injury carry a high risk of admission to an institution.[19]

Fear of falling

Restriction of activity after a fall is common. One study found that more than 50 per cent of fallers limited their activity either because of the fall itself, because of injury or because of a fear of further falls.[20] Fear of falls may also result in being unable to get up off the floor following a fall. This is a particularly frightening experience and is the consequence of physical frailty, muscle weakness and poor balance rather than serious injury. Those suffering a long lie on the floor are at increased risk of pressure sores and hypothermia and usually have a raised serum creatine kinase level which can lead the unwary to erroneously diagnose a myocardial infarct. About 40–50 per cent of fallers are unable to get up after the fall without help, with 3 per cent lying on the floor for more than 20 min.[20,21] Fallers that are unable to get up are more likely to suffer a lasting decline in activities of daily living.[21]

Falling is associated with an increased risk of long term institutionalization. Recurrent fallers have a 13 per cent risk of admission over 3 years, compared with 4 per cent for non-fallers. There is a consistent increase in risk of admission each year for both single and recurrent fallers and this applies to both sexes and all age groups. The association between single falls and admission to care suggests that the perceived risk to single fallers may be exaggerated and perhaps reflects more the anxieties of relatives. Fall rates for individuals vary considerably from year to year and those old people that have a single fall are more likely to have either no further falls or only very occasional falls rather than progressing to become a recurrent faller.[18] There are important practical issues for single and recurrent fallers, which are discussed below.

Fear of falling occurs in up to 50 per cent of fallers,[7,20] but may be present even if no falls have actually occurred.[33] Fear of falls is a relatively recent research area and much still needs to be clarified. Although fallers can simply be asked whether they are afraid of further falls, a single question cannot detect whether there are variations in the level of fear. The Falls Efficacy Scale is a continuous measure designed to measure fear of falling based on the definition of fear as 'low perceived self efficacy or confidence at avoiding falls'.[23] The scale has been used to measure the extent to which fear of falling causes functional decline. Although many fallers report fear, the majority feel confident in their ability to perform usual daily activities such as housework or walking without falling. Confidence in not falling (i.e. self efficacy) is strongly correlated with activities of daily living (ADL), social and physical function, whereas fear of falling has only a marginal association with ADL and no association with social or physical functioning.[24] However, other studies have shown that fear of falling in nursing home patients is an important predictor of functional decline[25] and in a prospective study of community volunteers fear of falling was associated over time with worsening gait and balance and increasing cognitive impairment resulting in reduced mobility[26] Although those that have had a fall are more likely to express fear of falling, neither the fall nor the fear are associated with activity restriction. Reducing activity appears to depend mainly on lack of social support. This support may encourage the elderly faller to remain active since they know that they can rely on others for help and this may help them maintain independence and reduce the risk of institutionalization. Reducing fear of falls and improving self efficacy may be important goals in rehabilitation.[27]

A cross-sectional study has emphasized the relationship between fear of falling, mood, function and handicap[28] but was unable to show whether fear of falling was the cause or the result of impaired physical function.

The effect of fear of falling on balance and gait is still not entirely clear. The cautious gait characterized by reduced stride length and speed, and increased double support time appears to be associated with fear, but increased stride width, although also associated with fear, may not necessarily increase stability but instead seems to predict an increased likelihood of falls.[29] During quiet standing, fear of falling is associated with larger amplitudes of postural sway when blindfolded and poorer scores when timed on a one-leg stance test. However, the causal relationship is not clear: does fear directly cause the poor balance or is fear and poor performance the result of a true deterioration in postural control?[30] It seems likely that fear of falls has a direct effect on control of balance since even in young adults the amplitude of center of pressure (COP) displacement decreases and the frequency of center of pressure displacement increases linearly as postural threat increases. In other words the central nervous system (CNS) adopts tighter control of posture under conditions of increased postural threat and this control is precisely scaled to the level of postural threat. Moreover, the control of posture is influenced by the order in which the threat to posture is experienced. Those that experience a high postural threat initially show increased amplitude of COP displacement compared with those that receive a low postural threat initially. The implication is that psychological factors such as fear of falling need to be taken into account when assessing gait and balance (M. G. Carpenter et al. 1999, unpublished data).

BALANCE AND GAIT CHANGES IN OLD AGE

Balance

During normal quiet standing, balance is maintained when the vertical projection of the center of mass (COM) on the ground (often called the center of gravity) is kept within the support base provided by the feet. Maintenance of this upright position is associated with body sway mainly in the anterior–posterior (A/P) direction and this sway may be measured either as degrees of angular movement or by using force platforms as the excursions of the COP. The COP is independent of the COM and represents the pressure over the surface of the feet in contact with the ground. There are separate COPs under each foot and when both feet are in contact with the ground the net COP lies somewhere between the two feet, depending on the relative weight taken by each foot.[31] Both A/P sway velocity and area increase in normal elderly subjects (i.e. those who report that their balance is normal and are functionally independent) and this difference is more obvious if the difficulty of the test is increased by using a moving platform or when eyes are closed.[32] Further increases in A/P sway have been correlated with spontaneous falls, but a better predictor of falls is mediolateral sway.[33,34] Falls depend on the relationship between the COM and the base of support. In the elderly, postural reactions controlling the COM are slowed and there appears to be particular difficulty in controlling lateral instability. Moreover, unexpected perturbations require an adjustment of the base of support through compensatory stepping and elderly fallers often have problems initiating and controlling these compensatory stepping movements. The elderly are much more likely to take additional steps to regain lateral stability. These compensatory steps may be very rapid in normal elderly subjects, indicating that simple aging changes in musculoskeletal capacity is not a problem in generating movement speeds.[35] The biomechanical requirements of a stepping response are different from the requirements for standing upright and are still poorly understood, but it does appear that measuring standing balance does not usefully predict the recovery from a perturbation such as a trip.[36] In normal older subjects, sway increases over time and sway is greater in older subjects with deteriorating balance than in those with normal balance. For the individual, increased sway is not a good predictor of falls and it seems unlikely that posturography has a useful place in the clinic, although simple clinical tests of balance may be valuable.

Gait

There has been a long running debate on what constitutes a normal gait in old age and the cause of the senile gait (idiopathic gait disorder). There are undoubtedly some elderly people who maintain a normal gait with a speed greater than 1 m/s[37] and a normal gait has been observed in 18 per cent of a community-living sample aged between 88 years and 96 years.[38] However, gait laboratory studies show subtle changes even in carefully screened healthy elderly subjects. Gait slowing is due to a decreased stride length and cadence (steps per minute) remains unaltered. Stance time and double support time increase and there is a less vigorous push-off. Whether this represents an early degeneration of the balance control system or an adaptation to make the gait safer is unclear.[39] The single best predictor of falling is stride to stride variability in velocity, but variability in stride width also appears to be predictive of falling.[29]

It is now apparent that the senile gait disorder, which is characterized by caution and shorter and more frequent strides, for which there is no apparent cause and is said to occur in 15–24 per cent of the elderly is not due to age, but to underlying neurodegenerative syndromes and stroke.[40] These patients have a twofold increased risk of cardiovascular death compared with age-matched subjects with a normal gait, further supporting the view that senile gait is caused by subclinical cerebrovascular disease.[41] The considerable confusion over the etiology of different gait disorders in the elderly has been clarified to a certain extent by the classification suggested by Nutt et al.[42] This proposed three broad categories of gait disorder: lower level due to peripheral skeleto-muscular or sensory problems; a middle level causing distortion of appropriate postural and locomotor synergies; and higher level disorders. The last category includes five gait types, which are essentially apraxias in that the walking difficulties are much greater than one would expect from a simple neurological examination. However, even this classification has not resolved the muddle and a clearer conceptual framework has recently been suggested, which divides vascular higher level gait disorders into ignition apraxia, equilibrium apraxia and a mixed gait apraxia.[43] This will be further discussed in the clinical section.

AGING OR DISEASE?

Aging is a complex process resulting from intrinsic and extrinsic damage to the organism at a rate dependent on each individual's genetic background and environment. From about 30 years of age a functional decline in performance can be detected in most organs and body systems, especially when faced with a challenge. However, the organs and systems age differentially so that the variation both within and between individuals increases with age. The chronological age of an old person may therefore bear little relation to their functional age and the response of an old person to the stress of illness will be more unpredictable than that of a young adult. There is therefore no stereotype of old age. An abrupt decline in any system should always be regarded as caused by underlying disease rather than by normal aging and the concept of 'healthy old age' is not a paradox.[44] There is growing recognition that functional disability in old age is a result of pathological processes rather than mere physiological decline.[45] There is a decline in sensorimotor function with increasing age. However, for peripheral nerve function this appears to be relatively slight and although there is a gradual decline in maximal muscle strength from the fourth decade onwards, and muscle wasting may be seen even in healthy old persons, it is not accompanied by significant weakness. Reflex inhibition of anterior horn cells secondary to joint pathology may well account for some of the muscle wasting seen in old age.[46] Reduced leg strength, however, does not appear to be the explanation for the reduced speed in stepping over an object seen in elderly women.[47]

In addition to peripheral mechanisms, balance depends on cognitive processes and attention, which may be affected by anxiety and depression or subclinical pathology. The ability to recover balance after a perturbation is more attentionally demanding even for healthy elderly compared with young adults.[48] Older people appear less able to weigh and select appropriate responses quickly when the environment changes suddenly. This slower processing of central information contributes to the increased risk of falling in patients with stroke, those with Alzheimer's disease and those who have been over-sedated with hypnotics. A 10 per cent increase in mean response times could result in a fivefold to sixfold increase in falls.[49] Even healthy elderly subjects appear to have a reduced central processing capacity so that reaction times are increased when sensory postural information is reduced. In other words, older people have to devote more attention to maintaining posture.[50] However, significant cognitive decline in elderly people cannot be attributed to age alone and is probably related to pervasive risk factors such as hypertension and cardiovascular disease.[51]

In summary, modest changes in sensorimotor function and central cognitive processes may be observed even in healthy old people but would be insufficient to explain significant functional impairment. Falls and obvious gait and balance impairment result from underlying pathological processes, which are likely to affect multiple organ systems.

RISK FACTORS FOR FALLS

Fallers can be broadly divided into two groups depending on whether they have had a simple trip or accident (an extrinsic fall) or whether they have had a spontaneous, intrinsic fall. The first group tends to be younger, fitter and more active and the second group is likely to be frail and at risk of further falls with evidence of multiple pathology including mental impairment. Patients in the second group will often attribute their falls to giddiness loss of balance, turning the head, their legs giving way or after rising from a chair.[52] In a community prospective study that looked at types of falls 55 per cent were extrinsic, 39 per cent were intrinsic (including loss of consciousness), 8 per cent were falls from a non-bipedal stance (e.g. fall out of bed or of a chair) and 7 per cent were unclassified.[53]

The importance of environmental hazards in the home has long been debated. There is some evidence that home hazards may increase the risk of falling in vigorous but not frail old people,[54] but a longitudinal study has found no increased risk of falls associated with environmental hazards.[55] The current view is that there is no clinical trial evidence that supports the benefit of home safety assessments and modifying the individual by addressing intrinsic risk factors is likely to be a more effective falls prevention strategy than modifying the environment.[56]

Several studies have identified risk factors for falls[20,57,58] and these highlight the constant themes of ill health and the multiplicity of defects in the balance system. Analysis of risk factors identified in 16 studies has shown that the most important are: lower limb muscle weakness, history of falls, gait deficit, balance deficit, use of assistive device, visual deficit, arthritis, impaired activities of daily living, depression, cognitive impairment and age over 80 years.[59] Recurrent falls are a better predictor of further falls than a single falls and recurrent fallers can be identified by a battery of tests, which include visual contrast sensitivity, proprioception in the lower limbs, quadriceps strength, reaction time and sway on a compliant surface with the eyes open.[60]

The inclusion of falls prevention in the UK National Service Framework for Older People[2] has meant that many health districts in the UK are introducing fall-prevention programs and the question arises as to how best to target limited resources most effectively. The likelihood of falling increases with the number of intrinsic risk factors present rising from an 8 per cent risk of a fall in those with no risk factors to 78 per cent for those with four or more risk factors.[57] The risk of recurrent falls also rises with increasing number of risk factors[20] but some people fall despite having no risk factors and it has been argued that single fallers should not be excluded from preventive services. However, epidemiological surveys have shown that falls do not fit a Poisson distribution, indicating that they do not occur in a purely random manner over time. Instead, there appear to be two populations which can be effectively separated by the number of falls that they experience. Patients most susceptible to falls (i.e. 'true fallers') are most likely to fall frequently, but patients recorded as having fallen once during the year will, by chance, include a substantial number of 'non-fallers'. Thus, from the pragmatic point of view, targeting those that have fallen twice or more in the past year is more likely to identify true fallers.[61,62] A checklist that identifies people at risk of falls should be simple if it is to be widely used in the community by carers or relatives as well as health professionals (Table 21.1) and there need to be clear referral pathways to falls assessment clinics (Table 21.2), which could be nurse led.

Table 21.1 *Falls risk assessment*

'yes' to question 1, or two or more 'yes' answers to question 2 indicates high risk.

Q.1 Two or more falls in the last year.
Q.2 Age 80+ years
Difficulty rising from a chair
Dizziness or fear when standing
Impaired balance or gait
Urge incontinence twice or more per week
History of single fall in the last year
Impaired memory or judgement
Agitation
Taking four or more drugs regularly
History of stroke
Parkinson's disease

A simple falls risk checklist for use in the community (based on ref 7, 20 and 57). People at high risk need a referral to the primary health care team or falls clinic with onward referral, as appropriate, to community therapy services and specialist clinics. In all patients there should be a review of remedial factors (see falls clinic checklist in Table 21.2).

Single fallers that attend accident and emergency departments as a result of an injury or are admitted with a fracture are high-risk groups and should be targeted for intervention.

CLINICAL APPROACH

The starting point is a careful history to establish as precisely as possible what the patient was doing at the time of the fall. One aim is to see whether the fall was a simple accident caused by a trip or slip (extrinsic fall) which generally carries a good prognosis or whether the patient has been having spontaneous intrinsic falls, which indicates the need for a more comprehensive assessment. It is important to establish early on whether the patient lost consciousness, which immediately limits possible diagnoses (see 'funny turns' and drop attacks below). Without a reliable witness this can often be difficult to establish since patients may deny loss of consciousness even when there is no doubt that it occurred.[63] Patients that can recall hitting the ground probably did not lose consciousness and those that are unable to remember the circumstances of the fall probably did (assuming that they are not cognitively impaired).

Points to note are whether there was a loss of concentration at the time of the fall, whether there was a change of posture, such as standing up or turning quickly, whether there was vertigo associated with head movement, deafness or tinnitus, cardiac symptoms (e.g. palpitations, breathlessness or chest pain), the direction of the fall and whether there was any difficulty arising afterwards.

Drugs

Drugs are often implicated in causing falls and should be critically reviewed. There is strong circumstantial evidence linking psychotropic drugs, particularly hypnotics and antidepressants with an increased risk of falls. Patients receiving two psychotropic drugs concomitantly have a more than threefold increased risk of falling than controls and those taking three drugs have a ninefold increased risk.[64] Benzodiazepines that are significantly associated with falls include temazepam, alprazolam, diazepam and lorazepam, but not triazolam, chlordiazepoxide or chlorazepate. Fall rates per dose dispensed by the pharmacy are highest for lorazepam and alprazolam and similar large fall rates are seen with nortriptyline and sertraline.

It was first realized in the 1970s that benzodiazepines, and other hypnotics could result in confusion, disorientation, incontinence and falls in elderly people.[65] In healthy old persons the pharmacokinetics of nitrazepam are unchanged, but in those that are sick the elimination half-life is significantly increased because of the larger

Table 21.2 *Falls clinic checklist*

	Action/comment
Inappropriate drugs (e.g. psychotropics)	Stop or reduce dose
Fear of falling	Refer occupational therapist
Depression	Treat
Urge incontinence	Examine abdomen (? palpable bladder or pelvic mass) PV, PR (exclude severe prolapse/fecal impaction) test urine (? infection/diabetes). Start bladder retraining and prescribe tolterodine or oxybutynin or refer nurse continence advisor
Cognitive impairment (AMTS less than 7/10, MMSE less than 24/30)	Refer community psychiatric nurse/old age psychiatry service
Loss of consciousness	Consider syncope, epilepsy or hypoglycemia. Refer to specialist to exclude arrhythmia, aortic stenosis, OH, carotid sinus sensitivity
Osteoporosis risk high if:	Take blood to exclude hypercalcemia
Previous low impact fracture	Start osteoporosis treatment (e.g. bisphosphonate or calcium and vitamin D)
Frail	
Housebound	
Nursing home resident	
Taking steroids	
Age 80+ years	
Body mass index less than 20 (weight in kg/height in m²)	Refer dietician
Visual impairment or refractive error	Refer optician/ophthalmologist
Lying and standing blood pressure (BP) (systolic BP falls of greater than 20 mm or diastolic BP falls of greater 10 mm after 2 min)	Review drugs. ? Specialist referral
Postural vertigo? Hallpike positive	Refer specialist/physiotherapist and occupational therapist
Parkinson's disease if poorly controlled	Refer specialist/PD nurse, physiotherapist and occupational therapist
Stroke	Refer physio and occupational therapist
Foot abnormalities	Refer chiropody
Inappropriate footwear	Advise
Painful hips or knees	Analgesia? Orthopedic referral
Difficulty arising from chair	Refer physiotherapist and occupational therapist
Impaired standing balance	
Abnormal gait	
Positive Romberg	Consider peripheral neuropathy or posterior column impairment
Social or housing problems	Refer social worker
Lives alone	? Install alarm

AMTS, Abbreviated Mental Test Score; MMSE, Mini Mental State Examination, OH, orthostatic hypotension.

volume of distribution.[66] Since steady-state plasma concentrations and total clearance time are unaltered it indicates that, for nitrazepam, increased receptor sensitivity is the main reason for the altered response seen in old age. The dangers of hypnotics in elderly people have been constantly emphasized by geriatricians and a good deal of publicity resulted from a report showing that over 90 per cent of elderly patients with a femoral fracture from a nocturnal fall had been taking barbiturates.[67] This was probably a freak result since a contemporary survey of femoral fractures found that 80 per cent of patients were not taking any hypnotic and only 9 per cent were on barbiturates.[68] These, and a number of related studies, had three main effects. First was the realization that psychotropic drugs with long elimination half-lives (greater than 24 h) were the ones most likely to cause troublesome side-effects. Second, the problem became widely recognized by doctors who changed their prescribing habits so that a prescription of an hypnotic to an elderly person is now the exception rather than the rule and when they are used a short-acting drug is chosen and prescribed only for a limited period. Third, it was recognized that side-effects depend on the size of the dose and the general health of the old person. Small doses of a short-acting hypnotic in a fit old person are relatively safe but may not be in someone who has other fall risk factors such as a peripheral neuropathy or cerebrovascular disease. Withdrawing psychotropic medication significantly reduces the risk of falling[69] but in nursing home residents who take an antidepressant there is an increased risk of falls and this risk is not reduced by changing from a tricyclic antidepressant to a selective serotonin reuptake inhibitor (SSRI) despite the fact that the SSRIs are generally free of the side-effects associated with tricyclics.[70]

However, none of the studies describing the association between psychotropic drugs and falls has been a randomized controlled trial and observational studies have fundamental deficiencies, including the possibility that the underlying condition for which the psychotropic drug was prescribed contributes to the risk of falling. Nonetheless, a critical meta-analysis recently concluded that there is a small but consistent association between the use of most classes of psychotropic drugs and falls. The odds ratio for one or more falls with any psychotropic use is 1.73 and fall risk is increased in those taking more than one psychotropic drug or having other risk factors for falls.[71] Another meta-analysis looked at cardiac and analgesic drugs, which have often been linked to falls. Again, only observational data are available, but there is a weak association between falls and digoxin, type 1A anti-arrhythmics (e.g. quinidine and disopyramide) and diuretics. Other cardiac drugs and analgesics are not associated with falls but there is an increased risk of recurrent falls in old people who take more than three or four medications of any type.[72]

Cognitive impairment

Patient examination should include an assessment of cognitive function using the Abbreviated Mental Test score[73] or the Mini Mental State Examination.[74] Recognizing cognitive impairment is important in its own right for subsequent patient management, but it is also an important risk factor for falls[7,75] and for injury following a fall[14,76] Patients with dementia have reduced walking speed and stride length, but stride length variability appears to be the best predictor of falls.[77] Patients with Alzheimer's disease appear to have no difficulty in maintaining balance on a stationary flat surface but they are unable to maintain stability in challenging situations that require a complex or longer-duration postural response and because they are more likely to catch the heel of their swing foot on an obstacle they are more likely to stumble.[78]

Vision

The association between impaired vision and a tendency to fall has long been recognized. Sheldon[79] found that 47 per cent of his elderly sample had difficulty in the dark. Some stated that 'they could not see where they were putting their feet and … they would lose their balance and stumble unless they could reinforce their postural senses by actually seeing the ground'. Early observations on postural sway during quiet standing showed that closing the eyes increases sway and no amount of practice can overcome this deficit. Peripheral vision appears to be particularly important for maintaining stability,[80] although some research has shown that the central area of the visual field, as compared with the peripheral retina, dominates postural control.[81] Experiments where the visual surroundings are manipulated indicate that misleading visual information is even more disruptive than no vision at all.[82,83] Falls have been associated with impaired visual acuity,[84,85] reduced depth perception,[20] reduced contrast sensitivity,[60] reduced visual fields and the presence of posterior subcapsular cataract.[85]

Visual input is particularly important in posturally challenging conditions, which in the laboratory are obtained by standing the subject on a compliant foam surface. In these circumstances, the most important visual functions are depth perception and stereopsis (i.e. perception of spatial relationships).[86] Quadriceps strength is also important in this situation to maintain stability.[87] What this means for the clinician is that even minor degrees of peripheral neuropathy which impair peripheral sensation will increase the patient's reliance on vision, and this can be most conveniently detected by the Romberg test. A positive Romberg test is not normal in old age and its finding means that the clinician should warn the patient of the importance of turning on the light at night when visiting the toilet, and check to see whether visual acuity can be improved. Foot position awareness declines with age because of loss of plantar tactile sensitivity and for patients with significant loss of sensitivity it is worth suggesting that they try wearing thin-soled shoes.[88] As already noted, faulty vision can be worse than no vision and bifocal spectacles are sometimes to blame. Half of patients admitted to hospital with an acute medical illness have visual impairment; 79 per cent have a reversible cause, mainly correctable refractive errors and cataracts. Patients admitted as a result of a fall are much more likely to have visual impairment (i.e. binocular visual acuity with or without distance glasses equal to or worse than 6/18) than those admitted for other reasons.[84]

Orthostatic hypotension

Orthostatic hypotension (OH) is undoubtedly a cause of falls in some old people.[89] In a randomized controlled trial assessing the value of a comprehensive post-fall assessment in a long-term residential care facility OH was found to be the primary cause of a fall in 16 per cent of patients and a possible contributory risk factor in a further 26 per cent.[90] However, a cross-sectional study involving nearly 10 000 ambulatory women found postural dizziness was more strongly associated than OH with a history of falling, syncope and impaired functional status. Orthostatic hypotension and postural dizziness are both common and found in 14 per cent and

19 per cent of subjects respectively. However, they are not highly correlated with each other. Orthostatic hypotension is strongly associated with age, history of parkinsonism, abnormal pulse rate (resting bradycardia or tachycardia) and systolic and diastolic hypertension. There is no significant relation with diuretic use. Postural dizziness, however, is associated with use of diuretics, antiepileptics, anxiolytics and hypnotics, parkinsonism, diabetes mellitus and stroke.[91] A prospective study among residents of apartment-style residential facilities found that neither the presence of OH nor the use of diuretics and sedative hypnotic drugs were related to risk of falls but antidepressant drugs were associated with falls.[92]

There are several definitions of OH, but the one most commonly used is a drop in systolic blood pressure of greater than 20 mmHg or diastolic blood pressure of greater than 10 mmHg after standing the patient for 2 min after 20-min supine rest. This will identify a symptomatic drop in the majority of patients. The significance of an asymptomatic drop is still unclear. Although, in population terms, OH may not be a good predictor of falls, for the individual patient with a history of falls and symptomatic OH the clinician should have no hesitation in stopping culprit drugs and if that does not help go on to start treatment (see Management section).

Dizziness

Chronic dizziness is a common symptom and occurs in one-quarter of community-living elderly people.[93] Close questioning usually reveals that these patients are describing a sense of unsteadiness or fear of falling rather than true vertigo. Those with vertigo and tinnitus and hearing loss should be referred to an otolaryngologist. Those who have a brief period of vertigo provoked by head movements, typically sitting up in bed in the morning or rolling over in bed at night, probably have benign positional vertigo. They should be tested with the Hallpike maneuver. For this, the patient is moved from the sitting to the supine position with the head extended over the edge of the couch and the head rotated 45° to one side, the maneuver is then repeated with the head rotated to the other side. In benign positional vertigo a rotational nystagmus appears after a short latent period when the head is turned to the affected side. The nystagmus may last for a few seconds to almost a minute and is accompanied by the sensation of vertigo, which fatigues on repeat testing.[94] Another common cause of acute episodic vertigo in this age group when accompanied by focal neurological signs such as diplopia or bilateral sensory motor symptoms is vertebro-basilar ischemia. Vertigo in isolation is not considered a focal neurological symptom and, therefore, is not classified as a transient ischemic attack (TIA).[95]

Dizziness in most patients is multifactorial and 85 per cent of chronically dizzy patients have more than one diagnosis. The most common are cerebrovascular disease (with signs of arteriosclerotic parkinsonism), cervical spondylosis (symptoms on head or neck movement with reduced range of neck movement), anxiety or hyperventilation and poor vision. Patients with dizziness have significantly poorer balance than control subjects. Extensive investigation is rarely helpful and in most patients the diagnosis can be made on the basis of the neurological and locomotor system examination supplemented by simple dizziness provocation testing.[96] A 1-year follow up of chronically dizzy elderly people living in the community showed that there was no increase in mortality or hospitalization or deterioration in activities of daily living. However, there was an increased risk of falls and syncope.[93] The classification of falls, syncope and dizziness is likely to overlap among patients seen in a tertiary referral syncope clinic. Half have syncope alone or syncope and dizziness and over 40 per cent have recurrent unexplained falls and dizziness. A few patients complain of dizziness alone and deny syncope but witness accounts confirm syncopal episodes in all.[97]

Lower limb disability

Lower limb disability and foot problems are significant risk factors for falls.[7] The problem may be recognized from seeing that the patient has difficulty rising from a chair,[58] or has evidence of arthritis, muscle weakness, absent tendon reflexes or sensory loss.[20,60] Quadriceps weakness and wasting is a common finding and is usually due to a combination of factors: arthrogenous myopathy resulting from arthritis affecting the hips or knees, lumbar spondylosis and disuse atrophy. Impaired proprioception and vibration sense in the feet is associated with falls and is common especially in diabetics.[33,98] Foot problems, particularly calluses, hallux valgus and digital deformities such as retracted toes are common in the elderly and may contribute to the risk of falls. Quite how they do this is speculative, but it has been suggested that reduced joint mobility and displacement of the center of gravity may impair postural stability.[99] Gross foot deformity, which can still be seen in elderly Chinese women that had their feet bound in childhood, results in an increased risk of falls and a reduced ability to get up from a chair without help. These women have impaired balance, as shown by a reduced functional reach.[100]

Gait and balance

Neurological and locomotor system examination of the patient lying on a couch is of limited value; directly assessing the patient's gait and balance is more informative.[57,101,102] One should watch to see whether the patient has to use their arms to rise from a chair, suggesting quadriceps weakness and possibly arthritis of hips or knees. The bradykinesia of Parkinson's disease may be apparent at this stage. Once the patient is upright note whether there are signs of fear or postural dizziness. Observe whether the patient can stand steadily with eyes open and feet apart and then ask them to bring the feet together. Inability to do this indicates severe unsteadiness due to cerebellar disease or a central or peripheral vestibular lesion. If the patient is steady with feet together tell them that you are ready to catch them and ask them to close their eyes. If they are now unsteady the Romberg test is positive and suggests either a posterior column lesion (e.g. cervical spondylosis, vitamin B_{12} deficiency or tabes dorsalis) or a peripheral neuropathy. Heel/toe walking may expose a mild ataxia. Difficulty walking on the heels indicates footdrop, which may be caused by a lesion of the common peroneal nerve, L5 radiculopathy or a pyramidal lesion. Inability to walk on the toes indicates weakness of gastrocnemius.

Now ask the patient to walk a short distance observing the width of the gait. This may be normal, wide-based (suggesting fear or vascular parkinsonism) or wide-based and incoordinated, suggesting cerebellar disease. Note any tendency to veer to one side (suggesting a vestibular lesion). Note any start or turn hesitation, the length of the step, any difficulty turning, the arm swing, the presence of tremor, a limp due to a painful foot or joint, whether the patient is stooped and their general demeanor.

A number of assessments of gait and balance have been described, including the Tinetti balance and gait evaluation,[103] the get up and go test,[104,105] functional reach[106] and one-leg balance.[107] The AGS/BGS Panel on Falls Prevention[1] recommends that all older persons reporting a single fall should be observed as they stand up from a chair, walk several paces and return (i.e. the get up and go test). Those showing no difficulty or unsteadiness need no further assessment. Those that have difficulty or demonstrate unsteadiness require multidisciplinary assessment.

COMMON CLINICAL CONDITIONS ASSOCIATED WITH FALLS

It is worth emphasizing again that recurrent falls in elderly people are usually multifactorial and a comprehensive assessment is likely to result in a better management plan than becoming preoccupied with searching for a single etiology. Nonetheless, precipitating factors are often implicated, usually in the setting of a frail patient who is prescribed a new drug or who develops an acute illness such as a chest infection or heart failure and falls as a result. Even with chronic progressive conditions it can be worth clarifying the diagnosis, which in the case of vascular parkinsonism may mean that the L-dopa can be stopped and some patients with cervical myelopathy

benefit from decompression surgery. Excluding those patients with joint disease, the commonest cause of gait disturbance in the elderly is parkinsonism, usually vascular or drug induced. Other common causes are: multiple sensory impairment, usually involving a degree of peripheral neuropathy and visual loss, Parkinson's disease and cervical myelopathy.[108,109]

Patients that have recovered from a stroke and are living at home are more than twice as likely to fall than other elderly people living in the community.[110] These patients may have perceptual difficulties or ataxia and the hemiplegia itself affects balance by causing an asymmetric stance. Attentional deficits resulting either from the cerebral injury or from depression also contribute.

Although it is not an early sign of idiopathic Parkinson's disease, postural instability causing unsteadiness when standing and walking is one of the cardinal features and is particularly associated with disease onset after the age of 70 years. Older patients are more likely to have balance impairment both at onset and after 5 years of treatment and its presence as the major criterion for Hoehn and Yahr stage III[111] marks a significant shift from mild to more disabling disease. There are a number of reasons why patients with Parkinson's disease may fall. There is a reduction in the normal toe raise at the end of leg swing, increasing the risk of trips, step length is reduced and stride to stride variability increase. Freezing when turning is often blamed by patients for causing a fall and dyskinesias and dystonias further impair the normal gait pattern in late disease. Cognitive impairment, which may be drug related, adds to the risk of falls but OH is not associated with falls.

Vascular parkinsonism

This is frequently misdiagnosed as idiopathic Parkinson's disease but there are a number of clinical features that point to the correct diagnosis. The condition is often called lower half parkinsonism since the symptoms and signs are predominantly in the legs. The gait is wide-based and short-paced (marche à petits pas). Start and turn hesitation is seen in more than half the patients and is even more common than in idiopathic Parkinson's disease.[112] The trunk is upright, the facies normal and the arm swing is preserved. Pyramidal tract signs and pseudo-bulbar palsy are common, but the typical rest tremor of idiopathic Parkinson's disease is absent. Cognitive impairment, symptoms of overactive bladder (frequency and urgency with or without urge incontinence) and disequilibrium can be more marked than in idiopathic Parkinson's disease.

A number of neuropathological changes have been associated with the clinical picture, including frontal lobe infarct, diffuse cerebral disease, multiple lacunar infarcts, basal ganglia infarcts and subcortical ischemia.

Magnetic resonance imaging (MRI) scanning of a largely healthy elderly population has shown that white matter lesions are strongly associated with stroke, but even in the absence of a history of stroke, 95 per cent of subjects have white matter lesions, most commonly in the periventricular area. Their presence is associated with greater age, evidence for a clinically silent stroke on MRI, hypertension, cognitive impairment and abnormal gait.[113,114] Typically, these patients have a cautious gait (wide-based and short-paced) and are at increased risk of falling.[115] Lacunar strokes and white matter lesions are better predictors of the development of parkinsonism than territorial strokes. However, white matter lesions are also more likely to be found in patients with idiopathic PD than in healthy subjects and are a marker for more severe disease, particularly bradykinesia, postural instability and gait difficulties. These patients have a shorter disease duration and their bradykinesia responds less well to L-dopa.[116] What is striking about this is that the characteristics of the more severe disease associated with white matter lesions are precisely those associated with late age of onset of Parkinson's disease.[117] In other words, elderly patients with idiopathic Parkinson's disease may also develop vascular parkinsonism and when they do, the problems with gait, balance and cognitive impairment become prominent.

Although impaired balance is a characteristic of idiopathic Parkinson's disease it tends to be a late feature and is often less marked than that seen in vascular parkinsonism. However, in both conditions there is an increased reliance on visual cues. Current views on the role of the basal ganglia suggest two main functions. First, they contribute to cortical motor set (i.e. the tonic discharge in motor cortical neurons that keeps the motor plans in a state of readiness). Motor set allows the motor plan to start and run automatically to completion with the correct amplitude. The second function is to provide internal cues to ensure that the motor plans, which are thought to be a predetermined set of submovements, run precisely and accurately with correct timing between the submovements. When a well-learned automatic movement such as walking is initiated the basal ganglia provide an internal cue to the supplementary motor area (SMA) where the correct submovement sequence is selected, which in turn triggers the motor cortex to produce the movement. Phasic activity from the basal ganglia provides a non-specific internal cue that turns off the preparatory activity of one submovement in the SMA, thus triggering the motor cortex and at the same time activating the next pre-movement sequence. Thus, abnormal internal cues would impair submovement preparation and interrupt the smooth action of walking.[118]

For externally cued movements, however, the process is different. The basal ganglia–SMA loop is bypassed and visual or auditory signals from the sensory cortex go directly to the premotor area, which activates the motor cortex. This model of basal ganglia function has been used by Liston and Tallis[43] to clarify the confusion surrounding higher-level gait disorders. Symptoms of Parkinson's disease such as start and turn hesitation and bradykinesia result from loss of internal cues from the basal ganglia to the SMA. However, the pathway between the sensory cortex, the premotor area and the motor cortex is intact and this allows Parkinson's disease patients to walk normally, either as the result of a visual cue or simply by concentrating on the correct size of step to take.[119] In vascular parkinsonism and other vascular higher-level gait disorders the periventricular white matter lesions disrupt the pathways from the basal ganglia to the SMA and this produces the characteristic problems of start and turn hesitation and reduced stride length. However, some patients with vascular higher-level gait disorders do not have difficulty with gait ignition or turn hesitation and instead suffer mainly from disequilibrium.[42] It is suggested that these patients have vascular lesions affecting the sensory cortex, premotor area, motor area pathway. Their ability to use visual, auditory and proprioceptive information is impaired but because their basal ganglia SMA pathway is intact, their walking remains reasonably normal. These patients would not be expected to benefit from visual or other environmental cues.

Based on this hypothesis, the following classification has been suggested. Ignition apraxia is characterized by ignition failure, shuffling and freezing. The site of the lesion is in the SMA, basal ganglia or its connections and patients are able to respond to visual or auditory cues. Equilibrium apraxia is characterized by poor balance and falls, and the site of the lesion is in the premotor area or its connections and there is no response to visual or auditory cues. Finally, there is mixed gait apraxia characterized by gait ignition failure, shuffling, freezing, poor balance and falls. The lesions are in the premotor area or connections and the SMA, basal ganglia or connections and there would be a response to visual or auditory cues.[43]

Cervical myelopathy

This is a common cause of gait disorder in the elderly and is caused by degenerative arthritis of the cervical spine. In advanced cases there is spasticity and hyperreflexia in the legs with posterior column signs, urinary urgency and frequency. Severe neck pain is usually absent and there may or may not be sensory symptoms in the distribution of C5, C6 and C7 with wasting of the small muscles of the hand. However, before these patients develop the typical stiff-legged, para-spastic gait there is impairment of balance apparent to the patient, who compensates by producing a protective gait pattern. Gait velocity, step length and cadence are reduced and step width is increased. Improvement follows decompressive surgery.[120]

'Funny turns'

The reason for questioning the patient and a reliable witness closely about whether the fall was associated with loss of consciousness is that for practical purposes there are only three possible diagnoses. The first is syncope (see Chapter 22), although as already noted some of these patients may deny loss of consciousness or complain only of dizziness or simply have unexplained falls. Hypoglycemia may cause loss of consciousness particularly with long-acting oral hypoglycemic drugs but the diagnosis is usually obvious. Loss of consciousness is rarely a feature of transient ischemic attacks and then only if there are accompanying focal neurological symptoms. Epilepsy, however, is a not infrequent cause of 'funny turns' although falls are uncommon. The type that cause diagnostic difficulty are complex partial seizures. A large number of symptoms may occur although in the individual patient the attacks are often stereotyped. Autonomic symptoms such as nausea and an unpleasant sensation rising from the stomach to the throat are common and there may be psychic features such as déjà vu or a feeling of being in 'another world'. Again, a reliable witness can be invaluable, particularly if they report automatisms such as lip-smacking or grimacing and a glazed look to the eyes as if there was 'nobody at home' for a few seconds. Post-ictal sleepiness and a feeling of being 'out of sorts' is typical. The usual etiology of epilepsy in the elderly is cerebrovascular disease and when choosing an antiepileptic drug it is best to pick one with a low rate of side-effects.[121] It is important to reconsider the diagnosis if patients with apparent epilepsy respond poorly to treatment. They should be referred for tilt-table testing to exclude convulsive vasovagal syncope.[122]

Drop attacks

These are falls characterized by their dramatic suddenness when one minute the old person is on their feet and apparently all right and the next moment is full-length on the floor without knowing why. There is no loss of consciousness. They have been reported to occur in a number of conditions including cervical spondylosis, normal pressure hydrocephalus and vestibular disorders (see Chapter 9). For these, and other unexplained falls it is important to consider the possibility of cardiac syncope and refer the patient for tilt-table testing and carotid sinus massage. If this is normal it will often be concluded that these are spontaneous falls occurring in a frail patient. Their balance will be impaired due to various combinations of somatosensory or visual impairment, weakness of the legs or slowing of central processes that monitor and react to sensory information. The old person simply has to pay more attention to maintaining balance, and momentary absent-mindedness particularly during postural changes may be sufficient to cause them to fall, apparently without explanation.

MANAGEMENT

The fit old person with normal balance and gait who has simply had an accidental fall needs only reassurance, encouragement to keep active, an advice leaflet such as the one recently issued by the Department of Trade and Industry[123] and to be considered for osteoporosis prevention. Avoiding fractures is an important part of the management plan for all fallers. Those at high risk (see Table 21.2) should routinely be given a treatment known to reduce the risk of hip fracture, such as alendronate, risederonate or calcium and vitamin D.[124] It is prudent to check the calcium level beforehand to exclude hypercalcemia.

It has already been stressed that the frail, recurrent faller needs comprehensive assessment and appropriate intervention. This includes drug review and efforts to improve treatment of other problems such as painful joints or shortness of breath caused by pulmonary disease or heart failure. Referral may be needed to: optician, ophthalmologist, orthopedic surgeon or chiropodist. The community psychiatric nursing service should be alerted to the patient with cognitive impairment. Urge incontinence and other overactive bladder symptoms should prompt an abdominal examination to exclude a palpable bladder or pelvic mass. A vaginal and rectal examination are needed to exclude severe prolapse or fecal impaction, and the urine should be tested to exclude infection, blood and diabetes. Advice on bladder retraining should be combined with a prescription of an antimuscarinic drug, such as tolterodine or oxybutynin and follow-up arranged with the nurse continence advisor. Patients with cerebrovascular disease should have vascular risk factors identified and controlled and be prescribed an anti-platelet drug. Management of Parkinson's disease may require some specialist input. *De novo* patients would normally be started on co-beneldopa or co-careldopa or an agonist drug or possibly selegiline. It is still not clear which drug is best and a large multicenter trial (PD MED) is in progress trying to clarify the issue.[125]. Severe dyskinesias must be controlled either by adjusting medication or stereotactic surgery if the physiotherapist is to have any chance of improving the gait pattern. Orthostatic hypotension should be managed by modification of medication, elastic stockings,[126] increased fluid intake and raising the head of the patient's bed. If these measures are unsuccessful fludrocortisone (initially 100 μg) should be tried.

Exercise

There is broad agreement that exercise is beneficial not only in maintaining mobility and reducing falls and functional decline, but also in reducing mortality.[127] Unfortunately, physical activity is now uncommon amongst many older adults in Western countries. In the UK, 40 per cent of all men and women aged over 50 years are sedentary, that is, they participate less than once a week in activity lasting for 30 min and of sufficient intensity to produce a health benefit. One-quarter of men and one-third of women aged over 70 years are unable to walk a quarter of a mile on their own.[128] Isometric strength and leg extensor power declines by 1–2 per cent per annum[129] and this results in increased difficulty stepping up onto a bus, holding on to a handrail when climbing stairs or rising from a chair.

There is now good evidence that exercise can improve functional ability in elderly people. An 8-week training period of moderately intense exercise undertaken at a weekly exercise class and twice-weekly unsupervised home exercise improves isometric knee extension strength, flexibility, balance and various functional abilities such as chair rise time and time to walk up and down a staircase.[130] The improvements in lower limb muscle strength also result in increased walking speed, cadence and stride length, and are associated with increased confidence.[131,132] Weight-bearing exercise also has a beneficial effect on improving bone mineral density.[133] Important as these benefits are, it is, however, essential to demonstrate that exercise results in reduced fall rates. There is now research to support this[69,134,135] but there are still unanswered questions about the best type of exercise, the degree of intensity and whether exercise should be prescribed on its own or be part of a multifaceted intervention. The evidence to date suggests that multiple interventions are best. A study looking at the effect of different interventions found that exercise was the single most effective intervention in reducing falls but that falls were further reduced by the addition of home hazard management and treatment of poor vision.[136] Even very elderly people will adhere to and benefit from an exercise program[137] but there are real problems in persuading people to take up activity programs because of the mistaken belief that they already do enough exercise to keep fit. Women tend to use the excuse that they lack an exercise partner; men blame a lack of interest in leisure time physical activity.[138] There is little evidence that 'prescription for exercise' schemes whereby general practitioners refer patients to a local leisure center are effective. The key components among successful schemes appear to be personal instruction with frequent on-going professional contact, programs that are home-based and unsupervised, of moderate intensity and which can be performed either alone or with others. The program should be enjoyable, convenient and completed in three sessions per week. Walking is the simplest solution to meet these criteria.[139] However, a note of caution has been sounded by the finding that brisk walking may be associated with an increased risk of falls.[140] A moderate impact activity such as walking has not been shown to

increase ultrasound attenuation at the heel (and by implication does not reduce hip fracture risk). High-impact activities such as aerobics or jogging, which could reduce the rate of bone loss, are not appropriate for all elderly people and exercise prescription needs to be tailored to the individual.[141] Tai chi, which stresses balance control mechanisms while increasing awareness of the position of the body in relation to the environment, has been shown to reduce the risk of falls by 47.5 per cent.[142] Moreover an exercise such as tai chi, which can be enjoyable, is likely to be adhered to because of the perception that it improves mental, as well as physical control and increases the general sense of well being.[143]

Falls prevention programs

It has long been recognized that the causes of falls are multifactorial and frequently indicate considerable frailty and 'failure to thrive'. The approach to prevention has therefore been multidisciplinary, aiming to tackle underlying causes of ill-health as well as addressing the more immediate problem of improving balance and gait. This is an effective strategy for at-risk patients identified in primary care[136,144] and accident and emergency departments,[145] but there is little evidence that falls prevention programs work in hospital.[146] There is a growing interest in providing a district-wide, coordinated approach, which identifies people at risk of falling using a simple checklist in all community and hospital settings and referring on to a nurse-led clinic[147] with appropriate support from physiotherapy and occupational therapy. General practitioners are good at implementing recommendations resulting from this kind of assessment, although patient adherence to exercise programs is poor.[148] A consultant-led falls clinic with access to tilt-table testing and Holter monitoring should be available to investigate unexplained falls and 'funny turns'.

Although interventions aimed at high-risk groups are effective, it is recognized that not all fallers have identifiable risk factors and it is not clear what strategy would be best suited to this group. It may be better to aim at improving physical function and mobility rather than reducing falls as such, but although this is a consistent public health message there is little evidence that it is working.

Therapist's approach to fallers

Although encouraging a brisk daily walk may be an adequate approach to the relatively fit older patient, for those that are frail and poorly mobile an individually tailored program of physiotherapy is necessary.[149,150] Muscle strengthening exercises may be needed before the therapist judges that it is safe to work on improving gait and balance. The management plan will also address specific neurological problems such as foot-drop, stroke or parkinsonism. Because physiotherapists are often in short supply, studies have been performed to determine whether other health professionals previously untrained in prescribing exercise are effective. These have shown that a trained district nurse can deliver a home exercise program which reduces falls by 46 per cent.[151] Physiotherapists have made considerable progress in structuring their approach to the more complex gait and balance disorders. Higher-level gait disorders[42] are characterized as previously noted, by either ignition apraxia, equilibrium apraxia or a combination of both, resulting in a mixed-gait apraxia.[43] Although the commonest cause is vascular, as a result of cerebral multi-infarcts, there are other causes and the therapist's approach is the same regardless of the etiology. A schedule of 31 interventions has been described aimed at improving gait ignition failure and turning (e.g. stepping over lines on the floor), improving postural alignment and balance reactions (e.g. training the patient to respond to an externally produced perturbation), improving postural alignment and pelvic control, and addressing other problems such as slow walking and short step length, *en bloc* turning, a tendency to fall backwards, shuffling gait, inadequate foot clearance and loss of arm swing.[152]

This conventional physiotherapy approach has been compared with treadmill walking in patients with higher level gait disorders caused by cerebral multi-infarct states. Treadmill retraining using a safety harness improves coordinated stepping in paraplegic patients as a result of activation of spinal locomotor centers[153] and patients with hemiplegia have also been shown to benefit. No difference has been shown between treadmill retraining and conventional physiotherapy for patients with higher-level gait disorder, but it is encouraging that both treatments show significant improvement in the time taken to complete the sit to stand test, time taken to walk 10 m, number of steps over 10 m, walking velocity and right and left step lengths.[154]

A similar structured approach has also been developed for Parkinson's disease,[155,156] which is characterized mainly by ignition apraxia, with patients still able to respond to visual or auditory cues. Using the Hoehn and Yahr scale,[111] specific interventions are recommended for different levels of disability. The therapist's job is to identify the main intrinsic (e.g. gait ignition failure, freezing, dyskinesias and postural imbalance) and extrinsic factors (e.g. the environment and the task in hand) that predispose patients to falling. Patients are also encouraged to keep a falls diary, recording both falls and near-falls, where they occurred and what the person was doing at the time. Certain patterns may emerge, such as the person falling when they try to do more than one task at once (walking and carrying a tray or walking and talking at the same time) or falling when turning in a narrow, confined space. Patients have difficulty performing complex dual tasks and the aim is to teach patients to break down these complex activities into simple parts and concentrate on performing each part separately. The approach to start and turn hesitation and freezing has three parts. First, the therapist teaches the use of auditory or visual cues such as white lines on the floor or large colored circles placed on the wall that keep the patient focusing ahead rather than at their feet. Second, the patient is taught to mentally rehearse the movement and imagine themselves going through the action before they actually attempt to do it. Interestingly, such visualization can result in Parkinson's disease patients walking with a normal step length without any visual aids. Finally, alterations are made to the environment, such as widening doorways or placing footprints on the floor of the toilet, which the patient steps on in order to smoothly maneuver in and out.

The occupational therapist clearly has an important role to play in manipulating the environment of patients with parkinsonism and other causes of ignition apraxia. What the occupational therapists should be doing with other elderly fallers is more open to debate. Traditionally the occupational therapist home visit has focused on improving home safety by removing hazards such as trailing wires and loose slip mats but the evidence from most studies is that environmental hazards make little or no contribution to the fall.[55,56] People become accustomed to their cluttered and apparently unsafe homes and, indeed, can frequently be seen using furniture as secure handholds when crossing a room. Patients often resist exhortations to tidy things up and may well be more vulnerable in wide open spaces. What is more useful is for the occupational therapist to teach the patient safe behavior within the home, especially with bed to chair transfers, avoiding climbing on to chairs to reach high cupboards and fitting appropriate aids and rails in areas such as the toilet and bathroom. It has been suggested that the change in behavior resulting from such an intervention reduces falls both within and outside the home by 36 per cent.[157]

Footwear

Advice is often given to patients on suitable footwear, although this is frequently ignored and there is only partial agreement on what constitutes best advice. High-heeled shoes impair balance[158] but older women are reluctant when going out to exchange their smart court shoes for low-heeled walking shoes, which they feel are not only unattractive but may mark them out as being disabled. Maximizing foot and ankle proprioception is desirable. Foot position awareness is impaired in the elderly and it has been argued that thin, hard soles provide better stability than those with thick, soft midsoles.[159] In younger men, ankle taping improves proprioception[160] and this may explain why shoes with a high collar (i.e. boots) improve postural stability compared with low collar shoes or being barefoot.[161]

However, this study also found that sole hardness was not related to balance. Although low-heeled boots can be confidently recommended it is still not clear whether these should be hard- or soft-soled.

Hip fracture prevention

In addition to osteoporosis treatment and prevention there is growing interest in mechanical methods of reducing the force of the impact when a person falls. Hip protectors used in a nursing home reduce the risk of fracture by over 50 per cent but only one-quarter of those given hip protectors actually wear them.[162] The low compliance rate means that hip protectors are not a universal solution but they are a very useful way of boosting confidence in those patients that recognize that they have a problem with balance but wish, nonetheless, to mobilize out of doors. Because the protectors reduce fear of falling, users feel more confident that they can complete tasks safely and this encourages more physical activity and independence.[163] Although effective in high-risk populations it is not yet clear how helpful they will be for general use.[164] Indoor carpeting can reduce the impact of a fall, but a safety floor consisting of two layers of polyurethane separated by a series of high elastic polymer columns may halve the rate of fall-related hip fractures. Despite its high cost, use of the flooring in nursing homes would be cost effective.[165]

SUMMARY

Recurrent falls are an important cause of disability in older persons and increase the risk of admission to an institution. Risk factors for falls reflect widespread pathological processes in different parts of the balance control system, which may be aggravated by drug side-effects, but rarely by environmental factors. Recurrent falls should be regarded as a cue for comprehensive assessment of the patient and multidisciplinary intervention. Much can be achieved by simple nurse-led falls clinics, supported by physiotherapy and occupational therapy, which can identify remediable factors such as use of inappropriate medications, refractive errors, fear of falling, urge incontinence, inappropriate footwear and muscle weakness. Physiotherapy and occupational therapy techniques for treating patients with parkinsonism and idiopathic Parkinson's disease are promising developments, and the role of the occupational therapist in the home visit is now largely concerned with improving safe behavior rather than removing environmental hazards. Falls associated with loss of consciousness need specialist assessment and usually tilt-table testing. Falls prevention programs which emphasize increased exercise are effective and should be targeted locally at patients who are identified as being at high risk and

nationally to all older persons through public health education.

REFERENCES

1. AGS/BGS Panel on Falls Prevention. Guidelines for the prevention of falls in older persons. *J Am Geriatr Soc* 2001;**49**:664–72.
2. Department of Health. *National service framework for older people 2001*. London: Department of Health, 2001(Website: http:/www.doh.gov.uk/nsf/olderpeople)
3. Evans JG. Disability in the elderly. *Lancet* 1997;**350**:1779.
4. Melzer D, McWilliams B, Brayne C, et al. Profile of disability in elderly people: estimates from a longitudinal population study. *BMJ* 1999;**318**:1108–11.
5. Tinetti ME, Inouye SH, Gill TM, Doucette JT. Shared risk factors for falls, incontinence and functional dependence. *JAMA* 1995;**273**:1348–53.
6. Blake AJ, Morgan K, Bendall MJ, et al. *Age Ageing* 1988;**17**:365–72.
7. Tinetti ME, Speechley, M, Ginter SF. Risk factors for falls among elderly persons living in the community. *N Engl J Med* 1988;**319**:1701–707.
8. Campbell AJ, Borrie MJ, Spears GF, et al. Circumstances and consequences of falls experienced by a community population 70 years and over during a prospective study. *Age Ageing* 1990;**19**:136–41.
9. Prudham, D, Evans JG. Factors associated with falls in the elderly: a community study. *Age Ageing* 1981;**10**:141–6.
10. Luukinen, H, Koski, K, Hiltunen, L, Kivela SL. Incidence rate of falls in an aged population in northern Finland. *J Clin Epidemiol* 1994;**47**:843–50.
11. Berg WP, Alessio HM, Mills EM, Tong C. Circumstances and consequences of falls in independent community-dwelling older adults. *Age Ageing* 1997;**26**:261–8.
12. Ashley, M. J, Gryfe, C. I, Amies, A. A longitudinal study of falls in an elderly population: some circumstances of falling. *Age Ageing* 1977;**6**:211–20.
13. Brown JS, Vittinghoff E, Wyman JF. Urinary incontinence: does it increase risk for falls and fractures. *J Am Geriatr Soc* 2000;**48**:721–5.
14. Tinetti ME, Doucette JT, Claus EB. The contribution of predisposing and situational risk factors to serious fall injuries. *J Am Geriatr Soc* 1995;**43**:1207–13.
15. Luukinen H, Koski K, Honkanen R, Kivela SL. Incidence of injury causing falls among older adults by place of residence: a population-based study. *J Am Geriatr Soc* 1995;**43**:871–6.
16. Luukinen H, Herala M, Koski K, et al. Rapid increase of fall-related severe head injuries with age among older people: a population-based study. *J Am Geriatr Soc* 1999;**47**:1451–2.
17. Cryer PC, Davidson, L, Styles CP, Langley JD. Descriptive epidemiology of injury in the South East: identifying priorities for action. *Public Health* 1996;**110**:331–8.
18. Donald IP, Bulpitt CJ. The prognosis of falls in elderly people living at home. *Age Ageing* 1999;**28**:121–5.
19. Tinetti ME, Williams CS. Falls, injuries due to falls and the risk of admission to a nursing home. *N Engl J Med* 1998;**337**:1279–84.
20. Nevitt MC, Cummings SR, Kidd, S, Black D. Risk factors for

recurrent non-syncopal falls. *JAMA* 1989;**261**:2663–8.

21. Tinetti ME, Liu WL, Claus EB. Predictors and prognosis of inability to get up after falls among elderly persons. *JAMA* 1993;**269**:65–70.

22. Downton JH, Andrews K. Postural disturbance and psychological symptoms amongst elderly people living at home. *Int J Geriatr Psychiatry* 1990;**5**:93–8.

23. Tinetti ME, Richman D, Powell L. Falls efficacy as a measure of fear of falling. *J Gerontol* 1990:**45**:239–43.

24. Tinetti ME, Mendes de Leon CF, Doucette JT, Baker DL. Fear of falling and fall-related efficacy in relationship to functioning among community-living elders. *J Gerontol* 1994;**49**, M140–7.

25. Franzoni S, Rozzini R, Boffelli S, et al. Fear of falling in nursing home patients. *Gerontology* 1994;**40**:38–44.

26. Vellas BJ, Wayne SJ, Romero LT, et al. Fear of falling and restriction of mobility in elderly fallers. *Age Ageing* 1997;**26**:189–93.

27. Howland J, Lachman ME, Peterson EW, et al. Covariates of fear of falling and associated activity curtailment. *Gerontologist* 1998;**38**:549–55.

28. Lightbody CE. *Preventing functional decline and further falls: the role of psychological factors.* MPhil thesis. Liverpool: University of Liverpool, 2000.

29. Maki B. Gait changes in older adults: predictors of falls or indicators of fear. *J Am Geriatr Soc* 1997;**45**:313–20.

30. Maki BE, Holliday PJ, Topper AK. Fear of falling and postural performance in the elderly. *J Gerontol* 1991;**46**:M123–31.

31. Winter DA. *ABC of balance during standing and walking.* Waterloo: Waterloo Biomechanics, 1995.

32. Baloh RW, Fife TD, Zwerling L, et al. Comparison of static and dynamic posturography in young and older normal people. *J Am Geriatr Soc* 1994;**42**:405–12.

33. Lord SR, Rogers MW, Howland A, Fitzpatrick R. Lateral stability, sensorimotor function and falls in older people. *J Am Geriatr Soc* 1999;**47**:1077–81.

34. Maki BE, Holliday PJ, Topper AK. A prospective study of postural balance and risk of falling in an ambulatory and independent elderly population. *J Gerontol Med Sci* 1994;**49**;M72–84.

35. McIlroy WE, Maki BE. Age-related changes in compensatory stepping in response to unpredictable perturbations. *J Gerontol* 1996;**51A**:M289–96.

36. Owings TM, Pavol MJ, Foley KT, Grabiner MD. Measures of postural stability are not predictors of recovery from large postural disturbances in healthy older adults. *J Am Geriatr Soc* 2000;**48**:42–50.

37. Immes FJ, Edholm OG. Studies of gait and mobility in the elderly. *Age Ageing* 1981;**10**:147–56.

38. Bloem BR, Haan J, Lagaay AM, et al. An investigation of gait in elderly subjects over 88 years of age. *J Geriatr Psychiatry Neurol* 1992;**5**:78–84.

39. Winter DA. *The biomechanics and motor control of human gait,* 2nd edn. Waterloo: Waterloo Biomechanics, 1991

40. Waite LM, Broe GA, Creasey H, et al. Neurological signs, aging and the neurodegenerative syndromes. *Arch Neurol* 1996;**53**:498–502.

41. Bloem BR, Gussekloo J, Lagaay AM, et al. Idiopathic senile gait disorders are signs of subclinical disease. *J Am Geriatr Soc* 2000;**48**:1098–101.

42. Nutt JG, Marsden CD, Thompson PD. Human walking and

higher-level gait disorders particularly in the elderly. *Neurology* 1993;**43**:268–79.

43. Liston R, Tallis RC. Gait apraxia and multi-infarct states. In: Meara J, Koller WC, eds. *Parkinson's disease and parkinsonism in the elderly.* Cambridge: Cambridge University Press, 2000;98–110.

44. Resnick NM, Marcantonio ER. How should clinical care of the aged differ. *Lancet* 1997;**350**:1157–8.

45. Mann DMA. Molecular biology's impact on our understanding of aging. *BMJ* 1997;**315**:1078–81.

46. Young A. Muscle function. In: Thomas PK, ed. *New issues in neurosciences.* Vol 1. New York: John Wiley and Sons, 1988;141–56.

47. Berg WP, Blasi ER. Stepping performance during obstacle clearance in women: age differences and the association with lower extremity strength in older women. *J Am Geriatr Soc* 2000;**48**:1414–23.

48. Woollacott, M, Shumway-Cook A. Attentional demands in postural tasks: changes in both healthy and balance impaired adults. *Gait Posture* 1999;**9**(S1);S12.

49. Stelmach GE, Worringham CJ. Sensorimotor deficits related to postural stability: implications for falling the elderly. *Clin Geriatr Med* 1985;**1**:679–94.

50. Teasdale N, Stelmach GE, Bard C, Fleury M. Posture and elderly persons: deficits in the central integrative mechanisms. In: Woollacott, M, Horak F, eds. *Posture and gait: control mechanisms,* Vol. 2. Portland: University of Oregon, 1992;203–207.

51. Starr JM, Deary IJ, Inch S, et al. Age associated cognitive decline in healthy old people. *Age Ageing* 1997;**26**:295–300.

52. Overstall PW, Imms RJ, Exton-Smith AN, Johnson AL. Falls in the elderly related to postural imbalance. *BMJ* 1977;i:261–268.

53. Lach HW, Reed AT, Arfken CL, et al. Falls in the elderly: reliability of a classification system. *J Am Geriatr Soc* 1991;**39**:197–202.

54. Northridge ME, Nevitt MC, Kelsey JL, Link B. Home hazards and falls in the elderly: the role of health and functional status. *Am J Publ Health* 1995;**85**:509–15.

55. Gill TM, Williams CS, Tinetti ME. Environmental hazards and the risk of falls in the home of community-living older persons. *J Am Geriatr Soc* 1999;**47**:S26.

56. Gill TM. Preventing falls: to modify the environment or the individual. *J Am Geriatr Soc* 1999;**47**:1471–2.

57. Tinetti ME, Ginter SF. Indentifying mobility dysfunctions in elderly patients. *JAMA* 1988;**259**:1190–3.

58. Campbell AJ, Borrie MJ, Spears GF. Risk factors for falls in a community based prospective study of people 70 years and older. *J Gerontol* 1989;**14**:M112–17.

59. Rubenstein LZ, Josephson KR. Assessment of falls risk. In: Overstall PW, ed. *Falls and bone health.* CD-ROM. Hereford: Kiss of Life Multimedia, 2002.

60. Lord SR, Ward JA, Williams P, Anstey KJ. Physiological factors associated with falls in older community-dwelling women. *J Am Geriatr Soc* 1994;**42**:1110–17.

61. Evans JG. Fallers, non-fallers and Poisson. *Age Ageing* 1990;**19**:268–9.

62. Campbell AJ, Spears GF. Fallers and non-fallers. *Age Ageing* 1990;**19**:345–6.

63. Shaw FE, Kenny RA. The overlap between syncope and falls in the elderly. *Postgrad Med J* 1997;**73**(864):635–9.

64. Mendelson WB. The use of sedative/hypnotic medication and

its correlation with falling down in the hospital. *Sleep* 1996;**19**(9):698–701.

65. Evans JG, Jarvis EH. Nitrazepam and the elderly. *BMJ* 1972;**4**:487.

66. Castleden CM, George CF, Marcer D, Hallett C1977. Increased sensitivity to nitrazepam in old age. *BMJ* **1**:10–12.

67. Macdonald JB, Macdonald ET. Nocturnal femoral fracture and continuing widespread use of barbiturate hypnotics. *BMJ* 1977;**2**:483–5.

68. Brocklehurst JC, Exton-Smith AN, Lempert Barber SM, Palmer MK. Barbiturates and fractures. *BMJ* 1977;**2**:699.

69. Campbell AJ, Robertson MC, Gardner MM, et al. Psychotropic medication withdrawal and a home-based exercise program to prevent falls: a randomised controlled trial. *J Am Geriatr Soc* 1999;**47**:850–3.

70. Thapa PB, Gideon, P, Cost TW. Antidepressants and the risk of falls among nursing home residents. *N Engl J Med* 1998;**339**:875–82.

71. Leipzig RM, Cummings RG, Tinetti ME. Drugs and falls in older people: a systematic review and meta-analysis: 1. psychotropic drugs. *J Am Geriatr Soc* 1999a;**47**:30–9.

72. Leipzig RM, Cummings RG, Tinetti ME. Drugs and falls in older people: a systematic review and meta-analysis: 2. cardiac and analgesic drugs. *J Am Geriatr Soc* 1999b;**47**:40–50.

73. Hodkinson HM. Evaluation of a mental test score for assessment of mental impairment in the elderly. *Age Ageing* 1973;**1**:233–8.

74. Folstein MF, Folstein SE. Mini mental state. A practical method for grading the cognitive state of patients for the clinician. *J Psychiatric Res* 1975;**12**:189–198.

75. van Dijk PTM, Meulenberg OGRM, van de Sande HJ, Habbema JDF. Falls in dementia patients. *Gerontologist* 1993;**33**:200–4.

76. Oleske DM, Wilson RS, Bernard BA, et al. Epidemiology of injury in people with Alzheimer's disease. *J Am Geriatr Soc* 1995;**43**:741–6.

77. Nakamura T, Meguro K, Sasaki H. Relationship between falls and stride length variability in senile dementia of the Alzheimer type. *Gerontology* 1996;**42**:108–13.

78. Alexander NB, Mollo JM, Giordani B, et al. Maintenance of balance, gait patterns and obstacle clearance in Alzheimer's disease. *Neurology* 1995;**45**;908–14.

79. Sheldon JH. *The social medicine of old age*. London: Oxford University Press, 1948.

80. Manchester D, Woollacott M, Zederbauer-Hilton N, Marin O. Visual, vestibular and somatosensory contributions to balance control in the older adult. *J Gerontol* 1989;**44**;M118–27.

81. Paulus WM, Straube A, Brandt T. Visual stabilisation of posture. *Brain* 1984;**107**:1143–63.

82. Lee DN, Lishman JR. Visual proprioceptive control of stance. *J Hum Mov Stud* 1975;**1**:87–95.

83. Horak FB, Shupert CL, Miska A. Components of postural dyscontrol in the elderly: a review. *Neurobiol Aging* 1988;**10**:727–38.

84. Jack CIA, Smith T, Neoh C, et al. Prevalence of low vision in elderly patients admitted to an acute geriatric unit in Liverpool. *Gerontology* 1995;**41**:280–5.

85. Ivers RQ, Cumming RG, Mitchell P, Attebo K. Visual impairment and falls in older adults: the Blue Mountains eye study. *J Am Geriatr Soc* 1998;**46**:58–64.

86. Lord S R, Dayhew J. Visual risk factors for falls. *J Am Geriatr Soc.* 2001;**49**:508–15.

87. Lord SR, Menz HB. Visual contributions to postural stability in older adults. *Gerontology* 2000;**46**:306–10.

88. Robbins E, Waked E, McClaran J. Proprioception and stability: foot position awareness as a function of age and footwear. *Age Ageing* 1996;**24**:67–72.

89. Lipsitz LA. Orthostatic and postprandial hypotension assessment and management. *Ann Long-Term Care* 2000;**8**:41–4.

90. Rubenstein LZ, Robbins AS, Josephson KR, et al. The value of assessing falls in an elderly population: a randomised clinical trial. *Ann Intern Med* 1990;**113**:308–16.

91. Ensrud KE, Nevitt MC, Yunis C, et al. Postural hypotension and postural dizziness in elderly women. *Arch Int Med* 1992;**152**:1058–64.

92. Liu BA, Topper AK, Reeves RA, et al. Falls among older people: relationship to medication use and orthostatic hypotension. *J Am Geriatr Soc* 1995;**43**:1141–5.

93. Tinetti ME, Williams CS, Gill TM. Health, functional and psychological outcomes among older persons with chronic dizziness. *J Am Geriatr Soc* 2000;**48**:417–21.

94. Lempert T, Gresty MA, Bronstein AM. Benign positional vertigo: recognition and treatment. *BMJ* 1995;**311**:489–91.

95. Hankey GJ, Warlow CP. *Transient ischaemic attacks of the brain and eye*. London: W. B. Saunders, 1994.

96. Colledge NR, Barr-Hamilton RM, Lewis SJ, et al. Evaluation of investigations to diagnose the cause of dizziness in elderly people: a community based controlled study. *BMJ* 1996;**313**:788–92.

97. McIntosh S, Da Costa D, Kenny RA. Outcome of an integrated approach to the investigation of dizziness, falls and syncope in elderly patients referred to a syncope clinic. *Age Ageing* 1993;**22**:53–8.

98. Lord SR, Caplan GA, Colagiuri R, et al. Sensori-motor function in older persons with diabetes. *Diabet Med* 1993;**10**:614–18.

99. Menz HB, Lord SR. Foot problems, functional impairment and falls in older people. *J Am Podiatr Assoc* 1999;**89**:458–67.

100. Cummings SR, Ling X, Stone K. Consequences of foot binding among older women in Beijing China. *Am J Public Health* 1997;**87**:1677–9.

101. Tinetti ME. Performance-orientated assessment of mobility problems in elderly patients. *J Am Geriatr Soc* 1988;**34**:119–26.

102. Topper AK, Maki BE, Holliday PJ. Are activity-based assessments of balance and gait in the elderly predictive of risk of falling and/or type of fall? *J Am Geriatr Soc* 1993,**41**.479–87.

103. Tinetti ME, Williams TF, Mayewski R. A fall risk index for elderly patients based on number of chronic disabilities. *Am J Med* 1986;**80**:429–34.

104. Mathias S, Nayak USL, Isaacs B. Balance in elderly patients: the 'get-up and go' test. *Arch Phys Med Rehabil* 1986;**67**:387–9.

105. Podsiadlo, D, Richardson S. The timed 'up and go': a test of basic functional mobility for frail elderly persons. *J Am Geriatr Soc* 1991;**39**:142–8.

106. Duncan PW, Weiner DK, Chandler J, Studenski S. Functional reach: a new clinical measure of balance. *J Gerontol Med Sci* 1990;**45**:M192–7.

107. Vellas BJ, Wayne SJ, Romero, L, et al. One leg balance is an important predictor of injurious falls in older persons. *J Am Geriatr Soc* 1997;**45**:735–8.

108. Sudarsky L. Geriatrics: gait disorders in the elderly. *N Engl J Med* 1990;**322**:1441–6.

109. Fuh JL, Lin KN, Wang SJ, et al. Neurologic disease presenting with gait impairment in the elderly. *J Geriatr Psychiatry Neurol* 1994;**7**:91–94.

110. Forster A, Young J. Incidence and consequences of falls due to stroke. *BMJ* 1995;**311**:83–6.

111. Hoehn MM, Yahr MD. Parkinsonism: onset, progression and mortality. *Neurology* 1967;**17**:427–42.

112. Giladi N, Kuo R, Fahn S. Freezing phenomenon in patients with Parkinsonian syndromes. *Mov Disord* 1997;**12**:302–5.

113. Longstreth WT, Manolio TA, Arnold A, et al. Clinical correlates of white matter findings on cranial magnetic resonance imaging of 3301 elderly people. *Stroke* 1996;**27**:1274–82.

114. Longstreth WT, Bernick C, Manolio TA, et al. Lacunar infarcts defined by magnetic resonance imaging of 3600 elderly people. *Arch Neurol* 1998;**55**:1217–25

115. Baloh RW, Yue Q, Socotch TM, Jacobson KM. White matter lesions and disequilibrium in older people. *Arch Neurol* 1995;**52**:970–4.

116. Piccini P, Pavese N, Canapicchi R, et al. 1995. White matter hyperintensities in Parkinson's disease. *Arch Neurol* **52**:191–4.

117. Blin J, Dubois B, Bonnet AM, et al. Does aging aggravate Parkinsonian disability. *J Neurol Neurosurg Psychiatry* 1991;**54**:780–2.

118. Georgiou N, Iansek R, Bradshaw JL, et al. An evaluation of the role of internal cues in the pathogenesis of Parkinsonian hypokinesia. *Brain* 1993;**116**:1575–87.

119. Morris ME, Iansek R, Matyas TA, Summers JJ. Stride length regulation in Parkinson's disease. *Brain* 1996;**119**:551–68.

120. Kuhtz-Buschbeck JP, Jöhnk K, Mäder S. Analysis of gait in cervical myelopathy. *Gait Posture* 1999;**9**:184–189.

121. Brodie MJ, Overstall PW, Giorgi L. Multi centre, double-blind randomised comparison between lamotrigine and carbamazepine in elderly patients with newly diagnosed epilepsy. *Epilepsy Res* 1999;**37**:81–7.

122. Zaidi A, Clough P, Scheepers B, Fitzpatrick A. Treatment resistant epilepsy or convulsive syncope. *BMJ* 1998;**317**:869–70.

123. Department of Trade and Industry. *Avoiding slips, trips and broken hips.* London: DTI, 1999.

124. Royal College of Physicians. *Osteoporosis: clinical guidelines for prevention and treatment.* London: Royal College of Physicians, 2000.

125. Overstall PW, Clarke CE. Uncertainties in the pharmacotherapy of Parkinson's Disease and how to solve them. *Gerontology* 2002;**48**:30–3.

126. Henry R, Rowe J, O'Mahony D. Haemodynamic analysis of efficacy of compression hosiery in elderly fallers with orthostatic hypotension. *Lancet* 1999;**354**:45–6.

127. Christmas, C, Andersen RA. Exercise and older patients: guidelines for the clinician. *J Am Geriatr Soc* 2000;**48**:318–24.

128. Skelton D, Young A, Walker A, Hoinville E. *Physical activity in later life.* London: Health Education Authority, 1999.

129. Skelton DA, Greig CA, Davies JM, Young A. Strength, power and related functional ability of healthy people aged 65–89 years. *Age Ageing* 1994;**23**:371–7.

130. Skelton DA, McLaughlin AW. Training functional ability in old age. *Physiotherapy* 1996;**82**:159–67.

131. Lord SR, Lloyd DG, Raymond NM, et al. The effect of exercise on gait patterns in older women: a randomised controlled trial. *J Gerontol Med Sci* 1996;**51**:M64–70.

132. Chandler JM, Duncan PW, Kochersberger, G, Studenski S. Is lower extremity strength gain associated with improvement in physical performance and disability in frail, community-dwelling elders. *Arch Phys Med Rehabil* 1998;**79**:24–30.

133. McMurdo MET, Mole PA, Paterson CR. Controlled trial of weight bearing exercise in older women in relation to bone density and falls. *BMJ* 1997;**314**:569.

134. Gardner MM, Robertson MC, Campbell AJ. Exercise in preventing falls and fall related injuries in older people: a review of randomised controlled trials. *Br J Sports Med* 2000;**34**:7–17.

135. Province M, Hadley E, Hornbrook M, et al. The effects of exercise on falls in elderly patients. A pre-planned meta-analysis of the FICSIT trials. *JAMA* 1995;**273**:1341–7.

136. Day L, Fildes B, Gordon I, et al. Randomised factorial trial of falls prevention among older people living in their own homes. *BMJ* 2002;**325**:128.

137. Shumway-Cook A, Gruber W, Baldwin M, Liao S. The effect of multi-dimensional exercises on balance, mobility and fall risk in community-dwelling older adults. *Phys Ther* 1997;**77**:46–57.

138. Satariano WA, Haight TJ, Tager IB. Reasons given by older people for limitation or avoidance of leisure time physical activity. *J Am Geriatr Soc* 2000;**48**:505–12.

139. Hillsdon M, Thorogood M, Anstiss T, Morris J. Randomised controlled trials of physical activity promotion in free living populations: a review. *J Epidemiol Community Health* 1995;**49**:448–53.

140. Ebrahim S, Thompson PW, Baskaran V, Evans K. Randomised placebo-controlled trial of brisk walking in the prevention of postmenopausal osteoporosis. *Age Ageing* 1997;**26**:253–60.

141. Jakes RW, Khaw KT, Day NE, et al. Patterns of physical activity and ultrasound attenuation by heel bone among Norfolk cohort of European Prospective Investigation of Cancer (EPIC Norfolk). *BMJ* 2001;**322**:140–43.

142. Wolf SL, Barnhart HX, Kutner NG, et al. Reducing frailty and falls in older persons: an investigation of Tai Chi and computerised balance training. *J Am Geriatr Soc* 1996;**44**:489–97.

143. Kutner NG, Barnhart H, Wolf SL, et al. Self-report benefits of Tai Chi practice by older adults. *J Gerontol Psychol Sci* 1997;**52**:P242–6.

144. Tinetti ME, Baker DI, McAvay G, et al. A multifactorial intervention to reduce the risk of falling among elderly people living in the community. *N Engl J Med* 1994;**331**:821–7.

145. Close J, Ellis M, Hooper R, et al. Prevention of falls in the elderly trial (PROFET) a randomised controlled trial. *Lancet* 1999;**353**:93–7.

146. Oliver D, Hopper A, Seed P. Do hospital fall prevention programs work? A systematic review. *J Am Geriatr Soc* 2000;**48**:1680–9.

147. Dyer C, Watkins C, Gould C, Rowe J. Risk factor assessment for falls: from written checklist to the penless clinic. *Age Ageing* 1998;**27**:569–72.

148. Shah PN, Maly RC, Frank JC, et al. Managing geriatric

syndromes: what geriatric assessment teams recommend, what primary care physicians implement, what patients adhere to. *J Am Geriatr Soc* 1997;**45**:413–19.

149. Campbell AJ, Robertson MC, Gardner MM, et al. 1997. Randomised controlled trial of a general practice programme of home based exercise to prevent falls in elderly women. *BMJ* 315:1065–9.

150. Herbert RD, Maher CG, Moseley AM, et al. Effective physiotherapy. *BMJ* 2001;**323**:788–90.

151. Robertson MC, Devlin N, Gardner MM, et al. Effectiveness and economic evaluation of a nurse delivered home exercise programme to prevent falls. 1. Randomised controlled trial. *BMJ* 2001;**322**:697–701.

152. Mickelborough J, Liston R, Harris B, et al. Physiotherapy for higher-level gait disorders associated with cerebral multi-infarcts. *Physiother Theor Pract* 1997;**13**:127–38.

153. Dietz, V, Colombo G, Jensen L. Locomotor activity in spinal man. *Lancet* 1994;**344**:1260–3.

154. Liston R, Mickelborough J, Harris B, et al. Conventional physiotherapy and treadmill re-training for higher-level gait disorders in cerebrovascular disease. *Age Ageing* 2000;**29**:311–18.

155. Morris M, Huxham F, McGinley J. Strategies to prevent falls in people with Parkinson's disease. *Physiother Singapore* 1999;**2**:135–41.

156. Morris M. Movement disorders in people with Parkinson's disease: a model for physical therapy. *Phys Ther* 2000;**80**:578–97.

157. Cumming RG, Thomas M, Szonyi G, et al. Home visits by an occupational therapist for assessment and modification of environmental hazards: a randomised trial of falls prevention. *J Am Geriatr Soc* 1999;**47**:1397–402.

158. Lord SR, Bashford GM. Shoe characteristics and balance in older women. *J Am Geriatr Soc* 1996;**44**:429–33.

159. Robbins SE, Gouw G, McClaran J. Shoe sole thickness and hardness influence balance in older men. *J Am Geriatr Soc* 1992;**40**:1089–94.

160. Robbins S, Waked E, Rappel R. Ankle taping improves proprioception before and after exercise in young men. *Br J Sports Med* 1995;**29**:242–7.

161. Lord SR, Bashford GM, Howland A, Munroe BJ. Effects of shoe collar height and sole hardness on balance in women. *J Am Geriatr Soc* 1999;**47**:681–4.

162. Lauritzen JB, Petersen MM, Lund B. Effect of external hip protectors on hip fractures. *Lancet* 1993;**341**:11–13.

163. Cameron ID, Stafford, B, Cumming RG, et al. Hip protectors improve falls self-efficacy. *Age Ageing* 2000;**29**:57–62.

164. Parker MJ, Gillespie LD, Gillespie WJ. Hip protectors for preventing hip fracture in the elderly. *Cochrane Database Syst Rev* 2001;**2**;CD001255.

165. Zacker, C, Shea D. An economic evaluation of energy-absorbing flooring to prevent hip fractures. *Int J Technol Assess Health Care* 1998;**14**:446–57.

22

Syncope-related falls in the older person

ROSE ANNE KENNY AND LYNNE ARMSTRONG

INTRODUCTION

Syncope and falls have historically been regarded as two distinct clinical entities, presenting to different health-care professionals and having separate means of evaluation and management. Fallers traditionally were investigated and managed by health-care professionals with experience in multidisciplinary and rehabilitative working, while patients with syncope would often have been assessed almost solely by cardiologists.

Increasingly, there is evidence of an overlap between these syndromes with common underlying abnormalities being identified. This chapter explores the epidemiology of falls and syncope in the older person, the possible common underlying abnormalities, mechanisms of assessment and available interventions.

FALLS AND THE OLDER PERSON

A fall can be defined as an event whereby an individual comes to rest on the ground or on another level with or without loss of consciousness. Falls have traditionally been categorized as 'extrinsic', caused by environmental hazards, or as 'intrinsic', caused by age-related physiological changes and/or clinical disorders. Most falls, particularly in the very elderly are caused by a combination of extrinsic and intrinsic factors. In patients who are cognitively normal, falls can be classified according to their clinical characteristics. If a patient can clearly recall a trip or a slip, the fall is 'accidental'. If a patient has fallen and/or lost consciousness for no apparent reason, the episode is described as an 'unexplained' fall. It is increasingly acknowledged that presyncope and syncope can present as recurrent unexplained falls. The evidence for this will be discussed later.

EPIDEMIOLOGY OF FALLS

The reported incidence of falls varies with the population studied (community-dwelling, hospital patients, those with cognitive impairment or in long-term care facilities) and the methods of recording or ascertaining falls. Self-reporting is likely to be the most accurate method of reporting falls.[1] In one year, 30 per cent of people aged over 65 years living in the community will fall.[2] The figure rises to 40 per cent in those over 80 years and to over 60 per cent in some nursing home populations.[3,4] In studies estimating annual incidence of falls in persons with cognitive impairment or dementia, incidences of 60–80 per cent have been reported.[2,5]

CONSEQUENCES OF FALLS

Falls are of major concern not only to the older individuals affected but also to any health-care system dealing with the initial resultant injuries and the longer-term consequences of loss of independence or function. It is the interplay between the high incidence of falling and the prevalence of comorbid disease such as osteoporosis which results in the high morbidity and mortality associated with older fallers. Both the incidence of falls and the severity of fall-related complications rises steadily after age 60 years. Half of all attendances by adults aged over 50 years at an inner city accident and emergency department in the UK followed a fall.[6] Fall-related injuries recently accounted for 6 per cent of all medical expenditure for persons aged 65 years and older in the USA.[7,8] Approximately 5 per cent of older people that fall require hospitalization.[9] Unintentional injury is the fifth leading cause of death in older adults and falls are responsible for two-thirds of all deaths resulting from unintentional injuries.[10]

Hip fractures represent one of the most important consequences of falls in the older adult. Approximately half of previously independent, older hip-fracture patients become partly dependent and one-third ultimately become totally dependent. Hip fractures are associated with a reduction of 12–20 per cent in expected survival, and with 5–20 per cent excess mortality within the year of injury.

In addition to physical injury, falls can also have important psychological and social consequences. Recurrent falls are one of the commonest reasons cited for admission of previously independent elderly people to nursing homes or institutional care.[11] Fear of falling and the post-fall anxiety syndrome are also well recognized as negative consequences of falls. Loss of confidence can result in self-imposed functional limitations and dependence.[4,12] The negative impact of falls on quality of life, mood and functional capacity is even more apparent for subjects that experience unexplained recurrent falls than for those that have accidental falls.[13]

RISK FACTORS FOR FALLS

This chapter concentrates principally on syncope-related falls but it is important to remember that, as with almost all syndromes affecting older people, multiple pathology and comorbidity are common. There is frequently more than one possible cause of falling and intrinsic and extrinsic causes interact in susceptible individuals. Syncope-related falls are often the result of neurovascular instability. The main clinical diagnoses included in this broad category are carotid sinus hypersensitivity, orthostatic hypotension, vasovagal or neurocardiogenic syncope and post-prandial hypotension.

SYNCOPE IN THE OLDER ADULT

Syncope is a symptom defined as a transient, self-limited loss of consciousness, usually leading to a fall. The onset of syncope is usually rapid, and the subsequent recovery is spontaneous, complete and prompt.[14] Individuals that

describe syncope will often experience more frequent episodes of presyncope. Presyncope or near-syncope refers to a condition where the patient feels as though syncope is imminent. Symptoms may be non-specific (e.g. dizziness) and tend to overlap with those of the premonitory phase of true syncope.

Epidemiology of syncope

The epidemiology of syncope in old age has not been well studied. The greatest difficulty in assessing the magnitude of the problem is that it is only recently acknowledged that there is considerable overlap between syncope and falls. This is likely to have led to a significant underestimate of the frequency of syncope in the older person. From available data the incidence of syncope is at least 6 per cent per year, with a 10 per cent prevalence and a 30 per cent 2-year recurrence rate.[15]

Pathophysiology of syncope in the older adult

The temporary cessation of cerebral function that causes syncope is caused by transient and sudden reduction of cerebral blood flow to areas of the brain responsible for consciousness (reticular activating system). Cerebral perfusion pressure is largely dependent on systemic arterial pressure. Any factor that either decreases cardiac output or total peripheral vascular resistance diminishes systemic arterial pressure and cerebral perfusion.[16]

Age-related physiological impairments of heart rate, blood pressure, cerebral blood flow, in combination with comorbid conditions and concurrent medications account for an increased susceptibility to syncope in older adults. Baroreflex sensitivity is blunted by aging, manifesting as a reduction in heart rate response to hypotensive stimuli.[17–19] The elderly are prone to reduced blood volume due to excessive salt-wasting by the kidneys as a result of diminished renin–aldosterone activity,[20] a rise in atrial natriuretic peptide[21] and concurrent diuretic therapy. Low blood volume together with age-related diastolic dysfunction can lead to a low cardiac output, which increases susceptibility to orthostatic hypotension and neurocardiogenic syncope. Cerebral autoregulation, which maintains a constant cerebral perfusion pressure over a wide range of systemic blood pressures changes is altered in the presence of hypertension and possibly by aging.[17,19] As a result, sudden mild to moderate declines in blood pressure which would not cause any embarrassment of cerebral perfusion in a younger individual can markedly affect perfusion pressures in the older adult and leave them very vulnerable to presyncope or syncope.

Etiology of syncope

Table 22.1 provides a pathophysiological classification of the commoner causes of transient loss of consciousness.

Table 22.1 *Common causes of syncope*

Neurally mediated reflex syncopal syndromes[a]
Neurocardiogenic/vasovagal syncope (common faint)
Carotid sinus syndrome

Situational syncope	Gastrointestinal stimulation (swallow, defecation, visceral pain)
	Micturition (post-micturition)
	Cough
	Glossopharyngeal and trigeminal neuralgia

Orthostatic[b]

Autonomic failure	Primary autonomic failure syndromes
	Secondary autonomic failure syndromes
	Drugs and alcohol

Volume depletion

Cardiac arrhythmia as primary cause[c]
Sinus node dysfunction (including tachycardia/bradycardia syndrome)
Atrioventricular conduction system disease
Paroxysmal supraventricular and ventricular tachycardias
Inherited syndromes (e.g. long QT syndrome, Brugada syndrome)
Implanted device (pacemaker) dysfunction

Structural cardiac or cardiopulmonary disease[d]
Cardiac valvular disease
Acute myocardial infarction/ischemia
Obstructive cardiomyopathy
Atrial myxoma
Acute aortic dissection
Pericardial disease or tamponade

Cerebrovascular
Vascular steal syndromes[e]

---

[a]Neurally mediated reflex syncopal syndrome refers to the Bezold–Jarisch reflex that when triggered gives rise to inappropriate vasodilatation and bradycardia.
[b]Orthostatic syncope occurs when the autonomic nervous system is incapacitated, resulting in failure of vasoconstrictor mechanisms thereby resulting in hypotension.
[c]Cardiac arrhythmias resulting in reduced cardiac output.
[d]Structural heart disease can cause syncope when circulatory demands outstrip the heart's ability to increase its output.
[e]Steal syndromes rarely can cause syncope when a blood vessel has to supply both part of the brain and an arm.

The commonest causes of syncope in older adults are orthostatic hypotension, neurally mediated syncope and cardiac arrhythmias.[22–24] Orthostatic hypotension is an attributable cause of syncope in 20–30 per cent of events.[23,24] Carotid sinus hypersensitivity is rare before the age of 40 years but the prevalence increases with age and with cardiovascular, cerebrovascular and neurodegenerative comorbidity.[25–27] Cardio-inhibitory carotid sinus syndrome has been recognized as an attributable cause of syncope in older adults in up to 20–30 per cent of cases.[23,28] Vasodepressor carotid sinus syndrome is likely to be equally prevalent.[23,24] Up to 15 per cent of syncope in the elderly is neurocardiogenic while 20 per cent is due to cardiac arrhythmias.[22,23]

OVERLAP OF FALLS AND SYNCOPE

The traditional view of syncope and falls is to regard them as separate conditions with different etiologies. It has been suggested that an accurate history of the event from the patient and an available witness will allow the differentiation between syncope and falls and will point to the diagnosis in over 40 per cent of cases.[22,29] This approach is problematic in older adults for a variety of reasons. Up to one-third of cognitively normal older adults have retrograde amnesia for witnessed loss of consciousness.[30] Similarly over one-third of community-dwelling older adults did not recall having fallen 3 months after a documented fall event.[31] In addition, witness accounts of syncopal events are only available in 40–60 per cent of older people attending a syncope clinic with recurrent symptoms.[23] In patients with cognitive impairment the differentiation between falls and syncope is likely to be even more difficult.

Experience from dedicated syncope and falls facilities would reinforce the evidence of an overlap between these syndromes. A review of three studies, which included a total of 109 patients for whom cardio-inhibitory carotid sinus syndrome was an attributable cause of falls, 38 per cent of patients presented with falls alone or falls and dizziness but denied syncope. Of the fallers, 51 per cent demonstrated amnesia for loss of consciousness during diagnostic testing. Two-thirds of patients with orthostatic hypotension as an attributable cause of symptoms presented with falls only, or falls and dizziness.[32,33] In a further case series of 169 patients that attended a dedicated syncope and falls clinic, over one-third presented with a history of unexplained falls; two-thirds of these had an attributable cardiovascular diagnosis, of which the majority were carotid sinus syndrome, orthostatic hypotension, cardiac arrhythmias and neurocardiogenic syncope.[23]

More recently there is emerging evidence from falls intervention studies that treatment of identified attributable cardiovascular causes of syncope and falls resulted in reduced subsequent frequency of falling[28,34] and have demonstrated that treatment of cardio-inhibitory carotid sinus syndrome with a rate drop demand pacemaker resulted in a 70 per cent reduction in the number of falls in the subsequent year of follow-up. Similarly preliminary data from SAFE-COG, a study of multifactorial intervention strategies in cognitively impaired fallers, suggests that treatment of cardiovascular abnormalities may reduce fall frequency in patients with dementia living in the community. Another possible explanation for the overlap between syncope and falls is that moderate hemodynamic changes insufficient to cause true syncope may result in falls in individuals already compromised by gait and balance instability and slow protective reflexes. It seems that syncope in older adults and falls are often indistinguishable and are manifestations of similar pathophysiological processes.

CAROTID SINUS SYNDROME

Carotid sinus syndrome (CSS) is a frequently overlooked cause of syncope in the elderly. Exaggerated baroreceptor-mediated reflexes result in episodic bradycardia/asystole and/or hypotension. Three subtypes of reflex hypersensitivity and hence CSS are currently recognized: cardio-inhibitory, vasodepressor and mixed. The three subtypes occur with equal frequency.[23]

Pathophysiology

The carotid sinus is located at the bifurcation of the internal and external carotid arteries. Afferent sensory nerve endings are embedded in the elastic tissue of the sinus wall. The nerves emerge as the nerve of Hering to join the glossopharyngeal nerve, with some fibers travelling with the hypoglossal, vagal and sympathetic nerves. The afferent limb of the carotid sinus reflex terminates at the nucleus of the tractus solitarius in the medulla. The efferent limb comprises the sympathetic

nerves supplying the heart, the vasculature and the cardiac vagus nerve. Physiological rises in arterial blood pressure generate the stretch necessary to activate the reflex. In patients with CSS, baroreflex sensitivity, which normally declines with age, is enhanced compared with age-matched controls.[35] The exact location of the pathological lesion in CSS is unknown. Although there is excessive clustering of atherosclerotic comorbidities with CSS, the abnormal response does not seem to be a purely local effect. Afferent pathways of the reflex appear to be intact, and the often dissociated response of pure vasodepressor or pure cardio-inhibition, would suggest that the lesion is centrally located. It seems likely that the central damage is ischemic in origin. It has been suggested that up regulation of postsynaptic α_2-adrenoceptors may cause exaggerated baroreflex efferent responses resulting in profound hypotension and bradycardia.[36]

Symptoms

Recent studies suggest that CSS is not a feature of normal aging.[25,37] Patients present with recurrent falls, drop attacks, presyncope and syncope. Unlike neurocardiogenic syncope, there is little or no prodroma: syncope and falls are sudden and unpredictable.[38] The symptoms are usually precipitated by mechanical stimulation of the carotid sinus; that is, by head turning, tight neckwear, shaving, neck pathology and by vagal stimuli such as prolonged standing.

Diagnosis

Carotid sinus syndrome is diagnosed when carotid sinus hypersensitivity is documented in a patient with otherwise unexplained dizziness, falls, presyncope or syncope in whom carotid sinus massage reproduces presenting symptoms. The cardio-inhibitory subtype is diagnosed if carotid sinus massage produces asystole exceeding 3 s, the vasodepressor subtype if there is a fall in systolic blood pressure exceeding 50 mmHg in the absence of significant bradycardia and a mixed subtype if both are present. Carotid sinus massage is a crude and unquantifiable technique prone to both intra- and inter-operator variation.

Treatment

Treatment strategies depend on the clinical subtype.

CARDIO-INHIBITORY CAROTID SINUS SYNDROME

Treatment of choice for cardio-inhibitory CSS is a permanent pacemaker. Recurrent syncope caused by CSS, producing greater than 3 s of asystole in the absence of medication that depresses the sino-atrial or the atrioventricular conduction, is a class I indication for pace-maker implantation. Recurrent syncope without clear provocative events and with a hypersensitive cardio-inhibitory response is a class IIa indication according to ACC/AHA guidelines.[39] Dual-chamber pacing signifi-cantly reduces syncope, falls, injury and hospital admis-sions.[28,40,41]

VASODEPRESSOR CAROTID SINUS SYNDROME

Management of vasodepressor CSS is much more diffi-cult. Dihydroergotamine and fludrocortisone have been used with limited effect.[42] The side-effects of these med-ications in the elderly negate their long-term usefulness. Midodrine, a peripheral α-adrenergic agonist, may yield some benefit but randomized controlled studies are not yet available.

ORTHOSTATIC HYPOTENSION

Orthostatic hypotension (OH) is a reduction in systolic blood pressure by at least 20 mmHg or diastolic blood pressure of at least 10 mmHg within 3 min of standing.[43] The prevalence of OH varies between 4 per cent and 33 per cent among community-dwelling elderly.[17,44] The prevalence and magnitude of falls in systolic blood pres-sure increase with age and are associated with general frailty and excessive mortality.[45]

Pathophysiology

Orthostasis refers to physiological stress related to the upright posture. Standing induces venous pooling, reduces venous return and decreases ventricular filling pressures. In health, cardiac output and arterial pressure are maintained by raising the heart rate and increasing peripheral vasoconstriction. These powerful compen-satory responses are initiated by the carotid and aortic arch baroreceptors. The baroreceptor input to the brain stem centers leads to inhibition of cardiac vagal tone and a brisk increase in sympathetic outflow. Norepinephrine

Table 22.2 *Etiology of orthostatic hypotension in older adults referred to a regional syncope service*

Etiology	Prevalence (%)
Drug induced	28
Autonomic failure	27
Age-related	20
Multiple system atrophy	13
Parkinson's disease	5
Unclassified	2

Data from Stout N., Kenny R. A. Causes of orthostatic hypotension in older adults referred to a regional syncope service. *Clin Auton Res* 1998;8:71–2.[33]

Table 22.3 *Commonly used drugs causing orthostatic hypotension*

Class of drug	Mechanism of orthostatic hypotension
Antihypertensives	
Calcium channel blockers	Vasodilatation
ACE inhibitors	Inhibition of angiotensin II production
Adrenergic nerve blocking agents	α-Adrenergic blockade
α-Adrenoceptor antagonists	α-Adrenergic blockade
Coronary vasodilators	
Nitrates	Vasodilatation
Diuretics	
Thiazide or loop	Volume depletion
Psychotropic drugs	
Phenothiazines	α-Adrenergic blockade
Tricyclic antidepressants	α-Adrenergic blockade
Anti-parkinsonian drugs	
Levodopa	Not clearly understood
Bromocriptine	Activate vascular dopaminergic receptors
CNS depressants	
Ethanol	Vasodilatation

(noradrenaline) released from sympathetic nerve end-ings, has a positive chronotropic and inotropic effect on the heart but also causes venous and arteriolar vasocon-striction.[46] Orthostatic hypotension results from failure of the arterial baroreflex.

Several pathological conditions are associated with OH. Stout and Kenny[33] describe a consecutive series of 70 patients with OH. The results are shown in Table 22.2.

Drug-induced OH is common. Table 22.3 outlines likely culprit medication.

A number of non-neurogenic conditions are also associated with or exacerbate pre-existing OH. They include hemorrhage, diarrhea, vomiting, burns, hemodialysis, diabetes insipidus, adrenal insufficiency, fever and extensive varicose veins.

Primary autonomic failure

The three main clinical entities are pure autonomic fail-ure, multiple system atrophy and autonomic failure associated with idiopathic Parkinson's disease. Pure autonomic failure is a relatively benign condition previ-ously known as idiopathic OH. It presents with OH, defective sweating, impotence and bowel disturbance. No other neurological defect is found. Multiple system atrophy is associated with the poorest prognosis. Clinical features include dysautonomia and motor disturbances due to striatonigral degeneration, cerebellar atrophy or pyramidal lesions. Orthostatic hypotension associated with Parkinson's disease can be caused by factors other than dysautonomia such as drug side-effects, other comorbidity and associated medication and the accompanying effects of aging.

Secondary autonomic failure

Secondary autonomic failure may be associated with diabetes, chronic renal and hepatic failure, connective tissue disorders, amyloidosis, demyelinating polyneuropathies, multiple sclerosis and brainstem lesions. In the absence of well-recognized conditions causing primary or secondary autonomic failure, aging can also be considered a cause of OH.

Symptoms

The classical history of OH is posture-induced dizziness or collapse within 3 min of rising from sitting or lying. Symptoms are generally worse in the morning when getting out of bed. A coat-hanger distribution of pain across the neck and shoulders often accompanies OH.[47]

Diagnosis

Diagnosis of OH involves demonstration of a postural fall in blood pressure after standing. Reproducibility of OH depends on the time of measurement and on autonomic function.[32] The measurement should be carried out as early in the morning as is practical after maintaining a supine posture for at least 10 min. Phasic beat-to-beat blood pressure measurements are more sensitive than sphygmomanometer measurements.

Treatment

Treatments to reduce the effects of venous pooling are particularly useful in OH. These include physical maneuvers (compression stockings and calf exercises) and vasoconstriction (adrenergic agonist midodrine). Increasing circulating blood volume, by increased salt and fluid intake and by the use of fludrocortisone, reduces the effects of venous pooling. Desmopressin has been used in resistant cases of OH for its antidiuretic and mild pressor effects. Since drugs are commonly indicated in the causation of OH it is paramount that all efforts be made to ensure rational drug prescribing, minimizing all non-essential therapy.

Hypertension and orthostatic hypotension

Aging is associated with an increased risk of hypertension. Hypertension is known to impair baroreflex-sensitivity and restricts ventricular filling.[48,49] Paradoxically, hypertension increases the risk of episodic hypotension.

A strong relationship between supine hypertension and OH has been reported among unmedicated, institutionalized older subjects.[15] Hypertension also alters the thresholds at which cerebral autoregulation occurs. Older subjects with hypertension are thus more likely to experience intermittent hypotension and be less able to compensate for its effects, with the result that they are exposed to cerebral ischemia. In addition, with increasingly aggressive blood pressure control targets, patients are likely to be taking two or three antihypertensive medications, which all impair cardiovascular reflexes and further increase the risk of OH.

NEURALLY MEDIATED SYNCOPE

Neurally mediated syncope or vasovagal syncope is the simple faint. It was previously believed that it was a rare phenomenon in older adults but more recently it has been estimated to be the cause of 20 per cent of recurrent syncopal events.[50] In older adults referred to a syncope clinic over a 6-month period, 11 per cent had neurally mediated syncope which commonly coexisted with CSS and OH.[23] In an unselected sample of older patients presenting to an accident and emergency department with unexplained or recurrent falls, neurally mediated syncope was present in 16–18 per cent.[6,50]

Pathophysiology

The normal physiological response to orthostasis, as described earlier, is to increase heart rate and raise peripheral vascular resistance to maintain an adequate cardiac output, thus maintaining cerebral perfusion in the upright position. In patients with neurally mediated syncope, these responses are replaced after a variable period by parodoxical withdrawal of sympathetic tone and increased parasympathetic activity. This results in the hallmark changes of neurally mediated syncope: hypotension and/or bradycardia sufficient to produce cerebral ischemia and loss of neural function. The precise sequence of events leading to neurally mediated syncope is not fully understood. A possible mechanism involves the stimulation of cardiac mechanoreceptors and activation of the Bezold–Jarisch reflex leading to peripheral vasodilatation (hypotension) and bradycardia. This is likely to arise in situations where a sudden fall in venous return causes a rapid fall in ventricular volume; compensatory mechanisms attempt to respond with vigorous ventricular contraction but produce virtual collapse of the ventricular wall.[52] This postulated mechanism has driven the choice of drug used in the treatment of neurally mediated syncope (negative inotropic agents such as beta-blockers and disopyramide). Other mechanisms of activation are also likely as syncope can be associated with fear and emotional upset, implying that higher central nervous centers can initiate the response. Several neurotransmitters, namely serotonin, endorphins and arginine vasopressin, play an important role in the pathogenesis of neurally mediated syncope, possibly by central sympathetic inhibition. Their exact role is not yet well established.

Symptoms

In most patients, manifestation of neurally mediated syncope occurs in three distinct phases: a prodrome or aura, loss of consciousness, and post-syncopal phase.[53] A precipitating situation is identified in most patients. These include anxiety, pain, anticipation of pain, warm environments, air travel and, most commonly, prolonged standing. The most common triggers in the older adult are prolonged standing and vasodilating medication.[23] Patients commonly experience slowly progressive lightheadedness, sweating, nausea, yawning and visual and auditory distortion. The syncopal period is usually brief, during which some patients develop involuntary movements from tonic–clonic movements to myoclonic jerks. These involuntary movements are more usual if there is prolonged bradycardia or asystole and can lead to confusion with epilepsy. Recovery is usually rapid, but some patients can experience protracted symptoms of nausea, headache, dizziness and general ill health probably related to excessive vagal activity. Rarely, neurally mediated syncope can be sudden, with no prodroma, and occur in unexpected situations: this is termed malignant neurally mediated syncope.

Diagnosis

There is no accepted 'gold-standard' diagnostic test for neurally mediated syncope but an appropriate clinical history in association with a positive head-up tilt test currently provides the cornerstone for the diagnosis of neurally mediated syncope.[54,55] The head-up tilt-table test mimics orthostatic stress, resulting in maximal venous pooling, central hypovolemia and peripheral provocation of neurally mediated syncope. While the initial response to the assumption of upright posture is similar in healthy subjects and syncopal patients, namely maintenance of arterial normotension through increasing cardiac inotropy and chronotropy, and vasoconstriction of splanchnic and skeletal vascular beds, patients eventually exhibit the hallmark of the vasovagal event. The head-up tilt table test should only be judged positive if symptoms are accompanied by arterial hypotension, bradycardia or both.[55] Neurally mediated syncope is classified according to heart rate response to tilt-table testing (Table 22.4).

Treatment

In those with recurrent neurally mediated syncope, treatment should be aimed initially at withdrawal of any culprit medications. In older patients, with serious comorbidity this may not be possible. An explanation of the cause of the syncope, along with clear guidelines on avoidance techniques may be all that is required. Various medications have been tried in the treatment of resistant neurally mediated syncope, each directed at various points in the abnormal reflex. Midodrine may reduce symptom frequency by preventing peripheral vasodilation and venodilation.[57] Fludrocortisone will increase plasma volume but is poorly tolerated in the elderly. Trials of the use of β-adrenergic antagonists have shown some benefit in uncontrolled trials but these effects have not been demonstrated in long-term follow-up studies and are not currently recommended for neurally mediated syncope.[14] There is some preliminary evidence that paroxetine, through its effects on central sympathetic outflow, may have some role in the management of neurally mediated syncope but this is not currently widely accepted.[58] Cardiac pacing is a potentially useful tool in the management of highly selected patients. Two major multicenter, randomized controlled trials have demonstrated effectiveness in individuals that have predominantly cardio-inhibitory faints.[59,60]

Table 22.4 *Classification of neurally mediated syncope*

Response	Classification	Heart rate	Blood pressure
Mixed	Type 1	> 40 b.p.m. or falls to < 40 b.p.m. for < 10 s	Falls before HR drops
Cardio-inhibitory	Type 2A	< 40 b.p.m. for > 10 s	Falls before HR drops
Cardio-inhibitory	Type 2B	< 40 b.p.m. for > 10 s 3 s asystole	Falls after HR drops
Vasodepressor	Type 3	Falls by < 10% of peak HR	Falls and produces syncope

Data from ACC/AHA guidelines for implantation of cardiac pacemakers and anti-arrhythmic devices. A report of the American College of Cardiology and the American Heart Association. Taskforce on practical guidelines (Committee on Pacemaker Implantation). *J Am Coll Cardiol* 1998;**31**:175–209;[39] Sutton R, Petersen M, Brignole M, Raviele A, Menozzi C. Proposed classification for tilt-induced syncope. *Eur J Cardiac Pacing Electrophysiol* 1992;**3**:180–3.[56]

POSTPRANDIAL HYPOTENSION

In healthy older adults, systolic blood pressure falls by 11–16 mmHg and heart rate rises by five to seven beats within 60 min of eating. In the majority of fit as well as frail older adults, most hypotensive episodes go unnoticed. In patients with hypertension, orthostatic hypotension and autonomic failure, the postprandial blood pressure fall is much greater and occurs without a corresponding heart rate rise.[61]

Pathophysiology

Vasodilating effects of insulin, and other gut peptides such as vasoactive intestinal peptide (VIP), are thought to be responsible for postprandial hypotension, although the precise mechanism is uncertain.[62]

Symptoms

The clinical significance of a fall in blood pressure after meals is difficult to quantify. Postprandial hypotension has been causally linked to recurrent syncope and falls in the elderly.[63] Symptoms are similar to those experienced with OH varying from dizziness, blurred vision, lethargy, generalized weakness to syncope, typically occurring approximately 60 min after meals. It should be remembered that postprandial hypotension is often associated with other hypotensive syndromes. In the experience of the author, postprandial hypotension occurs in at least 20 per cent of patients with orthostatic hypotension.

Treatment

Dietary adjustments may be sufficient to manage postprandial hypotension. Simple carbohydrate should be replaced by complex carbohydrate and smaller, more frequent meals should be substituted. Additional options include treatment with a non-steroid anti-inflammatory agent such as indometacin,[64] the somatostatin analogue octreotide[65] or caffeine. Caffeine, taken along with food, prevents hypotensive symptoms in fit as well as frail older adults.[66,67]

COGNITIVE IMPAIRMENT, NEUROVASCULAR INSTABILITY AND FALLS

Falls are exceptionally common in older subjects with dementia or cognitive impairment. Annual incidences of between 60 per cent and 80 per cent have been reported, irrespective of the study population.[68,69] This represents an approximate doubling of fall risk compared with cognitively normal older people.

Patients with cognitive impairment and dementia who fall are also at increased risk of sustaining a significant injury. Approximately 10 per cent of falls in patients with dementia living in institutional care will result in a fractured neck of femur.[5]

The major factors implicated in producing this increased risk of falls are neurovascular instability, postural instability, environmental hazards, medication and the type of dementia.

As described previously neurovascular instability refers to the broad category of disorders including CSS, OH and neurocardiogenic syncope. All of these conditions are known to cause recurrent falls or syncope-related falls. Ballard et al.[70] demonstrated the high prevalence of neurovascular instability in subjects with neurodegenerative dementias. At least one form of neurovascular instability was present in 77 per cent of subjects with Lewy body dementia (LBD) and in 57 per cent of subjects with Alzheimer's dementia. Abnormal autonomic function has been reported in subjects with Lewy body dementia and Alzheimer's dementia and this may explain this high prevalence of OH. An interesting, and as yet unpublished, study from our unit[71] examined cognitive function in a consecutive series of patient with OH compared with healthy controls. Subjects with OH had evidence of significant cognitive impairment compared with controls. The greater the measured drop in systolic blood pressure the greater the associated cognitive impairment. Subjects with OH had evidence of areas of watershed ischemia on cerebral magnetic resonance imaging. This work suggests that it may be the OH/autonomic dysfunction which is the primary defect; with cognitive impairment developing as a consequence of accumulated periventricular white matter damage caused by repeated episodes of cerebral hypoperfusion.

This is a controversial view but is an important area for further research to assess the importance of neurovascular instability in the pathogenesis and progression of dementias.

CARDIAC DISEASE–RELATED SYNCOPE

Table 22.1 lists cardiac diseases that commonly present with syncope.

Arrhythmias causing syncope

Bradyarrhythmias and tachyarrhythmias may cause a sudden decrease in cardiac output and cause sudden syncope. Initially, bradycardias may be partly compensated for by prolonged ventricular filling resulting in increased stroke volume and maintained cardiac output. As the heart rate slows this compensatory mechanism is overwhelmed and cardiac output falls and presyncope or syncope occurs. Similarly, mild to moderate tachycardias increase cardiac output while faster heart rates result in decreased ventricular diastolic filling, reduced cardiac output, hypotension and syncope. It has also been recognized that supraventricular and paroxysmal atrial fibrillation may activate cardiac mechanoreceptors and induce neurally mediated syncope (rapid, vigorous, ventricular contraction in the setting of a relatively empty ventricle).[71]

Physiological impairments associated with aging, the effects of multiple medications and comorbidity may predispose older adults to syncope even in the setting of brief arrhythmias, while similar arrhythmias may not produce any symptoms in a younger individual.

Arrhythmias cause approximately 20 per cent of syncopal episodes in older adults.[23] Sick sinus syndrome and ventricular tachycardias are the most common arrhythmic causes identified.[22] Syncope is a central manifestation of sick sinus syndrome and is reported in 25–70 per cent of patients. Electrocardiographic features include sinus bradycardia, atrial pauses, arrest or exit block. When bradycardias are associated with episodic supraventricular tachycardias, tachycardia/bradycardias syndrome is said to be present. Ventricular tachycardias generally occur in the setting of known organic heart disease, especially in those with poor left-ventricular systolic function. The severity of associated symptoms is related to the rate, the duration and myocardial pump function. Torsades de pointe and syncope in older adults occurs in those with the acquired long QT syndrome. Acquired long QT syndromes are often secondary to electrolyte disturbance or anti-arrhythmic drugs such as amiodarone, procainamide, disopyramide and flecainide.

Structural cardiac and cardiopulmonary disease causing syncope

Syncope with exertion is commonly a manifestation of organic heart disease in which cardiac output is fixed. Syncope is reported in up to 42 per cent of patients with severe aortic stenosis, commonly with exercise. A number of possible mechanisms of syncope have been proposed: (1) neurally mediated via cardiac mechanoreceptor stimulation; and (2) inability to increase cardiac output in response to exercise because of severe left-ventricular outflow tract obstruction, coupled with peripheral vasodilatation associated with exercise, resulting in hypotension and syncope.

Syncope is an important prognostic indicator in aortic stenosis. In the absence of valve replacement the average survival is 2–3 years. Exertional syncope is also commonly associated with hypertrophic cardiomyopathy. The mechanism of syncope is similar to that of aortic stenosis. In addition, approximately 25 per cent of subjects with hypertrophic cardiomyopathy have ventricular tachycardias, which may induce syncope.[72]

Older adults with acute myocardial infarction may present atypically; 5–12 per cent may present with syncope. Various mechanisms may cause this syncope, such as rhythm disturbance or acute pump failure leading to hypotension (e.g. extensive infarction, papillary muscle rupture and interventricular septal rupture). Rare abnormalities such as atrial myxoma, pericardial disease and tamponade or aortic dissection may present with syncope. Pulmonary embolism should also be considered as a cause of syncope.

DIAGNOSTIC EVALUATION OF SYNCOPE IN OLDER ADULTS

A major issue in the use of diagnostic tests is that syncope is a transient symptom. Typically, patients are asymptomatic at the time of assessment and the opportunity to capture a spontaneous event during diagnostic testing is rare. Multiple illness are common in older adults: subjects over the age of 65 years have an average of 3.5 illnesses.[73] It is important to carefully attribute a diagnosis rather than to assume that the presence of an abnormality known to produce syncope or hypotensive symptoms is the causative factor. In order to attribute a diagnosis with certainty, patients must have symptom reproduction during investigation and preferably alleviation of symptoms with specific intervention during follow-up. In addition, various hypotensive disorders often coexist in the same patient, making a precise diagnosis of the symptom more difficult.[74] The most important elements in the evaluation of syncope in older adults are to establish whether the patient has actually experienced syncope and to select the appropriate cardiovascular investigations to define the cause. Table 22.5 shows conditions that may be confused with syncope.

Table 22.5 *Causes of non-syncopal attacks*

Disorders of impairment or loss of consciousness	
Metabolic disorders	Hypoglycemia, hypoxia, hyperventilation with hypocapnia
Epilepsy	
Vertebrobasilar ischemia	Associated with specific neurological deficits
Disorders resembling syncope without loss of consciousness	
Cataplexy	
Psychogenic 'syncope'	Somatization disorders

History and physical examination

A detailed history and physical examination can result in a diagnosis in up to 40 per cent of cases.[22] An accurate witness account should always be sought but this is likely to be available in only 40 per cent of cases.[23] Important elements of the history are shown in Table 22.6. These should be key features in the diagnostic work-up.

Clinical features suggestive of specific causes of syncope are shown in Table 22.7.

Table 22.6 *Important historical feature of possible syncope*

Circumstances just prior to attack
Position (supine, sitting, standing)
Activity (rest, change in posture, exercise associated, micturition, cough, swallowing, defecating)
Predisposing factors (crowds, warm places, prolonged standing, fear, pain, neck movement)

Onset of attack
Nausea, vomiting, feeling cold, sweating, pain in neck or shoulders, blurred vision

Attack (witness)	Way of falling (slumping over)
	Color (pallor, cyanosis)
	Duration of loss of consciousness
	Movements and duration (tonic, clonic, tonic-clonic, myoclonic, automatisms)

End of attack
Nausea, vomiting, sweating, confusion, muscle aches, skin color, injury, chest pain, incontinence

Background
Family history of sudden death
Previous cardiac disease
Neurological history (Parkinson's disease, epilepsy, narcolepsy)
Metabolic disorders
Medication (vasoactive drugs, anti-arrhythmics, diuretics, QT prolonging agents)
Frequency of episodes
Driving history

Dizziness is a frequent accompanying symptom in subjects that have unexplained falls, presyncope and syncope. Clinical features of dizziness can further help to identify an underlying cause of symptoms. Four types of dizzy symptom have been recognized: vertigo, disequilibrium, lightheadedness and others (or non-specific).[75] Lightheadedness is often associated with an underlying cardiovascular cause of symptoms, vertigo with peripheral vestibular or central lesions and unsteadiness or disequilibrium with central degenerative disease.[76] In addition, dizziness is most likely to be attributed to a cardiovascular cause if there is associated pallor, syncope, history of prolonged standing or a feeling of the need to sit or lie down when symptoms occur.[76] Physical examination is used to diagnose specific entities and exclude others. Orthostatic blood pressure recording, cardiovascular findings and neurological examination are crucial in this regard. Assessment of gait, mobility, muscle strength and the use of walking aids are important in patients complaining of unexplained falls and possible syncope. Assessment of vision is also important.

Orthostatic blood pressure measurement

Supine blood pressure measurements should be taken after a minimum of 10 min at rest. Blood pressure should be recorded for up to 3 min while standing unaided. Measurements may be continued for longer if blood pressure is still falling after 3 min. A decrease in systolic blood pressure of greater than 20 mmHg, a 10 mmHg fall in diastolic blood pressure, or a fall in the systolic blood pressure to 90 mmHg or less is considered diagnostic of

Table 22.7 *Clinical features suggestive of specific causes of real or apparent loss of consciousness*

Symptom or finding	Possible cause
After sudden unexpected, unpleasant sight, sound or smell	Neurocardiogenic
Prolonged standing or crowded warm place	Neurocardiogenic or autonomic failure
Nausea or vomiting associated with syncope	Neurocardiogenic
After meals	Postprandial
After exertion	Neurocardiogenic or autonomic failure
With head rotation, pressure on carotid sinus	Carotid sinus syndrome
Within seconds or minutes of standing	Orthostatic hypotension
Temporal association with start or change of dose of medication	Drug induced
During exertion or when supine	Cardiac
Preceded by palpitation	Tachyarrhythmia
Family history of sudden death	Long QT syndrome
	Brugada syndrome
	HCM
Associated with vertigo, dysarthria, diplopia	Brainstem ischemia
With arm exercise	Subclavian steal
Confusion after attack lasting more than 5 minutes	Seizure
Tonic-clonic movements, automatism, blue face	Seizure
Frequent attacks associated with somatic symptoms and no organic heart disease.	Psychiatric illness

orthostatic hypotension, regardless of whether or not symptoms occur. In patients with unexplained syncope or falls an attributable diagnosis of orthostatic hypotension depends on symptom reproduction.

BASELINE ELECTROCARDIOGRAM

An abnormal electrocardiogram (ECG) may be found in up to 50 per cent of patients presenting with syncope.[77] When abnormal, the ECG may disclose an arrhythmia associated with syncope (2–11 per cent of patients), or more commonly an abnormality that may predispose to arrhythmia development and syncope.[77] An abnormality of the baseline ECG is an independent predictor of cardiac syncope and it is associated with increased mortality. Equally important, a normal ECG is associated with a low risk of cardiac syncope.

Prolonged electrocardiographic monitoring and electrophysiological testing

In patients where an arrhythmic cause of syncope is strongly suspected, the main tools of investigation are prolonged ambulatory electrocardiograms, patient-activated recorders, implantable loop recorders and electrophysiological studies. Diagnostic yield from 24-h Holter monitoring remains very low: only 4 per cent of patients have correlation of symptoms and arrhythmia. Extending monitoring to 72 h does not significantly improve diagnostic yield. Patient-activated external loop recorders have a higher diagnostic yield compared with prolonged ambulatory monitoring but do not have good rhythm–symptom correlation in more than one-third of subjects.[78] Older patients must have sufficient manual dexterity and cognitive function to use these systems. Prospective recording is useful in those with presyncope, but of no benefit in patients with sudden collapse who do not have warning to enable them to activate the recorder. Continuous external loop recorders are more useful in this situation. These recorders will save a variable period prior to activation, as well as a short period of post-event recording. Implantable loop recorders offering extended ECG monitoring over an 18-month period have recently become available. Using an activation device, the patient, a family member or carer 'freezes' the loop during or after a typical syncopal episode, thus storing the preceding segment, which can be retrieved later using a standard pacemaker programmer. The clinical usefulness and cost effectiveness of this device has been described in younger subjects with unexplained syncope but this is not established for older adults.[79,80] Initial experience using an implantable loop recorder in subjects over the age of 60 years with suspected arrhythmic causes of syncope suggest that it may prove a valuable diagnostic tool.[81]

Ambulatory blood pressure monitoring

Ambulatory blood pressure monitoring is predominantly used in the management of hypertension. However, it can play a role in the diagnosis and management of hypotensive disorders. Information such as the pattern of diurnal blood pressure behavior, postprandial dips in blood pressure and blood pressure changes after medication are useful in patients suffering from syncope and dizziness. A reversal of the diurnal blood pressure pattern is frequently observed in subjects with symptomatic orthostatic hypotension.[82]

Carotid sinus massage

The subject should lie supine on a footplate-type tilt-table for a minimum of 5 min with continuous surface ECG and blood pressure monitoring (where possible, phasic beat-to-beat monitoring is preferred as the blood pressure nadir in response to carotid sinus massage occurs around 18 s and returns to baseline at 30 s). Firm, longitudinal massage should be performed for 5 s at the site of maximal pulsation at the right carotid sinus, located between the superior border of the thyroid cartilage and the angle of the mandible.[83] Massage is repeated over the left carotid sinus supine and then repeated right and left erect (70° head-up tilt). Only performing carotid sinus massage in the supine position will fail to demonstrate an abnormal response in 20–40 per cent of those with CSS.[37]

Table 22.8.shows contraindications to carotid sinus massage

Table 22.8 *Contraindications to carotid sinus massage*

Absolute	Myocardial infarction within 3 months
	Transient ischemic accident within 3 months
	Stroke within 3 months
Relative	Previous ventricular fibrillation
	Previous ventricular tachycardia
	Presence of carotid bruit*

*Known to be a poor predictor of presence or severity of carotid artery stenosis; carotid Doppler studies may help to stratify risk of proceeding.

Adherence to these exclusion criteria results in a very low complication rate of two persistent neurological defects and nine transient ischemic events per 16 000 episodes of carotid sinus massage.[84]

Head–up tilt-table testing

Head-up tilt-table testing has been used as tool to investigate the pathophysiology of orthostatic stress for over 50 years but it was not until the 1980s that its clinical utility in the diagnosis of unexplained syncope was recognized.[54] Kenny et al.[54] found that 67 per cent of patients with otherwise unexplained syncope demonstrated a neurocardiogenic reaction during head-up tilting, compared with only 10 per cent of healthy controls. Head-up tilt testing has since evolved into the diagnostic test of choice in assessing neurocardiogenic and related disorders. Many authors have proposed different protocols for diagnostic, investigative and therapeutic purposes. A detailed description and justification of various tilt protocols is available elsewhere.[85] Protocols principally vary with respect to the angle of tilting, time duration and the associated use of provocative agents such as glycerol trinitrate and isoprenaline. The angle and duration of the test are the most powerful determinants of its diagnostic utility. Evidence suggests that tilt angles between 60° and 80° are optimal in creating sufficient orthostatic stress without increasing the number of false positives or negative tests.[50,55,86] The duration of the test also varies between centers, but it is suggested that prolonged tilting for 30–45 min is optimal.[54] Longer periods of tilting produce unacceptably high proportions of false positive results. Our own practice is to use a 70° tilt angle for 40 min.

Conditions where tilt–table testing is warranted

Conditions where tilt-table testing is warranted are:

- when evaluating older adults with recurrent unexplained falls
- the evaluation of recurrent syncope or a single syncopal event in a high-risk patient (syncope has resulted in injury or determination of cause has significant occupational consequences; e.g. pilot or machine operator) whether or not the history is suggestive of neurally mediated syncope and (1) no evidence of structural cardiovascular disease, or (2) structural cardiovascular disease is present, but other causes of syncope have been excluded by appropriate testing.
- further evaluation of patients in whom an apparent cause has been established (e.g. asystole, atrioventricular block) but in whom demonstration of susceptibility to neurally mediated syncope could alter treatment choice
- part of an evaluation of exercise-associated syncope.

Relative contraindications to tilt testing include proximal coronary stenosis, critical mitral stenosis, clinically severe left-ventricular outflow obstruction and severe known cerebrovascular disease.

Equipment, monitoring and environment

The laboratory environment in which tilt testing is undertaken is important. To minimize stimuli affecting autonomic function, the test should be carried out in a quiet, dimly lit room at a comfortable temperature and should be as non-threatening as possible.

Patients should be fasted for 2 h prior to the procedure (in order to minimize the confounding effects of postprandial hypotension) and then rested supine for 20–45 min. Longer periods may be necessary if intravascular instrumentation is used. This is known to increase the risk of false positive tests.[87] Drugs affecting cardiovascular or autonomic function should be discontinued 5 half-lives pretest, unless they are etiologically implicated. During the test the patient should be instructed to avoid movements of the lower extremities to maximize venous pooling. The tilt-table should be of the footplate support variety and should allow rapid achievement of the upright position and allow calibrated angles of between 60° and 80° (Fig. 22.1). A minimum of three ECG leads should be recorded simultaneously and continuously throughout the study. Blood pressure recording should ideally be the non-invasive continuous beat-to-beat method (e.g. digital photoplethysmography, Finapres, Ohmeda, WI, USA or Portapres, TNO Biomedical, Amsterdam, The Netherlands).

Advanced resuscitation equipment should be immediately available and to the standard required in exercise testing facilities. The test should be continuously supervised by a physician, nurse or technician experienced in the management of the test and its possible complications.

The hemodynamic responses that can occur in a positive tilt-table test are as previously shown in Table 22.4. Brignole et al.[88] proposed exceptions to these categories: 'Chronotropic Incompetence', with no heart rate rise during the tilt test (less than 10 per cent rise from the pre-tilt rate); and 'Excessive Heart Rate Rise', with an excessive heart rate rise both at the onset of the upright position and throughout its duration before syncope (greater than 130 b.p.m.).

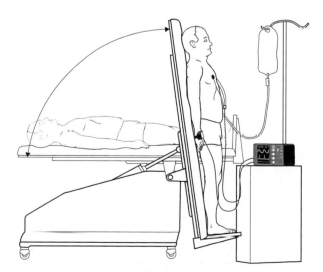

Figure 22.1 *Head-up tilt-table test with footplate support type table (Akron) and continuous electrocardiogram and photoplethysmographic blood pressure monitoring (Finapres).*

The decision of the supervisor when to terminate the test influences the type of response.[89] Some suggest that the test should continue until the precise occurrence of loss of consciousness with simultaneous loss of postural tone.[88] Premature interruption of testing underestimates, and delayed interruption overestimates cardio-inhibitory responses, and exposes the patients to the risks of prolonged hypotension and loss of consciousness. There is no consensus of when to stop the tilt but many physicians consider a steadily falling blood pressure, accompanied by usual symptoms sufficient reason to stop the test.

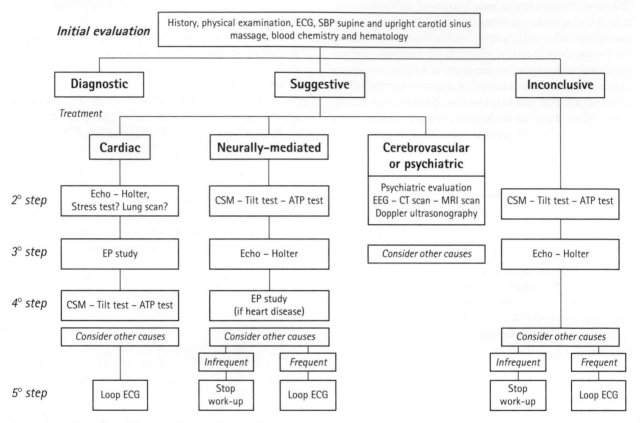

Figure 22.2 *Algorithm of assessment and management of patients referred to a dedicated syncope, falls and dizziness clinic.*

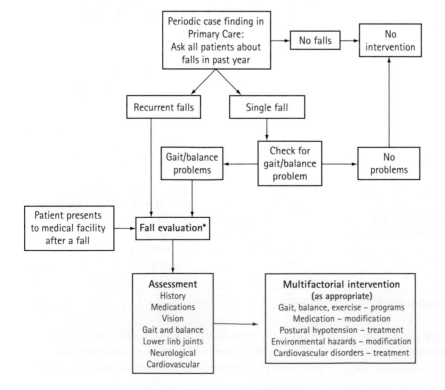

Figure 22.3 *Algorithm of assessment of falls (UK/US Falls Guidelines).*

Figures 22.2 and 22.3 are algorithms of our current preferred clinical assessment and management of patients referred to our syncope and falls clinic.

Figure 22.2 demonstrates the complexity of managing these challenging patients. It is apparent that a physician who undertakes assessment of older subjects with falls/syncope requires a broad range of skills, with particular expertise in cardiovascular investigation in older adults, neurological training and knowledge of multi-professional functional assessment. Our decade of experience running a dedicated falls and syncope service suggests that appropriate investigation and management of these patients has key benefits, namely higher diagnostic rates[23] and shorter hospital admissions with more efficient use of health service resources.[28]

SUMMARY

Accurate diagnosis of syncope in an older patient requires a high degree of clinical suspicion, thorough physical examination and carefully directed and interpreted investigations, including repeated measurement of orthostatic blood pressure, carotid sinus massage and head-up tilt testing. The importance of identifying a cause of syncope is vital if there is to be appropriate treatment to reduce associated falls, fractures and hospital admissions.

REFERENCES

1. Kantern DN, Mulrow CD, Gerety MB, Lichenstein MJ, Aguilar C, Cornell JE. Falls: an examination of three reporting methods in nursing homes. *J Am Geriatr Soc* 1993;**41**:662–6.
2. Tinetti ME, Speechley M, Ginter SF. Risk factors for falls among elderly persons Living in the community. *N Engl J Med* 1988;**319**:1701–7.
3. Kellog International Work Group. Prevention of falls in the elderly. *Dan Med Bull* 1987;**34**(Suppl I4):1–24.
4. Clark RD, Lord SR, Webster IW. Clinical parameters associated with falls in the elderly population. *Gerontology* 1993;**39**:117–23.
5. van Dijk PTM, Meullenberg OGRM, van de Sande HJ, et al. Falls In dementia patients. *Gerontologist* 1993,**33**.200–4.
6. Richardson DA, Bexton RS, Shaw FE, et al. Prevalence of cardioinhibitory carotid sinus hypersensitivity (CICSH) in accident and attendances with falls or syncope. *Pace* 1997;**20**:820–3.
7. Berstein AB, Schur CL. Expenditure for unintentional injuries among the elderly. *J Aging Health* 1990;**2**:157–78.
8. Rubenstein LZ, Powers C. *Falls and mobility problems: potential quality indicators and literature review (the ACOVE project)*. Santa Monica: Rand Corporation, 1999;1–40.
9. Bezon J, Echevarria KH, Smith GB. Nursing outcome indicator:Preventing falls for elderly people. *Outcomes Manag Nurs Pract* 1999;**3**:112–116.
10. American Geriatrics Society, British Geriatrics Society, and American Academy of Orthopaedic Surgeons Panel on Fall Prevention. Guideline for the prevention of falls in older persons. *J Am Geriatr Soc* 2001;**49**:664–672.
11. Donald IP, Bulpitt CJ. The prognosis of falls in elderly people living at home. *Age Ageing* 1999;**28**:121–25.
12. Brown AP. Reducing falls in elderly people: a review of exercise interventions. *Physiother Theory Pract* 1999;**15**:59–68.
13. Davies AJ, Steen N, Kenny RA. Carotid sinus hypersensitivity common in older patients presenting to an accident and emergency department with unexplained falls. *Age Ageing* 2001;**30**:289–93.
14. Brignole M, Alboni P, Benditt D, et al. Task Force on Syncope, European Society of Cardiology. Guidelines on management (diagnosis and treatment) of syncope. *Eur Heart J* 2001;**22**(15):1256–306
15. Lipsitz LA, Storch HA, Minaker KL, Rowe JW. Intra-individual variability in postural blood pressure in the elderly. *Clin Sci* 1985;**69**:337–41.
16. Hainsworth R. Syncope and fainting: classification and pathophysiological basis. In: Mathias CJ, Bannister R, eds. *Autonomic failure: a textbook of clinical disorders of the autonomic nervous system*, 4th edn. Oxford: Oxford University Press, 1999;428–36.
17. Lipsitz LA. Abnormalities in blood pressure homeostasis that contribute to falls in the elderly. *Clin Geriatr Med* 1985;**1**(3):637–48.
18. Lipsitz LA, Pluchino FC, Wei JY, Rowe JW. Syncope in an elderly institutionalized population: prevalence, incidence and associated risk. *Q J Med* 1985;**55**:45–54.
19. Lipsitz LA. Altered blood pressure homeostasis in advanced age: clinical and research implications. *J Gerentol* 1989;**44**:179–83.
20. Crane MG, Harris JJ. Effect of ageing on renin activity and aldosterone secretion *J Lab Clin Med* 1976;**87**:947–959.
21. Epstein M, Hollenberg MK. Age, a determinant of renal sodium conservation in normal man. *J Lab Clin Med* 1976;**87**:411–17.
22. Kapoor W, Snusted D, Petersen J, et al. Syncope in the Elderly. *Am J Med* 1986;**80**:419–28.
23. McIntosh SJ, da Costa D, Kenny RA. Outcome of an integrated approach to the investigation of dizziness, falls and syncope in the elderly referred to a syncope clinic. *Age Ageing* 1993;**22**:53–58.
24. Allcock LM, O'Shea D. Diagnostic yield and development of a neurocardiovascular investigation unit for older adults in a district general hospital. *J Gerontol A Biol Sci Med Sci* 2000;**55**(8):M458–62.
25. Brignole M, Gigli G, Almonte F, et al. The cardioinhibitory reflex evoked by carotid sinus stimulation in normal and in patients with cardiovascular disorders. *G Ital Cardiol* 1985;**15**:514–19.
26. Brignole M, Menozzi C, Gianfranchi L, et al. Carotid sinus massage and head-up tilt testing in patients with syncope of uncertain origin and in healthy control subjects. *Am Heart J* 1991;**122**:1644–51.
27. Brignole M, Oddone D, Cogorno S. et al. A long term outcome in symptomatic carotid sinus hypersensitivity. *Am Heart J* 1992;**123**:687–692.
28. Kenny RA Richardson DA, Steen N, et al. Carotid sinus syndrome: a modifiable risk factor for nonaccidental falls in

older adults (SAFE PACE). *J Am Coll Cardiol* 2001;**38**(5): 1491-7.

29. Kapoor WN. Syncope in older persons. *J Am Geriatr Soc* 1994;**42**:426-436.

30. Kenny RA, Traynor G. Carotid sinus syndrome – clinical characteristics in elderly patients. *Age Ageing* 1991;**20**:449-54.

31. Cummings SR, Nevitt MC, Kidd S. Forgetting falls: the limited accuracy of recall falls in the elderly. *J Am Geriatr Soc* 1988;**36**:613-16.

32. Ward C, Kenny RA. Reproducibility of orthostatic hypotension in symptomatic elderly. *Am J Med* 1996;**100**:418-22.

33. Stout N, Kenny RA. Causes of orthostatic hypotension in older adults referred to a regional syncope service. *Clin Auton Res* 1998;**8**:71-72.

34. Close J, Ellis M, Hooper R, et al. Prevention of falls in the elderly trial (PROFET): a randomised controlled trial. *Lancet* 1999;**353**:93-7.

35. Dehn TCB, Morley CA, Sutton R. A scientific evaluation of the carotid sinus syndrome. *Cardiovasc Res* 1984;**18**:746-51.

36. O'Mahony D. Pathophysiology of carotid sinus hypersensitivity in elderly patients. *Lancet* 1995;**346**:950-2.

37. McIntosh SJ, da Costa D, Lawson J, et al. Heart rate and blood pressure responses to carotid sinus massage in healthy elderly subjects. *Age Ageing* 1994;**23**:317-9.

38. Davies AJ, Kenny RA. Syncope in older patients. *Rev Clin Gerontology* 1999;**9**:117-26.

39. Gregoratos G, Cheitlin MD, Conill A, et al. ACC/AHA Guidelines for implantation of cardiac pacemakers and antiarrhythmia devices: executive summary - a report of the American College of Cardiology/American Heart Association Task Force on Practice Guidelines (Committee on Pacemaker Implantation). *Circulation* 1998;**97**(13):1325-5

40. Bexton RS, Davies A, Kenny RA. The rate drop response to carotid sinus syndrome The Newcastle experience. *Pac Clin Electrophysiol* 1997;**20**:840.

41. Crilley JG, Herd B, Khurana CS, et al. Permanent cardiac pacing in elderly patients with recurrent falls, dizziness and syncope and a hypersensitive cardio-inhibitory reflex. *Post Grad Med J* 1997;**73**:415-18.

42. da Costa D, McIntosh S, Kenny RA. Benefits of fludrocortisone in the treatment of symptomatic vasodepressor carotid sinus syndrome. *Br Heart J* 1993;**69**:308-310.

43. Anonymous. Consensus statement on the definition of orthostatic hypotension, pure autonomic failure, and multiple system atrophy. The Consensus Committee of the American Autonomic Society and the American Academy of Neurology. *Neurology* 1996;**46**(5):1470

44. Palmer KT. Studies of postural hypotension in elderly patients. *N Z Med J* 1983;**96**:43-5.

45. Schatz IJ, Masaki KH, Burchfield CM, et al. Orthostatic hypotension (OH) as a predictor of 2-year mortality in elderly men, the Honolulu Heart Program. *Clin Auton Res* 1995;**5**:321.

46. Rowe JW, Troen BR. Sympathetic nervous system and ageing in man. *Endocrinol Rev* 1980;**1**:167-79.

47. Mathias CJ, Mallipeddi R, Bleasdale-Barr K. Symptoms associated with orthostatic hypotension in pure autonomic failure and multiple system atrophy. *J Neurol* 1999;**246**(10):893-8.

48. Gribben B, Pickering TG, Sleight P, Peto R. Effect of age and blood pressure on baroreflex sensitivity in man. *Circ Res* 1971;**29**:424-31.

49. Lakatta EG. Do hypertension and aging have a similar effect on myocardium. *Circulation* 1987;**75**:169-77.

50. Fitzpatrick A, Theodorakis G, Vardas P. et al. The incidence of malignant vasovagal syndrome in patients with recurrent syncope. *Eur Heart J* 1991;**12**:389-94.

51. Davies AJ, Kenny RA. Falls presenting to the accident and emergency department; types of presentation and risk factor profile. *Age Ageing* 1996;**25**:362-66.

52. Samoil O, Grubb BP. Vasovagal (neurally-mediated) syncope: pathophysiology, diagnosis and therapeutic approach. *Eur J Cardiac Pacing Electrophysiol* 1992;**2**:234-41.

53. Wayne HH. Syncope: physiological considerations and the analysis of the clinical characteristics of 510 patients. *Am J Med* 1961;**30**:418-38.

54. Kenny RA, Ingram A, Bayliss J, et al. Head-up tilt: a useful test for investigating unexplained syncope. *Lancet* 1986;**1**:1352-4.

55. Benditt DG, Ferguson DW, Grubb BP, et al. Tilt table testing for assessing syncope. ACC Expert Consensus Document. *J Am Coll Cardiol* 1996;**28**:263-75.

56. Sutton R, Petersen M, Brignole M, et al. Proposed classification for tilt-induced syncope. *Eur J Card Pacing Electrophysiol* 1992;**3**:180-3.

57. Ward CR, Gray JC, Gilroy JJ, Kenny RA. Midodrine:a role in the management of neurocardiogenic syncope. *Heart* 1998;**79**(1);45-9.

58. Di Gerolamo E, Di Iorio C, Sabatini O, et al. Effects of paroxetine hydrochloride a selective serotonin uptake inhibitor, on refractory vasovagal syncope: a randomised, double blind, placebo controlled study. *J Am Coll Cardiol* 1999;**33**:1227-30.

59. Connolly SJ, Sheldon R, Roberts RS, Gent M. Vasovagal pacemaker study investigators. The North American Vasovagal Pacemaker Study (VPS): a randomised trial of permanent cardiac pacing for the prevention of vaso-vagal syncope. *J Am Coll Cardiol* 1999;**33**:16-20.

60. Sutton R, Brignole M, Menozzi C, et al. Dual-chamber pacing in the treatment of neurally-mediated tilt-positive cardio-inhibitory syncope: pacemaker versus no therapy: a multicentre randomised study. *Circulation* 2000;**102**:294-9.

61. Jansen RWMM, Penterman BJM, van Lier HJ, Hoefnagels WHL. Blood pressure reduction after oral glucose loading and its relation to age, blood pressure and insulin. *Am J Cardiol* 1987;**60**;1087-91.

62. Mathias CJ, da Costa DF, Fosbraey P, et al. Hypotensive and sedative effects of insulin in autonomic failure. *BMJ Clin Res* 1987;**295**:161-3.

63. Jonsson PV, Lipsitz LA, Kelly M, Koestner J. Hypotensive responses to common daily activities in institutionalised elderly. *Arch Intern Med* 1990;**150**:1518-24.

64. Robertson D, Wade D, Robertson RM. Postprandial alterations in cardiac vascular hemodynamics in autonomic dysfunctional states. *Am J Cardiol* 1981;**48**:1048-52.

65. Raimbach SJ, Cortelli P, Kooner JS, et al. Prevention of glucose induced hypotension by the somatostatin analogue octreotide (SMS201-995) in chronic autonomic failure, hemodynamic and hormonal changes. *Clin Sci* 1989;**77**:623-8.

66. Lenders JWM, Morre HLC, Smit P, Thien TH. The effect of caffeine on the postprandial fall in blood pressure in the elderly. *Age Ageing* 1988;**17**:236-40.

67. Heseltine D, Dakak M, Woodhouse K, et al. The effect of

caffeine on postprandial hypotension in the elderly. *J Am Geriatr Soc* 1991;**39**:160–4.

68. Visser H. Gait and balance in senile dementia of Alzheimer's type. *Age Ageing* 1983;**12**:296–301.

69. Tinetti ME, Speechley M, Ginter SF. Risk factors for falls among elderly persons living in the community. *N Engl J Med* 1994;**331**:821–7.

70. Ballard C, Shaw F, McKeith I, Kenny R. High prevalence of neurovascular instability in neurodegenerative dementias. *Neurology* 1998;**51**(6):1760–2.

71. Leitch JW, Klein GJ, Yee R, et al. Syncope associated with SVT: an expression of tachycardia rate or vasomotor response? *Circulation* 1992;**22**:1123.

72. Kowey PR, Eisenberg R, Engel TR. Sustained arrhythmias in hypertrophic obstructive cardiomyopathy. *N Engl J Med* 1984;**310**:1566–9.

73. Besdine RW. Geriatric medicine: an overview. *Ann Rev Gerontol* 1980;**1**:135–53.

74. McIntosh SJ, Lawson J, Kenny RA. Clinical characteristics of vasodepressor, cardioinhibitory and mixed carotid sinus syndrome in the elderly. *Am J Med* 1993;**95**:203–8.

75. Drachman DA, Hart CW. An approach to the dizzy patient. *Neurology* 1972;**22**:323–4.

76. Lawson J, Fitzgerald J, Birchall J, et al. Diagnosis of geriatric patients with severe dizziness. *J Am Geriatr Soc* 1999;**47**:12–17.

77. Kapoor W. Evaluation and outcome of patients with syncope. *Medicine* 1990;**69**:160.

78. Kenny RA, Krahn AD. Implantable loop recorder: evaluation of unexplained syncope. *Heart* 1999;**81**:431–3.

79. Krahn AD, Klein GJ, Yee R, et al. Use of extended monitoring strategy in patients with problematic syncope: reveal investigators. *Circulation* 1999;**99**:406–10.

80. Krahn AD. Klein GJ, Yee R, Manda V. The high cost of syncope: cost implications of a new insertable loop recorder in the investigation of recurrent syncope. *Am Heart J* 1999;**137**:870–7.

81. Armstrong VL, Lawson J, Kamper AM, et al. The use of an implantable loop recorder in the investigation of unexplained syncope in older people. *Age Ageing* 2003;**32**(2):185–8.

82. Senard JM, Charmontin B, Rascol A, Montastruc JL. Ambulatory blood pressure in patients with Parkinson's disease without and with orthostatic hypotension. *Clin Auton Res* 1992;**2**:99–104.

83. Kenny RA, O'Shea D, Parry SW. The Newcastle protocols for head up tilt testing and carotid sinus massage, initial diagnosis of vasovagal syncope and related disorders. *Heart* 2000;**83**(5):564–69

84. Davies AJ, Kenny RA. Frequency of neurologic complications following carotid sinus massage. *Am J Cardiol* 1998;**81**:1256–57.

85. Parry S.W, Kenny R.A. Tilt table testing. In: Malik M, ed. *Clinical guide to cardiac autonomic tests.* Dordrecht: Kluwer Academic Publishers, 1998;67–99.

86. Fitzpatrick A, Sutton R. Tilting towards a diagnosis in recurrent unexplained syncope. *Lancet* 1989;**1**:658–70.

87. McIntosh SJ, Lawson J, Kenny RA. Intravenous cannulation alters the specificity of head-up tilt testing for vasovagal syncope in elderly patients. *Age Ageing* 1994;**23**:317–19.

88. Brignole M, Menozzi C, Del Rosso A, et al. New classification of haemodynamics of vasovagal syncope: beyond the VASIS classification. Analysis of the pre-syncopal phase of the tilt test without and with nitroglycerin challenge. *Europace* 2000;**2**:66–76.

89. Weiling W, van Lieshout JJ, ten Harkel ADJ. Dynamics of circulatory adjustments to head up tilt and tilt back in healthy and sympathetically denervated subjects. *Clin Sci* 1998;**94**:347–352.

Index

Notes: page numbers in **bold** denote figures and/or tables